YOU AND YOUR CANCER

A Child's Guide

Lynda Cranston
Medical Writer

Chantal LeBlanc
Child Life Specialist

Maria Restivo
Child Life Specialist

Ronald Barr
Pediatric Oncologist

Children's Hospital, Hamilton Health Sciences Corporation
and McMaster University, Hamilton, Ontario, Canada

2001

BC Decker Inc

Hamilton • London

BC Decker Inc
20 Hughson Street South
P.O. Box 620, L.C.D. 1
Hamilton, Ontario L8N 3K7
Tel: 905-522-7017; 1-800-568-7281
Fax: 905-522-7839
E-mail: info@bcdecker.com
Website: www.bcdecker.com

Illustrations by Cynthia Watada

01 02 03 04 / CAD / 6 5 4 3 2 1

ISBN 1–55009–147–6
Printed in the United States

Sales and Distribution

United States
BC Decker Inc
P.O. Box 785
Lewiston, NY 14092-0785
Tel: 905-522-7017;
1-800-568-7281
Fax: 905-522-7839;
1-888-311-4987
E-mail: info@bcdecker.com
Website: www.bcdecker.com

Canada
BC Decker Inc
20 Hughson Street South
P.O. Box 620, L.C.D. 1
Hamilton, Ontario L8N 3K7
Tel: 905-522-7017;
1-800-568-7281
Fax: 905-522-7839
E-mail: info@bcdecker.com
Website: www.bcdecker.com

Foreign Rights
John Scott & Company
International Publishers' Agency
P.O. Box 878
Kimberton, PA 19442
Tel: 610-827-1640
Fax: 610-827-1671

**U.K., Europe, Scandinavia,
Middle East**
Harcourt Publishers Limited
Customer Service Department
Foots Cray High Street
Sidcup, Kent
DA14 5HP, UK
Tel: 44 (0) 208 308 5760
Fax: 44 (0) 181 308 5702
E-mail: cservice@harcourt_brace.com

Australia, New Zealand
Harcourt Australia Pty. Limited
Customer Service Department
STM Division
Locked Bag 16
St. Peters, New South Wales, 2044
Australia
Tel: (02) 9517-8999
Fax: (02) 9517-2249
E-mail: stmp@harcourt.com.au
Website: www.harcourt.com.au

Japan
Igaku-Shoin Ltd.
Foreign Publications Department
3-24-17 Hongo
Bunkyo-ku, Tokyo, Japan 113-8719
Tel: 3 3817 5680
Fax: 3 3815 6776
E-mail: fd@igaku.shoin.co.jp

**Singapore, Malaysia,
Thailand, Philippines,
Indonesia, Vietnam,
Pacific Rim, Korea**
Harcourt Asia Pte Limited
583 Orchard Road
#09/01, Forum
Singapore 238884
Tel: 65-737-3593
Fax: 65-753-2145

Notice: The authors and publisher have made every effort to ensure that the patient care recommended herein, including choice of drugs and drug dosages, is in accord with the accepted standard and practice at the time of publication. However, since research and regulation constantly change clinical standards, the reader is urged to check the product information sheet included in the package of each drug, which includes recommended doses, warnings, and contraindications. This is particularly important with new or infrequently used drugs.

**RONALD MCDONALD
HOUSE CHARITIES**

Ronald McDonald House Charities provide comfort and care to children and families through their network of local Chapters currently serving in 32 countries. The Charities make grants to non-profit organizations, primarily for programs that provide services aimed at improving the health and wellness of children, and provide support to Ronald McDonald Houses worldwide. Their grant of US $281,437.00 to Children's Hospital of Hamilton Health Sciences Corporation underwrote the printing costs of two cancer resource guides. These will be used to educate the 50,000 families of children who are newly diagnosed with cancer in North America over the next five years.

My name is _____

and I have cancer. It's called

_____.

I am _____ years old.

I live in _____.

My hospital is called

_____.

DEDICATION

This book is dedicated to kids who are meeting the challenge of cancer. From the time of diagnosis, through active treatment and beyond, there are many hurdles for you to face. With the help of your families and friends, the staff at the hospital, and others who care about you, those problems can be overcome. It is our hope that *your* book will be a guide and support as you take this difficult journey. Let us know if it is useful and if it could be better. Make *your* book special by adding your own ideas. This will help to make *your* cancer and its treatment less scary and take out some of the bumps on your journey to a cure.

Ronald Barr, MB, ChB, MD
for the authors
June 2001

ACKNOWLEDGMENTS

We wish to thank Cynthia Watada for the illustrations; Teri Grad for the advice on nutrition; and Paula Presutti, Debbie Maraldo, and Rochelle Decker at BC Decker Inc for making our dream a reality.

Lynda Cranston
Chantal LeBlanc
Maria Restivo
Ronald Barr

CONTENTS

Marcus

Heather

Tommy

These are the names of the people who take care of me at the hospital.

_____

_____

_____

_____

_____

What Do You Want to Know?

What is cancer?

Your body is made up of millions and millions of cells. These cells are like building blocks that work together to help your body do all the things it needs to. When you have cancer, some healthy cells get out of control and change into sick cells. These sick cells push your healthy cells out of the way. They become strong, grow, and can spread into the rest of your body. When sick cells clump together, they make a lump in your body. This is called a tumor. Sick cells stop your body from working the way it should. That's why you start to feel tired and achy.

How did I get cancer? Did I catch it from someone else?

We don't know how you got cancer, but we do know that you can't catch it from another person. It's not like a cold or the flu. And you didn't get cancer because you did something wrong. Nothing you or your family did made you get cancer.

Finding out you have cancer can be scary. You might feel mad or worried or all mixed up. Knowing more about cancer and how to get better can make it easier. To help, here are answers to some questions from other kids with cancer.

"Hi, my name's Marcus and I have leukemia. If you have leukemia too, keep an eye out for me in this book. Together, we can learn more about cancer and how to feel less afraid of it."

Will I get better?

Most kids with cancer are cured — this means their cancer is gone and will never come back. The doctors will use the best treatment they can for your kind of cancer. We know this treatment does a good job so you can feel better and have more energy.

If I need an operation, will I wake up in the middle of it?

No, you will not wake up during your operation. While one doctor is doing the operation, there is another doctor, called an anesthetist (a-nees-tha-tist), whose only job is to give you the medicine that makes sure you stay asleep. When the operation is over, this doctor will stop giving you the medicine so you can wake up again.

Why do some kids need chemo (kee-mo) medicine?

Sick cells can be in more than one place and sometimes they're even hiding. Chemo is needed for only some kinds of cancer when it is the only way to find all the sick cells and to get rid of them.

How will the chemo get into my body?

There are different ways to get chemo — taking pills through your mouth or by injection through a needle in your leg or back or under your skin. Another way is through a special tube that is put into your body. There are two types of tubes — Port and Hickman tubes.

A Port tube is put under your skin during an operation while you get sleeping medicine. You can't see it. Chemo is put into the Port tube by a needle through your skin. This needle won't hurt because the nurse will put some cream on your skin to make it numb.

If you have a Hickman tube, part of it is put under your skin and the other part stays outside your body on your chest. A bandage will cover the tube so it will stay in place. Chemo is then put into the tube by a needle. This will not hurt because the needle goes in the tube, not through your skin.

How will the chemo make me feel?

It might not make you feel different at first, but later it might make your body feel tired, cranky, angry, sad, or other feelings you'll read about. Sometimes your tummy might feel upset and you might throw up, but we do have medicine that can help you feel better.

Will I lose my hair when I'm taking chemo? Will it ever grow back?

Some kids only lose some of their hair. Others lose all of their hair. That's because the medicine can hurt your healthy cells (like hair cells) while it's trying to get rid of the sick cells. Your hair will fall out slowly — you might find it on your pillow or sometimes it gets in your mouth. You can leave your hair to fall out on its own or you can get a short haircut right away. It's your choice. Once you've finished taking chemo, your hair will grow back. It might look a little different — more curly, more straight, or even a slightly different color.

"Hey…Tommy here. What's your name, kiddo? I have a tumor in my brain. Stick with me and we'll find out everything we can about it."

My school doesn't let kids wear hats. Will I be able to wear one?

Usually schools don't let kids wear hats, but in your case they will. And sometimes your teacher might have a special hat day, so that all your classmates can wear one too.

What is radiation (ray-dee-ay-shun)?

Radiation is one way to treat cancer. When you have this treatment, a machine sends invisible rays into your body that you can't feel. These rays zap the sick cells and stop them from growing. If you're going to have radiation, you will visit the hospital a few times before treatment starts. That's so the hospital staff can decide exactly where the rays need to go to zap the sick cells. Once this is done, the radiation treatment only takes a few minutes each time.

"Hi ya. I'm Heather and I have a tumor in my leg. You might have one there too or somewhere else on your body. If you're like me you've got lots of questions. Let's find the answers together, okay?"

Will I have to stay at the hospital the whole time?

No. At first, you will stay at the hospital to get your chemo so the doctors and nurses can see how your body is feeling. Then you can go home. When you need to come back, you will visit the hospital clinic to get your chemo. You might have to sleep over in the hospital from time to time.

What does neutropenic (new-tro-pee-nic) mean? Why can't I leave my room?

In the same way the chemo can hurt your other healthy cells, it can hurt your white blood cells — we call them your fighter cells. When you're neutropenic, you don't have enough fighter cells and your body can't fight infections very well. During this time, it's important to stay away from other people who might have infections. That's why you'll need to stay at home or in your room if you're in the hospital until your fighter cells are strong again.

Can I go to school during my treatment?

If your fighter cells are strong, then you can go to school as long as kids in your school don't have an infection like chicken pox. But, if you don't have enough fighter cells, you might have to stay at home. There are teachers at the hospital who can talk to your school to have your work sent home. Sometimes short visits to your school can be planned for you. And when you're not at school, your parents, teachers, and the hospital staff can find ways for you to still be part of your class.

What if other kids at school make fun of me?

Usually kids make fun of people when they don't understand or if they're scared. If there are kids at school who say things that hurt your feelings, you can say something back to them or you might not pay any attention. If the person is mean more than once, tell someone you trust about it. Remember, you have lots of people who care about you.

Is there something else you want to know?

Write down other questions you might have about your cancer, treatment, tests… anything you want to know. Then ask your parents, doctor, child life specialist, nurse, or other kids with cancer for their answers. The more you know, the better you'll feel.

1. _____

_____

_____

2. _____

_____

_____

3. _____

_____

_____

4. _____

_____

_____

What Kinds of Cancer Are There?

There are many different kinds of cancer. Your doctor will tell you and your family all about the kind of cancer you have and how it will be treated to help you get better.

Let's talk about some of the cancers that kids get.

Leukemia (lu-kee-mee-ah)

Leukemia means you have cancer of your blood.

Blood is made up of different things, like white blood cells. We call white blood cells the fighter cells because they help you to fight infections. Your fighter cells are made in the bone marrow, which is the soft part inside your bones. That's where leukemia starts.

"Leukemia means you have cancer in your blood. You're probably feeling tired. You might have lots of bruises too. But don't worry, you're not alone. We're in this together!"

Cancer is just one word but it isn't only one thing. It's made up of many things that affect different kids in different ways. There are lots of different kinds of cancer. You'll find out what kind of cancer you have. Sometimes you might hear words that you don't understand. Always ask if you don't know what they mean.

When you have leukemia, your body makes sick fighter cells that don't do their job right. You get so many of these sick cells that there's not enough room for your healthy cells to grow. That's why you start feeling differently. You might:

- be more tired

- get a lot of bruises

- have pain in your bones

- have a fever

Brain tumors (too-mers)

Sometimes sick cells in your brain get out of control and can clump together to make a lump. This lump is called a tumor. A brain tumor can grow and push against other parts of your brain. That's why you start feeling differently. You might:

- have headaches

- be clumsy — you might fall over or drop things more often

- be moody — you might be angry or sad or cranky more than usual

- be sick to your stomach

- be sleepy more often

- have fits — they're called seizures (seez-yures)

"A brain tumor can make you feel lousy. Believe me, I know! But radiation can help you get better. Radiation is pretty cool. It's just like you're in a Star Wars movie."

Tumor in another part of your body

Sometimes cancer cells can clump together to make a lump in another part of your body, like your kidneys, stomach, muscles, bones or eyes. This tumor can grow and make it hard for that part of your body to do its job. That's why you may notice different things about your body. You might:

- find a lump in your body

- find it hard to walk, swallow, or see

- not want to eat

- feel pain where the tumor is

"Having a tumor in your leg can be scary and it might hurt. But I'm going to help you learn more about cancer. The more you know about it, the better you're going to feel."

Find the cancer words.

Find and circle the cancer words that are listed at the side of the page.

k	o	p	w	s	h	r	d	y	i	j	n	q	a
f	h	e	k	o	e	u	g	s	j	l	e	w	c
g	z	c	h	l	p	l	m	l	p	t	u	d	h
l	f	h	p	k	p	t	w	g	k	o	t	l	e
e	c	h	o	c	a	r	d	i	o	g	r	a	m
u	q	g	r	j	p	a	d	l	f	d	o	v	o
k	s	y	t	x	v	s	h	k	l	s	p	f	t
e	a	s	n	j	k	o	s	f	j	k	e	e	h
m	z	f	h	j	r	u	k	l	o	g	n	x	e
i	v	n	m	c	a	n	c	e	r	e	i	c	r
a	f	g	n	s	d	d	f	d	x	w	c	k	a
q	u	p	f	l	i	d	g	m	v	s	r	w	p
h	i	c	k	m	a	n	s	u	r	g	e	r	y
v	s	f	b	j	t	e	j	l	p	r	s	f	m
e	r	j	i	o	i	s	w	t	y	u	o	p	j
f	o	t	u	m	o	r	d	w	b	n	p	y	f
q	g	o	p	d	n	s	h	l	o	r	d	r	b

cancer

chemotherapy

echocardiogram

hickman

leukemia

neutropenic

port

radiation

surgery

tumor

ultrasound

Answers can be found on page 55.

3

At the Hospital

During your first visit to the hospital, your doctors will find out what type of cancer you have.

While you're there, you'll have a special tube put into a vein in your arm, hand, or leg. It's called an IV — that's short for intravenous (in-tra-veen-us). An IV looks like a long, clear straw. At one end is a bag of liquid (it looks like water) and at the other end is a tube that's put into your arm, hand, or leg. Don't worry, the tube won't hurt because some cream will be put on your skin to make it numb.

Most medicine that needs to go into your body for tests and treatment will be put through this IV. You'll stay in the hospital for a little while to start your treatment and make sure you're doing okay on it. After that, the IV will be taken out and you can go home. Then you'll come back to the hospital clinic during the day to get your chemo.

By Sabrina Fortino

I like watching movies

We all know one thing — nobody loves going to the hospital. If you've never been there before, it can be pretty scary at first. But being at the hospital is a big part of getting rid of your cancer. And don't forget that all the people at the hospital are there to help you get better and answer your questions.

Sometimes you might need a special treatment or you might get sick with a bad infection like chicken pox. At these times, you'll have to sleep over in the hospital for a few days until your doctor decides that you can go home.

"At first I didn't know anyone in the hospital and I felt really lonely. All I wanted was to go home. But then I got to know some of people who work in the hospital. They're so nice. They're my friends and help me feel better when I'm upset."

When you're first at the hospital, you might feel scared or lonely. Good news! Your Mom or Dad can stay overnight with you if you want. Sometimes they might sleep on a small bed right in your own room. You might pretend it's a special sleepover or that you're sleeping in a tent together deep in the forest.

Who's at the hospital?

The hospital is full of new people you've never met before. Let's talk about some of them.

Doctors

There will be many different doctors who will take care of you. There's a doctor who knows all about your cancer and how to treat it, a doctor who does operations, a doctor who keeps you asleep during operations and a doctor who will give you radiation if you need it.

Nurses

Nurses work with your doctors to help take care of you. They give you your medicine. No matter what time of day or night, there will always be a nurse there if you need one. You might wonder how all the nurses know about you. Well, there's a story written about you. All the nurses read it, so they learn everything they need to know to take good care of you.

Child Life Specialists (spesh-a-lists)

These people will help you feel less scared or lonely when you're at the hospital. They will talk to you about tests and operations that you will have, how you're feeling inside or anything else that happens at the hospital. Child life specialists even play with you. That's their job. Fun, isn't it?

Social (so-shull) Workers

The social worker helps you and your family to be strong during this time and can help with any worries that your Mom or Dad might have about things like money or their jobs.

Nutritionists (new-trish-on-ists)

These people make sure that you will be eating the right food when you have cancer, so that your body can stay strong. Sometimes you might have an upset tummy and not even want to eat. The nutritionist will help you feel better by choosing foods and ways of eating that will make it easier.

Pharmacists (farm-a-sists)

Every hospital has its own pharmacists. They put together the medicine that you need to get better. They will tell you and your family how the medicine works. And they will make sure your medicine is safe and working right.

Physiotherapists (fiz-ee-o-ther-a-pists)

These people help keep your body strong when you have cancer by keeping it moving. They might give you exercises to do.

School Teacher

If you have to miss school, teachers may be at the hospital to help you keep up with your schoolwork. Your teachers can help find ways for you to keep learning while you are taking your medicine.

Other People

There are many other people you'll meet in the hospital who do a bunch of things, like take pictures of the inside of your body or poke your finger to get blood. Remember, everyone at the hospital is there to help you get well again. Many of them might become your friends too.

What parts of the hospital will you see?

Your Room

You'll probably share a room with another child when you're in the hospital. This is someone to talk to and get to know. Sometimes when you don't have enough fighter cells, you will have a room all to yourself. Each room has its own TV, so you can watch your favorite shows. You might want to bring your special blanket or stuffed animal from home, so that your hospital room doesn't feel so strange.

"The hospital playroom is the best. I get to paint and draw and do lots of things that help me forget that I have cancer."

The Playroom

This is a fun place where you can play with toys, draw, do crafts, or even play computer games. Often there are other kids there too, so you can play with them if you want to.

The School Room

This is where you'll do your schoolwork. A teacher will be there to help you.

14

Radiology (ray-dee-all-o-jee)

This is where pictures are taken of the inside of your body. There are big machines here called CAT scanners and MRIs. These big machines are noisy but they won't hurt you or touch you.

Operating Room

If you need an operation (op-er-ay-shun), you will go to an operating room. Everyone in there will be wearing special gowns, hats, masks, and gloves to keep everything clean.

Recovery Room

This is where you go to wake up after an operation. There are nurses there to take care of you. Once you're awake, you'll go back to your room.

Clinic

This is the place you'll visit a lot once you've gone home. At the clinic you'll have check ups and medicine. The clinic has a room where you'll wait with your Mom or Dad. There's also a place where you can play. Waiting can be boring so why not bring a game or your favorite toy with you?

"There's lots of things about the hospital I don't like. But what I do like is that I never have to make my bed or help wash the dishes."

Find your way back to your room.

Recovery Room

Radiology

Playroom

Your Room

Clinic

School Room

Operating Room

Answers can be found on page 56.

4

What Tests Will You Have?

When your doctor thinks you have cancer, you'll need to have tests to find out which type of cancer you have, where it is, and what kind of treatment you need. Then, tests can help your doctor see how well the treatment is working. At the beginning, you'll have most of the tests while you stay in the hospital. Later, you'll have them when you visit the clinic from home.

So…let's talk about some of the tests you might have.

"I got so tired of having my finger poked. Sometimes I would get really mad at the nurse because it hurt. Then I started telling her jokes. It helped me forget the pain and made her laugh."

Finger Poke

Testing your blood is one of the best ways for your doctor to tell how you're doing. That's why your finger will be poked and blood taken often when you're in the hospital and on every visit to the clinic. Your finger will be cleaned very well, then poked with a needle. The poke will hurt for a second, but then the hurt goes away.

Tests are a big part of having cancer because they're the best way for your doctor to find out how you're doing. Let's face it — tests aren't much fun and sometimes they can hurt. It's okay to feel afraid or mad or bored. But, remember, there are things you can do to make the tests easier, help the time go faster … and even have some fun.

17

Then the nurse will gently squeeze your finger so that the blood goes into a tube. Your job is to hold still. You can watch while the nurse is doing it or you might want to look away. You can tell stories to your Mom or Dad, or even cry out if you want to. Do whatever makes you feel better. And don't worry about the blood that's taken. Your body makes more right away, so you won't miss what's gone.

CAT Scan

A CAT scan uses a computer to take pictures of the inside of your body. You will need to lie very still so that the pictures aren't blurry. Sometimes you will be given medicine to help you sleep.

"I was scared for my first ultrasound, but it was really neat to see my insides on that TV screen. I bet none of my friends at school get to see that."

For this test, you will lie down on a table with a belt or strap over your tummy. The table will gently move through a large machine shaped like a circle. The machine will never touch your body and it won't hurt you. Sometimes you will drink a special liquid or the nurse will put fluid into your IV so that different parts of your body will show up on the picture. You might not be able to eat or drink before your CAT scan. Your Mom or Dad can be in the room, but they will have to wear a special apron to protect themselves. While you're having the CAT scan, you might pretend you're in a time machine. Travel back in time and imagine what it would be like to be a pioneer in the wild west.

Ultrasound

An ultrasound helps your doctor see the organs in your body, like the kidneys or liver. First, the person doing the test will put gel on your tummy and then will move a wand over the gel. This makes pictures of the inside of your body show up on a TV so your doctor can see it. If you want, you can look too.

An ultrasound doesn't hurt, but you must lie very still. Your Mom or Dad can be in the room with you while you're having an ultrasound. While you're waiting for the test to finish, why not think about doing something you've always dreamed of, like going to Disneyland or meeting your favorite music star?

MRI

MRI is a machine that takes very clear pictures of the inside of your body. You must lie very still while the machine is taking these pictures so they won't be blurry. If the test is going to take a long time, you will be given some medicine to make you sleep.

This is me having a CAT scan. The medicine tastes so good, I wanted to drink 3 cans

Zachary age 5

For this test, you will lie down on a table, which moves gently backwards into a machine shaped like a tunnel. This machine makes loud noises while it's taking pictures. But don't worry, the machine never touches you and it doesn't hurt you. You can wear earplugs to help block out the noise, but you'll still be able to hear the nurse who will be talking to you during the test.

Your Mom or Dad might be able to be in the room with you and can even hold on to your feet while you're having the test. When you're in the machine, you might like to imagine you're someplace else, like in a spaceship flying to Mars or walking through a tunnel to find hidden treasures.

Echocardiogram (ec-o-car-dee-o-gram)

An echocardiogram is often called an 'echo'. It takes a picture of your heart to see how it's working. You must lie still during this test. You might be given medicine to help you sleep. Like the ultrasound, there will be gel on your chest and a wand is moved back and forth. A picture of your heart then shows up on a TV — you can look if you want to. Sometimes you can actually hear your heart beating. This test doesn't hurt. While you're having the test, your Mom or Dad can be with you. If you're afraid, take slow, deep breaths in and out to help you feel better.

Lumbar Puncture (punk-chur)

A lumbar puncture is sometimes called a spinal tap or an LP. Using a needle, a doctor takes fluid from the spine in your back to check if sick cells are there and may inject chemo through the same needle. For this test, you will be given medicine to make you sleep until the test is done. You will be asleep during the whole test and should not feel anything. After the test is over, you might feel a little sore where the needle was put in. And you will need to lie down for a while so you don't get a headache.

"Waiting at the clinic to have my tests done was so boring. But then my Mom said I should write a different story during each visit. She collected them and we made a scrapbook. I took the scrapbook with me every time I went to the clinic and showed it to the nurses and doctors — they even wrote in it."

Bone Marrow Exam

A bone marrow exam takes a sample of your bone marrow through a needle. Bone marrow is the soft part inside your bones where your blood is made. Your doctor will give you medicine to sleep. You will be asleep during the whole test and will not feel anything.

Bone Scan

A bone scan takes pictures of the bones inside your body. Before the test, some liquid will be put into your IV. This makes sure the pictures we take of your bones come out clearly. For this test, you lie on a table, which is moved under the camera machine. This machine will never touch you and it won't hurt you. Your Mom or Dad can be in the room with you. You will be awake for this test. Listen to this ... there might be even a movie for you to watch until the test is over. Yippee!

Philip age 8

I don't mind needles, except I.V. needles ... OUCH!!!

Lung Function (fung-shun) Test

Sometimes your doctor needs to see how well you're breathing. For this test, you will sit down and then take a deep breath. Then a tube is placed in your mouth and you will blow all of the air out as fast as you can. You will do this a few times. That's all there is to it.

ACTIVITY PAGE

The worst and best of your tests.

Write or draw the worst part of a test you've just had. Then tell us about the best part.

_____

_____

_____

_____

_____

_____

_____

_____

_____

_____

_____

5

How Will Your Cancer be Treated?

Operation (op-er-ay-shun)

When sick cells clump together, they make a lump in your body. This is called a tumor. Your doctor will want to look at the tumor and take some or all of it out. But how? Your doctor makes a cut in your body and looks inside. This is called an operation. Don't worry, you won't feel anything during the operation because you'll be fast asleep.

To get ready for an operation, you might need some tests. These are done to make sure the operation is as safe as it can be.

Before the operation, you won't be able to eat or drink anything. The nurse may give you some medicine that makes you sleepy and helps you to feel calm and relaxed.

Then you'll be put on a stretcher — that's a skinny bed with wheels — and you'll be taken to the operating room. In there, all the nurses and doctors will be wearing special gowns, hats, masks, and gloves. They might look like they're dressed up for Halloween! They do it so that everything is kept clean during your operation.

Treatments that get rid of sick cells might make you feel lots of different things, like tired, cranky or mad. Sometimes your hair will fall out. With all these things happening to you, it might be hard to remember that the treatments are working hard to help you get better. It's true, they are.

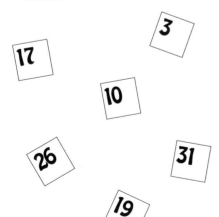

"I was getting tired of all the treatments and visits to the clinic. There seemed to be s-o-o-o many of them and I was getting confused about when I was having them. Then the nurse said I should make my very own calendar and mark all the days that I have my treatments. It's fun keeping track and now I know when I'm coming in. Sometimes I even have to remind my Mom!"

One doctor you'll see is the anesthetist — remember, that's the doctor who makes sure you stay asleep during the operation. This doctor will give you medicine through your IV or through a mask that's put over your nose and mouth. Before you know it, you'll be fast asleep. And you'll stay asleep during the whole operation. You won't feel anything.

During an operation, the doctor might put a plastic tube inside your body. It's called a catheter and it collects your pee during the operation. Sometimes the catheter will stay in your body for a few days after your operation. That's so that your doctor can see if your body is doing okay.

If you're having an operation on your head, your doctor will shave off some of your hair. That's so that there is a clean, clear spot to do the operation.

At the end of the operation, your doctor will sew up the cut with stitches. Then, in what seems like a second or two, you'll wake up and the operation will be over. By now you're in the recovery room. This is the room where you stay until you're wide awake. Hurrah! — your Mom and Dad can come into the recovery room to see you.

You might be a little sore after the operation when you move or when you cough. If you feel a lot of pain, your doctor can give you medicine to help you feel better. After several days, the doctor or nurse will take your stitches out. There will be a scar left over that shows where your doctor looked inside your body. You'll always have this scar but you'll notice it less and less as time goes on.

Your medicine tube

You will have an operation where a special tube is put into your body. Then, medicines are put into your body through that one tube. This makes it much easier for you and for the people working at the hospital. Once all treatments are finished, the doctor takes the tube out.

There are two kinds of tubes — Port and Hickman tubes.

A Port tube is put under your skin. You can't see it. Medicine is put into the Port tube by a needle through your skin. This needle won't hurt because the nurse will put some cream on your skin to make it numb.

If you have a Hickman tube, part of it is put under your skin and the other part stays outside your body on your chest. Medicine is then put into the tube by a needle or by connecting an IV to your Hickman. This will not hurt. To help keep the tube in place, a bandage is put over it. Then the tape on the end of the Hickman is pinned to your clothing.

You can help take good care of your tube. Try not to bump the area where the tube is. And keep an eye on the skin around your tube. If it looks red, tell your Mom, Dad, or the nurse.

If you have a Hickman tube, it will need a bit more care. That's because part of it is outside your body on your chest. Don't get it wet while you're taking a bath. And make sure that the bandage stays in place over the tube and the tube stays pinned to your clothing.

Chemotherapy (kee-mo-ther-a-pee)

You'll probably hear everyone call this treatment "chemo" (kee-mo). Sick cells can be in more than one place and sometimes they're even hiding. For some kinds of cancer, chemo is the only way to get rid of the sick cells.

There are different ways to get chemo. One way is taking pills through your mouth. Another way is through a Port or Hickman tube. Some children have chemo put in their back, leg or under their skin through a needle.

Chemo will work hard to help you get better, but it can make you feel lots of different things.

- It might make your body feel tired, cranky, angry, sad or any other feelings which you'll be told about.

- Your tummy might feel upset and you might throw up, but we do have medicine that can help you feel better.

- You might get sores in your mouth, which may make it hard to eat food. Remember to take good care of your teeth and gums when you're taking chemo.

- You might get a rash on your skin.

- You will lose some or all of your hair. That's because the medicine can hurt your healthy cells (like hair cells) while it's trying to get rid of the sick cells. The good news is that your hair will grow back once you've finish taking chemo.

Radiation (ray-dee-ay-shun)

Radiation sends invisible rays into your body that you can't feel, smell, touch, or see. These rays zap the sick cells and stop them from growing and spreading.

"I felt sad when my hair started falling out. But it was fun to pick out scarves to wear. The ones with flowers are my favorite — I have a different one for every day of the week. You know the best part? I never have to wash my hair."

You will visit the radiation department a few times before treatment starts. That's so the radiation doctor can decide exactly where the rays need to go to zap the cancer cells. If you're having radiation to your head, neck, or tummy, a plastic mould will usually be made. You'll wear this mould every time you have radiation. Special markings will be put on the mould so that the radiation can go to the right part every time.

If you're having radiation on another part of your body, color marks may be drawn right on your body — just like a cool tattoo. Be sure not to wash those marks off — they have to stay on until your treatment is finished.

You'll come in every day for some weeks to have radiation. You'll only get a little bit each time. Too much radiation at once wouldn't be good for you.

When you have radiation, you'll lie on a table and the rays will be aimed at the marks on your mould or other part of your body. The machine makes noises but it never touches you and never hurts you. All it does is send invisible rays into your body. You must lie very still but only for a few seconds. You'll be alone for these few seconds. Don't worry, your Mom or Dad or nurse can talk to you through a special speaker. Then it's all over and you didn't even feel a thing!

Radiation might give you an upset tummy for a little while. We can give you medicine to help you feel better. And you might feel tired and sleepy. Try to take it easy and do things that don't take a lot of energy — like watching TV or playing video games. Sometimes the skin where the invisible rays go is red and sore for a bit — your nurse can give you something to take the itch or sting away.

If you have radiation to your head, your hair will fall out. That means it's working! Sometimes it doesn't all grow back. Think about all the different kinds of wigs, hats, and scarves you can wear.

"When I put on my mask for the radiation, I pretend I'm a pilot in outer space. I'm getting ready to fight the aliens. The radiation machine is my weapon that shoots invisible rays at the alien troops."

How the cancer medicine goes to work.

We did the pictures. You fill in the words.

Introducing:

Super Med
The Cancer Medicine Hero

Sick Cell

Healthy Cell

6

How Are You Feeling?

You

There are lots of feelings that go along with cancer. Sad, mad, lonely, afraid, bored, and upset feelings. Then there are hope, joy, and strong feelings. You might feel like you're a yo-yo with all the different things that you'll feel inside.

"I try to be very brave. Sometimes I don't want anyone to know that I feel really scared inside. The other day I asked my Dad if he's afraid about me having cancer. He said yes. I told him I am too. It helps to know he feels the same way I do."

Whatever you're feeling, it's okay. Try not to hide it. Sometimes hiding your feelings can make you feel more scared. There are lots of people you can talk to, like your Mom and Dad. In the hospital, there are doctors, nurses, child life specialists, and many others who can listen to you and answer your questions. Or you might choose to talk to other kids with cancer — they might understand better than anyone how you're feeling.

When you have cancer, you'll have many different feelings — so many that it might be hard to sort them out. Maybe you'll feel scared and want to cry. Or you might feel mad and want to stamp your feet. Remember, one of the best things you can do is to tell someone else how you're feeling. Sure, there are times to be quiet, but there are also times not to be!

Your parents

Your Mom and Dad love you, so they're upset that you have cancer. They might feel afraid about what's happening to you or they might be angry because they feel there's nothing they can do to make you better.

It might be hard for your Mom and Dad to talk to you about cancer because they think it might upset you. Why not ask them to talk to you about it? If you talk together, there's a good chance that you'll all feel much better.

"The worst part for me is when I feel like I'm never going to get better. So mostly I try to think about today and how everyone is working hard to get me well again. I know it's okay to feel bad sometimes. But I still keep telling myself I'm going to get through it and I dream about what I'll do when I'm older...when I don't have cancer anymore."

Brothers and sisters

If you have a brother or sister, they might feel mixed up about what's happening to you. Because your parents need to spend so much time with you, your brother or sister might feel jealous or angry. It might be hard for them not to get the cards and presents that you might be getting. They might be worried about you being sick. Or maybe they're worried about getting sick too. The more they know about what's happening to you, the better they'll feel. If you want, talk to your brother or sister and ask them if they have questions. That helps them to feel included.

30

Friends

Some friends will always be your friends, no matter what. They'll stick by you and help you when you need it. Other kids might tease you and hurt your feelings. They might be doing that because they feel scared. You can say something to them, you can pretend not to hear them or you can see that they're scared too.

Sometimes kids might ask questions about why you're sick. If you want to, you can answer them, or you can tell them you don't want to talk about it. It's up to you.

UPSET **MAD** Cranky

"Right after my operation, I was mad because I couldn't be out playing with my best friend, Suzy. I yelled at the nurse but then I felt so bad because maybe I'd hurt her feelings. She said not to worry about it. And she said it's good to yell and let your mad feelings out. Then they go away."

How are you feeling?

Write or draw how you're feeling today. Then do the same for tomorrow and the day after that. You'll find out that cancer makes you feel many different things.

7

What About Your Life?

Eating

Some treatments for cancer can make eating a real chore. You might not even feel like having your favorite pizza or a Big Mac. Eat the best you can because it's important to get enough food so your body can be strong and keep growing. Try to eat healthy foods that give you lots of energy. The hospital nutritionist can tell you what the best foods are to eat.

Here's what to do if it's hard to eat.
If your mouth is sore or dry:

- suck on your favorite hard candy or even a piece of cold ice

- drink some water or juice

- put lots of yummy gravy and butter on your food

- spread some vaseline on your lips — it will make them smooth and soft

It seems that cancer turns your life upside down. You might wonder if you can still do the things you used to do — like play with your friends, eat your favorite foods or go to your favorite places. It's true that some things in your life will change — for now anyway — but you can still do many of the things you've always done.

H₂O

GingerAle

33

If your tummy is upset or you're throwing up:

- try not to eat too much

- eat lots of small meals or snacks

- don't eat hot and cold food together

- have ginger ale, popsicles (yum!) or crackers

- try not to eat too many sweet foods

- don't lie down right after you eat

"My tummy gets so upset after the radiation. I just can't eat. Sucking on my favorite candy —hard toffee— helps. My Mom gives me a lot of apple juice too."

Sometimes you just can't eat enough food on your own, so you might need extra help to put more food into your body. That's done with a special tube. A tube might be put into your nose and then down into your tummy. When the tube is put in, you might feel upset but it only takes a few minutes to do. Even with the tube in, you can still eat and drink on your own. At first, you will feel the tube but then you'll get used to it.

You can also get extra food through your Port or Hickman tube. This food looks like milk or juice and will help you get stronger.

Other times, a tube is put right into the tummy if your body needs help for a long time. This will be done during an operation. When your nutritionist thinks you're eating enough food, the feeding tube will be taken out.

Your mouth

Some medicines can make your mouth feel sore. One of the best things you can do is take good care of what's inside your mouth — your teeth and gums.

"My friends and I have fun riding our bikes but some days I feel too tired to do it. That's when I have my best friend Suzy over to paint or play video games. Just because I'm tired doesn't mean I can't have fun!"

- Have your Mom or Dad buy you a new, soft toothbrush. Pick your favorite color. Then brush your teeth after every meal. Remember to brush gently.

- Your doctor might give you a mouth rinse to keep your mouth clean and make the pain go away. How long can you gargle for?

- Your lips might get dry a lot. Get your own tube of vaseline and spread it on your lips whenever you need to.

Being active

There will be some days, like after your treatments, when you will be tired and sleepy. That's the time to take it easy until you feel better. There are lots of things you can do when you're feeling tired. Pretend there's a big storm outside and you can't go out — what would you do? Write a story, do a puzzle or maybe watch your favorite video.

The good news is there are other days when you'll feel full of energy. On those days, do all the things you like to do. Being active is good for your body and your feelings.

Infections (in-fek-shuns)

An infection is a sickness that can spread from one person to another. The cold, flu, measles, and chicken pox are all infections. If you're having chemo, your body can catch infections more often. That means that you will have to stay away from school if someone there has an infection that could be passed on to you.

"I was mad when one of my friends got the chicken pox. I know it wasn't his fault, but I had to stay away from school. It's good that he's better now so I can go back to school."

Fun recipes for good eating

Ask your Mom or Dad to help you try these recipes — they're yummy and will give you lots of energy!

Fruit Milkshake

1/2 cup (125mL) whole milk
1/4 cup (50mL) skim milk powder
3/4 cup (200mL) vanilla ice cream
1/2 cup (125mL) fresh strawberries

Blend all ingredients until smooth.

Try adding:
1 small ripe banana
Or 1/2 cup (125mL) peaches
Or 1/4 cup (50mL) peanut butter
Or 1/4 cup (50mL) chocolate/butterscotch syrup

Trail Mix

1 cup (250mL) sunflower seeds
1/2 cup (125mL) raisins
1 cup (250mL) shredded coconut
1/2 cup (125mL) peanuts (chopped)
1/2 cup (125mL) dried dates (chopped)
1/2 cup (125mL) almonds
1/2 cup (125mL) brazil nuts

Mix well. Store in airtight containers.

Rice Pudding

1/2 cup (125mL) uncooked rice
1 egg, beaten
1/4 cup (50mL) sugar
pinch of salt
1 cup (250mL) whole milk
1/4 cup (50mL) skim milk powder
1 tsp (5mL) vanilla
1 cup (250mL) raisins

Add rice to boiling water. Cover and reduce heat. Simmer for 10 minutes. Combine egg, sugar, salt, whole milk and skim milk powder. Add to cooked rice and mix well. Continue cooking over low heat for 5 minutes until mixture thickens. Remove from heat. Stir in vanilla and raisins and enjoy!

What About School?

While you're being treated for cancer, there may be times when you have to stay in the hospital or at home. You might be worried about falling behind in your school work and you might miss being with your friends. When you have to stay away from school, you can still do the work your friends are doing in class. And ask your friends to write you letters, call or visit when they can. That way you won't feel left out.

When you're in the hospital

There is a school room in the hospital where you can go and do your schoolwork. There is a teacher there especially for you. This person will talk to your own teacher to find out what you've been doing in school and will help you keep up with the rest of your classmates. There might be times when you don't feel well enough to do your homework. That's okay. When you're better, you'll catch up.

When you go back to school

Some kids are nervous about going back to school. That's natural. Remember that your parents and people from the hospital will talk to your teacher, principal, and school nurse about why you've been away.

When you have cancer, you might miss some — or a lot — of school. After you've been away from school, you might have mixed-up feelings about going back. You might be excited but you might be worried about how the other kids will treat you. Don't forget, you're not alone. Your Mom, Dad, teacher, even the hospital staff will make it easier for you to go back to school.

39

"I love school, so it's hard to be in the hospital and be away from it for so long. I was so happy when I saw the school room at the hospital. Now I go as often as I can to see the teacher there. She's helping me keep up with my schoolwork."

When you go back, the kids might ask you questions. You don't have to answer them if you don't want to. But if you do, why not talk with your Mom and Dad about how to answer any questions? That way you'll be ready. Some kids do a special project on cancer for the whole class. Sometimes people from the hospital can go to your school to explain to your classmates what it's like to have cancer.

Some kids might tease you and hurt your feelings. They might be doing that because they feel scared or are worried about you. You can say something to them, you can pretend not to hear them or you can see that they're scared or worried too.

Sometimes you will need to take your medicine at school. Don't worry. Your Mom or Dad will talk to the school nurse and your teacher about your medicine and when you need to take it. Some kids might ask why you're taking medicine. If you want to, you can explain that it's helping you get better.

"When I went back to school, the bully in our class stole my hat and ran away with it. Luckily, I had an extra one in my pocket. I put it on and went and stood with my friends. I didn't pay any attention to the bully and he left me alone."

At school, you can probably do all the activities you did before you got cancer. Sometimes you might feel tired because of the treatment you're having. If you do, try to take it easy until you have more energy.

One of the best parts of going back to school is being with your best friends again.

"I was feeling embarrassed about going back to school because I look different. So it's good that before I went back, my teacher explained to the whole class why I'd been gone. I'm glad I didn't have to tell them. And everyone is so nice now that I'm back."

41

School hats — choose your own.

Here's a collection of fun hats you might want to wear to school. Color them in and then choose your favorite one.

Where Can You Get Help and Have Fun?

As we've told you, there's lots of help for you and your family from people at the hospital. But there are also other people around you, where you live, who can offer extra things that you might need. If you need to know how to find these other people, ask the staff at the clinic or the social worker. They can help.

"I'd never been to camp, but I've always wanted to go. Then we heard about Camp Trillium — it's just for kids with cancer. So I went and you know what, I loved it. I even got to paddle a canoe. And I made lots of friends."

Camps

Have you ever been to camp? Have you ever thought about going? Water, sun, crafts, trees, canoe trips, hiking … there's lots of fun to be had at camp. When you have cancer, you might not be able to go to regular camps, but hold onto your hats … there are special camps just for kids with cancer. Yup, that's right. And some of them are even free. At these camps, you can meet, play, have fun and talk to other kids with cancer. And at some of the camps, your family can even go with you.

Cancer is tough and it can take a lot out of kids and their families. There will be lots of time when you need help and kindness to be okay. Remember, you're not alone and there is plenty of help out there. All you need to do is ask for it.

Help groups

There are many groups that help you and your family in all kinds of ways when you have cancer. They have lots of books, videos and other things to help you learn more about what's happening to you. Some groups help your parents find a nice place to stay, like a Ronald McDonald house, if you're having treatment far from home. Others help you and your family talk about your worries with people who are going through the same thing.

Making wishes come true

Have you ever made a wish? Has it ever come true? Believe it or not, there are groups that make wishes come true for kids with cancer. They grant wishes — like going to Disneyland or meeting a famous person — so that kids with cancer and their families can feel really happy.

"If I had one wish, it would be to fly to the moon. I don't think anyone can make that wish come true. But maybe I could go and see the space shuttle take off. I've seen it on TV but it would be really cool to see it in real life."

44

The internet

Have you ever 'surfed' the internet? Well, if you can, why not give it a try? You can get a ton of information about kids and cancer on the internet. And you can even get in touch with other kids with cancer from faraway countries, like Japan or Australia.

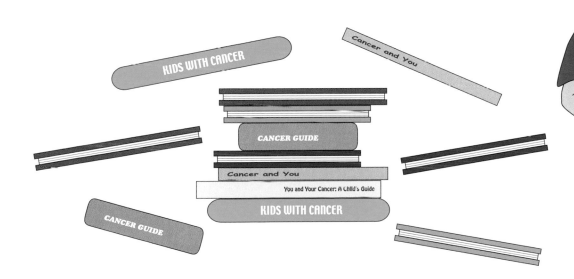

"You know, I really want to know more about cancer. I was worried because I couldn't find any books just for kids, but then the child life specialist told me about Candlelighters — they have lots of books for kids my age. My mother is going to call next week to check it out."

When you wish upon a star

If you could have or do anything, what would it be? Make one wish, or two or three. Then draw or write them down here.

_____

_____

_____

_____

10

Why Do Some Kids Die?

We know that most kids with cancer get better. But, for a few kids, the treatment can't do its job or the cancer comes back again later. Sometimes these kids die. It's important to remember that death is natural — it just happens sooner for some people than for others. Some kids worry that death might be painful. But it doesn't have to be — if there's any pain, doctors give medicine to make it go away. After death, there's no pain at all.

"My best friend in the hospital was Charlie. One day I went into his room and he wasn't there. My Mom told me Charlie died. I felt mad and sad all at the same time. Later, my Mom and I looked at all the pictures Charlie and I had done together. I got a scrapbook for the pictures. That way I'll always remember him."

by Marcus   by Charlie

It's natural to want to know what death means — to want to know what happens to us when we die. Everyone has his or her own ideas about it. For instance, some people think that when a person's body dies, their spirit goes up to heaven to be with all the other spirits who have gone there before.

Life is like a circle. Everything that lives must also die sometimes. That goes for people, animals, trees, plants …everything and everyone. It's okay to think about death and it's even better to talk about it with someone else. Talking can give you courage and help you feel less afraid.

47

When someone we know dies, it hurts. That's because we miss them very much. It's okay to cry or shout or whatever you need to do. If you can, try not to keep your feelings inside. Let them out — you'll feel better that way. Someday you'll be able to think about the person who has died and not feel so sad. You see, a person who dies always lives on because we remember them.

"I've been thinking a lot about death lately. Sometimes I worry that I might die sooner because I think about it so much. But then, Grace, my child life specialist, said it's natural to think about death — she said it's good to talk about it too. And I felt much better when she said that thinking about death doesn'tmake it happen."

If you have questions about death or if you feel scared, talk about it with someone you trust. Some moms and dads might not want to talk about death to their kids. That's because it makes them sad. If you want, you might talk to someone who works at the hospital, like your nurse or child life specialist. Some kids say it's easier to talk to other kids and find out what they think about death.

If you don't want to talk about death, keeping your own journal might be a good way of letting your feelings out. Put whatever you want in your journal — words, poems, pictures… anything at all. You can keep your journal private or you can show it to people who are close to you. Sharing your feelings will help you feel better.

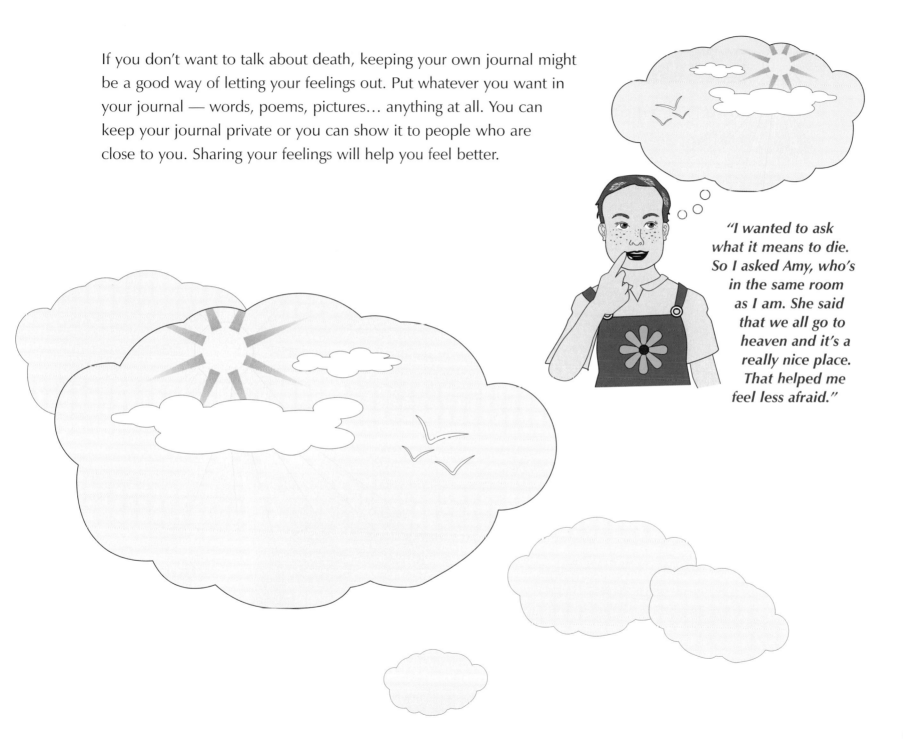

"I wanted to ask what it means to die. So I asked Amy, who's in the same room as I am. She said that we all go to heaven and it's a really nice place. That helped me feel less afraid."

Why not write a letter?

Have you known a person who has died? Or a pet? Try writing a letter to them. Tell them what you're thinking about death and what you imagine it to be like. Then, if you want, show this letter to someone and see what they think about death too.

_____

_____

_____

_____

_____

_____

_____

_____

_____

_____

11

When You're All Better

When your doctors know that the sick cells have gone away, your treatments will finish. They will still watch you regularly and will do tests to check how your body is doing. As time goes on and you're doing well, these visits will happen less often. One day, you will need to go only once a year.

It's a funny thing. When you have cancer, all you might think about is getting better. So how will you feel when you are better? Kids are usually happy, but sometimes they're scared too — scared of what will happen next or scared that they're not going to stay better.

"I'm going to miss Peter, he gave me my radiation. We saw a lot of each other and he really helped me feel less scared. I've been seeing so much of him and now I won't see him at all. Then the other day, Peter asked for my address so he could send me a birthday card. I'm going to send him one on his birthday too!

Some kids even miss having cancer. Let's face it — when you have cancer, lots of people pay attention to you. You may have gotten lots of gifts and cards, and made lots of friends. That might change now and you might miss it.

Think of all the changes that happened in your life when you found out you had cancer. Now that you're better there may be other, different changes to get used to. For some kids, everything goes back to the way it was before they got sick; for others, life will be different...but maybe even better.

You've met lots of new people at the hospital. And you've probably made friends with some of them. You might miss them — they're going to miss you too. Why not send photos and cards to your favorite people at the hospital? That way they will know how you're doing.

"I'm only 8 years old, but after having cancer, I feel older. I think about how great it is to be alive. Maybe someday I'll be a cancer doctor, so I can help kids just like me."

Some kids have a big party when they've finished their treatments, with cake, balloons, music and friends. Maybe you'll have one too — this will be one party you'll always remember.

Think about how cancer has changed you inside and out. Maybe there have been lots of changes; maybe there haven't been any. Some kids say they feel more grown up; others say they love life more because their bodies aren't sick anymore.

I'm Smiling Because I Feel Better

Jackson Larouche (7)

One thing's for sure. You're alive and you beat cancer. And while you might have changed in some ways, you're still you. That's what counts. Now it's time to start to enjoy being you again; time to live your own special life, whatever it may bring.

"Good and bad things happen to everyone. Cancer was a bad thing that happened to me. Sometimes I'd like to forget that I ever had it. But, you know, remembering that I had cancer helps me like life even more. I feel really lucky to be alive."

Have you changed?

Everything changes in life — like the leaves changing color in fall. How has cancer changed you — inside or out?

Changes you like the most.   **Changes you don't like.**

_____	_____
_____	_____
_____	_____
_____	_____
_____	_____
_____	_____
_____	_____
_____	_____
_____	_____
_____	_____

Answer Key

for word search, page 10.

k	o	p	w	s	h	r	d	y	i	j	n	q	a
f	h	e	k	o	e	u	g	s	j	l	e	w	c
g	z	c	h	l	p	l	m	l	p	t	u	d	l
l	f	h	p	k	p	t	w	g	k	o	t	l	e
e	c	h	o	c	a	r	d	i	o	g	r	a	m
u	q	g	r	j	p	a	d	l	f	d	o	v	o
k	s	y	t	x	v	s	h	k	l	s	p	f	t
e	a	s	n	j	k	o	s	f	j	k	e	e	h
m	z	f	h	j	r	u	k	l	o	g	n	x	e
i	v	n	m	c	a	n	c	e	r	e	i	c	r
a	f	g	n	s	d	d	f	d	x	w	c	k	a
q	u	p	f	l	i	d	g	m	v	s	r	w	p
h	i	c	k	m	a	n	s	u	r	g	e	r	y
v	s	f	b	j	t	e	j	l	p	r	s	f	m
e	r	j	i	o	i	s	w	t	y	u	o	p	j
f	o	t	u	m	o	r	d	w	b	n	p	y	f
q	g	o	p	d	n	s	h	l	o	r	d	r	b

Answer Key

for maze, page 16.

Recovery Room

Radiology

Playroom

Your Room

Clinic

School Room

Operating Room

BUSINESS REPLY MAIL
FIRST-CLASS MAIL   PERMIT NO. 25   LEWISTON, NY

POSTAGE WILL BE PAID BY ADDRESSEE

B C DECKER INC

ORDER DEPARTMENT

P O BOX 785

LEWISTON NY 14092-9956

BUSINESS REPLY MAIL
FIRST-CLASS MAIL   PERMIT NO. 25   LEWISTON, NY

POSTAGE WILL BE PAID BY ADDRESSEE

B C DECKER INC

ORDER DEPARTMENT

P O BOX 785

LEWISTON NY 14092-9956

NATION
OF NATIONS
Volume II: Since 1865

Here is not merely a nation but a teeming nation of nations.
—WALT WHITMAN

NATION
OF NATIONS

A NARRATIVE
HISTORY
OF THE AMERICAN REPUBLIC

VOLUME II: SINCE 1865

JAMES WEST DAVIDSON

WILLIAM E. GIENAPP
The University of Wyoming

CHRISTINE LEIGH HEYRMAN
Brandeis University

MARK H. LYTLE
Bard College

MICHAEL B. STOFF
The University of Texas, Austin

McGRAW-HILL PUBLISHING COMANY
New York   St. Louis   San Francisco   Auckland   Bogotá   Caracas   Hamburg   Lisbon
London   Madrid   Mexico   Milan   Montreal   New Delhi   Oklahoma City   Paris
San Juan   São Paulo   Singapore   Sydney   Tokyo   Toronto

NATION OF NATIONS: A NARRATIVE HISTORY OF THE AMERICAN REPUBLIC
Volume II: Since 1865

2 3 4 5 6 7 8 9 0   VNH   HNV   VNH   9 4 3 2 1 0

ISBN   0-07-557202-8

This book was set in Caledonia by York Graphic Services, Inc.
The editors were Christopher J. Rogers and Judith Kromm; the designer was John Lennard; the
production supervisor was Laura Lamorte. Von Hoffmann Press, Inc., was printer and binder.

Cover and Title Page Photo:
John Sloan, "Election Night," 1907, oil on canvas, 26⅜ × 32¼ inches. Memorial Art Gallery of
the University of Rochester, Marion Stratton Gould Fund. Photo by James M. Via.

Library of Congress Cataloging-in-Publication Data

(Revised for vol. 2)

Nation of nations.

  Includes bibliographical references.

  Contents: v. 1. To 1877.--v. 2. Since 1865.
  1. United States--History. I. Davidson, James West.
E178.1.N346 1990   973   89-14592
ISBN 0-07-557198-6 (v. 1)

Permissions Acknowledgments

921 Reprinted from *Smithsonian Collection of Classic Jazz*. © Smithsonian Institution, Washington,
D.C., pp. 4–5; **923** Excerpt from Claude McKay, "If We Must Die" from *White Shadows*. Copyright ©
1981 Twayne Publishers, a division of G. K. Hall & Co., Boston. Reprinted with permission; **942** From
Gordon Thomas and Max Morgan-Witts, *The Day the Bubble Burst: The Social History of the Wall
Street Crash of 1929*, Doubleday & Co., 1979; **1106** Taken from Frank Levy, *Dollars and Dreams: The
Changing American Income Distribution*. © 1987 Russell Sage Foundation. Used with permission of
the Russell Sage Foundation; **1143** Adapted from Richard Day, "The Economics of Technological
Change and the Demise of the Sharecropper," *American Economic Review* 57 (1967) [Figure 3], with
additional data from the U.S. Department of Agriculture, Economic Research; **1206** Excerpt from
Nikki Giovanni, "The True Import of Present Dialogue: Black vs. Negro" from *Black Feeling, Black
Talk, Black Judgment,* William Morrow & Co., © 1968, 1970 by Nikki Giovanni; **1259** Taken from
Frank Levy, *Dollars and Dreams: The Changing American Income Distribution*. © 1987 Russell Sage
Foundation. Used with permission of the Russell Sage Foundation; **1260** From "I Am Changing My
Name to Chrysler" by Tom Paxton. © Copyright 1980 Accabonac Music. All Rights Reserved. Used by
permission.

CONTENTS

CHAPTER 33   The Vietnam Era   1192

LIST OF MAPS AND CHARTS

PREFACE

History is both a discipline of rigor, bound by rules and scholarly methods, and something more: the unique, compelling, even strange way in which we humans define ourselves. We are all the sum of the tales of thousands of people, great and small, whose actions have etched their lines upon us. History supplies our very identity—a sense of the social groups to which we belong, whether family, ethnic group, race, class, or gender. It reveals to us the foundations of our deepest religious beliefs and traces the roots of our economic and political systems. It explores how we celebrate and grieve, sing the songs we sing, weather the illnesses to which time and chance subject us. It commands our attention for all these good reasons and for no good reason at all, other than a fascination with the way the myriad tales play out. Strange that we should come to care about a host of men and women so many centuries gone, some with names eminent and familiar, others unknown but for a chance scrap of information left behind in an obscure letter.

Yet we do care. We care about Sir Humphrey Gilbert, "devoured and swallowed up of the Sea" one black Atlantic night in 1583, about George Washington at Kips Bay, red with fury as he takes a riding crop to his retreating soldiers. We care about Octave Johnson, a slave fleeing through Louisiana swamps trying to decide whether to stand and fight the approaching hounds or take his chances with the bayou alligators, about Clara Barton, her nurse's skirts so heavy with blood from the wounded, she must wring them out before tending to the next soldier. We are drawn to the fate of Chinese laborers, chipping away at the Sierras' looming granite; a Georgian named Tom Watson seeking to forge a colorblind political alliance; and desperate immigrant mothers, kerosene in hand, storming Brooklyn butcher shops that had again raised prices. We follow, with a mix of awe and amusement, the fortunes of the quirky Henry Ford ("Everybody wants to be somewhere he ain't"), turning out identical automobiles, insisting his factory workers wear identical expressions ("Fordization of the Face"). We trace the career of young Thurgood Marshall, crisscrossing the South in his own "little old beat-up '29 Ford," typing legal briefs in the back seat, trying to get black teachers to sue for equal pay, hoping to get his people somewhere they weren't. The list could go on and on, spilling out as it did in Walt Whitman's *Leaves of Grass:* "A southerner soon as a northerner, a planter nonchalant and hospitable, / A Yankee bound my own way. . . . a Hoosier, a Badger, a Buckeye, a Louisianian or Georgian. . . ." Whitman embraced and celebrated them all, inseparable strands of what made him an American and what made him human:

> In all people I see myself, none more and not one a barleycorn less,
> And the good or bad I say of myself I say of them.

To encompass so expansive an America Whitman turned to poetry; historians have traditionally chosen *narrative* as their means of giving life to the past. That mode of explanation permits them to interweave the strands of economic, political, and social history in a coherent chronological framework. By choosing narrative, they affirm the multicausal nature of historical explanation—the insistence that events be portrayed in context. By choosing narrative, they are also acknowledging that, while long-term economic and social trends shape societies in deep and significant ways, events often take on a logic (or illogic) of their own, jostling one another, being deflected and redirected by unpredictable successions of personal decisions, sudden deaths, natural catastrophes, and chance. There are literary reasons, too, for preferring a narrative approach, since it supplies a dramatic force usually missing from more structural analyses of the past.

In some ways, surveys like this one are the natural antithesis of narrative history. They strive, by definition, to be comprehensive: to furnish a broad, orderly exposition of their chosen field. Yet to cover so much ground in so limited a space necessarily deprives readers of the pacing and context of more detailed accounts. Then, too, the resurgence of social history—with its concern for class and race, patterns of rural and urban life, the spread of market and industrial economies—lends itself to more analytic, less chronological treatments. The challenge facing historians is to incorporate these areas of research without losing the narrative drive that propels the story or sacrificing the chronological flow that orients readers to the more familiar events of our past.

Lately there has been increased attention to the worldwide breakdown of so many nonmarket economies, and by inference, to the greater success of the market societies of the United States and other capitalist nations. As our own narrative makes clear, American society and politics have indeed come together centrally in the marketplace. What Americans produce, how and where they produce it, and the desire to buy cheap and sell dear have been defining elements in every era. That market orientation has created unparalleled abundance and reinforced striking inequalities, not the least a society in which, for two centuries, human beings themselves were bought and sold. It has made Americans powerfully provincial in protecting local interests and internationally adventurous in seeking to expand wealth and opportunity.

It goes without saying that Americans have not always produced wisely or well. The insistent drive toward material plenty has levied a heavy tax on the global environment. Too often quantity has substituted for quality, whether we talk of cars, education, or culture. When markets flourish, the nation abounds with confidence that any problem, no matter how intractable, can be solved. When markets fail, however, the fault lines of our political and social systems become all too evident.

In the end, then, it is impossible to separate the marketplace of boom and bust and the world of ordinary Americans from the corridors of political maneuvering or the ceremonial pomp of an inauguration. To treat political and social history as distinct spheres or hostile camps is counterproductive. The primary question of this narrative—how the fledgling, often tumultuous confederation of "these United States" managed to transform itself into an enduring republic—is not only political, but necessarily social. In order to survive, a republic must resolve conflicts between citizens of different geographic regions and economic classes, of diverse racial and ethnic origins, of competing religions and ideologies. The resolution of these conflicts has produced tragic consequences, perhaps, as often as noble ones. But tragic or noble, the destiny of these states cannot be understood without comprehending the social dimension of the story.

A word about organization and strategies. The narrative is divided into six parts, each beginning with a brief essay setting American events of the period in a global context. We believe it important to make clear that the United States did not develop in a geographic or cultural vacuum and that the broad forces shaping it also influenced other nations. Thus we compare the extraordinary demographic growth of colonial America with the worldwide eighteenth-century rise in population; the effects of democratic and industrial revolutions here with those abroad; the massive voluntary migrations of the nineteenth century to many parts of the globe. We examine the rise of industrial societies of the twentieth century and the environmental constraints to growth as we approach the twenty-first. Each essay ends with a time line comparing political and social events in the United States with developments elsewhere.

Throughout the book we have sought to sustain a narrative approach, starting with introductory episodes for each chapter. Complementing the narrative for each chapter is a two-page essay, "Daily Lives," focusing on one of five topics that give insight into the lives of ordinary Americans: clothing and fashion; time and travel; food, drink, and drugs; political culture; public and private spaces. These topics recur regularly throughout the book, providing additional thematic continuity. Each chapter concludes with a summary of significant events; full and up-to-date bibliographies can be found at the back of the book.

For each of the book's six parts, we have included an essay, "Generations of th Republic," which takes one generation of Americans and charts its progress from birth, childhood, and adolescence through courtship, marriage, adulthood, and old age. In moving from the first Anglo-Americans (Part 1) to the baby-boomers born in the 1940s and 50s (Part 6), we have sought to integrate recent research on family structure and demographics with a sense of how national events affected the lives of ordinary citizens. In effect, we are applying a narrative approach to illuminating the intersection of biography and history.

Any account of a republic with a global reach must be geographically grounded. We have taken particular care in developing the maps for this book, working closely with the cartographers to create geographically detailed yet clear renderings. Full captions are provided whenever necessary; a number of maps are unique to this book, while many others include unusual information. In addition, six geographic essays explore such topics as the commercial and subsistence regions of the young republic, the economics of cotton in the post–Civil War South, and the geographic aspects of the war in Vietnam.

In addition to characterizing the American experience through a complement of paintings, photographs and drawings, we have tried to convey a sense of change over time by incorporating into the book's design contemporary printers' ornaments. The initial blocks opening each chapter have been taken from type specimen books of different eras; similarly, the decorative drawings have come from contemporary engravings.

Many people proved indispensable to the completion of this effort. In the editorial department, first at Alfred A. Knopf and then McGraw-Hill, Edna Shalev and Niels Aaboe somehow managed to keep control of the project's many facets, as did Project Manager Judith Kromm, Production Manager Laura Lamorte, and Photo Manager Safra Nimrod during production. John Lennard took our often inchoate suggestions of how this book might look and transformed them into a clean, elegant design. We are grateful, as well, to a host of readers whose comments and suggestions helped improve an earlier draft of this manuscript. They include Carol Berkin, Baruch College and the Graduate Center of the City University of New York; Roger W. Biles, Oklahoma State University; Carol Brown, Houston Community College; Victor Chen, Chabot College; Mario S. DePillis, University of Massachusetts, Amherst; Lynn Dumenil, Claremont McKenna College; Robert Elam, Modesto Junior College; Robert G. Fricke, West Valley College; James L. Gormly, Washington and Jefferson College; Peter Iverson, Arizona State University; George Juergens, Indiana University; Mark H. Leff, University of Illinois at Urbana-Champaign; John McCardell, Middlebury College; Gerald W. McFarland, University of Massachusetts, Amherst; Dennis C. Rousey, Arkansas State University; James C. Schneider, University of Texas, San Antonio; Lewright B. Sikes, Middle Tennessee State University; Gregory Holmes Singleton, Northeastern Illinois University; David Sloan, University of Arkansas, Fayetteville; Donna J. Spindel, Marshall University; Thomas E. Terrill, University of South Carolina; Stephen G. Weisner, Springfield Technical Community College; Frank J. Wetta, Galveston College; and William Bruce Wheeler, University of Tennessee, Knoxville. In addition, many friends and colleagues contributed their advice and constructive criticism in ways both small and large. These included Michael Bellesiles, Lawrence A. Cardoso, Dinah Chenven, James E. Crisp, R. David Edmunds, Drew McCoy, James McPherson, Stephen E. Maizlish, Harold Silesky, David J. Weber, and Virginia Joyner.

For a book to be successful, of course, the dialogue between readers and authors should continue. We welcome comments, criticisms, or suggestions, any of which will reach us addressed care of McGraw-Hill, College Department (History), 1221 Avenue of the Americas, New York, N.Y. 10020.

The division of labor for this book was determined by our respective fields of scholarship: Christine Heyrman, the colonial era, in which Europeans, Africans, and Indians participated in the making of both a new America and a new republic; William Gienapp, the ninety years in which the young nation first flourished, then foundered on the issues of section and slavery; Michael Stoff, the post–Civil War era, in which industrialization and urbanization brought the nation more centrally into an international system constantly disrupted by depression and war; and Mark Lytle, the modern era, in which Americans finally faced the reality that even the boldest dreams of national greatness are bounded by the finite nature of power and resources both natural and human. Finally, because the need to specialize inevitably imposes limits on any project as broad as this one, our fifth author, James Davidson, served as a general editor and writer, with the intent of fitting individual parts to the whole, as well as providing a measure of continuity, style, and overarching purpose. In producing this collaborative effort, all of us have shared the conviction that the best history speaks to a larger audience.

We began the writing of this book as friends; what is perhaps more unusual, given the strains of such undertakings, is that over the years our friendship deepened. The responsibility for such a happy outcome no doubt rests squarely on the shoulders of our editor, Christopher Rogers. He conceived the project, brought the authors together, consistently pushed us to make this the best book it could be, and marshalled the unstinting support of our publisher for its completion and production. Authors could ask for no more from an editor.

JAMES WEST DAVIDSON
WILLIAM E. GIENAPP
CHRISTINE LEIGH HEYRMAN
MARK H. LYTLE
MICHAEL B. STOFF

17

Reconstructing the Union

On November 19, 1866, Joseph Davis sold his plantations Hurricane and Brierfield, located on a large bend of the Mississippi River south of Vicksburg. In one sense, there was nothing unusual in this transaction. Like other southern planters financially ruined by the war, Davis had decided to quit agricultural operations. Yet the sale was bound to attract attention, since Joseph Davis was the elder brother of Jefferson Davis. In fact, before the war the Confederate president had operated Brierfield as his own plantation, even though his brother retained legal title to it. In truth, however, this sale was so unusual that the two parties agreed to keep it secret, and with good reason. The purchasers, Benjamin Montgomery and his sons, were black, and Mississippi law prohibited blacks from owning land.

Though a slave, Montgomery had been the business manager of the two Davis plantations before the war. Displaying unusual talent and ambition, he had also obtained Joseph Davis' permission to open a store on Hurricane Plantation and had developed considerable business expertise, operating on his own line of credit in New Orleans and dealing with white as well as black customers. In 1863, when the fighting reached the area around Vicksburg, Montgomery fled to Cincinnati, where his mechanical ingenuity landed him a job in a boatyard. With the coming of peace, however, he returned to Davis Bend, where the federal government had established a settlement of independent black farmers to whom it leased plots of land on confiscated plantations—Joseph Davis' among them. Reopening his plantation store, as well as beginning planting operations, Montgomery emerged as the leader of the African-American community at the Bend.

Then, in 1866, President Andrew Johnson pardoned Joseph Davis and restored his lands. Black hopes of creating a permanent settlement of independent farmers at Davis Bend were thrown into doubt. But when Joseph Davis took possession of Brierfield and Hurricane, he was over 80 years old. He lacked the will and stamina to rebuild and start over again. Unlike many one-time slaveholders, however, Davis still felt bound by obligations to his former slaves, and he remained deeply interested in their welfare. Convinced that with proper encouragement African-Americans could succeed economically in freedom, he sold his land secretly to Benjamin Montgomery in order to promote black self-help. Only when the law prohibiting blacks from owning land was overturned in 1867 did Davis publicly confirm the sale to his ex-slave.

A Visit from the Old Mistress, by Winslow Homer, captures the conflicting, often awkward emotions felt by both races after the war.

For his part, Montgomery undertook to fulfill the dream of his former master to create a model society at Davis Bend where African-Americans could prosper through mutual cooperation. Moving with his family into what had once been the home of Jefferson Davis, Montgomery guided the settlement with a paternalistic hand, much like Joseph Davis had earlier. He rented land to black farmers, hired others to work his own fields, sold supplies on credit, and ginned and marketed the crops. To the growing African-American community, he constantly preached the gospel of hard work, self-reliance, and education.

Severe difficulties, including the destruction caused by the war, several disastrous floods, insects, droughts, and declining cotton prices, dogged these farmers. Yet before long, cotton production exceeded that of the antebellum years. In 1870 the black families at Davis Bend produced 2500 bales, more than twice the amount produced by whites on a neighboring plantation with the same acreage. In fact, in that year the Montgomerys accounted for over half of all the cotton bales produced by African-Americans in the state's 20 richest cotton counties. The following year they bought Ursino Plantation, which adjoined their holdings. The addition of 1500 acres to the 4000 they had purchased from Joseph Davis made them reputedly the third largest planters in the state, and they won national and international awards for the high quality of their cotton. Their success was an inspiration and example of what African-Americans, given a fair chance, might accomplish.

The experiences of Benjamin Montgomery during the years after 1865 were not those of most southern blacks, who did not own land or have a powerful white benefactor. Yet Montgomery's dream of economic independence was shared by all African-Americans. As one black veteran noted, "Every colored man will be a slave, and feel himself a slave until he can raise him own *bale of cotton* and put him own mark upon it and say dis is mine!" Blacks could not gain effective freedom simply through a proclamation of emancipation, no matter how well intentioned. They also needed to live in a society where they had economic power of their own—to become the largest cotton planter in the district, like Montgomery, or simply a farmer with a plot of land no one could unfairly take away.

For nearly two centuries, the laws had prevented slaves from possessing such economic power. Inevitably, if such conditions were to be overturned, blacks needed political power too. The whole theory that underlies a democratic republic is that social conflict—between different classes, economic groups, or regions—may be peacefully resolved if all groups share power in the political arena. For 200 years, African-Americans lacked that power, and the conflict and inequality that had built up in American society had led to civil war. In political terms, the Republic would have to be reconstructed in order to share power with a major group of Americans who had been previously denied it.

To achieve that goal in a land where racism had distorted society for so long in both the North and the South would be a major task. War, in its blunt way, had roughed out the contours of a solution, but only in broad terms. Clearly, African-Americans would no longer be slaves. The North, with its industrial might, would be the driving force in the nation's economy and retain the dominant political voice. It had the power to set the terms for admitting the defeated Confederate states back into the Union. But beyond that, the outlines of a reconstructed Republic remained vague. How much effective power would blacks receive? How would the North and South readjust their economic and social relations? These questions lay at the heart of the problem of Reconstruction.

PRESIDENTIAL RECONSTRUCTION

Even in the early months of the war, Abraham Lincoln had considered Reconstruction his responsibility. In devising a program, Lincoln never lost sight of its political consequences. Elected with less than 40 percent of the popular vote in 1860, he was acutely aware that the Republican party had no real strength in the South. Once the states of the Confederacy were restored to the Union, they would again have 22 senators and 63 representatives, as well as 85 votes in the Electoral College. The Republicans inevitably would be weakened unless they evolved into more than a sectional party. Lincoln looked to the old Whigs, who supported many of the Republicans' economic programs, to build up a southern wing of the party. By a generous peace, he hoped to attract white southerners and assure his party's continuing national supremacy.

Lincoln's Plan

As the Union army conquered parts of the Confederacy, Lincoln set up a flexible program of Reconstruction in a Proclamation of Amnesty and Reconstruction, issued in December 1863. A minimum of 10 percent of the qualified voters from 1860, having taken a loyalty oath to the Union, could organize a state government. The new state constitution had to be republican in form, abolish slavery, and provide for black education. High-ranking Confederate leaders were not eligible to take the loyalty oath, although Lincoln did not require that the new state government bar them from public life. Once these requirements had been met, the president would recognize the new civilian state government.

Lincoln also assured southerners that there would be no mass arrests, trials, and executions, for he had no desire to create any Confederate martyrs. He indicated that he would be generous in granting pardons and did not rule out compensation for slave property. Moreover, while he suggested to the Unionist governor of Louisiana that it would be wise to permit a few black men to vote, "as for instance, the very intelligent and especially those who have fought gallantly in our ranks," Lincoln did not demand social or political equality for blacks. Nor did he envision any long-term federal assistance to former slaves. Although he seemed to be moving toward requiring limited black suffrage in the disloyal southern states, he recognized pro-Union governments in Louisiana, Arkansas, and Tennessee that allowed only white men to vote.

The Radical Republicans, who constituted the most militant antislavery wing of the party, found Lincoln's approach much too lenient. Radical members of Congress like Charles Sumner and George W. Julian had been openly condemning slavery and the Slave Power for over a decade. They had led the struggle to make emancipation a war aim and now were in the forefront in advocating rights and privileges for the freedmen. They were also disturbed that Lincoln had not enlisted Congress in devising Reconstruction policy. Lincoln argued that the rebellious states had never left the Union because secession was illegal. Therefore, the executive branch should bear the responsibility for restoring proper relations with the former Confederate states. The Radicals, on the other hand, believed that in seceding, these states had ceased to exist; consequently, it was Congress' duty to set the terms under which they would regain their rights in the Union. Though the Radicals often disagreed with each other on matters of detail, they were united in a determination to readmit southern states only after slavery had been ended, black rights protected, and the power of the planter class destroyed.

Led by Senator Benjamin Wade of Ohio and Representative Henry Winter Davis of Maryland, Congress proposed that Confederate states would be ruled temporarily by a military governor. Under the Wade–Davis bill, state conventions could meet to draft a new state constitution only when fully half the white adult males took an oath of allegiance. The constitution had to renounce secession as illegal, abolish slavery, and repudiate all debts incurred by the Confederate government, ensuring that those who bought Confederate bonds and loaned money to finance the rebellion would not be repaid. To qualify as a voter or to serve as a delegate to the constitutional convention required a second oath, the so-called ironclad oath, attesting that a person had never voluntarily aided or supported the Confederacy. Since only a small minority of white southerners could take this oath in good conscience, this bill would have given political power to the hard-core Unionists in each state.

When the Wade–Davis bill passed on the final day of the 1864 congressional session, Lincoln exercised his right of a pocket veto and the bill died.* The Radicals bitterly assailed the president, but if anything, their strident objections won him wider popular support. Still, his own program could not succeed without the assistance of Congress, which refused to count the electoral votes of the reconstructed states in the 1864 election or seat Unionist representatives who had been elected to Congress from Louisiana or Arkansas. By April 1865, with the war in its last days, Lincoln appeared willing to make concessions to the Radicals. He suggested that he might favor different—and conceivably more rigorous—Reconstruction plans for different states. At his final cabinet meeting, he acknowledged that perhaps he had gone too fast on Reconstruction and approved in principle a proposal by Secretary of War Edwin Stanton to place the defeated South temporarily under military rule.

But only a few days later Booth's bullet found its mark, and Lincoln's final approach to Reconstruction would never be known. Would he have continued to push for moderation? Or being a practical politician, would he have made peace with the Radicals and pushed ahead with a firmer hand? How would the South respond to any plan of "Reconstruction"?

The Mood of the South

Northerners worried about the attitude of ex-Confederates at war's end. During Lincoln's visit to Richmond, he had ridden along deserted, rubble-strewn streets past charred buildings, to be greeted by a dusty silence. Hundreds of white southerners peered out windows, "but it was a silent crowd," recalled one of his guards. "There was something oppressive in those thousands of watchers without a sound, either of welcome or hatred." In the wake of defeat, the immediate reaction among whites was one of shock, despair, and hopelessness. Some southerners, of course, were openly antagonistic. A North Carolina innkeeper remarked bitterly that Yankees had stolen his slaves, burned his house, and killed his son, leaving him only one privilege: "to hate 'em. I git up at half-past four in the morning, and sit up till twelve at night, to hate 'em." Most Confederate soldiers were less defiant, having had their fill of war; and even among hostile civilians there was a pervasive feeling that the South must accept northern terms. A South Carolina paper admitted that "the conqueror has the right to make the terms, and we must submit."

This psychological moment was critical. To prevent a resurgence of resistance, the president needed to lay out in unmistakable terms what white southerners had to do to regain their old status in the Union. A confusion in policy, or a wavering on the terms of how political power was to be shared in the reconstructed Union, could only increase the likelihood that southerners would resist the logic of the war's victory. Perhaps even a clear and firm policy would not have been enough. But Lincoln was no longer president, and as events would prove, the executive power now rested in less capable hands.

Johnson's Program of Reconstruction

Andrew Johnson, the new president, had been born in North Carolina and eventually moved to Tennessee, where he supported himself as a tailor. His wife taught

*If a president does not sign a bill after Congress has adjourned, it has the same effect as a veto.

him to read and write. Something of a demagogue, he rose to political power in eastern Tennessee, where there were few slaves, by portraying himself as the champion of the people against the wealthy planter class. "Some day I will show the stuck-up aristocrats who is running the country," he vowed as he began his political career. "A cheap purse-proud set they are, not half as good as the man who earns his bread by the sweat of his brow." In Tennessee, he campaigned for a free, tax-supported public school system, and when he went to Congress, he led the fight for a homestead act to grant free land from the public domain to small farmers. He had not opposed slavery before the war—in fact, he hoped to disperse slave ownership more widely in southern society. Although he accepted emancipation as one of the consequences of the war, Johnson remained an inveterate racist with no concern for the welfare of blacks. "Damn the negroes," he said during the war, "I am fighting these traitorous aristocrats, their masters."

Johnson had been the only southerner to remain in the Senate when his state seceded in 1861. In Congress, he had joined with the Radicals in calling for stern treatment of southern rebels. "Treason must be made odious and traitors must be punished and impoverished," he proclaimed in 1864. After serving as military governor of Tennessee following its occupation by Union forces, Johnson, a Democrat, was tapped by Lincoln in 1864 as his running mate on the rechristened "Union" ticket.

The Radicals expected Johnson to uphold their views on Reconstruction, and upon assuming the presidency he spoke of trying Confederate leaders and breaking up planters' estates. In reality, the grounds of agreement between Johnson and the Radicals were quite narrow. Unlike most Republicans, Johnson strongly supported states' rights and decentralization. He opposed government aid to business and romanticized the self-sufficient yeoman farmer he had championed in Tennessee politics. Given such differences, conflict between the president and the majority in Congress was inevitable. But Johnson's abrasive personality and politi-

Andrew Johnson was a staunch Unionist, but his contentious personality and inflexibility masked a deep-seated insecurity, which was rooted in his humble background. As a young man, he worked and lived in this rude tailor shop in Greenville, Tennessee.

cal shortcomings made the situation worse. Scarred by his humble origins, he remained throughout his life an outsider. When challenged or criticized, he became tactless and inflexible, alienating even those who sought to work with him.

At first, Johnson seemed to be following Lincoln's policy of quickly restoring the southern states to their rightful place in the Union. Like Lincoln, he prescribed a loyalty oath southern whites would have to take to receive pardon and amnesty. Those who took the oath would have their property, except for slaves, restored and would regain their civil and political rights. Like Lincoln, Johnson excluded high Confederate officials from this group, but he added those with property worth over $20,000, which included his old foes in the planter class. These groups had to apply to the president for individual pardons.

Loyal state governments could be formed after a provisional governor, appointed by the president, called a state convention and supervised the election of delegates. Voters and delegates had to qualify under the 1860 state election laws and take the new loyalty oath. Once elections were held to choose a governor, legislature, and members of Congress, Johnson announced he would recognize the new state government, revoke martial law, and withdraw Union troops. Again, the plan was similar to Lincoln's, though more lenient. Johnson did not require southern states to repeal their ordinances of secession, repudiate the Confederate debt, or ratify the proposed Thirteenth Amendment abolishing slavery. He only recommended that they do so.

The Failure of Johnson's Program

The southern delegates who met to construct new governments soon demonstrated that they were in no frame of mind to follow mere recommendations. Several states, instead of repudiating their ordinances of secession, merely repealed them, refusing to yield in principle the right to secede. Mississippi and Texas rejected the Thirteenth Amendment, while Georgia ratified it with the provision that slaveholders be compensated. South Carolina and Mississippi refused to repudiate the Confederate debt.

Most damaging, however, was that none of the new governments allowed blacks any political rights, and none made any effective provision for black education. Mississippi was the first to act in August 1865, but Johnson, instead of pressing harder for change, telegraphed the provisional governor with suggestions on how to appear to comply with his terms without provoking northern public opinion. Give the vote only to the tiny minority of literate black males and those who owned property worth more than $250, he advised. "This you can do with perfect safety and, ... as a consequence, the radicals, who are wild upon negro franchise, will be completely foiled." But the new southern governments refused to make even that gesture. In addition to denying black political rights, each state passed a series of laws, often modeled on the earlier slave code, that applied only to African-Americans.

The black codes did grant African-Americans some rights they had been denied as slaves. They legalized marriages from slavery and allowed blacks to hold and sell property and to sue and be sued in state courts. Yet their primary intent was to keep African-Americans as propertyless agricultural laborers without political rights and with inferior legal rights. The new freedmen could not serve on juries, could not testify against whites, and could not marry whites. And their freedom to work as they pleased was severely limited. South Carolina forbade

13th Amend –
Abolish
slavery

blacks from engaging without a special license in anything other than agricultural labor; Mississippi prohibited them from buying or renting farmland; Louisiana required that agricultural laborers make contracts within the first 10 days of January that bound them for the entire year. Most states ominously provided that blacks who were vagrants could be arrested and hired out to landowners.

Although several northern states had narrowly defeated their own proposals to give black men the vote, most northerners were incensed by the restrictive black codes. "We tell the white men of Mississippi that the men of the North will convert the State of Mississippi into a frog pond before they will allow such laws to disgrace one foot of the soil . . . over which the flag of freedom waves," proclaimed the Chicago *Tribune*. Carl Schurz, a Radical Republican orator and politician who toured the South at Johnson's request, wrote that the black codes were "a striking embodiment of the idea that although the former owner has lost his individual right of property in the former slaves, the blacks at large belong to the whites at large."

Southern voters under Johnson's plan defiantly elected governors and members of Congress who were by and large prominent Confederate military and political leaders, headed by Alexander Stephens, the vice president of the Confederacy, who was elected senator from Georgia. At this point, Johnson faced a critical decision. He could have called for new elections or admitted that a different program of Reconstruction was needed. Yet for all his rabble rousing, he recoiled from the prospect of social and economic upheaval in the South. Although he had smarted for years at "the taunts, the jeers, the scowls" of upper-class planters, at the same time, he craved their respect. When they began flocking to the White House, begging for pardons and praising his conduct, he found it enormously gratifying. He began to issue special pardons almost as fast as they could be printed; in the next two years he pardoned some 13,500 Confederates. Confronted with southern defiance, Johnson capitulated and failed to follow through on his original goals.

In private, Johnson warned southerners against a reckless course. Publicly he put on a bold face, announcing that Reconstruction had been successfully completed. But many in the new Congress thought it a failure, and the stage was set for a serious confrontation.

Johnson's Break with Congress

The new Congress was by no means of one mind. The most conservative element, a small number of Democrats and conservative Republicans, backed the president's program of immediate and unconditional restoration. At the other end of the spectrum, a larger group of Radical Republicans, led by Thaddeus Stevens, Charles Sumner, Benjamin Wade, and others, was bent on fundamentally restructuring southern society and making it over on a northern model. Reconstruction must "revolutionize Southern institutions, habits, and manners," thundered Representative Stevens. "The foundations of their institutions must be broken and relaid, or all our blood and treasure have been spent in vain."

As a minority, the Radicals could accomplish nothing without the aid of the Moderate Republicans, the largest bloc in Congress. Led by William Pitt Fessenden, Lyman Trumbull, and John Sherman, the Moderates hoped to avoid conflict

Thaddeus Stevens, Radical leader in the House.

This drawing by Thomas Nast expresses northern condemnation of the black codes enacted in the South after the war. On the left, a black man accused of crime is sold as punishment, while on the right another freedman is whipped in front of a blindfolded justice.

with the president, and they had no desire to foster social revolution in the South. But they wanted to keep Confederate leaders from reassuming power and readmit southern states only after they had fulfilled certain conditions. Finally, while they had no sympathy for the idea of racial equality promoted by many Radicals, the Moderates saw the need to extend federal protection to the freedman, who, Trumbull declared, would "be tyrannized over, abused, and virtually reenslaved without some legislation by the nation for his protection."

The central issue dividing Johnson and the Radicals was the place of African-Americans in American society. Johnson, along with other racists, accused his opponents of seeking "to Africanize the southern half of our country." The Radicals, on the other hand, championed civil and political rights for blacks, particularly the right to vote. Convinced that southern white Unionists were too small a nucleus to build a party around, Radicals believed that the only way to maintain loyal governments and develop a Republican party in the South was to give black men the ballot. Moderates, however, feared too much of an emphasis on black rights would alienate northern voters. But they agreed with Radicals that the new southern governments were too harsh toward blacks and too defiant toward the victorious North. In December 1865, when southern representatives to Congress appeared in Washington, a majority in Congress voted to exclude them. They also appointed a joint committee, chaired by Moderate William Fessenden, to look into Reconstruction.

The growing split with the president became clearer when Congress passed a bill extending the life of the Freedmen's Bureau. Created in March 1865 during the last days of the war, the Bureau provided emergency food, clothing, and medical care to war refugees (including whites) and took charge of settling freedmen on abandoned lands. The new bill not only continued these duties, but also called for the Bureau to supervise special courts to resolve disputes involving freedmen and to set up and support schools for southern blacks. This bill passed with virtually unanimous Republican support, but to the surprise of Moderates, Johnson vetoed the measure, charging that the Bureau's military courts lacked the fundamental guarantees of juries and rules of evidence. (African-Americans, of course, could neither sit on the juries nor testify against whites under the state laws approved by Johnson.) Even more alarming, the president claimed the bill was unconstitutional because southern representatives had been excluded from Congress, which if accepted would mean that any legislation passed by Congress was unconstitutional. Still, Congress failed to override the veto.

Johnson also vetoed a civil rights bill designed to overturn the more flagrant provisions of the black codes. The law made African-Americans citizens of the United States and granted them the right to own property, make contracts, and have access to courts as parties and witnesses. It also provided that federal courts could take jurisdiction if state courts discriminated against blacks. Johnson vetoed the bill on the grounds that it granted greater safeguards to blacks than whites. For most Republicans, Johnson's action was the last straw. In April 1866 Congress overrode his veto, the first major legislation to be enacted into law over a presidential veto in American history. Congress then approved a slightly revised Freedmen's Bureau bill in July and promptly overrode the president's veto. Only three Republicans in the Senate supported the president. "He has broken the faith, betrayed his trust, and must sink from detestation to contempt," observed Senator Fessenden. Johnson's refusal to compromise drove the Moderates into the arms of the Radicals.

The Fourteenth Amendment

To prevent unrepentant Confederates from taking over the reconstructed state governments and denying blacks basic freedoms, the Joint Committee on Reconstruction proposed an amendment to the Constitution, which passed both houses of Congress with the necessary two-thirds vote in June 1866. In effect, the amendment, coupled with the Freedmen's Bureau and civil rights bills, represented the Moderates' terms for Reconstruction.

The amendment put a number of matters beyond the control or discretion of the president. It guaranteed repayment of the national war debt and prohibited repayment of the Confederate debt, which Johnson had not insisted on. To counteract the president's wholesale pardons, the amendment disqualified prominent Confederates from holding office and provided that only Congress by a two-thirds vote could remove this penalty. Radicals had pushed for a provision giving the franchise to blacks, but Moderates balked, convinced that many white northerners would oppose such a provision. Instead, the amendment merely gave Congress the right to reduce the representation of any state that did not have impartial (male) suffrage. The practical effect of this provision, which Radicals labeled a "swindle," was to allow northern states to continue a policy of white suffrage if they wished, for they had few blacks and would not be penalized. Southern states, on the other hand, had significant African-American populations and risked losing part of their representation in Congress by adhering to white suffrage.

The most important provision of the amendment, Section 1, defined an American citizen as anyone who had been born in the United States or naturalized. Blacks thereby automatically became citizens, effectively repealing the Supreme Court's ruling in the *Dred Scott* case. Section 1 also prohibited states from abridging "the privileges or immunities" of citizens, depriving "any person of life, liberty, or property, without due process of law," or denying "any person . . . equal protection of the laws." The framers of the amendment probably intended to prohibit laws that applied to one race only, such as the black codes; or that made certain acts felonies when committed by blacks but not whites; or that decreed different penalties for the same crime when committed by whites and blacks. The framers probably did not intend to prevent African-Americans from being excluded from juries or segregated in schools and public places.

Still, Section 1 used general phrases for the rights it enumerated: "privileges and immunities," "due process of law," and "equal protection of the laws." The authors deliberately made those guarantees broad, to cover unanticipated abuses. And indeed, the first section of the Fourteenth Amendment has been the basis for more litigation than the rest of the Constitution combined, and one of the greatest safeguards of individual liberty and equal rights.

Ratification of a constitutional amendment does not require the president's approval; still, Johnson denounced the proposed amendment and urged southern states not to ratify it. Ironically, the president's own state ignored his advice, and one gleeful foe sent Congress a telegram announcing Tennessee's approval, which concluded, "Give my respects to the dead dog in the White House." Congress readmitted the state with no further restrictions. All the other seceded states rejected the amendment.

The Election of 1866

With Congress and the president at loggerheads, Johnson took his case to the people. In the election of 1866, he hoped to build a new National Union party, rallying Democrats, southern whites, and conservative Republicans on the platform of immediate readmission of the southern states. When a national convention in Philadelphia in August attracted few Republicans, Johnson became a man virtually without a party.

News that summer of major race riots in Memphis and New Orleans heightened northern concern. Forty-six blacks died when white mobs invaded the black section of Memphis, burning homes, churches, and schoolhouses; about the same number were killed in New Orleans when whites attacked both black and white delegates to a convention supporting black suffrage. "The negroes now know, to their sorrow, that it is best not to arouse the fury of the white man," boasted one Memphis newspaper. In the face of such attitudes, Johnson, who launched a tour of the East and Midwest to drum up support for his cause, found it difficult to convince audiences that white southerners were fully repentant. To make things worse, he conducted his campaign "swing around the circle" as if he were stumping the backwoods of Tennessee, trading insults with hostile crowds, responding in kind when they heckled him, and ranting that the Radicals were traitors. Even his supporters found the performance humiliating.

Not to be outdone, the Radicals vilified Johnson as a traitor aiming to turn the country over to rebels and Copperheads. Resorting to the tactic of "waving the bloody shirt," they appealed to voters by reviving bitter memories of the war and sectional distrust. In a classic example of such rhetoric, Governor Oliver Morton of Indiana proclaimed that "every bounty jumper, every deserter, every sneak who ran away from the draft" was a Democrat; everyone "who murdered Union prisoners," every

> New York rioter in 1863 who burned up little children in colored asylums, who robbed, ravished and murdered indiscriminately . . . called himself a Democrat. In short, the Democratic party may be described as a common sewer and loathsome receptacle, into which is emptied every element of treason North and South.

Such rhetoric became a Republican campaign staple for many years.

The voters soundly repudiated Johnson, as the Republicans won over a two-thirds majority in both houses of Congress, every northern gubernatorial contest, and control of every northern legislature. The Radicals had reached the height of their power, propelled by genuine alarm among northerners that Johnson's policies would lose the fruits of the Union's victory and leave the ruling class of the South undisturbed.

CONGRESSIONAL RECONSTRUCTION

With a clear mandate in hand, Republicans devised their own program of Reconstruction. The first Reconstruction Act was passed in March 1867 and, like all other subsequent pieces of Reconstruction legislation, was promptly repassed over Johnson's veto. The 10 unreconstructed states were divided into five military districts, each under a military commander with authority over the provisional state governments. In enrolling voters, officials were to include black adult males but not those former Confederates who were barred from holding office under the Fourteenth Amendment. Delegates to the state conventions would frame constitutions that provided for black suffrage and disqualified prominent ex-Confederates from office; the first state legislatures to meet under the new system were required to ratify the Fourteenth Amendment. Once these steps were completed and Congress approved the new state constitution, a state could send representatives to Congress.

Southern whites found these requirements so obnoxious, they preferred to remain under military rule; thus officials took no steps to register voters. Congress then enacted a second Reconstruction Act, also in March, ordering the local military commanders to enroll voters and put the machinery of Reconstruction into motion. Johnson's efforts to limit the power of military commanders produced a third act, passed in July, which upheld their superiority in all matters and confirmed their power to remove officials and reject voters' loyalty oaths. Southerners then adopted a strategy of delay, hoping that a Democratic victory in the 1868 presidential election would lead to repeal of all the Reconstruction acts. When elections were held to ratify the new state constitutions, southern whites boycotted them in large numbers. In Alabama, the first state to vote on a new constitution, only 43 percent of registered voters participated, less than the required majority. Congress was not to be daunted. It passed the fourth Reconstruction Act

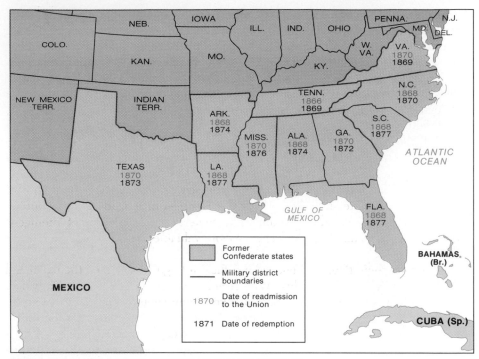

THE SOUTHERN STATES DURING RECONSTRUCTION

(March 1868), which required ratification of the constitution by only a majority of those voting rather than those who were registered. (Congress applied this act retroactively to Alabama and readmitted the state under its new constitution.)

By June 1868, Congress had readmitted the representatives of seven states. Georgia's state legislature expelled its black members once it had been readmitted, granting seats to those barred by Congress from holding office. Congress ordered the military commander to reverse these actions and Georgia was then admitted a second time in July 1870. Texas, Virginia, and Mississippi did not complete the process until 1869.

The Land Issue

While the political process of Reconstruction proceeded, Congress confronted the question of whether it was sufficient to give former slaves political and civil rights alone. Radical Republicans argued that without economic independence, blacks would enjoy only nominal freedom. Certainly many blacks felt that way. At a meeting with Secretary of War Edwin Stanton near the end of the war, African-American leaders declared, "The way we can best take care of ourselves is to have land, and till it by our own labor." Since slaves had been deprived of the right to own property before the war, Congress debated whether they should now be compensated.

During the war, the Second Confiscation Act had authorized the government to seize and sell the property including land of supporters of the rebellion. General Sherman had also issued his Special Order No. 15 in January 1865, granting blacks 40-acre homesteads on abandoned lands along the South Carolina and

Georgia coasts inland for 30 miles. In June 1866 President Johnson ruled that the Second Confiscation Act of 1862 applied only to wartime, and he also overturned Sherman's order. But Congress continued to debate the matter of confiscation from December 1865 until early 1867.

Thaddeus Stevens, the leader of the Radical Republicans in the House, advocated confiscating 394 million acres of land from about 70,000 of what he termed the "chief rebels" in the South, who comprised less than 5 percent of the South's white families. He proposed to give 40 acres to every adult male freedman and then sell the remaining land, which would amount to nine-tenths of the total, to pay off the public debt, compensate loyal southerners for losses they suffered during the war, and fund veterans' pensions. "How can republican institutions, free schools, free churches, free social intercourse exist in a mingled community of nabobs and serfs?" Stevens asked. "If the South is ever to be made a safe Republic, let her lands be cultivated by the toil of the owners or the free labor of intelligent citizens." Land, he insisted, would be far more valuable to blacks than the right to vote.

But even some Radicals believed it sufficient to give black men the ballot and pass laws protecting black rights. With Americans' strong belief in self-reliance, little sympathy existed for the idea that government should support any group or that blacks deserved special consideration. In addition, land redistribution represented an attack on property rights, another cherished American value. "A division of rich men's lands amongst the landless," argued the *Nation*, a Radical journal, "would give a shock to our whole social and political system from which it would hardly recover without the loss of liberty."

By 1867 land reform was dead. Except for property that had already been sold during the war under the Confiscation acts, seized land was returned to its former owners. Few freedmen acquired land after the war, a development that severely limited African-Americans' economic independence and left them vulnerable to white coercion. Certainly the failure to provide an economic foundation for black freedom helped undermine Reconstruction. That this decision was the basic cause of the failure of Reconstruction, however, is doubtful. In the face of white hostility and institutionalized racism, African-Americans probably would have been no more successful in protecting their property than they were in maintaining the right to vote, especially once the federal government refused to use its power to protect them. Southern whites no doubt would have devised ways to dispossess most black landowners.

Impeachment

Throughout 1867 the battle between the executive and legislative branches settled into a predictable rhythm: Congress would pass a bill, the president would veto it, Congress would override. But Johnson had other ways of undercutting congressional Reconstruction. He interpreted the new laws as narrowly as possible. He removed military commanders who vigorously enforced the laws, and his belligerence alarmed even Moderates. "Is the President crazy . . . ?" asked one. "I am afraid his doings will make us all favor impeachment." Congress fought back, directing the president to issue orders to the five military commanders in the southern states only through the general of the army, Ulysses S. Grant. Congress even limited Johnson's control of his cabinet through the Tenure of Office Act, which forbade him from removing any member without the Senate's consent. The

Facsimile of a ticket of admission to the impeachment trial of President Andrew Johnson.

intention of this law was to prevent him from firing Secretary of War Edwin Stanton, the only remaining Radical in the cabinet.

When Johnson tried to dismiss Stanton in February 1868, the determined secretary of war barricaded himself in his office (where he remained night and day for about two months). On February 24, the House of Representatives angrily approved articles of impeachment. The articles focused on the violation of the Tenure of Office Act, but the charge with the most substance was that Johnson had conspired to systematically obstruct Reconstruction legislation. In the trial before the Senate, his lawyers argued that a president could be impeached only for an indictable crime, which Johnson clearly had not committed. They also claimed that the president had fired Stanton merely to test the constitutionality of the Tenure of Office Act, while simultaneously they argued inconsistently that the Tenure of Office Act did not apply to Stanton, since he had been appointed by Lincoln and not Johnson. The Radicals countered that impeachment applied to political offenses and not merely criminal acts, a position James Madison had supported during the drafting of the Constitution.

In May 1868, after a three-month trial at which Johnson did not appear, the Senate voted 36–19 to convict, one vote short of the two-thirds majority needed. The seven Republicans who had joined the Democrats in voting for acquittal were uneasy about using impeachment as a political weapon. In addition, the president pro tempore of the Senate, Benjamin Wade of Ohio, was in line to succeed Johnson, and his Radical views on Reconstruction as well as women's rights and the currency frightened Moderates. Their vote against conviction established the precedent that a president could be removed from office only for indictable offenses, which greatly lessened the effectiveness of the threat of impeachment.

Reconstruction and the Constitution

Impeachment represented an attempt by Congress to establish its supremacy in the federal government. The Supreme Court also became a target of congressional pressure and control. Democrats, who were a hopeless minority in Congress, increasingly looked to the Court to overthrow the Reconstruction acts. For their part, Republicans worried that the *Milligan* decision (page 583), which struck down military trials for civilians during wartime, was a sign that the Court might declare the Reconstruction acts unconstitutional, since they provided for military rule and trials in the southern states. Republicans' fears crystallized when the

Court agreed to hear the appeal of an editor from Mississippi named William McCardle, who had been arrested under the Reconstruction acts and tried by a military commission. The first Reconstruction Act had given federal courts jurisdiction over certain cases, to protect freedmen from state courts. Congress responded by retroactively denying federal courts jurisdiction in such appeals and the Court, unwilling to challenge Congress, ruled in *Ex parte McCardle* (1868) that it had no jurisdiction.

Indeed, throughout this era the Court decided several relevant cases on very narrow grounds and declined to rule on the constitutionality of the Reconstruction acts. In *Texas v. White* (1869) it ruled that secession was illegal and the Union perpetual, and asserted that it was up to Congress to guarantee a republican government in each state. But it perceived, properly, that Reconstruction was an extraordinary situation, one the Constitution had never anticipated. Had the Court challenged Congress on such a highly political matter, it would have precipitated a constitutional crisis that would have led to a concerted effort to restrict the Court, if not destroy its power. Restraint on the Court's part proved wise.

RECONSTRUCTION IN THE SOUTH

The waning power of the Radicals in Congress, evident in the failure to remove Johnson, meant that the success or failure of Reconstruction increasingly hinged on developments in the southern states themselves. Power in these states rested with the new Republican parties, representing a coalition of southern blacks, southern whites, and transplanted northerners.

Black Officeholding

Black men formed the bulk of the Republican voters in the South—perhaps as much as 80 percent. Almost from the beginning, they insisted that they were the only sizable loyal population in the South and lobbied for the right to vote. When they finally received the franchise, they were not about to support the Democratic party and its appeal to white supremacy. As one Tennessee Republican explained, "The blacks know that many conservatives [Democrats] hope to reduce them again to some form of peonage. Under the impulse of this fear they will roll up their whole strength and will go entirely for the Republican candidate whoever he may be."

Yet, even though African-American males eagerly accepted the ballot, they never held office during Reconstruction in proportion to their voting strength. They lacked a majority in any southern legislature; only in South Carolina, where they constituted over 60 percent of the population, did they control even one house of the legislature. No African-American was ever nominated or elected governor. Only in South Carolina did a black judge serve on a state supreme court. Between 15 and 20 percent of the state officers and 6 percent of the congressmen in Reconstruction were black. Two blacks from Mississippi served in the U.S. Senate, and 15 blacks served in the House. In reality, only in South Carolina, where they held 52 percent of all state and federal elective offices, did black officeholding approach their proportion of the population.

This engraving shows a black politician addressing former slaves at a political meeting in the South during the 1868 presidential campaign. Although only men could vote, black women are also in the audience. Commented *Harper's Weekly* when this picture appeared, "Does any man seriously doubt whether it is better for this vast population to be sinking deeper and deeper in ignorance and servility, or rising into general intelligence and self-respect?"

Those who held office came from the top levels of African-American society. Among state and federal officeholders, perhaps four-fifths were literate, and over a quarter had been free before the war, both marks of distinction in the black community. Their occupations also set them apart: two-fifths were professionals (mostly clergy), and of the third who were farmers, nearly all owned their own land. Others were skilled workers or ran small businesses. Among blacks in Congress, all but three had a secondary school education, and four had gone to college. Jonathan Gibbs, the Florida secretary of state, was a graduate of Dartmouth and the Princeton Theological Seminary, and Francis Cardozo, who served as secretary of state and treasurer in South Carolina, had attended several colleges in England. Senator Blanche Bruce of Mississippi was the son of a white planter and had been educated on his father's plantation. In their political and social values, African-American leaders were more conservative than the rural black population, and they showed little interest in land reform. Like whites, they ranged from the talented to the incompetent.

Southern White Republicans

The failure of Congress to disfranchise Confederates meant that the Republican party had to secure white votes to stay in power. Blacks were a majority of the voters only in South Carolina, Mississippi, and Louisiana. Opponents labeled southern whites who allied with the Republican party scalawags, a pejorative term referring to scrubby cattle. An estimated quarter of southern whites at one time voted Republican, including prominent southerners like General James Longstreet, one of Robert E. Lee's key commanders, and James Lusk Alcorn, a wealthy Mississippi planter. Although the party appealed to some wealthy southern Whigs, they were outnumbered by Unionists from the upland counties and hill areas who were largely yeoman farmers. Such voters were attracted to Republican promises to rebuild the South, restore prosperity, create public schools, and open isolated areas to the market with railroads.

The other group of white Republicans in the South hailed originally from the North: carpetbaggers, they were derisively called, allegedly poor and ignorant men who arrived with all their worldly possessions stuffed in a carpetbag, ready to loot and plunder the defeated South. Some did, certainly, but northerners who moved south came for a variety of reasons. Those in political office were especially well educated and, although they constituted only a small percentage of Republican voters, they controlled almost a third of the offices, especially the higher ones. More than half of all southern Republican governors and nearly half of Republican congressmen and senators were originally northerners.

The Republican party in the South had difficulty agreeing on a program or maintaining unity. Scalawags were especially susceptible to the race issue and social pressure. "Even my own kinspeople have turned the cold shoulder to me because I hold office under a Republican administration," testified a Mississippi Republican. As blacks pressed for more recognition and a greater share of the offices, southern whites increasingly defected to the Democrats. Carpetbaggers, by contrast, were less sensitive to race and more strongly committed to the party. A number had previously worked for black rights and education, although most felt that blacks needed guidance and should be content with minor offices. The friction between carpetbaggers and blacks was minor compared to scalawags' resentment of carpetbaggers, intruders who in their eyes had seized offices that rightfully belonged to native southerners. As a result, southern Republicanism was riven by growing factionalism.

The New State Governments

The new state constitutions in the South included a number of significant reforms. In older states the earlier inequitable legislative apportionment, which discriminated against the interior counties, was replaced by a fairer system. Many previously appointive offices were made elective, and property requirements for office-holding were abolished. In South Carolina, for the first time, voters were allowed to vote for the president, governor, and other state officers.* The Radical state governments also assumed some responsibility for social welfare and established the first statewide systems of public schools in the South. The new governments also substantially increased state aid to the insane, the handicapped, and the poor. Women's rights were also enlarged, and divorce was finally legalized in South Carolina.

Although the Fourteenth Amendment prevented high Confederate officials from holding office, virtually all the new state constitutions refused to place any additional penalties on them. Only Alabama and Arkansas temporarily forbade some ex-Confederates from voting. Understandably, the strongest advocates of harsh penalties were southern Unionists, who often had suffered at the hands of

*Previously, presidential electors as well as the governor had been chosen by the South Carolina legislature.

their Confederate neighbors and who believed that political power in the reconstructed South rightfully belonged to them. African-American delegates, on the other hand, generally opposed any penalties. They argued that blacks and whites had to live together in the South, and such penalties could lead only to growing bitterness between the races.

All of the new constitutions proclaimed the principle of equality and granted black adult males the right to vote, but on social relations they were much more circumspect. No state outlawed social segregation, and South Carolina and Louisiana were the only states requiring integration in public schools. Even so, that requirement was ignored except in New Orleans and at the University of South Carolina. Sensitive to status, mulattoes were more insistent on eliminating social discrimination, but white Republicans refused to adopt such a radical policy.

Economic Issues and Corruption

The problems of economic reconstruction were as difficult as those of politics. Major sections of the South lay in ruins; its people, white and black, faced dire poverty. Charred and gutted buildings scarred cities like Columbia, Atlanta, and Richmond; rail networks were broken up; central South Carolina, where Sherman's army had struck, was described as "a broad black streak of ruin and desolation."

The Republican governments in the South sought to encourage industry by providing subsidies, loans, and even exemption from taxes for a certain number of years. These governments also largely rebuilt the southern railroad system, often offering lavish aid and privileges to railroad corporations. In the two decades after 1860, the region doubled its manufacturing establishments, and centers like the Birmingham iron and steel industry became symbols of a new industrial South. Yet the harsh reality was that the South steadily slipped further behind the economy of the North, which had boomed throughout the war. Between 1854 and 1879, 7000 miles of railroad track were laid in the South, but in the same period 45,000 miles were constructed in the rest of the nation. Social disorder also discouraged outside investment, and southern energy and capital initially were devoted simply to rebuilding what the war had destroyed. The Radical governments could not create the prosperity that they unrealistically promised in hopes of gaining the support of upper-class southerners.

The expansion of government services and the cozy relationship with business leaders offered sometimes irresistible temptations for corruption. In many southern states, officials regularly resorted to fraud and received bribes and kickbacks for their award of railroad charters, franchises, and other contracts. The tax rate grew as expenditures went up, so that by the 1870s it was four times the rate of 1860. By 1872, the debts of the 11 states of the Confederacy had increased $132 million. In Florida between 1868 and 1874 the state debt grew tenfold; in South Carolina in only three years it increased to almost six times its previous size.

Corruption, however, was not only a southern problem. The decline in morality was nationwide, as scandals in the federal administration and in northern state governments revealed. During these years, the Democratic Tweed Ring in New York City stole more money than all the Radical Republican governments in the South combined. Moreover, corruption in the South was hardly limited to Republicans. Many Democrats and white businessmen participated in and profited from the corrupt practices, both before and after the Radical governments were in power. In Louisiana, where corruption had flourished long before Reconstruction, Governor Henry Warmoth, a carpetbagger, told a congressional committee the legislature was as good as the people it represented. "Why, damn it," he testified, "everybody is demoralizing down here. Corruption is the fashion."

While fraud contributed to the public debt in the South, most of the increase came from the cost of rebuilding. In fact, most of the debt represented grants to railroads. In addition, freeing millions of slaves greatly increased the number of citizens eligible for government services. The new public school systems, even if inadequately funded, meant that state taxes were bound to increase.

Corruption in Radical governments undeniably existed, but southern whites exaggerated its extent for partisan purposes. Conservatives as bitterly opposed the Radical regime in Mississippi, which was untainted by any significant financial scandal, as they did the notoriously corrupt Republican governments in Louisiana and South Carolina. In the eyes of most southern whites, the real crime of the Radical governments was that they recognized blacks in the distribution of offices and tried to protect the civil rights of black Americans. Race was the conservatives' greatest weapon and would prove the most effective means to undermine Republican power in the South.

BLACK ASPIRATIONS

Emancipation came to slaves in different ways. For some it arrived during the war when Union soldiers entered an area; for others it came some time after the Confederacy's collapse when Union troops or officials announced that they were free. On some plantations the news set off a wild celebration—a "Day of Jubilee" and thanksgiving—while other slaves received the news with no outward reaction. But after the initial celebration, what did freedom mean to people who had been in bondage all their lives?

Experiencing Freedom

The first impulse was to think of freedom as a contrast to slavery, to understand the new state of affairs in terms of limitations on white behavior and a release from the most oppressive aspects of bondage—the whippings, the work routine, the breakup of families. Above all, freedom meant that African-Americans were now their own masters and that their labor would be for their own benefit. One Arkansas freedman, who earned his first dollar working on a railroad, recalled that when he was paid, "I felt like the richest man in the world."

Freedom also meant movement, the right to travel without a pass or white permission. In the first months after the war, former slaves clogged the roads of the South. For some, this was a way to experience the thrill of moving about freely. For others, it was an attempt to find lost family members, to visit relatives, or to return to the place where they had grown up either to resettle or just to visit. Some never found the kin they sought, while others wept when reunited at last with husbands, wives, and children.

Freedom also included finding a new place to work. Changing jobs was a concrete way to break the psychological ties of slavery. Blacks especially deserted masters who had been harsh and cruel, but even planters with reputations for kindness and fairness sometimes found most of their former hands had departed. The cook who left a South Carolina family, even though they offered her higher

Daily Lives

PUBLIC SPACE/PRIVATE SPACE
The Black Sharecropper's Cabin

On the plantations of the Old South, slaves had lived in cabins along a central path in the shadow of the white master's "big house" or the overseer's dwelling. These quarters were the center of their community, where marriages and other festivals were celebrated, family life went on, and slaves shared a sense of kinship. With the coming of emancipation, however, freedmen looked to rid themselves of the old quarters, which stood as a symbol of bondage and of close white supervision. Hence when white landowners switched to a system of sharecropping or tenant farming, African-Americans either dismantled their old cabins and hauled them to the plots of land they rented or simply built new housing. This enabled them to live on the land they farmed, just as white farmers and tenants did. It also provided a greater measure of privacy.

In selecting a cabin site, freedmen tried to locate within a convenient distance of their fields, but close to the woods as well, since cutting wood was a year-round task for boys. To improve drainage, cabins were often built on a knoll or had a floor raised above the ground; in low-lying areas, stone or log piers were used. A nearby stream, spring, or well provided not only water but a place to cool butter and other perishable dairy products.

Like slave cabins, sharecroppers' dwellings were one story high with a gable roof, about 16 feet square, and built usually of logs chinked with mud. The few windows had shutters to protect against the weather; glass was rare. Though the inside walls normally lacked plaster or sheeting, they were given a coat of white-wash annually to brighten the dark interior and make the room seem larger. To provide a bit of cheer, the womenfolk often covered the walls with pictures from seed catalogues and magazines. The floor, packed dirt that was as smooth and hard as concrete, was covered with braided rugs made from scraps of cloth and worn-out clothing.

The main room served as kitchen and dining room, parlor, bathing area, and the parents' bedroom. To one side might be a homemade drop-leaf table (essential because of cramped space), which served as a kitchen work counter and a dining table. The other side of the room had a few plain beds, their slats or rope bottoms supporting corn shuck or straw mattresses. (Featherbeds were considered a remarkable luxury.) The social center of the room was the fireplace, the only source of heat and the main source of light after dark. Pots and pans were hung on the wall near the fireplace, and the mother and daughters did the cooking stooped over an open fire. Since the family usually could not afford to buy matches, the fire was rarely extinguished. Some earthen or tin dishes, steel eating utensils, assorted containers, a rifle or shotgun, and a few prized possessions (usually displayed on the mantlepiece over the fireplace) rounded out the family's furnishings. Clothing was hung on pegs in the wall. If the family owned a trunk, the parents' Sunday clothes and valuables would be stored in it.

The fireplace was constructed of smooth stone; the chimney was made of small logs notched together and covered with several layers of clay to protect it from the heat. It often narrowed toward the top, and sometimes its height was extended by empty flour barrels, for a taller chimney drew better. That made for a hot-

Daily Lives

Chimneys on share-croppers' cabins were often tilted deliber-ately, so they could be pushed away from the house quickly if they caught fire.

ter fire and kept smoke from blowing back down into the house and sparks away from the roof. After the evening meal, the family gathered around the fireplace, the children to play with homemade dolls and toys, the mother to sew, and the father perhaps to play the fiddle. At bedtime, a trapdoor in the ceiling offered access up a ladder to the loft beneath the gabled roof. Being cold and dark, it was used only for sleeping. Normally the parents and infants slept downstairs, older children upstairs until the girls reached puberty, after which they slept downstairs too. The children often slept on pallets on the floor, as had been the case in slavery.

In the summer, cooking was done outdoors over an open fire. Women preferred to cook under a tree, which offered some protection from rain as well as relief from the sun and the high humidity. Sharecropper families rarely had separate cooking rooms attached to or next to the cabin. Separate kitchens, which were a sign of prosperity, were more common among black landowners and white tenant farmers.

Gradually, as black sharecroppers were able to scrape together some savings, the quality of their homes improved. By the end of the century, frame dwellings were more common, and many older log cabins had been covered with wood siding. The newer homes were generally larger, with wood floors, and often had attached rooms such as a porch or kitchen. In addition, glass panes covered the windows, roofs were covered with shingles instead of planking, and stone and brick chimneys were less unusual. A narrow stairwell, often with a door to shut out cold drafts, provided access to the loft; underneath it was a closet for additional storage. Ceramic dishes were more frequently seen, and wood-burning stoves made cooking easier for women and provided a more efficient source of heat.

Without question, the cabins of black sharecroppers provided more space than the slave quarters had, and certainly more freedom and privacy. Still, they lacked many of the comforts that most white Americans took for granted. Such housing reflected the continuing status of black sharecroppers as poverty-stricken laborers in a caste system based on race.

wages than her new job, explained, "I must go. If I stays here I'll never know I'm free." And a black preacher told a group of freedmen in Florida: "So long as the shadow of the great house fall across you, you ain't going to feel like no free man and no free woman. You must all move to new places that you don't know, where you can raise up your head without no fear of Master This and Master The Other."

Symbolically, freedom meant, too, having a full name. As slaves, African-Americans often had no surname, but with the coming of freedom, more than a few took the name of some prominent individual, such as Washington or Jefferson, or else some leading figure in the community. More common, however, was to take the name of the first master in the family's oral history as far back as it could be recalled. Most freedmen, on the other hand, retained their first name in slavery, especially if they had been named by their parents (as most slaves were). It had been their form of identity in bondage, and for those separated from their family it was the only link with their parents. But whatever name they took, it was important to blacks that they made the decision themselves without white interference.

The Black Family

African-Americans also sought to strengthen the family in freedom. Since slave marriages had not been recognized as legal, thousands of former slaves insisted on being married again by proper authorities. Although not required by law, these wedding ceremonies represented a reaffirmation of commitments made earlier. This new right created a dilemma for those who had been forcibly separated from a spouse in slavery and subsequently remarried. Should they return to their first spouse or remain with the current one? The Freedmen's Bureau urged blacks in this predicament to take the spouse with whom they had the greatest number of dependent children, but the final decision rested with the individuals. Laura Spicer, who had been separated from her slave husband, received a series of wrenching letters from him after the war. He had thought her dead, had remarried, and had a new family. "I would come and see you but I know you could not bear it," he wrote.

> You know it never was our wishes to be separated from each other, and it never was our fault . . . I had rather anything to had happened to me most than ever have been parted from you and the children. As I am, I do not know which I love best, you or Anna . . . I do not think I would die satisfied till you tell me you will try and marry some good, smart man that will take good care of you and the children; and do it because you love me; and not because I think more of the wife I have got than I do of you. The woman is not born that feels as near to me as you do.

A family decision that had major economic repercussions for agricultural labor was the insistence of black men that their wives would not work in the fields as they had in slavery. As in white families, black fathers deemed themselves the head of the family and the breadwinner and acted legally for their wives. "The [black] women say they never mean to do any more outdoor work," one planter reported, "that white men support their wives and they mean that their husbands shall support them." African-American families also often withdrew their children from labor. In negotiating contracts, a father demanded the right to discipline his children. All these changes were designed to insulate the black family from white control.

Making the rounds of the parish, a black minister shares a meal with some of his parishioners. Such meals were a welcome supplement to a clergyman's scanty salary. Black ministers were important leaders of the African-American community in freedom.

The Gospel and the Primer

In freedom, the schoolhouse and the black church became essential institutions in the black community. Next to ownership of land, African-Americans saw education as the best hope for advancement. "My Lord, Ma'am, what a great thing learning is!" a South Carolina freedman told a northern teacher. "White folks can do what they likes, for they know so much more than we." Initially, northern churches and missionaries, working with the Freedmen's Bureau, set up black schools in the South. The Bureau also spent over $400,000 to support black colleges, including Howard University in Washington, which were founded to train future African-American leaders and teachers to staff black schools.

The freedmen's schools were not free and required a substantial commitment on the part of the family of those who enrolled. Tuition represented 10 percent or more a laborer's monthly wages, yet these schools were full. Blacks eagerly came; one school official reported they were simply "crazy to learn." Many parents sent their children to school by day and attended classes themselves at night. Eventually, the freedmen's schools were replaced by the new public school systems, which by 1876 had enrolled 40 percent of African-American children.

Black adults had good reasons for seeking literacy. They wanted to be able to read the Bible, to defend their newly gained civil and political rights, and to protect themselves from being cheated. Slavery had bred a deeply ingrained suspicion of whites, and as one elderly Louisiana freedman explained, giving children an education was better than giving them a fortune, "because if you left them even

$500, some man having more education than they had would come along and cheat them out of it all." White resistance stimulated this desire for education. Black schools were often destroyed, and white teachers threatened and even murdered. Both races saw in the postwar South that education would undermine the old servility that slavery had fostered. More than other Americans, blacks knew that education would overthrow the legacy of slavery.

For the first time in the South, blacks were allowed to establish their own churches. Most slaves had attended white churches or services supervised by whites, and northern organizations like the African Methodist Episcopal Church had been banned. Once free, African-Americans quickly established their own congregations led by black preachers. In the first year of freedom, the Methodist Church South lost fully half of its black members. By 1870, the Negro Baptist Church had increased its membership threefold compared to 1850, and the African Methodist Episcopal Church expanded at an even greater rate.

Indeed, black churches were so important because they were the only social organization in the African-American community actually controlled by blacks. Black ministers were respected leaders. An officer of the American Missionary Association reported that "the Ebony preacher who promises perfect independence from White control and direction carried the colored heart at once." Many of the black men elected to office during Reconstruction were preachers. Just as in slavery, religion offered African-Americans a place of refuge in a hostile white world and provided them with hope, comfort, and a means of self-identification.

New Working Conditions

For blacks, freedom involved more than just receiving pay for labor performed; they sought to remove all the emblems and habits of servitude. Owning land would have best provided them with economic independence, but the few feeble attempts at land reform failed. Blacks remained a largely propertyless class, forced to work for former masters and landowners. Whites insisted, as they had before the war, that blacks would not work without compulsion. Except for paying wages, they tried to retain the old system of labor, including close supervision, gang labor, and discipline by the whip or other physical punishment. African-Americans, however, not only refused to work under this system; they demanded time off to devote to their own work and leisure interests. Convinced that working at one's own pace was part of freedom, they simply would not work as long or as hard as they had in slavery. Because of shorter hours and the withdrawal of children and women from the fields, work output declined by an estimated 35 percent. Blacks also refused to live in the old slave quarters located near the master's house. Instead, they erected cabins on distant parts of the plantation. Wages initially were $5 or $6 a month plus provisions and a cabin; by 1867, they had risen to an average of $10 a month.

Such changes in the labor system eventually led to the rise of the sharecropping system. Under this arrangement, African-American families farmed separate plots of land and then at the end of the year divided the crop with the owner. The farmer's share depended on whether he supplied the seeds, animals, and implements, but the normal arrangement was an equal division of the crop between the sharecropper and the landowner. Although sharecropping was not the same as owning a farm, blacks believed it offered higher status and greater personal freedom than being a wage laborer. One black defended his right to leave the planta-

A GEORGIA PLANTATION AFTER THE WAR

After emancipation, sharecropping became the dominant form of agricultural labor in the South. Black families no longer lived in the old slave quarters, but dispersed themselves to separate plots of land that they farmed themselves. At the end of the year each sharecropper turned over part of the crop to the white landowner.

tion at will without permission of the owner. "I am not working for wages," he declared, "but am part owner of the crop and as I have all the rights that you or any other man has I shall not suffer them abridged." Actually, black per capita agricultural income increased 40 percent between 1857 and 1879, since white landlords were unable to expropriate as large a share of black earnings as they had in slavery.

The Freedmen's Bureau

The task of supervising the transition from slavery to freedom on southern plantations fell to the Freedmen's Bureau, a unique experiment in social policy supported briefly by the federal government. Created as an agency of the War Department, the Bureau provided relief for refugees, helped settle freedmen on abandoned lands, and put them back to work. During the summer of 1865 the Bureau provided 150,000 daily rations, a third of which went to whites; from 1865 to 1870 it issued 2 million rations, built 40 hospitals, and treated 450,000 patients. But the Bureau's major task was to protect the freedmen's economic rights. Approximately 550 local agents supervised and regulated working conditions in an attempt to bring order to southern agriculture after the war. The racial attitudes of Bureau agents varied widely, as did their commitment and competence. Since their guidelines were vague, they used their own judgment to settle cases, and they depended on the army to enforce their decisions.

Most agents encouraged or required written contracts between white planters and black laborers, specifying not only wages, but the conditions of employment. Agents adjudicated disputes, sometimes intervening to protect freedmen from unfair treatment. But agents also used their power to get African-Americans who had migrated to the cities back on the plantations. They preached to the freedmen the gospel of work and the need to be orderly and respectful. Given such attitudes, blacks increasingly complained that Bureau agents were mere tools of the planter class. "They are, in fact, the planters' guards, and nothing else," claimed the New Orleans *Tribune*, a black newspaper. Agents did provide important help to planters. They insisted that blacks not desert at harvest time; they arrested as vagrants those who violated their contracts or refused to sign new ones at the beginning of the year. One observer reported, "Doing justice seems to mean seeing that the blacks don't break contracts and compelling them to submit cheerfully."

The primary means of enforcing working conditions were the Freedmen's Courts, which Congress created in 1866 because of persistent discrimination against African-Americans in the state courts. These new courts functioned as military tribunals and often the agent was the entire court, hearing testimony and then rendering a verdict. These courts were more sympathetic to freedmen in some states than others. In 1867 one agent summarized the Bureau's experience with the labor contract system: "It has succeeded in making the freedman work and in rendering labor secure and stable—but it has failed to secure to the Freedman his just dues or compensation."

In 1869, with the Bureau's work scarcely under way, Congress ordered it to prepare to shut down. Even the Radical Republicans did not want to create a permanent welfare agency. By 1872 the Bureau had gone out of business, leaving behind a mixed record. Its major accomplishment was freedmen's schools, but the absence of any program for significant land redistribution ensured that its contributions would be limited. The disbanding of the Bureau, the most effective and efficient agency that protected blacks' civil and political rights, signaled the beginning of the northern retreat from Reconstruction.

Planters and a New Way of Life

Planters and other southern whites faced emancipation with dread. Unwilling to live with free blacks, some planters fled to the North, the West, or even to foreign countries like Mexico and Brazil. Most, however, stayed, searching for a system to replace slavery. "All the traditions and habits of both races had been suddenly overthrown," a Tennessee planter recalled, "and neither knew just what to do, or how to accommodate themselves to the new situation."

The old ideal of a paternalistic planter, which required a facade of black subservience and affection, gave way to an emphasis on strictly economic relationships. Mary Jones, a Georgia slaveholder before the war who did more for her workers than the law required, complained of their disrespectful language, imper-

Black education was one of the significant changes freedom brought during the era of Reconstruction. Here a group of black students pose with their books outside their crude schoolhouse.

tinent gestures, and poor work. But her patience snapped when two workers accused her of trickery and hauled her before a Freedmen's Bureau agent, with whom she won her case. Upon returning home, she announced to the assembled freedmen that "in doubting my word they offered me the greatest insult I ever received in my life; that I have considered them friends and treated them as such but now they were only laborers under contract, and only the law would rule between us." The subservience that planters had demanded and taken for granted—touching one's hat, the obsequious, smiling demeanor, the fawning guise of gratitude—now melted away in freedom. Only with time did planters develop new norms and standards to judge black behavior. What in 1865 had seemed insolence was viewed by the 1870s as the normal attitude of freedom.

Slavery had been a complex institution that welded blacks and whites together in intimate relationships, but under the new system planters increasingly embraced the ideology of segregation. Planters kept dealings with African Americans to a minimum. Since emancipation significantly reduced the social distance between the races, whites sought psychological separation. Segregation—the legal separation of the races—became an institution to buttress white status. By the time Reconstruction ended, white planters had developed a new set of values to replace those of slavery. Their new way of life was reflected in the institutions of sharecropping and segregation and undergirded by a militant white supremacy. Planters endured, but with emancipation, they lost their pride, confidence, and some of their identity.

Nor did planters regain the economic prosperity of the antebellum years.

Rice plantations, which were not suitable to tenant farming, largely disappeared after the war. The cotton crops in 1865 and 1866 failed, and it was not until 1877 that cotton production consistently exceeded the prewar level. Furthermore, cotton from new areas such as India, Egypt, and Brazil now competed with American cotton, while the world demand grew at a much slower rate after 1865 than it had earlier. Cotton prices began a long decline, and southern per capita income suffered as a result. Cotton plantations continued to dominate southern agriculture, but many planters' income declined sharply. Most escaped total collapse, but by 1880 the value of southern farms had slid 33 percent below the level of 1860.

THE ABANDONMENT OF RECONSTRUCTION

The Radical Republicans had failed to impeach Johnson by one vote—a narrow margin, but effective nevertheless. The Radicals' influence was waning and the Republican party was being drained of the crusading idealism that had stamped its early years. Ulysses S. Grant was hardly the cause of this change, but he certainly came to symbolize it.

The Election of Grant

Grant had not identified with the Radical wing of the party until Johnson used the general as a pawn in his struggle with Congress. In relieving Stanton, Johnson had tried to maneuver Grant to take his place, and in the process drove the general into an alliance with the Radicals. Afraid of sinking into obscurity, Grant yearned to be president, the only office that would be a promotion for him. Immensely popular, he was the natural choice of Republicans in 1868. Since the Republican platform called for repayment of the national war debt in gold, which pleased businessmen but hurt workers and farmers, the Democrats proposed a more inflationary monetary policy. That appealed to many debtor farmers (who were helped by inflation), and the Democrats also hoped to pick up votes of whites who disapproved of Republican policies on behalf of the freedmen.

Grant easily defeated his opponent, former governor Horatio Seymour of New York, in the Electoral College, but his popular margin was only 300,000 votes. With a ticket headed by a great military hero, the close vote shocked Republican leaders. Although Grant would have won in the Electoral College even without the estimated 450,000 votes he received from southern blacks, a majority of whites had voted for Seymour. The 1868 election helped convince Republicans that an amendment securing black suffrage throughout the nation was necessary.

In February 1869 Congress sent the Fifteenth Amendment to the states for ratification. It forbade any state from denying the right to vote on grounds of race, color, or previous condition of servitude. Some Radicals had hoped to forbid literacy or property requirements, to protect blacks further; others wanted a simple declaration that all adult male citizens had the right to vote. But the Moderates feared that only a conservative version could be ratified, since many northerners were increasingly worried about the number of immigrants who were again enter-

Declining to adopt her husband's name, Lucy Stone (right) was a major figure in the women's rights movement after the Civil War. Northern women who had worked for emancipation during the war protested the failure to grant them the right to vote along with male freedmen during Reconstruction.

ing the country. As a result, the final amendment left loopholes that eventually allowed southern states to disfranchise African-Americans.

Radicals saw the Fifteenth Amendment as an antidote to the hypocrisy of the Fourteenth Amendment, which fastened black suffrage only upon the South (and even there, only by indirection). "We have no moral right to impose an obligation on one part of the land which the rest will not accept," one Radical leader declared. Party leaders also felt that the small black vote might be critical to the Republicans in closely contested northern states. The amendment was ratified in March 1870, in part with the votes of the four southern states that had not completed the process of Reconstruction and thus were also required to endorse this amendment before being readmitted to Congress.

Proponents of women's suffrage were gravely disappointed at the refusal of Congress to prohibit voting discrimination on the basis of sex as well as race. Many of the women's suffrage supporters had been associated with the abolitionist movement earlier and had worked hard to get the Thirteenth Amendment ratified. The Women's Loyal League, led by Elizabeth Cady Stanton and Susan B. Anthony, had pressed for first the Fourteenth and then the Fifteenth Amendment to recognize women's public role, but even most Radicals, contending that black rights had to be assured first, were unwilling to back women's suffrage. The Fifteenth Amendment ruptured the feminist movement. While disappointed that women were not included in its provisions, Lucy Stone and the American Woman

Suffrage Association urged ratification of the amendment. Anthony and Stanton, on the other hand, broke with their former allies among the Radicals, denounced the amendment, and organized the National Woman Suffrage Association to work for passage of a new amendment giving women the ballot. This division continued to hamper the women's rights movement in the future.

The Grant Administration

Grant lacked the moral commitment to make Reconstruction succeed. Unsure of himself socially, he gravitated toward the wealthy elements in American society, the businessmen and financiers that the party increasingly aided. He was ill at ease with the political process, lacked trustworthy advisers, and, haunted by his undistinguished career before 1861, had an abiding fear of failure. Grant's simple and taciturn style, while superb for commanding armies, did not serve him as well in politics, and his well-known resolution withered when he was uncertain of his purpose or goal. His bewilderment over the complex political problems he confronted made him appear pathetic, a handicap that even his good intentions could not overcome.

A series of scandals wracked Grant's presidency, so much so that "Grantism" soon became a code word in American politics for corruption, cronyism, and venality. Although Grant did not profit personally, those close to him dipped freely into the public till. Loyal to his friends, he displayed little zeal to root out corruption or bring the guilty to justice. His relatives were implicated in a scheme to corner the gold market, his private secretary escaped conviction for stealing federal whiskey revenues only because Grant interceded on his behalf, and his secretary of war, who was selling Indian trading post contracts, resigned to avoid impeachment. James W. Grimes, one of the party's founders, denounced the Republican party under Grant as "the most corrupt and debauched political party that has ever existed."

Nor was Congress immune from the lowered tone of public life. The Crédit Mobilier, a corporation established to build the Union Pacific Railroad, siphoned huge profits from the coffers into its directors' hands, but a number of bribed congressmen successfully headed off an investigation. In such a climate ruthless state machines, led by men who favored maintaining the status quo, came to dominate the Republican party. Office and power became ends in themselves, and party leaders worked in close cooperation with northern industrial interests.

At the same time, the Radicals who had spearheaded the movement for a rigorous program of Reconstruction were passing from the scene. Thaddeus Stevens died in August 1868, shortly after Johnson's impeachment trial. Benjamin F. Wade and George Julian were defeated, and Charles Sumner, who got into a tug of war with the Grant administration over an attempt to annex the island of Santo Domingo, was stripped of his chairmanship of the foreign relations committee by the Senate. The few Radicals still active in public life increasingly repudiated Grant and the Republican governments in the South. Congress in 1872 passed an amnesty act, removing the restrictions of the Fourteenth Amendment on office holding, except for about 200 to 300 ex-Confederate leaders.

As corruption in both the North and South worsened, reformers in the party became more interested in cleaning up government than in protecting black rights. These liberal Republicans, who considered themselves "the best men," opposed the continued presence of the army in the South, denounced the corrup-

Grant swings from a trapeze while supporting a number of associates accused of corruption. Among those holding on are Secretary of the Navy George M. Robeson (top center), who was accused of accepting bribes in the awarding of navy contracts; Secretary of War William W. Belknap (top right), who was forced to resign for selling Indian post traderships; and the president's private secretary Orville Babcock (bottom right), who was implicated in the Whiskey Ring scandal. Though not personally involved in the scandals during his administration, Grant was reluctant to dismiss supporters accused of wrongdoing from office.

tion of southern governments as well as the national government, and advocated free trade and civil service reform. In 1872 they broke with the Republican party and nominated for president Horace Greeley. The editor of the New York *Tribune* and a one-time Radical, Greeley was disillusioned with Reconstruction and urged a restoration of home rule in the South. Democrats decided to back the Liberal Republican ticket. The Republicans renominated Grant, who, despite the defection of Radicals such as Sumner, Carl Schurz, and E. L. Godkin of the *Nation*, won an easy victory with 56 percent of the popular vote.

Growing Northern Disillusionment

During Grant's second term, Congress passed the Civil Rights Act of 1875, the last major piece of Reconstruction legislation. Up until this time, Congress had refused to challenge segregation and racial discrimination practiced by individuals and corporations. The 1875 law prohibited racial discrimination in all public accommodations, transportation, places of amusement, and juries. Congress, however, rejected a ban on segregation in public schools, which was almost universally practiced in the North as well as the South. While some railroads, streetcars, and public accommodations in both sections were desegregated after the law passed, the federal government made little attempt to enforce the law, and it was ignored throughout most of the South. In 1883 the Supreme Court struck down its provisions except that relating to juries.

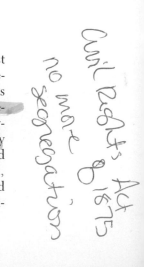

Civil Rights Act 1875, no more segregation

Despite passage of this law, northern public opinion was, in fact, growing increasingly disillusioned with Reconstruction. Northerners were bothered by the corruption and dishonesty of the southern governments and tired of the violence and disorder in the South. Even at the height of Reconstruction, the support for black rights owed more to antisouthern than problack motives. "People are becoming tired of abstract questions," one Republican paper commented. "The negro question, with all its complications, and the reconstruction of the Southern states, with all its interminable embroilments, have lost much of the power they once wielded."

At the same time, a number of Republicans were attracted to Lincoln's old strategy of forging an alliance with southern whites. Influential northern business leaders were particularly eager to establish conditions favorable to investment in the South. They began to look to southern conservatives, many of whom were proponents of the idea of a New South based on urbanizaton and industry, to restore order and political stability. William Dodge, a wealthy New York capitalist, wrote in 1875: "What the South now needs is capital to develop her resources, but this she cannot obtain till confidence in her state governments can be restored, and this will never be done by federal bayonets." It had been a mistake, he went on, to make southern blacks feel "that the United States government was their special friend, rather than those with whom their lot is cast, among whom they must live and for whom they must work. We have tried this long enough," he concluded. "Now let the South alone."

As the agony of the war became more distant and Republicans got less mileage out of waving the bloody shirt, economic matters drew public attention away from Reconstruction. The Panic of 1873 marked the beginning of a severe depression that lasted for four years. Some 3 million people were thrown out of work, and much of the wrangling in Congress about how to revive the economy centered on the question of the currency. In 1874 Grant vetoed a bill to increase the supply of greenbacks, and the next year Congress adopted the policy of requiring greenbacks to be convertible to gold by 1878. The question of inflation and the gold standard would remain a central political issue for the remainder of the century (page 782).

But in its immediate political consequences, the depression led to a surge in Democratic strength. Battered by the panic and the corruption issue, the Republicans lost a shocking 77 seats in Congress in the 1874 elections, and along with them control of the House of Representatives for the first time since 1861. The Democrats scored striking gains in every region of the country, even winning the Massachusetts governorship for the first time in 40 years. "The truth is our people are tired out with the worn out cry of 'Southern outrages'!!" one Republican concluded. "Hard times and heavy taxes make them wish the 'ever lasting nigger' were in hell or Africa." Republicans spoke more and more about cutting loose the southern governments to enhance the party's strength in the North.

The Triumph of White Supremacy

As northern commitment to Reconstruction declined, southern Democrats set out to overthrow the remaining Radical governments. Already white southerners were deserting the Republican party by the thousands. A white Republican in Mississippi justified his decision to leave the party on the grounds that otherwise, his children had no future. "No white man can live in the South in the future and act with any other than the Democratic party unless he is willing and prepared to live a life of social isolation and remain in political oblivion."

To poor whites who lacked social standing, the Democratic appeal to racial solidarity offered great comfort. As one explained, "I may be poor and my manners may be crude, but I am a white man. And because I am a white man, I have a right to be treated with respect by Negroes. That I am poor is not as important as that I am a white man; and no Negro is ever going to forget that he is not a white man." The large landowners and other wealthy groups that led southern Democrats objected less to blacks voting, in part because they did not face social and economic competition from them, but also because they were confident that if outside influences were removed, they could control the black vote. When Wade Hampton, a wealthy planter, ran for governor in South Carolina in 1876, he pledged that if elected he would "observe, protect, and defend the rights of the colored man as quickly as any man in South Carolina."

Democrats also resorted to economic pressure to undermine Republican power. The lack of a secret ballot strengthened the hand of white conservatives. White landlords refused to hire or take on as sharecroppers African-Americans who voted Republican. In heavily black counties, white observers at the polls took down the names of blacks who cast Republican ballots and published them in local newspapers. A Mississippi paper urged planters to "discharge . . . every laborer who persists in the diabolical war that has been waged against the white man and his interest ever since the negro has been a voter."

But terror and violence proved the most important means used to overthrow the radical regimes in the South. A number of paramilitary organizations, of which the Ku Klux Klan was the most famous, broke up Republican meetings, terrorized white and black Republicans, assassinated Republican leaders and candidates, and prevented blacks from voting. Founded in 1866 in Tennessee, the Klan represented all social classes, although the leaders were often locally prominent planters. Most of the members were young men in their twenties and thirties, and many were Confederate veterans. The Klan and similar organizations functioned as an unofficial arm of the Democratic party.

Congress finally moved to break the power of the Klan with the Force Act of 1870 and the Ku Klux Klan Act of 1871. These laws made it a felony to interfere with the right to vote; they also authorized use of the army, suspension of the writ of habeas corpus, and removal of Klan supporters from juries. The Grant administration eventually suspended the writ of habeas corpus in nine South Carolina counties and arrested hundreds of suspected Klan members throughout the South. Although these actions weakened the Klan, terrorist organizations continued to operate underground.

What became known as the Mississippi Plan was inaugurated in 1875, when Democrats decided to use as much violence as necessary to carry the state election. Several local papers trumpeted, "Carry the election peaceably if we can, forcibly if we must." Democratic clubs, organized into irregular military companies, paraded in black areas to intimidate voters, dispersed Republican meetings, and assassinated Republican leaders. When Republican Governor Adelbert Ames requested federal troops to stop the violence, Grant's advisers warned that sending troops to Mississippi would cost the party the Ohio election. In the end, the administration told Ames to depend on his own forces. As the attorney general

Two Ku Klux Klan members pose in full regalia. Violence played a major role in overthrowing the Radical governments in the South. One South Carolina paper openly praised Klan attacks on blacks and the Republican Union Leagues:

> Born of the night, and vanish by day;
> Leaguers and niggers, get out of the way!

explained, "The whole public are tired out with these annual autumnal outbreaks in the South, and the great majority are now ready to condemn any interference on the part of the government."

Bolstered by this terrorism, the Democrats swept the election. Violence and intimidation prevented as many as 60,000 black and white Republicans from voting, converting the normal Republican majority into a Democratic majority of 30,000. The victors boasted that Mississippi had been "redeemed."

The Disputed Election of 1876

With the Republican party on the defensive across the nation, the 1876 presidential election was crucial to the final overthrow of Reconstruction. Only three states—Louisiana, South Carolina, and Florida—still remained in Republican hands, and Democrats were prepared to use the Mississippi Plan to carry them in 1876.

The Republicans nominated Ohio governor Rutherford B. Hayes to oppose Samuel Tilden, a Democrat who had won fame by prosecuting the corrupt Tweed Ring in New York City. Once again, violence prevented an estimated quarter of a million Republican votes from being cast in the South, and the outcome was in doubt. Tilden had reported majorities in South Carolina, Florida, and Louisiana, but Hayes' supporters also claimed them. Hayes needed all three states to be elected, for even without them, Tilden had amassed 184 electoral votes, one short of a majority. Tilden also had a clear majority of 250,000 in the popular vote. Although the Democrats also claimed to have carried the governorships and legislatures in South Carolina, Louisiana, and Florida, the Republican canvassing boards in power disqualified enough Democratic votes to give each state to Hayes.

To arbitrate the disputed returns, Congress established a 15-member electoral commission: 5 members each from the Senate, the House, and the Supreme Court. As originally constituted, the commission divided evenly between 7 Republicans and 7 Democrats, with Supreme Court Justice David Davis, who had been a Republican and was now a political independent, as the swing vote. But when Davis was elected to the Senate from Illinois, he declined to serve on the commission and was replaced by a Republican member of the Court. By a straight party vote of 8–7, the commission awarded the disputed electoral votes—and the presidency—to Hayes.

When angry Democrats threatened a filibuster to prevent the electoral votes from being counted, Republicans scrambled to head off a stalemate. On February 26, key Republicans met with southern Democrats at the Wormley Hotel in Washington and reached an informal understanding, later known as the Compromise of 1877. Hayes' supporters agreed to withdraw the troops and not oppose the new white state governments if Democrats would drop their opposition to Hayes' election. Southerners, for their part, pledged to treat blacks fairly and respect their rights. Hayes was quite happy with this deal, for he hoped to rebuild his party in the South by appealing primarily to whites who were former Whigs. Assurances that Republicans would help pass federal aid for a number of southern internal improvement projects also helped in a minor way to ease Democratic objections.

Once in office, Hayes withdrew military support for the Republican governors in South Carolina and Louisiana, who had claimed victory. Those administrations promptly collapsed, and Democrats took control of the remaining two states of the Confederacy. By 1877, the entire South was in the hands of the Redeemers, as they called themselves, and Reconstruction and Republican rule had come to an end.

THE ELECTION OF 1876

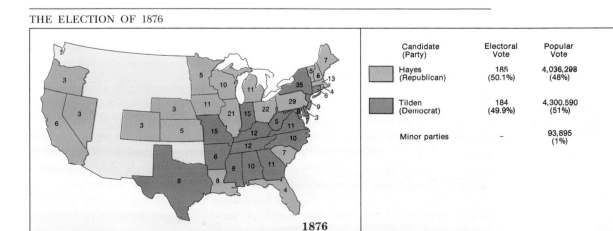

Candidate (Party)	Electoral Vote	Popular Vote
Hayes (Republican)	185 (50.1%)	4,036,298 (48%)
Tilden (Democrat)	184 (49.9%)	4,300,590 (51%)
Minor parties	–	93,895 (1%)

1876

In a crowded Supreme Court chamber, lawyers for both Hayes and Tilden present evidence to the electoral commission (seated on the rostrum at left) created to decide the outcome of the 1876 election. Members of all branches of government listen to the testimony, along with a number of socially prominent women, including Cornelia Adele Fassett, the artist who painted the scene from which this detail is taken.

Racism and the Failure of Reconstruction

Reconstruction failed for a multitude of reasons. The reforming impulse that had created the Republican party in the 1850s had been battered and worn down by the war. The new materialism of industrial America inspired in many a jaded cynicism about the corruption of the age and a desire to forget the uncomfortable issues of the past. In the South, African-American voters and leaders inevitably lacked a certain amount of education and experience; elsewhere, Republicans were divided over policies and options. Yet beyond all these obstacles, the sad fact remains that the ideals of the war and Reconstruction were most clearly defeated by a deep-seated racism that permeated American life. Racism was why the white South so unrelentingly resisted Reconstruction; racism was why most northern whites had little interest in black rights except as a means to an end, to preserve the Union or to safeguard the Republic; racism was why northerners were willing to write off Reconstruction, and with it the welfare of black Americans. Ever since the mid-seventeenth century, the system of slavery had been based on race. While Congress might pass a constitutional amendment abolishing the peculiar institution, it could not overturn at a stroke the social habits of two centuries.

Certainly the political equations of power, in the long term, had been changed. The North had fought tenaciously during the war to preserve the Union, and in doing so, had retained the power to dominate the economic and political destiny of the nation. With the overthrow of Reconstruction, the white South had won back in time of peace some of the power it had lost through war. But even with white supremacy triumphant across the land, African-Americans did not remain on the same social footing as before the war. They were no longer slaves, and blacks who walked dusty roads in search of family members, sent their children to school, or worshiped in churches they controlled, knew what a momentous change this was. Even under the exploitive sharecropping system, black income rose 40 percent in freedom. Then too, the principles of "equal protection" and "due process of law" had been written into the Constitution and would be available for later generations to use in resurrecting the Radicals' goal of racial equality.

But this was a struggle left to future generations. For the time being, the clear trend was away from change, reform, or hope—especially for blacks like Benjamin Montgomery and his sons, the owners of the old Davis plantation in Mississippi. In the 1870s bad crops, falling cotton prices and land values, and other misfortunes undermined the Montgomerys' financial position. At the same time, white violence against blacks made them more dependent than before on white goodwill, and in 1875 Jefferson Davis, who was now in dire economic circumstances himself, sued to have the sale of Brierfield invalidated. Davis acknowledged that he had never received legal title to the land, but he contended that his brother Joseph, who had died in 1870, had given him the plantation years ago to operate as his own.

In 1876, a lower court ruled against Davis, since he had executed his brother's will for four years without challenging its validity. But with the overthrow of Mississippi's Radical government, the political winds in the state shifted, and Davis appealed to the state supreme court, which now had a white conservative majority. The court, in a politically motivated decision, awarded Brierfield to Davis in 1878, and the Montgomerys lost Hurricane as well. The final outcome was not without bitter irony. In applying for restoration of his property after the war, Joseph Davis had convinced skeptical federal officials that he, and not his younger brother, held legal title to Brierfield. Had they decided instead that the plantation belonged to Jefferson Davis, it would have been confiscated.

But the waning days of Reconstruction were times filled with such ironies: of governments "redeemed" by violence, of Fourteenth Amendment rights designed to protect black people being used by conservative courts to protect giant corporations, of reformers searching elsewhere for other causes. Repudiated by its northern supporters and unmourned by public opinion, Reconstruction was over.

Benjamin Montgomery, together with his sons, purchased Jefferson Davis' plantation along the Mississippi River after the war. A former slave, Montgomery pursued the dream of black economic independence by renting land to black farmers at Davis Bend.

SIGNIFICANT EVENTS

1863	Lincoln outlines Reconstruction program
1864	Lincoln vetoes Wade–Davis bill; Louisiana, Arkansas, and Tennessee establish governments under Lincoln's plan
1865	Freedmen's Bureau established; Johnson becomes president; Presidential Reconstruction; Congress excludes representatives of Johnson's governments; Thirteenth Amendment ratified; Joint Committee on Reconstruction established
1865–1866	Black codes enacted
1866	Civil Rights bill passed over Johnson's veto; Memphis and New Orleans riots; Fourteenth Amendment passes Congress; Freedmen's Bureau extended; Ku Klux Klan organized; Tennessee readmitted to Congress; Republicans win decisive victory in congressional elections
1867	Congressional Reconstruction; Tenure of Office Act; Control of the Army Act
1867–1868	Constitutional conventions in the South; blacks vote in southern elections
1868	Johnson impeached but acquitted; Fourteenth Amendment ratified; Grant elected president
1869	Fifteenth Amendment passes Congress; *Ex parte McCardle*
1870	Last southern states readmitted to Congress; Fifteenth Amendment ratified; Enforcement acts
1871	Ku Klux Klan Act
1872	General Amnesty Act; Freedmen's Bureau dismantled; Liberal Republican revolt
1873–1877	Panic and depression
1874	Democrats win control of the House
1875	Civil Rights Act; Mississippi Plan
1876	Disputed Hayes–Tilden election
1877	Compromise of 1877; Hayes declared winner of electoral vote; last Republican governments in South fall

PART 4

THE UNITED STATES IN AN INDUSTRIAL AGE

The Statue of Liberty has now stood watch over New York harbor for more than a hundred years. In that time the tired, poor, huddled masses of immigrants who passed beneath her torch have become, to late-twentieth-century Americans, anonymous parts of a continuing stream, stretching back in the mind's eye to the English Pilgrims, the French fur traders along the St. Lawrence, and the Spanish friars of Old California. But the nineteenth-century stream of immigrants arriving at Ellis Island was different from the large majority of those who had traveled to America in an earlier age. Innovations in transportation, communications, and industry created an international network that made possible for the first time voluntary migration on a massive scale.

Before 1820 substantial numbers of people had moved to North and South America, but for the great majority the choice had hardly been voluntary. Perhaps 7.8 million Africans were brought to the Americas during those years, virtually all as slaves. That number was four to five times the number of Europeans who came during the same period. In contrast, between 1820 and 1920 nearly 30 million free immigrants arrived from Europe.

Nor was this flood directed only toward America. At least as many Europeans left their homelands for other regions of Europe or the world. While millions of immigrants were taking trains across the American plains in search of jobs and homesteads, millions more from eastern Europe followed the Trans-Siberian Railway (completed in 1905) into Asiatic Russia. The Canadian prairie provinces of

Manitoba and Saskatchewan competed for homesteaders with Montana and the Dakotas. And when cowboys began driving American steers to newly built railheads for shipment east, gauchos across the pampas of western Argentina were rounding up cattle to be shipped to Buenos Aires. Before 1900 two out of three emigrating Italians booked passage not for the United States but for Brazil and Argentina.

This broad movement could not have taken place without a widening global network of communication, markets, and transportation. Some of the effects of the industrial transformation had been felt well before the end of the nineteenth century. Indeed, the Civil War was a consequence, in part, of the conflicting ways in which the North and the South had evolved. Though still relatively rural, the northern economy had begun to urbanize by 1860, with textile mills clustered in factory towns along New England rivers, and railroads from the Midwest opening up commercial markets for grain and dairy products. The South remained overwhelmingly rural, but industry shaped it nonetheless, as New England and European factories clamored for southern cotton to spin into fabric and "ready-made" clothing. The demand for cotton ensured that the slave labor system firmly entrenched itself in the South, until at last the issue of whether the nation could endure half-slave and half-free was decided by force of arms.

By the end of Reconstruction, urbanization and industrialization were well under way, not only in America but also in Europe. The British, whose innovations had sparked the revolution in industry, also discovered its devastating side effects. Population swelled in urban areas of Great Britain, as rural workers flocked after factory jobs. Without efficient transportation, the workers were forced to live within walking distance of the factories. The resulting overcrowding and filth were almost stupefying: families jammed into dark, pungent row houses built with few windows along narrow alleyways and streets where open sewers flowed with garbage. In London one construction engineer reported that the overflow from privies had collected to the depth of three feet in the cellars of nearby houses.

Spurred on by a deadly cholera epidemic in 1848, British social reformer Edwin Chadwick completed a long and hard-fought campaign to install a system of cheap iron pipes and tile drains to provide running water and sewers throughout major cities. In addition, French and German research during the 1860s and 1870s established the germ theory of disease, which confirmed the need for better sanitation. Other urban planners took note of the radical renovation of Paris begun by Baron Georges Haussmann. Under Haussmann's direction, workers tore down the city's medieval fortress walls, widened its major streets into boulevards, and set aside land for green and pleasant parks. American cities had no ancient walls and fewer narrow roads, and since Americans were less tradition-bound, they were often more willing to rebuild and enlarge. Their innovations led Europeans to adopt horse-drawn streetcars and, later, electric trolleys. By establishing an intracity transportation network, the old "walking cities" were able to add suburbs, partially easing the crush of earlier industrial crowding.

As hubs of the new industrial networks, where immigrants and newcomers from the countryside flocked, cities needed efficient links to raw materials, as well as markets for their finished products. Much of the late nineteenth century can be seen as a scramble of Western nations for raw materials and markets. Miners combed the hills of California for gold in 1849, as they did two years later in Victoria, Australia. In South Africa, the rush was for diamonds discovered along the Vaal and Orange rivers and gold near present-day Johannesburg. In Canada, Australia, Argentina, and New Zealand, agriculture and stock-raising moved steadily toward larger, more commercialized operations. All of these enterprises extracted value from previously untapped natural resources, funneling commodities into the growing global network.

The end result of the scramble was the age of imperialism, as the European powers sought to dominate their newly acquired territories. The United States joined the rush somewhat late, in part because the nation had consumed so much of its energies extracting raw materials from its own "colonial" regions, the burgeoning West and the conquered South. Incorporating these two regions into a national industrial dominion raised unpleasant questions of power, just as imperialism itself did. European imperialists justified their rule over nonwhite races in Darwinian fashion, as the survival of the fittest. "The path of progress is strewn with the wreck . . . of inferior races," one English professor proclaimed in 1900. The British poet Rudyard Kipling even suggested that Europeans see themselves as making a noble sacrifice on behalf of their subject peoples. "Take up the White Man's Burden—," he exhorted them:

> Send forth the best ye breed—
> Go bind your sons to exile
> To serve your captives' need.

All too clearly, however, the needs being served were usually not those of the "captives." Imperialism certainly did not serve the needs of coolie laborers of Kipling's India, who died by the thousands clearing virgin jungles for tea plantations; or black miners in South Africa laboring for nearly slave wages; or Chinese workers in Australia and the United States, excluded and segregated after both gold rushes; or southern black sharecroppers, oppressed by a system of racism; or American Indians, driven off their lands by successive waves of prospectors, cowhands, and sodbusters.

The racist undercurrent of both European imperialism and American expansion was something most whites of the era ignored. But farmers in both the South and the West did lash out at industrial "robber barons" and railroad "monopolists," who seemed to epitomize the abuses of the new industrial order. The social strains arising out of these wrenching changes were reflected in the American political system, first in the Populist movement of the 1890s and then in the tide of progressivism that became prominent at the turn of the century. In Europe, too, industrializing nations responded to pressures for political reform, passing social legislation that included the first social security systems and health insurance.

Through imperialism, then, the modern industrial states spread their political dominion across the world, as migrants traveled in search of jobs and land, merchants sought new markets, industries explored and extracted raw materials, and nations established colonial regimes. The United States, too, joined this global order of commerce, political alliances, and rivalries—an order that finally collapsed with the coming of World War I.

CHRONOLOGY

AMERICAN EVENT	YEAR		GLOBAL EVENT
Commodore Perry visits Japan	1853		
	1859		Darwin's *On the Origin of Species* published
Transcontinental railroad completed	1869	GRANT	Suez Canal completed
Rockefeller founds Standard Oil	1870		Franco-Prussian War
			Britain produces half the world's pig iron
Bell invents telephone	1876		Refrigerated ships permit export of beef from Argentina
Battle of Little Bighorn			
Reconstruction ends	1877	HAYES	
	1880s		Pogroms against Russian Jews spur emigration
American Federation of Labor founded	1881	GARFIELD	
	1881	ARTHUR	
Twain's *Huckleberry Finn* published	1885	CLEVELAND	Berlin Conference concluded; European powers partition Africa
			Indian National Congress formed
	1888		Slavery abolished in Brazil
	1889	HARRISON	Germany enacts a social security system
			Japan establishes the Meiji Constitution
Sherman Antitrust Act	1890		
Three-year depression begins	1893	CLEVELAND	
Plessy v. Ferguson upholds segregation	1896		
First U.S. subway opens (Boston)	1897	MCKINLEY	
Spanish-American War	1898		Germany modernizes navy
Carnegie Steel produces more steel than all Great Britain	1900		Boxer Rebellion in China
			Freud's *Interpretation of Dreams* published
J. P. Morgan creates U.S. Steel	1901	ROOSEVELT	
	1904		Outbreak of Russo-Japanese War
			Social welfare legislation in France
	1905		Trans-Siberian railroad completed; revolution in Russia
			Einstein begins work on relativity
Sinclair's *The Jungle* published	1906		
U.S. troops intervene in Nicaragua	1909	TAFT	
	1910		Mexican Revolution begins
Armory Show, New York City, introduces modern art	1913	WILSON	
Panama Canal opened	1914		World War I begins
United States enters World War I	1917		Russian Revolution
Senate rejects Versailles Treaty	1919		Treaty of Versailles signed
Women's suffrage ratified (Nineteenth Amendment)	1920		
	1921	HARDING	

18

The Rise of a
New Industrial Order

It was so dark that Robert Ferguson could not see his own feet. Inching along the railroad tracks, he suddenly pitched forward and felt his breath taken away as the ground vanished beneath him. To his dismay, he found himself wedged between two railroad ties, legs dangling in the air. That was enough. Scrambling back to solid ground, he retreated along the tracks to the railroad car, where he sat meekly until dawn.

Ferguson, a Scotsman visiting America in 1866, had been in Memphis only two days earlier, ready to take the "Great Southern Mail Route" from the Mississippi River east some 850 miles to Washington. Things had gone badly from the start. About 50 miles down the track, a broken bridge at the Hatchie River forced him from the train and onto a ferry across the river. Bumping along another 10 miles in a mule-drawn truck, he arrived at Brownsville, Tennessee, where he was told the rail line did not resume for at least 40 miles, a distance impossible to travel in less than two days. Disheartened, he decided to return to Memphis and try another rail route.

The "excursion" to Memphis, due to leave the town of Big Hatchie at 10 a.m., arrived at four in the afternoon, six hours late. By seven Ferguson had traveled half of the 50-mile journey when the train suddenly stopped. It was dinnertime, not for the passengers but for the conductor, engineer, and stoker. The crew left the engine idling while they ate. Barely three hours later came another wrenching stop as the train derailed several miles outside of Memphis.

A few passengers decided to hike the remaining distance to Memphis, banding together for mutual protection against any toughs who might be lurking beyond the city's gaslights. Ferguson followed but lagged farther and farther behind in the darkness. It was then that he fell between the tracks and retreated to the safety of the railcar. At dawn he discovered how narrow his escape had been: just ahead, the tracks led out onto a high river bridge, consisting of nothing more than cross rails supported on trestles. Ferguson had trouble managing them even in daylight.

Before he finally reached Washington, Robert Ferguson traveled six days more, with connections between lines that took anywhere from a few hours to an entire evening. Meals were not served "on board," nor were there any sleeping

In a fiery display giant egg-shaped Bessemer converters remove carbon from molten iron ore to make steel at Andrew Carnegie's steelworks in Pittsburgh.

cars. Railside inns were primitive and usually crowded. "It was certainly what the Americans would call 'hard travelling,'" he snorted; "—they do not make use of the word 'rough,' because roughness may be expected as a natural condition in a new country."

Southern rail lines had been hit hard by the Civil War, but northern travelers encountered similar difficulties. Bridges across major rivers were scarce. One line would end, and passengers and freight would be forced to transfer to another because rail gauges—the width of the track—differed from line to line. Accommodations were still fairly primitive. The Reverend Newman Hall, visiting from England in 1867, rode his first "sleeping car" from Niagara to Chicago and was roused at six in the morning for a "wash-up" of "towels, soap, &c." To eat, he had to purchase apples from a boy roaming the aisles, who cheekily stopped to finger Newman's diamond stickpin.

A mere 20 years later, rail passengers traveled in relative luxury. T. S. Hudson, another British tourist, launched a self-proclaimed "Scamper Through America" in 1882. It took him just 60 days to go from England to San Francisco and back. He traveled across the entire continent on a ticket booked by a single agent in Boston. Such centralization would have been unthinkable in 1866 when, in any case, the transcontinental railroad was still three years from completion. Hudson's trains had Pullman Palace cars with luxurious sleeping accommodations and a breakfast menu offering coffee, tea, and iced milk; broiled meats (including "game in their season"); hot breads and rolls; eggs prepared in every imaginable style; fried bacon, sausage, oysters, and trout; relishes, vegetables, fruits, even chocolate—all for 75 cents. Newly installed air brakes made the trains he rode safer and their stops less jarring. Bridges appeared where none had been before, including a "magnificent" span over the Mississippi at St. Louis, with three arches of "five hundred feet each, approached by viaducts, and, on the western shore, also by a tunnel."

Hudson also found himself in the midst of a communications revolution. Traveling west across the plains, he was struck by the number of telephone poles along the route. Salt Lake City, to his surprise, had launched its own phone exchange. The problem remained of adjusting to local times, for each town still set its clocks by the sun. (New York and Boston, for example, were 11 minutes and 45 seconds apart.) By 1882, there were some 50 rail systems of time, no two identical. To aid passengers, stations often had several clocks showing the time on different lines along with one showing "local mean time." Had Hudson waited another year for his "scamper," the railroads would have reinvented time for him. In 1883, independently of any government or court, the railroad companies divided the country into four standard time zones, called "railroad time," to which cities and towns soon adjusted. Congress did not get around to making the four zones official until 1916.

What made America in the 1880s so different from the 1860s was a new industrial order. The process of industrialization had begun much earlier, at least three decades before the Civil War. Small factories had produced light consumer goods like clothing, boots and shoes, and furniture. They catered largely to local markets in what was predominantly an economy of farmers and merchants. After the 1850s the industrial economy matured and a new industrial order flowered. The transformation, remarkable as it was, brought not only progress but pain. In 1882, the year T. S. Hudson scampered comfortably across America, an average of 675 workers were killed on the job every week.

THE DEVELOPMENT OF INDUSTRIAL SYSTEMS

The new industrial order can be best understood as the emergence of a host of complex industrial systems that became woven into the fabric of everyday life. Look, for example, at the industrial systems required to build the bridge across the Mississippi that Hudson so admired. When James B. Eads constructed his soaring 515-foot arches in 1874, he needed steel, which was refined from iron ore most likely from the Mesabi range in Minnesota. At Mesabi, giant mechanized shovels scraped up the ore and in a few swings loaded an entire freight car. A transportation revolution, in the form of heavy-duty railroads, ore boats, and ore carriers, then moved the ore and other materials to a manufacturing center, perhaps near Pittsburgh, Pennsylvania. High-quality anthracite coal, probably from the mines of western Pennsylvania, fired the blast furnaces. The factory system—in this instance, a steel mill—provided the machinery and manpower to finish the steel. The costs of creating such a system—buying giant shovels, financing transportation, underwriting steel plants, hiring labor—ran into the millions of dollars. Investment banks and stock markets in New York and Chicago furnished the money. Not just laborers but a national network of industrial systems built the Eads bridge.

The industrializing of America after the Civil War is not the story of one but of many processes, all linked, all acting together to forge an industrial nation. Americans tied the country's natural resources into an interlocking system. They used technological innovations to streamline communication and transportation networks. They organized complex bureaucracies and coordinated workers through new techniques of management. They generated capital and dispersed ever

STEEL PRODUCTION, 1880 AND 1914

Millions of Tons

France   Russia   Great Britain   Germany   United States

☐ 1880   ▨ 1914

greater amounts of it. Without the entwining of such facilities there would have been no Eads bridge—and no industrial America.

Natural Resources and Industrial Technology

The earliest European settlers had waxed eloquent about the "merchantable commodities" of America, whether the glittering silver mines of the Spanish empire or the hardwood forests that stretched from New England halfway across the continent. What set the new industrial economy apart from that older America was the scale, range, and efficiency of exploiting resources. New industrial technologies, most of them developed initially in Europe, made possible the use of natural riches in ways undreamed of only decades earlier.

Iron, for example, had been made into steel for use in the blades of fine swords as far back as the Middle Ages. In the 1850s, however, Henry Bessemer in England and William Kelly in Kentucky independently discovered a way to convert iron into steel in large quantities. To heat iron ore the new "Bessemer process" required egg-shaped converters, some the size of small houses and capable of holding five tons of molten metal. At precisely the right moment and in exactly the right places, the converters blew drafts of hot air through the mixture to burn out the carbon that made iron brittle.

By the late 1870s, the Bessemer process had reduced the price of steel from $100 to $40 a ton. Steel quickly became the construction material of the age. For railroads, steel rails were lighter than iron, could support 20 times as much weight, and lasted 20 years instead of 3. Steel girders replaced the old cast iron frames of buildings, and steel cables supported new suspension bridges. By the 1870s, steel shovels, saws, and nails were common at construction sites.

Under the impact of industrial technology some worthless natural resources became valuable. Petroleum had once been little more than an annoyance—a smelly, thick liquid that bubbled to the surface of springs and was used occasionally as patent medicine. By the middle of the nineteenth century, distillation processes changed it into paraffin for making candles and sealing jars, oil for lubricating machinery, and kerosene for lighting lamps. Within a few years, chemists added to the list of petroleum products varnish, grease, polish, and paint.

Such innovation made oil into an even bigger business. Two subsequent events turned it into a major industry. In 1859, near Titusville, Pennsylvania, Edwin M. Drake drilled an oil well that tapped pools of petroleum below the surface. Then, in 1859, the Frenchman Etienne Lenoir constructed the first practical internal combustion engine. By the late 1870s, George Selden, a lawyer from Rochester, New York, had begun experimenting with gasoline-driven engines that powered road vehicles. In the twentieth century these "automobiles" would transform social and economic life in America and would help, along with vast natural reserves of petroleum, to make the American oil industry preeminent in the world.

The environmental price of industrial technology soon became all too evident. Loggers cut down the forests of the Pacific Northwest with a ruthless efficiency that threatened to destroy them. Mining scarred the land, and industrial wastes befouled lakes and rivers. At the turn of the century the Monongahela River, site of the huge Homestead steel mill, was so polluted local residents doubted that even microbes could survive in it. After a cloudburst trees around the mill were gray with soot.

Systematic Invention

The United States had always lagged behind Europe in basic scientific research, but for sheer inventiveness, the 40 years following the Civil War have rarely been matched in American history. Between 1790 and 1860, 36,000 patents had been registered with the government. Over the next three decades, the U.S. Patent Office granted more than 500,000; and in one year, 1897, the office issued over 21,000 patents, more than the total number recorded during the 1850s.

Even the process of invention became systematized. In the first half of the nineteenth century new inventions usually had come from practical tinkerers, operating by trial and error. While such lone operators continued to make important contributions, the process of industrialization required more orderly innovation. Small-scale inventors experimenting in machine shops were replaced by "invention factories"—highly capitalized research labs. Inventing became not only a system but also a business.

No one did more to bring system and order to invention than Thomas Alva Edison. Born in 1847, Edison spent his adolescence tinkering with electricity and telegraphs. At the age of 21, he went to work for a New York brokerage house and promptly improved the design of the company's stock tickers. With the $40,000 bonus he received, he set himself up as an independent inventor. For the next five years, Edison patented a new invention almost every five months. Before he was 30 he had come up with a "quadraplex" (he also invented the word) capable of sending four messages over a single telegraph wire, an electric voting machine, an "electric pen," a mimeograph, and a host of other marketable items.

Thomas Edison's unkempt hair, often matted with oil and dust, his wrinkled suit, and acid-stained hands belied his meticulous intellect and devotion to the dollar. "Anything that won't sell," he said, "I don't want to invent."

Edison was not content with unstructured tinkering. In 1876 he moved 15 of his workers to Menlo Park, New Jersey, where he created the first "scientific" factory, determined to turn out "minor" inventions every 10 days and "a big thing every six months or so." Like a manufacturer, he subdivided the work among gifted inventors, engineers, toolmakers, and others, including a mathematical physicist. An orderly bureaucracy evolved, and in 1878 it became a full-blown business—the Edison Electric Light Company.

Edison aimed at nothing less than bringing electricity into the homes of America. Before Edison's innovations, the only electric alternatives for lighting streets were arc lamps, which tended to short-circuit and were far too bright for use indoors. For Edison, the solution was not merely technical but social, which meant solving the problem of marketing and distribution as well. What was needed, he realized, was a unified electric system: a central power station to send out electric current; a network of wires to every home; thousands of small lights to illuminate households.

To launch his enterprise, Edison enlisted the backing of several major banking houses. When his system became practical in 1882, Edison shrewdly chose to illuminate the Wall Street financial district first. It looked, said a reporter, "like writing by daylight." Potential investors were impressed, and soon Edison power plants, organized by his private secretary Samuel Insull, sprang up everywhere. Correcting a critical mistake Edison had made, inventor George Westinghouse relied on high-voltage alternating current instead of Edison's low-voltage direct current, which could travel only a mile or two. He then installed transformers to reduce voltage back to low levels for household use. Despite initial skepticism over safety (for years "to Westinghouse" meant to electrocute), the improvements worked. By 1898 there were nearly 3000 power stations in America, lighting some 2 million bulbs.

Electricity was more flexible than earlier sources of energy. Factories no longer had to be built near rivers and falls to make use of their power. Before the end of the century, electricity was running automatic looms, trolley cars, subways, and factory machinery. Electricity not only revolutionized industry; it also worked in the homes of ordinary citizens. The electric motor, developed commercially by Westinghouse and Nikola Tesla in 1886, ran everything from sewing machines to phonographs.

George Eastman revolutionized photography by developing a system that substituted the ordinary consumer for the skilled professional. In 1879 he patented the "dry plate," which replaced the hundred pounds of chemicals photographers had to carry to take pictures. He spent the next several years trying to find a way to get his product to consumers. In 1888 he marketed the "Kodak" camera, a black box containing a strip of celluloid film. It weighed just over two pounds and cost $25. After 100 snaps of the shutter, the owner simply sent the camera back to the store or factory and waited for the developed photos, along with a reloaded camera, to return by mail. "You press the button—we do the rest" was Eastman Kodak's apt slogan. By the mid-1890s the company had done the rest so often that it was worth $8 million.

What united these innovations was the notion of rationalizing inventions—of making a systematic business out of them. The Westinghouse Electric Company

Thomas Edison's gramophone, patented in 1877.

and the General Electric Company both set up their own research labs, as did E. I. Du Pont de Nemours & Company (1911), the U.S. Rubber Company (1913), the Standard Oil Company of New Jersey (1919), and the Bell Telephone Company (1925). Researchers themselves formed professional organizations like the American Chemical Society. By the middle of the twentieth century, the research laboratory had spread beyond business to the federal government, universities, trade associations, even labor unions.

Transportation and Communication

Abundant resources and new inventions such as electric motors remained worthless to industry until they could be moved to processing plants, factories, and offices. But with over three and a half million square miles of land, the distance from resources to factories to markets, negligible in Europe, was huge in the United States. Where 100 miles of railroad track would suffice for hauling raw or finished materials in Germany and England, 1000 miles was necessary in America. Furthermore, railroads in Europe usually appropriated existing roads and horse tracks for their rail lines; in America the routes more often broke new ground, opening areas to settlement and exploitation.

An efficient internal transportation network tied the country into an emerging international system. Steam-powered ships, introduced before the Civil War, assumed greater importance in the 1870s, pushing barge traffic on American rivers and carrying passengers and goods across the oceans. Ever larger ships with more powerful engines cut the time of transatlantic travel in half, to about 10 days. Between 1870 and 1900, the value of American exports tripled. Eventually the rail and water transportation systems became entwined. By 1900 railroad companies owned nearly all of the country's domestic steamship lines.

Goods could be transported efficiently across large distances only with an effective communications network in place. First put into service in 1844, by the end of the Civil War the telegraph had 76,000 miles of line in the United States as well as a transatlantic cable. By the 1870s cables stretched underwater to Japan and China, and before the turn of the century they reached Africa and South America. In the United States the telegraph developed side by side with railroads, which allowed poles and wires to be set up along their rights of way in exchange for free telegraphic service. By the turn of the century a million miles of wire crisscrossed the continent, handling some 63 million messages a year.

A second innovation in communication, the telephone, vastly improved on the telegraph. Alexander Graham Bell, a Scot who emigrated to Boston in 1871, was teaching the deaf when he began experimenting with the electrical transmission of speech. Using pairs of telegraph instruments with receiving and transmitting reeds to get the right pitch, he and his young assistant, Thomas Watson, succeeded in sending a "twang" across the wires in 1875. Nine months later, on March 10, 1876, Bell's "telephone" finally transmitted the first intelligible words at their true pitch.

The telephone transformed communications. In 1878, when President Rutherford B. Hayes installed one in the White House, the instrument was still a curiosity. The same year, New Haven, Connecticut, opened the first telephone exchange in America. By 1895 there were 310,000 telephones in America; five years later there were 1.5 million. The telephone patent, issued in 1876, proved to be the most valuable ever granted. In the scramble for profits, the Bell Telephone

Daily Lives

TIME AND TRAVEL
The Rise of Information Systems

"Mr. Watson, come here. I want you." With those seven words, transmitted to his assistant on March 10, 1876, Alexander Graham Bell ended years of frustrating experimentation and ushered in the age of the telephone. At first Bell's electrical toys were purchased by individuals who wanted to connect two places, perhaps their home and business or their factory and office. Within a year, however, the advantages of such direct communication led to the first intercity hookup, between New York and Boston. Before the turn of the century, the Bell-organized American Telephone and Telegraph Company had combined over 100 local telephone companies to furnish business and government with long-distance service. When rates began to drop after 1900, telephones found their way into more and more American homes. The number of telephones installed jumped from 1,355,000 in 1900 to 10,535,000 in 1915 to 20,200,000 in 1930.

During the first half of the nineteenth century, information had traveled largely through the mails, which meant that it moved slowly. It took as many as 10 days for newspapers from New York to reach Indiana in 1841. In 1844 Samuel F. B. Morse succeeded in sending the first message across electrical wires, thereby achieving instantaneous communication. By 1860 telegraph wires stretched across the nation and replaced the fastest existing means of communication—the pony express.

The telegraph had obvious drawbacks. Instantaneous communication was by no means direct. Messages had to be taken to a telegraph office, where trained

Systems of finance and communication intersected at Wall Street, New York City, where the nation's most important investment banks and markets were located. In 1888 a snowstorm blanketed the district.

clerks could translate them into "Morse code," an unwieldy language of dots and dashes developed by the inventor for transmission by electrical impulse. When they arrived at the receiving station, messages were recast into comprehensible language, then carried by hand to their precise destination. This was a far cry from the telephone, which was both instantaneous *and* direct. Callers could speak to each other immediately and without the aid of intermediaries.

Daily Lives

The "speaking telegraph," as Bell called his invention, revolutionized communication, cutting time and obliterating distances. The telephone and a host of other innovations were the basis of the information system required of any thriving industrial nation. Information was a precious commodity, every bit as essential to the functioning of the economy as natural resources, finance capital, factories, and labor. The increased specialization at all stages of production, with raw materials from one area being processed in an urban industrial center and then distributed widely to other regions, required information about markets, prices, and supply sources—and required it quickly. Just as the rail system came to overshadow the earlier nineteenth-century steamboats and canal packets as efficient means of moving commodities, the telephone gradually superseded the telegraph as an efficient means of moving information.

Another such device that helped businesses to grow and prosper was the typewriter. C. Latham Sholes, a Milwaukee printer and editor, had been tinkering with an automatic numbering machine when a friend suggested he develop a mechanical letter-writing device. In 1868 he patented the "Type-Writer," and by the 1870s the Remington Arms Company was mass-producing them. Decorated with floral designs, these early machines rested on a sewing machine stand with a treadle that operated the carriage return. By the early twentieth century the typewriter had taken its modern shape—a keyboard with upper- and lower-case letters and a carriage that allowed typists to see the output.

At first typewriters were used mainly by writers, editors, ministers, and others from the world of letters. (Legend has it that Mark Twain's *The Adventures of Tom Sawyer* was the first book manuscript to be typed.) Impressed by the speed, uniformity, and legibility of typewriting, business executives began using the machines. Early critics charged that "machine-made" letters were too impersonal, and when farmers complained about receiving them, Sears, Roebuck hired secretaries to write their business letters by hand. Nevertheless, machine writing soon became standard business practice. As it did, the value of elegant and distinctive handwriting declined. Colleges of penmanship began to disappear, replaced by new vocational schools that taught shorthand and typing.

The need for speed and efficiency in the office led to other innovations. Carbon paper, designed for making a typewritten copy along with the original, was patented in 1872. In 1890 Alfred Dick invented the mimeograph to reproduce many copies of a single document cheaply, a communications boon not only to businesses but also to churches, reform organizations, and political groups. By the mid-twentieth century, as the processes of photography were applied to the problem of reproducing documents, xerography, or photocopying, would advance the communications revolution still further. And when photocopying was combined with telephonic and satellite technology in the late twentieth century, fax machines would enable senders to transmit over the phone facsimiles of documents instantaneously across the globe from business to business or home to home. Communications, like the rest of the new industrial order, were steadily becoming more rationalized and efficient, permitting the rapid distribution of information to those who needed or desired it.

Company fought off challenges from competitors and suits from rivals who claimed that their contributions were worth a share of the rights.

Along with typewriters (1867), ticker tape machines (1867), and adding machines (1888), telephones modernized offices and eased business transactions. In 1915, when the American Telephone and Telegraph Company opened the first transcontinental line, a business executive in New York could speak instantaneously to someone in San Francisco. The telephone was also part of a social revolution in America. Like the railroad and the telegraph, it compressed distances and homogenized the country. In time, remote households on farms and in villages would be connected to distant neighbors and to vital services offered by hospitals and fire departments.

Finance Capital

As industry grew, so did the demand for investment capital—the money spent on land, buildings, and machinery. The sheer scale of enterprise required more funds than ever before. In the 1870s an average iron and steel firm employed fewer than 100 workers to produce just under 4000 tons of material a year. The capital invested amounted to about $150,000. In 1900 the same firm employed four times as many workers, produced over ten times as much steel, and required almost $1 million. Not surprisingly, the amount of invested capital increased twelvefold over those years.

The need for capital was great especially because so many new industrial systems were being put into place at the same time. In the old days, a steamboat could be set afloat for the price of the boat itself. A railroad, on the other hand, had enormous start-up costs before it could even begin to run. Miles of track had to be laid, engines and cars bought, depots constructed, and so on. Similarly, electric utilities had to string wires, make light fixtures available, and build generating plants before they could function. In other words, an industrial process involving so many expensive systems could not take shape until someone raised money to build the systems.

Where did the money come from? For the first three-quarters of the nineteenth century investment capital came primarily out of the savings of the firms that used it. In the last half of the century "capital deepening"—a process essential for industrialization—took place. Simply put, as national wealth increased people began to save and invest more of their money. This meant that greater amounts of capital were available to companies seeking to start up or expand.

Savings and investment grew increasingly attractive with the development of a sophisticated network of financial institutions. Commercial and savings banks, investment houses, and insurance companies all gave savers increased opportunities to channel money to industry. The New York Stock Exchange, in existence since 1792, became the major conduit for connecting eager investors with money-hungry firms. By the end of the century it had established itself as the primary instrument for exchanging securities and making capital available to industry.

The Corporation

Finance, like natural resources, technology, transportation, and communication, was just one piece of the industrial mosaic. For those business leaders with the skill to put all the pieces together, large profits awaited. This was the era of the notorious "robber baron," and to be sure, sheer ruthlessness and a disregard of legal niceties went far in the fortune-building game. "Law? Who cares about law!" railroad magnate Cornelius Vanderbilt once bellowed. "Hain't I got the power?"

To survive in the long term, however, business leaders could not depend on ruthlessness alone. The growing scale of enterprise and the money required to run it led them to adapt an old device, the corporation, to new needs. Corporations had existed since colonial times, when governments granted charters of incorporation to organizations that ran such public facilities as turnpikes, canals, and banks. After the Civil War the modern corporation came into being as an instrument for mobilizing capital and protecting business holdings.

The corporation had several advantages over more traditional forms of ownership, such as the single proprietorship and the partnership. A corporation could raise large sums quickly by selling "stock certificates," or shares in the enterprise, to the public. It could also outlive its owners because it required no legal reorganization if one of them died. It limited liability because owners were not personally responsible for corporate debts. And it separated owners or stockholders from the actual running of the company, which permitted professional managers to operate complex businesses with unprecedented efficiency. So overwhelming were these advantages that even before the turn of the century, two-thirds of all manufactured products in the United States were made by corporations.

A Pool of Labor

Last, but hardly least important for the success of the new industrial order, was a pool of labor. All industrializing nations required workers, but in the United States demand was so great that the native population alone could not fill it. In 1860 it took about 4.3 million workers to run all the factories, mills, and shops in the United States. By 1900 there were approximately 20 million industrial workers in America.

Gas company employee in Chicago, 1891.

Europe was a primary recruiting ground. In the late nineteenth century poverty, oppression, and mechanization conspired to push Europeans from farms into cities and finally off the continent entirely. Meanwhile, economic opportunity pulled them to America. The Labor Contract Law, repealed in 1885, allowed prospective employers to recruit laborers abroad, pay their passage, then deduct the cost from their wages. Industrialists were among the most aggressive recruiters, advertising in newspapers, distributing pamphlets, and sending agents to Europe. When iron workers arrived in the United States from Sweden in the 1880s, they often knew only three words of English: "Charlie—Deere—Moline" (Charlie being the president of the John Deere Plow Company in Moline, Illinois).

An unprecedented wave of immigration flooded American shores. Over 8 million people arrived between 1870 and 1890, another 14 million by 1914. Eastern and southern Europe, where mechanized agriculture and religious persecution simultaneously took hold, replaced northern and western Europe as the chief sources of immigration. Most of the new arrivals settled in industrial cities. Often unskilled, many of them peasants, they went to work in factories and mines or on construction and road gangs. In at least 21 major manufacturing or mining industries two out of every three employees were new immigrants from eastern and southern Europe or African-Americans from the South.

To get those jobs they relied on well-defined networks of friends and relatives, together with a new breed of labor brokers. Tough and savvy immigrants themselves, these contractors met newcomers at the dock, promising work and serving as a funnel to the new world. For their trouble they took a healthy cut of the immigrants' wages and overcharged them for goods. Among Italians they were known as "*padrones*," and by the end of the nineteenth century they controlled two-thirds of the labor in New York.

Following such prescribed paths tended to concentrate one group or another within certain industries or at specific jobs. Poles, Slavs, and Italians began to fill the mines of Pennsylvania; Greeks worked in the textile mills of New England. In

OCCUPATIONAL DISTRIBUTION, 1880 AND 1920

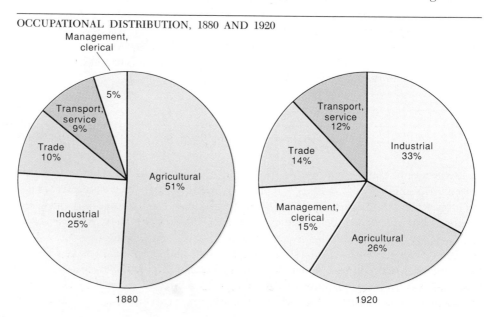

1880

1920

one Pittsburgh steel mill, Serbians clustered in the blooming mill, Poles in the hammer shop. Russian and Polish Jews, skilled tailors and seamstresses in the old country, went into needle trades of New York. But whatever they did, hard-pressed immigrants were willing to accept less pay and put in more hours than those they replaced. "Immigrants work for almost nothing," complained one native-born laborer, "and seem to be able to live on wind—something which I cannot do."

At the same time a massive migration of rural Americans—some 11 million between 1865 and 1920—provided a source of home-grown labor for industrial cities. Driven from the farm by machines and bad times or just following dreams of a new life, they moved first to small and then perhaps to larger cities. Unlike the vast majority of immigrants, they could often read and write English. At the very least they could speak the language and understand American ways. In iron and steel cities as well as coal-mining towns, they sometimes commanded better industrial jobs or served as supervisors and foreman. More often they lacked the skills for higher paying work. If they could get them, they found jobs instead in retail stores or offices and slowly entered the new urban middle class of white-collar workers.

Unless, of course, they were black. Most African-Americans continued to work the cotton fields of the South, but a small number, nearly 300,000, moved to northern cities between 1870 and 1910. Like the new immigrants, they sought to escape discrimination and find jobs. Unlike many of those immigrants, few blacks returned home. More often they stayed in the industrial cities and brought their families, one by one. They failed to escape discrimination but did find work—usually in low-paying jobs as day laborers and janitors or laundresses and domestic servants. By 1890 only 7 percent of all black men worked in industry.

The development of an industrial labor force extracted high human costs. The daily work rhythms of a European peasant, a black field hand, and a midwestern farmer were quite different from the 12-hour shifts of a Pittsburgh steelworker or a woman plucking tobacco from cigarette-rolling machines in North Carolina. Monotonous, alienating, and difficult, such work was as dangerous as it was dehumanizing. In the last third of the nineteenth century the United States had the highest rate of industrial accidents in the world, another component in the emerging industrial order. Labor would pay dearly for economic progress.

RAILROADS: AMERICA'S FIRST BIG BUSINESS

At the center of the new industrial systems were the railroads, helping to spread communications networks, efficiently moving freight, reinventing time. Steel rails even redefined the geography of America. Unlike canals, which ran only between bodies of water, railroads could move goods and raw materials wherever track was laid. Under their impact the commercial axis of the nation shifted from New York and New Orleans, with its heavy reliance on river and coastal shipping, to New York and Chicago. Railroads also stimulated economic growth, simply because they required so many resources to get things built. By the 1850s they furnished the largest single market in the country for iron and devoured large quantities of coal, wood, felt, glass, rubber, and brass. In the 1880s, three-fourths of all the steel made in the United States went into rails. By lowering transportation costs railroads allowed manufacturers to reduce prices and thereby attract more buyers. To control their far-flung operations, they pioneered new techniques of management, soon adapted to the needs of other business.

In time the railroad became a cultural symbol of American might, energy, and foresight. The poet Walt Whitman called the locomotive the "emblem of motion and power—pulse of the continent." Those who drove them, like the 6-foot, 4-inch John Luther "Casey" Jones (who really did drive the Cannonball Express between Memphis and Canton, Illinois), became folk heroes. Everyone along the New York-to-Chicago route knew that the New York Central and the Pennsylvania were making the run in 27 hours. Whole towns turned out to greet an incoming train, and the most impressive building in any hamlet was likely to be not a church or the city hall or the municipal court, but the railroad depot.

A Managerial Revolution

To the men who ran them, railroads were primarily businesses, and the railroad business was growing so fast that new ways of organizing and financing it were essential. With operations extending over hundreds of miles, railroad lines had to construct and maintain an immense inventory of engines, cars, tracks, shops, terminals, stations, warehouses, office buildings, bridges, and even telegraph lines. In the 1850s, one of the largest industrial enterprises in America, the Pepperell textile mills of Maine, employed no more than 800 workers. By the early 1880s the Pennsylvania Railroad had nearly 50,000 people on its payroll. Railroads serviced untold numbers of customers, and the facilities of any one line would take literally weeks to see. Each day managers had to make countless decisions involving the delivery of freight and the safety of passengers. From setting rates to determining costs and profits, everything required a level of coordination unknown in earlier businesses.

To achieve it, railroads found themselves forced to develop new systems of management. Here the so-called "trunk lines" were innovators. Scores of early companies had serviced local networks of cities and communities, often with less than 50 miles of track. During the 1850s four great trunk lines emerged east of the Mississippi to connect the shorter branch, or "feeder," lines. By the outbreak of the Civil War, the Erie, the Baltimore and Ohio, the Pennsylvania, and the New York Central all furnished roads under a single management that linked the eastern seaboard with the Great Lakes and western rivers. After the war, the South and West organized their own trunk lines, largely with capital from Europe and the North.

Simply keeping track of the money was a major task, since conductors, station agents, freight agents, and scores of other employees were involved in paying out or collecting cash. To supervise and account for the funds, the Baltimore and Ohio separated the management of finances from all activities involving the movement of trains. Accounting was handled by a special section called the controller's office, working directly with another new financial section, the treasurer's office. The treasurer watched over and helped allocate revenue raised by the sale of securities and from profits. Both offices came under the jurisdiction of a new vice president, whose sole duty was to oversee finances.

The operations of large lines spawned a business bureaucracy staffed by a new style of business executive. Typically these bureaucrats were not entrepreneurs who started or owned businesses but a class of managers, subordinate to owners but having wide authority over daily operations. By the first two decades of the twentieth century nearly a third of the prominent business executives born between 1861 and 1880 had climbed the bureaucratic ladder. A hundred years earlier, only 5 percent had reached the top by working through their organizations. Cautious by nature, this managerial elite preferred to negotiate and administer rather than compete.

Daniel McCallum, a talented engineer and inventor, was the prototype. As general superintendent of the New York and Erie in the 1850s, he drew up the first table of organization for an American company—a tree with roots representing the president and board of directors, five branches comprising the main operating divisions, and leaves standing for the local agents, train crews, and others. Information moved up and down the chain of command so that managers could get daily reports to and from the separate parts. Even within small units like the machine shop, hierarchy prevailed. The duties of each grade were carefully prescribed, and every employee wore an insignia on his uniform for easy identification of both grade and job.

Soon railroads were dividing their operations, giving local superintendents the power to move passengers and freight, while the "central office" concentrated on the broader problems of cost, competition, and expansion, based on information from the field. By the turn of the century, the railroads had led a managerial revolution in American industry. Central offices operated as corporate nerve centers, housing functional divisions responsible for purchases, production, transportation, sales, and accounting. A new class of "middle managers" ran them and imposed new order. What was going on, in other words, was a process of economic rationalization of business practices. Executives, managers, and laborers were being taught to work in increasingly precise and coordinated ways.

Competition and Consolidation

While managers made operations more systematic, the struggle among entrepreneurs to achieve dominance in the railroad industry was at times anything but precise and rational. In the 1870s and 1880s, competition to attract profitable business reached fierce proportions.

More than any other contemporary enterprise, railroads were saddled with enormous "fixed costs"—expensive equipment, huge payrolls, high debts. These remained constant regardless of the volume of traffic. To generate more revenue, railroads constructed more lines in hopes of increasing their traffic. Soon the railroads had overbuilt. (Recall that Robert Ferguson could choose from more than one line running from Memphis to Nashville.) With so much excess capacity, railroad owners schemed desperately to win new accounts. They gave free passes to favored shippers, promised them free sidings constructed at their plants, offered free land to bring businesses and traffic to their territory.

Nothing worked better than manipulating prices. Managers lowered rates for freight that was shipped in bulk, on long hauls, or on return routes (since the empty cars were coming back anyway). When those tactics failed, they used "rebates," secret kickbacks to preferred customers, which dropped prices below the posted rates of competitors. Losses were recouped by overcharging small shippers like farmers. Such competition could prove fatal to some railroads. When the economy plunged, or if a weak line sought to improve its position, savage rate wars broke out. In the shakeout caused by the depression of 1873, some 40 percent of all railroad bonds went into default; 65 lines declared bankruptcy by 1879.

One way to prevent the ravages of competition was to consolidate: buy up competing lines. But that could lead to even fiercer war. From 1866 to 1868 Cornelius Vanderbilt of the New York Central waged a futile battle to gain control of the Erie, headed by a trio of railroad sharks: the corporate buccaneer Daniel Drew, the flamboyant speculator James Fisk, Jr., and the subtle, calculating, and utterly unscrupulous Jay Gould (a "perfect eel," according to one railroad president). They fought Vanderbilt in the courts, where each side brought its own attorneys and bought its own judges. They fought him in the legislature, where both sides bribed legislators to vote their way. (The going rate, it was said, was $15,000 apiece.) They fought on the streets with gangs of hired toughs. They even patrolled the seas with Fisk serving as admiral of a Hudson River flotilla armed with riflemen.

Eventually the "Erie Wars" ended in a standoff. The Erie paid Vanderbilt a huge ransom; Gould and Drew retained effective control of the company until they turned against each other. By 1877, the Erie was bankrupt, mismanaged and drowned in a sea of "watered stock" (stock issued in excess of the company's true assets). Gould emerged unscathed. When he died of tuberculosis at the age of 56 in 1892, his estate totaled $74 million.

The strategies of consolidation developed by railroad managers were more productive. During the 1870s a number of regional railroad federations were created to pool traffic among their members and divide the profits equitably. Pooling was designed to remove the incentive for cutting rates. Without the force of law, however, these associations failed to control competition. In the end the rail wars subsided only when the strongest lines bought up their competitors.

In the East purchases, leases, and mergers accomplished the task. In the West new construction produced self-contained systems like the Atchison, Topeka and Santa Fe. By 1890 that rail line stretched from Chicago to the Pacific coast and operated over 9000 miles of track. But in the depression of 1893, it too went bankrupt, the victim of management's overambitious vision. Railroad executives learned a lesson: although they had gained some control through consolidation, they had also overexpanded. By the mid-1890s, a third of the mileage of American railroads was tied up in foreclosure or bankruptcy proceedings.

The Role of Finance

In the early days many railroads had relied on state governments for financial aid. When the depression of the late 1830s and early 1840s turned states stingy, promoters looked to counties, cities, and towns for bonds and other commitments. In the 1850s and 1860s western promoters went to Washington seeking federal assistance. Congress responded with loans of $65 million to six western railroads and lavish grants of land that totaled more than 131 million acres. Even so, federal support helped to build only about 8 percent of the nation's railroads.

So executives developed new ways of raising capital from private investors. At first people living near the ends of the rail lines, who stood to gain more from construction, received stock in exchange for their land or their labor. Investors in Europe or in eastern cities had more money, and promoters soon tapped them by offering bonds, the preferred instrument of nearly all American railroads for rais-

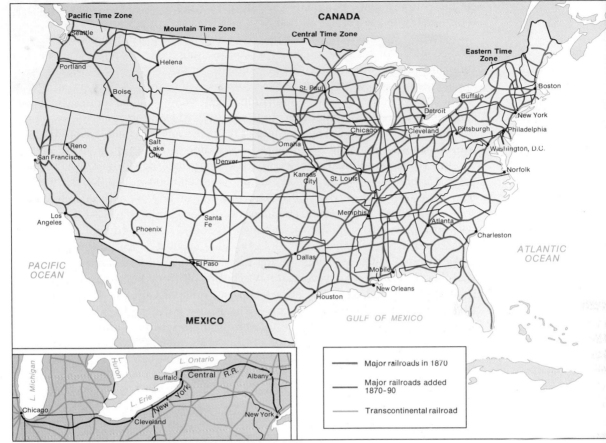

RAILROADS, 1870–1890

On the eve of the Civil War there were 31,000 miles of track in America, most of it east of the Mississippi. By the end of the century, the railroad network stretched from one end of the country to the other, with more miles of track than in all of Europe combined, including Russia. New York and Chicago, linked by the New York Central trunk line, became the new axis of commerce in America.

ing capital. These interest-bearing certificates promised regular payments to investors and involved no ownership of the line.

Beginning around 1850, the financial needs of railroads outreached the capacities of local banks and stock exchanges. The New York Stock Exchange, already growing, expanded even more rapidly as the securities of railroad corporations began to be listed and traded there. Over the same period, investment banking houses developed financial networks through which they found and distributed capital. The banks were soon marketing railroad and other industrial securities abroad as well as in the United States. As late as 1898 Europeans owned nearly a third of all American railroad securities. At home, life insurance companies became a prominent source of capital. Organized in the 1840s, when reliable mortality tables were first drawn up, the companies blossomed during the 1870s by introducing innovative group and industrial insurance contracts. By the turn of the century life insurance companies had over $1.5 billion to invest, and a third of their assets went into railroad bonds.

Because investment bankers played such prominent roles in controlling the flow of funds, they found themselves advising railroads about their affairs. If a company fell into bankruptcy, bankers sometimes served as the "receivers," who oversaw the property until the firm returned to financial health. By absorbing smaller lines into larger ones, eliminating rebates, and stabilizing rates, the bankers helped to reduce competition. In the process, they often came to control the companies they advised. Their system of financing not only underwrote the network of transportation; it also imposed new order and centralization.

By 1900, the application of industrial systems had transformed the railroads. With a capital investment of $11 billion, some 200,000 miles of track were in operation, with six groups of railroads owning over 80 percent of those miles. Time zones allowed for coordinated schedules on a national level; standard track gauges permitted easy cross-country freighting. Passengers were traveling 16 billion miles every year. To that total could be added wheat, corn, and hogs, which moved from the Great Plains, cotton and tobacco from Mississippi and North Carolina, lumber from Oregon and Wisconsin, oil from Pennsylvania, and coal from West Virginia to the great factories and mills of Chicago, Pittsburgh, and Birmingham. Finished products made the return trips, and everything moved with a predictable regularity that allowed businesses to plan and prosper.

THE GROWTH OF BIG BUSINESS

The process of system building continued to spread through other industries. Although most entrepreneurs still functioned on a small scale, many businesses grew big. Like the railroads, they adopted several operating strategies. Combination—a loose alliance of enterprises under a large national organization—helped to coordinate operations over vast distances. And consolidation—blending separate companies into one corporation—actually integrated operations under a single corporate headquarters and permitted unprecedented control.

These giant industrial organizations were put together in a number of ways. Some firms grew horizontally by absorbing several competitors engaged in the same activity. For other companies the issue was assuring access to raw materials and markets. These firms grew vertically, acquiring the successive stages needed to make and sell a product. Some combined the two strategies, spreading vertically up toward consumers and down toward raw materials as well as horizontally outward over competitors. By the end of the century, innovative instruments of control—the trust and the holding company—pumped big business to remarkable proportions. The overall aim was to create an environment that provided managers with greater predictability and more influence over materials and markets. In the process business leaders reorganized the economy, concentrated power, and laid the foundations of a modern business system.

Growth in Consumer Goods

By the 1860s salt producers in Michigan were locked in deadly competition. Salt processing and other industries that specialized in consumer products for ordinary home use had low start-up costs, so they often were beset by stiff competition. In Michigan the presence of too many salt makers had sent prices plummeting. Seeing salvation in combination, they drew together (like the railroads) in an informal pool, the Michigan Salt Association, in 1869. They voluntarily agreed to allocate production, divide markets, and set prices—at double the previous rate. Horizontal combination saved them. By the 1880s there was a whiskey pool, a cordage pool, and countless rail and other pools. Informal pools ultimately proved to be unenforceable and unsatisfactory (and after 1890 they were considered illegal restraints on trade), but other forms of horizontal growth, such as formal mergers, spread in the wake of an economic panic in the 1890s.

Some entrepreneurs, like Gustavus Swift, adopted a vertical growth strategy and ended up integrating several different activities under one company. Swift, a New England butcher, moved to Chicago in the mid-1870s. Aware of the demand for fresh beef in the East, he acquired new refrigerated railcars to ship meat from western slaughterhouses and a network of ice-cooled warehouses in eastern cities to hold the meat. By 1885 he had created the first national meat-packing company. Swift moved forward, even closer to consumers, by putting together a fleet of wagons to distribute his beef to retail butchers. He moved back toward his own raw materials, extending and coordinating the purchase of cattle at the Chicago stockyards. He built plants to make chemicals, fertilizers, and other by-products. By the 1890s the Swift Company was a fully integrated, vertically organized corporation operating on a nationwide scale. Other meat packers followed, and soon Swift, Armour and Company, and 3 other giants—together called the "Big Five"—controlled 90 percent of the beef shipped across state lines.

Carnegie Integrates Steel

Industrialization encouraged integration in heavy industry as well. Here Andrew Carnegie led the way. More than any of his contemporaries, Carnegie's life was entwined with the industrial revolution. His father, a hand weaver in Scotland, had been thrown out of work by machines. When the family emigrated to Allegheny, Pennsylvania, in 1848, 12-year-old Andrew found his first jobs in industry—as a bobbin boy in a textile mill and later as a machine wiper deep in the cellar of a factory. For the rest of his days, the scent of machine oil made him ill.

When the telegraph came to Pittsburgh, Carnegie became a messenger boy, then a skilled operator whose talent and hard work drew the attention of Thomas Scott, a local superintendent of the Pennsylvania Railroad. Scott needed a personal telegrapher and secretary; Carnegie got the job. Over the next 12 years, as Scott rose (ultimately to become president of the railroad), Carnegie followed along. In 1859, at the age of 24, he was appointed superintendent of the Pennsylvania's western division.

Under Scott's shrewd tutelage, Carnegie learned how to manage a railroad and how to make money from money. Through attention to detail, resourcefulness, initiative, and quick action, he made things work. When wrecked freight cars blocked service, Carnegie coolly ordered them burned. His colleagues swallowed hard, but the procedure soon became standard practice for the Pennsylvania Railroad. With a tip and a loan from Scott, Carnegie profited from investments in the first sleeping car, the first iron railroad bridge, a locomotive factory, and finally a local iron factory that became the nucleus of his steel empire.

In 1872, on a trip to sell railroad bonds in England, Carnegie chanced to see the Bessemer process in action. Awe-struck by the fiery display, he jumped aboard the first steamer home and announced his intention to build the biggest steel mill in the world. In 1875 he did, in the midst of a severe depression. Over the next 25 years, he added mills at Homestead and Keystone, Pennsylvania, moved from railroad building to city building, and won a contract for supplying steel for the Brooklyn Bridge in 1876. His structural steel went into New York City's elevated railway, the frames of early skyscrapers, and the Washington Monument.

Carnegie succeeded, in part, by taking advantage of the boom-and-bust business cycle of the late nineteenth century. He jumped in during hard times, building and buying when equipment and businesses came cheap. He also had a knack for finding skilled managers, like Henry Clay Frick and Charles M. Schwab, who employed the administrative techniques pioneered on the railroads. Carnegie set managers against each other in races to quicken the pace of production. The winners received handsome bonuses, the losers embarrassing telegrams: "Puppy dog Number Two has beaten puppy dog Number One on fuel." Competition was also Carnegie's way of dealing with rival steelmakers. To undercut contenders, he would scrap new machinery, a new mill, even his own workers for the sake of efficiency and low costs. A beneficent federal government helped too. The federal decision to build an all-steel navy in the mid-1880s furnished added demand for his product, while protective tariffs helped to keep British steel from the American market.

The final key to Carnegie's success was expansion and still more expansion: horizontally, by purchasing and constructing more and larger steel mills; and vertically, by buying up sources of supply, transportation, and sales. Beneath the Thomson, Homestead, and Keystone mills lay a supporting network of industries: giant furnaces for making pig iron and giant ovens for making coke; 40,000 acres of coal land; fleets of railway cars and ore-carrying steamers; a shipping company; a docking company; and nearly two-thirds of the Mesabi iron ore range. Controlling such an integrated system, Carnegie could assure a steady flow of materials from mine to mill and market as well as profitable investments at every stage along the way. In 1900 his company turned out more steel than Great Britain and made $40 million dollars in profits.

Integration of the kind Carnegie employed expressed the logic of the new industrial age. More and more, the industrial activities of society were being linked in one giant, interconnected process.

Rockefeller and the Great Standard Oil Trust

John D. Rockefeller accomplished in oil what Carnegie achieved in steel. And he went further, developing an innovative business structure—the trust—that promised even greater power. Rockefeller was as taciturn and cold as Carnegie was warm and charming. While Carnegie looked on religion with skepticism, Rockefeller was a devout believer who taught Bible classes at Cleveland's Erie Street Church. "God gave me my money," he once remarked. More earthly powers shaped his approach to business. In the rough-and-tumble commercial world of the late nineteenth century, his father had been an able tutor. "I cheat my boys

John D. Rockefeller.

every time I get a chance," the elder Rockefeller once explained. "I want to make them sharp."

In John's case, he succeeded beyond his wildest imaginings. After a stint of bookkeeping in commission houses, the young Rockefeller entered the refining business in 1862. Cleveland was just emerging as a commercial center on the shores of Lake Erie, owing to its location near one of the early oil fields and to the competition of railroads for its trade. By 1870 Rockefeller and his partners controlled nearly a fifth of all the city's refining facilities.

In 1870 Rockefeller and his associates incorporated their business as the Standard Oil Company (Ohio), looking for even greater gains. Unlike the competitive Carnegie, Rockefeller put his faith in combination, achieved through alliances, "voluntary" associations, and cooperation. But oil refining, like steelmaking, was a jungle of competitive firms, so Rockefeller proceeded to twist arms. In the name of higher cooperation, he used bribery, spying, railroad rebates, phony companies, and price-slashing to eliminate rivals or persuade them to join him. When necessary he undersold them with high-quality products. He moved horizontally to gain control of refining, succeeding so well that by 1880, a decade after Standard Oil had incorporated, he headed an alliance of companies that together commanded 90 percent of the nation's oil refining capacity. Rockefeller also grew vertically all the way back to drilling for oil and forward into selling its products.

How could he maintain and control such an empire? Through the 1870s Rockefeller relied on informal pools and other business combinations. Because they had no legal standing, they proved too weak. Corporations, though legal entities, were restricted by state law. In Ohio, where Rockefeller operated, corporations were forbidden from owning plants in other states or stock in out-of-state companies. Another device was called for, and Samuel C. T. Dodd, an ingenious lawyer who became chief counsel of Standard Oil, came up with one in 1879. The "trust," as Dodd conceived it, was a quasi-legal arrangement under which a corporation's stockholders surrendered their shares "in trust" to a central board of nine directors. The directors could "hold, control, and manage" all property. In exchange, stockholders received certificates of trust that paid dividends (a handsome 30 to 48 percent in the case of Standard Oil).

In 1882 the Standard Oil Company of Ohio formed the country's first great trust. For six years, until a New York state investigation unmasked it, the arrangement was kept secret. Since no one was any the wiser, Rockefeller and his associates could testify with straight faces that they had "harmonized" the industry rather than conspired to restrain it. Secret or not, the trust brought Rockefeller what he had so relentlessly sought—centralized management of the oil industry. The Standard Oil Trust, worked out over the next several years, included 14 companies and controlled 26 more.

Trusts surmounted the legal barriers states had erected to regulate corporations, and immediately the form was copied by businesses that dealt in copper, sugar, cottonseed oil, rubber, leather, and farm machinery. Just as quickly, trusts developed unsavory reputations for extortion and monopoly. In time most people came to regard any large combination of capital as a trust, whether it was a formal voting trust (like Standard Oil) or a looser affiliation of giant companies (like the "Big Five" Beef Trust). The average citizen, one observer noted sarcastically, was born to profit the milk trust and died to profit the coffin trust. In practice, no trust was a true monopoly that completely controlled an entire industry. Trusts generally were "oligopolies" in which a few large firms dominated an industry.

The Mergers of J. Pierpont Morgan

The voting trust was only a steppingstone to an even more effective means of avoiding competition, managing people, and controlling business: the corporate merger. The idea of two companies merging—one company buying out another—remained impractical until 1889, when New Jersey became the first of several states to permit corporations to own other companies. The following year, the need to find a substitute for the trust increased when that arrangement was outlawed by Congress under the Sherman Antitrust Act of 1890. So the ever-inventive Samuel Dodd came up with the "holding company," a corporation of corporations that had the power to hold shares of other companies. Many industries converted their trust arrangements into holding companies, and in 1899 Dodd created the Standard Oil Company of New Jersey, an immense holding company for Rockefeller's oil empire.

Two years later came the biggest corporate merger of the era, the creation not of a lawyer but of a financial wizard named J. Pierpont Morgan. After the Civil War Morgan had become head of the powerful investment house that bore his father's name. Born rich, he made the House of Morgan richer still by buying, holding, and merging companies. For 50 years after the Civil War Morgan had a hand in reorganizing almost every important American enterprise: railroads, coal, steel, steamships, electricity. His orderly mind abhorred chaotic competition, especially when it threatened the profitability of his investments. "I like a little competition," he was quoted as saying, "but I like combination more." Between 1892 and 1902 he was instrumental in creating such massive consolidations as General Electric, American Telephone and Telegraph, and International Harvester.

Morgan's greatest triumph was in steel, where for years Carnegie had refused to combine with his rivals. In January 1901, with the threat of a colossal steel war looming, Morgan convinced Carnegie to put a price tag on his company. When a messenger brought the scrawled reply back—over $400 million—Morgan merely nodded and said, "I accept this price." Within three months he had bought Carnegie's eight largest competitors and announced the formation of the United States Steel Corporation.

A mammoth holding company, U.S. Steel embraced every aspect of steelmaking from ore beds to finishing plants. It gobbled up over 200 manufacturing and transportation companies, 1000 miles of railways, and the whole Mesabi iron range. It employed over 170,000 workers and controlled 60 percent of America's steel capacity. U.S. Steel was the largest industrial combine the world had ever seen and America's first billion-dollar corporation. Capitalized at $1.4 billion, its value was greater than the national debt. All the same, it was a bloated giant with far too many costs ever to realize Morgan's dream of high profits.

What Morgan helped to create in steel was rapidly coming to pass in other industries. A wave of mergers swept through American business in the wake of the depression of 1893. As the economy plunged, cutthroat competition bled businesses until they were eager to sell out. Over 1200 companies "disappeared" in mergers in 1899 alone. Within industries, giants grew almost overnight. By 1904 a single firm came to account for 60 percent or more of the total output in each of 50 different industries. The economic results were mixed. Bigness helped to bring down prices. Economies of scale—the reduced cost of each item that resulted from the production of many—lowered prices and increased profits. Consolidation also eliminated the perils of cutthroat competition, which demoralized business leaders and threatened the benefits of industrialization. Yet the merger movement never succeeded in wholly ending competition. The market shares of the giants steadily declined as smaller and more aggressive firms stole business and as new companies entered the industry. Still, the big firms were there to stay.

Corporate Critics

Many Americans were not pleased about the development of corporate giants. Industrialization and the growth of big business might have helped to rationalize the economy, increase national wealth, and tie the country together, but they also exploited workers, concentrated power, corrupted politics, and widened the gap between rich and poor. According to the census of 1890, the richest 9 percent of the people held nearly three-quarters of all wealth in America. By the turn of the century, one American in eight (nearly 10 million people) lived below the poverty line.

In truth, the concentration of wealth was not much different from what it had been in 1850. What had changed was the rise of a visible new class of millionaires. They lived ostentatiously, and much of the country hated them for it. Two Vanderbilt mansions on New York's Fifth Avenue alone cost a total of $14 million. The family owned seven altogether, in addition to several country estates. The anger of ordinary people sometimes boiled over. When the kidnapper of Eddie Cudahy, the son of a prominent member of the beef trust, confessed to the crime, the jury acquitted him all the same.

New York's wealthy called their elaborate summer homes "cottages," but they were mansions by any standard. The Breakers, designed by Richard Morris Hunt for Cornelius Vanderbilt II, looks like an Italian palace and has this grand music room among its 70 rooms. Now open to the public, the mansion cost $5 million to build.

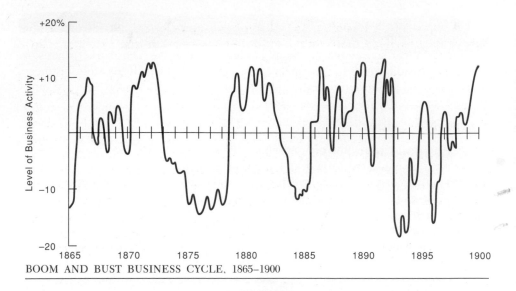

BOOM AND BUST BUSINESS CYCLE, 1865–1900

Industrialization also subjected the national economy to enormous disruptions. The banking system could not always keep pace with the demand for capital, and businesses failed to distribute enough of their profits to workers to sustain purchasing power. Supply often outstripped demand. A vicious cycle of boom and bust developed. Three severe depressions—1873–1879, 1882–1885, and 1893–1897—ravaged the country in the last third of the nineteenth century. With hard times came fierce competition as companies struggled to survive, collapsed, or were bought at bargain prices. Faced with shrinking markets, managers worked harder to cut costs, and the industrial barons earned their reputations for ruthlessness.

Corporate apologists justified the system by applying Charles Darwin's new theories of evolution to society at large. Distorting Darwin, British philosopher Herbert Spencer maintained that in society, as in biology, only the "fittest" survived. How prosperously they survived reflected how fit they truly were. His American apostle, William Graham Sumner, defended property and privilege by arguing that competition was natural and had to proceed without any restraints, including government regulation. Millionaires, in his view, were simply the "product of natural selection." Such "Social Darwinism" found ready adherents among businessmen, who applauded their own survival in the business jungle even as they worked to reduce the very competition they extolled.

For all the contemporary celebrations of wealth and big business, many Americans longed for a more promising future. A group of radical social prophets offered one by mounting a powerful attack on corporate capitalism. Henry George, a journalist and self-taught economist, advanced an arresting scheme to redistribute wealth in *Progress and Poverty* (1879). It became one of the best-selling books ever published in America. Trying to explain how poverty could continue when industrial progress had created great wealth, George pointed to greedy landowners who held their property until labor, technology, and speculation on nearby sites raised the price. He called the profit thereby reaped an "unearned increment." He proposed a "single tax" on all such property to bring an end to monopoly landholding and eliminate all other taxes. "Single-tax" clubs sprang up throughout the country, and with the support of labor, George nearly won the race for mayor of New York in 1886.

Edward Bellamy, a journalist turned novelist, tapped the same vein of popular resentment with his utopian novel *Looking Backward* (1888). The hero, a Boston millionaire, falls asleep in 1887 and awakens Rip Van Winkle–like in the year 2000. His competitive, caste-ridden society is gone. In its place he finds an orderly utopia, managed in military fashion by a vast, government-controlled trust. Cruel exploitation, class divisions, political corruption, and disparities in wealth have vanished. Instead abundance is shared equally, and "fraternal cooperation" has replaced competition. Bellamy called it "nationalism," and the idea soon spawned more than 160 clubs in 27 states. His followers called for redistribution of wealth, civil service reform, and nationalization of railroads and utilities.

Less popular but equally hostile to competitive capitalism was the Socialist Labor party, formed in 1877. Dominated for many years by Daniel De Leon, a West Indian immigrant, it advocated revolution through class conflict and worker control over the means of production. De Leon's unyielding emphasis on purity of theory attracted more intellectuals than workers. The Socialist Labor party found some adherents in the ethnic communities of the great industrial cities but never polled more than 82,000 votes. Party members, bent on gaining popular and trade union support, revolted and in 1901 founded the more successful Socialist Party of America. Here and elsewhere workers were beginning to organize their own responses to industrialism.

WORKERS RESPOND TO AN INDUSTRIAL CULTURE

The new systems of industrialization, far-reaching as they were, could hardly fail to shape the lives of ordinary workers. It was they who struggled most to adjust to the new industrial order and they who sought to bring the large processes within their control.

The vast steel mills, the cramped tenement sweatshops, the dank tunnels of the coal fields—all demanded workers, whether "greenhorns" from abroad, "hay seeds" from the countryside, children, adults, blacks, whites, Mexicans, or Asians. Furthermore, the new industrial systems required people to work in new and foreign ways. Farmers or peasants, accustomed to timing themselves by the daily position of the sun, now learned to live by the clock and work in the twilight of gaslit factories. Instead of being self-employed or paid by a boss whom they knew and could bargain with, industrial workers had to deal with foremen, were paid by the hour or the piece, and had the pace of their work set by relentless cycles of machines. Increasingly they bore the brunt of depressions, faced periodic unemployment, worked under dangerous conditions, and lived in substandard housing.

The Workers' World

By 1880 the number of nonagricultural laborers had risen above the number of farm workers for the first time in American history. Five million Americans toiled in manufacturing, construction, and transportation—more than three times the number employed a generation earlier. Though small shops could still be found at the end of the century, industrial work had grown big and harsh.

In 1881, for example, when the Pittsburgh Bessemer Steel Company opened its new mill in Homestead, Pennsylvania, nearly 400 men and boys went to work on its 60 acres of sheds. To keep the mill going 24 hours a day, they worked every day but Christmas and the Fourth of July, 12 hours a day one week, 12 hours a night the next, except for the weekly "swing shift." Then the Saturday night crew took Sunday off, and the Sunday swing worked 24 hours straight. In the furnace room, ovens and huge pits ("gaping like the mouth of hell," wrote novelist Hamlin Garland) emitted terrible heat that quickly exhausted men who tended them. The incessant vibration of machinery and the screeching of cold saws rang in the ears of workers, making some of them deaf. Shiny grains of steel covered their clothing and coated their lungs. There were no breaks of any kind, not even for lunch, and no shower rooms. "Home is just the place where I eat and sleep," one steelworker said. "I live in the mills."

Few industrial laborers had it quite so bad. Less than 1 percent of all jobs were in iron and steel mills in 1880. Still, Homestead reflected a common pattern of industrial work: mechanization and mass production, the dictatorship of the clock, subdivision of labor, intricate organization, and brutal conditions. By the turn of the century, most of those earning wages in industry worked 6 days a week, 10 hours a day. They held jobs that increasingly required more machines and fewer skills. Repetition of small tasks replaced fine craftsmanship. In the 1880s, for example, almost all the 40 different jobs that went into making a pair of shoes could be performed by a "green hand" with a few days of instruction at a simple machine.

New high-speed machines also brought danger to the workplace. If a worker succumbed to boredom, fatigue, or simple miscalculation, disaster could strike. Each year of the late nineteenth century some 35,000 wage earners were killed by industrial accidents. In Pittsburgh iron and steel mills alone, in one year 195 men died from hot metal explosions, asphyxiation, and falls, some into pits of molten metal. Men and women working in textile mills were poisoned by the thick dust and fibers in the air; similar toxic atmospheres injured those working in anything from twine-making plants to embroidery factories. Railways, with their heavy equipment and unaccustomed speed, were especially dangerous. In Philadelphia over half the railroad workers who died between 1886 and 1890 were killed by accidents. For injury or death, workers and their families could expect no payment from employers, since the idea of worker's compensation was unknown.

Industrial workers almost never saw an owner. The foreman exercised complete authority over the unskilled in his section, hiring and firing them and even setting their wages. A worker with a complaint, an industrialist observed, "stood just about as much chance to get in to see any one . . . as he would to get into the Kingdom of Heaven." Skilled workers had much greater freedom; yet in time even they yielded to technology and organization. Carpenters found that machine-made doors were replacing the ones they had before constructed at the site, while painters no longer mixed their own paints. More and more, labor became a commodity and workers cogs in a vast industrial machine. "I regard my people," one manager stated, "as I regard my machinery. So long as they can do my work for what I choose to pay them, I keep them, getting out of them all I can."

Higher productivity was the aim. It received a powerful boost from Frederick

W. Taylor, who revolutionized working conditions in the steel industry. Taylor was obsessed with efficiency. As a boy, he had invented the overhand pitch to deliver a baseball with new speed and precision. In steel plants during the 1870s and 1880s, he undertook careful time-and-motion studies of workers' movements, set up standard procedures, and offered pay incentives to those who surpassed his production quotas. In a famous application of his theories, he designed 15 ore shovels, each for a separate task to be performed in a specific way, so that 140 men were able to do what had previously required a crew of 600. The company cut its costs in half, and the remaining shovelers got a raise. By the early twentieth century "Taylorism" had become a full-blown philosophy, complete with its own professional society. "Management engineers" prescribed routines from which workers could not vary. Work itself was thus separated from the planning of work, and labor was managed as yet another part of an integrated system.

For all the high ideals of Taylorism, ordinary workers refused to perform as simple cogs. Many European immigrants, accustomed to celebrating numerous saints' holidays, continued to take those days off, regardless of factory work rules. (The Greek Orthodox church had more than 80 festivals a year, while Polish weddings lasted as long as five days.) When the pressure of six-day weeks became too stifling, workers took an unauthorized "blue Monday" off. Often they simply walked off the job, took another "greenhorn" opening in another industry, or packed up and moved to a new city. Come spring and warm weather, the turnover in factories rose significantly, just as it decreased in the fall. At the turn of the century, factories reported turnover rates of more than 100 percent in the course of a year. That meant that the Armour meat-packing plant in Chicago, for example, had to hire 8000 new workers in 1914 just to stay fully staffed.

Workers who stayed on the job earned low wages. Before 1900, an unskilled laborer could expect between $1.25 and $1.50 for 10 hours of work, a skilled one perhaps twice that amount. It took about $600 to make ends meet, but most manufacturing workers made just under $500 a year. Native white Americans tended to earn more than immigrants, those who spoke English more than those who did not, men more than women, and all others more than African-Americans and Asians. By 1900, some 1.7 million children worked in factories and fields, more than double the number 30 years earlier. On average, their paychecks were three times smaller than those of adult males. Parents often had no choice but to send their children to work. As one union leader observed of coal miners, "Absolute necessity compels the father in many instances to take the child into the mine to assist him in winning bread for the family."

Women worked outside the home too. Farm women had always labored on the family homestead, but by 1870 one out of every four nonagricultural workers was female. In general they earned one-quarter of what men did. Nearly all were single and young, anywhere from their mid-teens to their mid-twenties. Most lived in boarding houses or at home with their parents, where they usually contributed their wages to the family kitty. Once married, they took on a life of full-time housework and child rearing.

Only 5 percent of married women held paying jobs in 1900. That figure can be misleading, since home-bound women who needed money earned it by increasing their housework with extra laundry or sewing or by taking in boarders. And industrialization inevitably pushed women out of the traditional domestic women's sphere and into new jobs. The census of 1890 listed 369 occupations in America. Women worked in all but nine. Mainly they had jobs considered exten-

Clerks' jobs, traditionally held by men, increasingly came to be filled by women as inventions like the typewriter and telephone created new opportunities for office work.

sions of housework: food processing, textiles and millinery, and cigar making. By far the largest number of jobs available to women were in clothes manufacturing and domestic service. New methods of management and marketing opened new avenues of employment for some women as "typewriters," "telephone girls," bookkeepers, and secretaries. On rare occasions they entered the professions, though law and medical school administrators continued to see them as unworthy invaders. Instead, ambitious, educated women became nurses, librarians, and teachers. Their presence effectively "feminized" these pursuits, making them women's work and driving men upward into managerial slots or out of these occupations entirely.

African-Americans, even more than women, faced discrimination in the workplace. Paid less than whites and relegated to the most menial employment, blacks found their greatest opportunities in industry as "scabs" to replace striking white workers. Once a strike ended, they were themselves replaced—and hated by whites all the more. The service trades furnished the largest single source of jobs, though black craftsmen and a sprinkling of professionals could usually be found in cities. The pattern of black employment in Washington, D.C., was typical. In 1870 the population of the nation's capital included 410 black waiters, 133 black carpenters, and one black lawyer. Most single black women in the South worked for wages as laundresses and domestic servants. If married, they were five times more likely than married white women to work outside their homes.

Whatever their separate experiences, American workers did improve their lot, at least in the aggregate. Though the gap between rich and poor widened, ordinary laborers, with the exception of African-Americans, made measurable gains. Wages rose, prices fell, and the number of hours on the job declined. Not that workers rose from "rags to riches." Few could expect to repeat the experience of an Andrew Carnegie. But for most there was a chance to rise. About one-quarter of the manual laborers in one study entered the middle class in their own lifetimes. And most workers believed in the American dream of success, even if they did not fully share in it.

The Systems of Labor: Early Unions

Working longer to save a few pennies, walking off the job in exhaustion or disgust, taking in boarders—these were the ways most workers coped with the new systems of industrial America. Yet such responses were the actions of individuals against the complex structures being set in place around them. For ordinary workers to have any effect on the process of industrialization they had to combine, just as businesses had. They needed to integrate horizontally—which for workers meant organizing not just locally but on a national scale. And they needed to integrate vertically: to coordinate their actions along a wide range of jobs and skills, just as Andrew Carnegie coordinated the production of steel, all the way from the iron ranges of Minnesota to the delivery of finished steel girders. For workers, labor unions were their systematic response to industrialization.

In the United States the earliest unions had been formed before the Civil War among such craftsmen as iron molders, machinists, printers, and cigar makers. Railroad "brotherhoods" had also appeared, more in an effort to furnish insurance for those hurt or killed on the job than to exert economic leverage on bosses. Such organizations remained local, exclusively male, and weakened by small membership and divided power. Once in a while a nationwide craft organization such as the National Typographic Union emerged, but on the eve of the Civil War only six national unions existed in the whole country.

After the war, a group of craft unions, brotherhoods, and reformers banded together as the National Labor Union (NLU). Although national in scope, the goals of the organization looked backward. Using the language of abolitionism, the NLU called for an end to "wage-slavery" and spoke longingly of a mythic, simpler past when workers employed themselves. It vigorously opposed anything, including strikes, that encouraged members to think of themselves as a working class. By the early 1870s, the NLU claimed over half a million members, but it faded quickly once the depression of 1873 set in.

The Knights of Labor

Similarly nostalgic and visionary but much more successful was a national union born in secrecy, amid elaborate ritual. This was the Noble and Holy Order of the Knights of Labor. Founded by Uriah Stephens and a group of Philadelphia garment workers in 1869, the Knights remained small and fraternal for a decade. Their strongly Protestant tone repelled Catholics, who made up almost half the work force in many industries. Then in 1879, as the 1873 depression waned, the Knights elected Terence V. Powderly their Grand Master Workman. Handsome, dynamic, Irish, and Catholic, Powderly threw off the Knights' secrecy, dropped their religious rituals, and opened their ranks. He called for "one big union" that would embrace the "toiling millions"—skilled and unskilled, men and women, natives and immigrants, all religions and all races. Within half a dozen years, membership rose from 10,000 to 100,000; by 1886, it reached nearly 730,000.

Like the NLU, the Knights saw workers as producers, denied by monopoly and special privilege "the full enjoyment of the wealth they create." Nothing short of a radical reordering of society would do. "The aim of the Knights of Labor—properly understood—is to make each man his own employer," said Powderly. He hated the word "class," shunned labor violence, and urged harmony. His would be a cooperative economy of mines, factories, and railroads, owned and operated by workers. They would pool their resources and share their profits.

The Knights knew that such a radical vision might take years to realize. In the interim they set up over 140 cooperative workshops, sponsored political candidates in 200 cities and towns, and pressed for short-term reform. Their platform advocated the eight-hour workday, regulation of trusts, the prohibition of child and convict labor, and the abolition of liquor. They were, in fact, prescribing not only an economic system but also a social plan, guided by Christian moralism. Only when citizens put aside greed, sloth, and dishonesty, they argued, would class divisions and corruption fade away.

It was one thing to proclaim a united national organization but another to coordinate the activities of so many members. Powderly disapproved of strikes, but soon found his local members engaged in quite a few of them. During the mid-1880s, when such stoppages wrung concessions from the western railroads, the Knights attracted thousands of new recruits. But the organization soon became associated with unsuccessful strikes and violent extremists. And the gains against the railroads were wiped out when Jay Gould and his Texas and Pacific Railroad broke the locals striking against it. By 1890, the Knights of Labor teetered on the edge of extinction.

The American Federation of Labor

The Knights' position as the premier union in the nation was usurped by the rival American Federation of Labor (AFL). The AFL reflected the practicality of its leader, Samuel Gompers. Born in a London tenement, the son of a Jewish cigar maker, he had emigrated in 1863 with his family to New York's Lower East Side. Gompers had little use for Terence Powderly's radical vision of a cooperative commonwealth. Pragmatic and conservative, he accepted capitalism and the wage system. In his view, workers were "a distinct and practically permanent class." So he sought to organize those with the most leverage—craftsmen. Above all, Gompers wanted results: higher wages, fewer hours, improved safety, increased benefits. By bargaining with employers and using strikes or boycotts when necessary, his "pure and simple unionism" was designed to win better conditions for those with skills.

Using the Cigar Makers' Union as his base, Gompers helped found the first national federation of craft unions in 1881. In December 1886, when it was reorganized as the American Federation of Labor, 25 labor groups joined, representing some 150,000 mostly skilled laborers. It was labor's answer to the corporation and trust: a consolidated organization for controlling resources (in this case labor) and competition (for jobs). From 1886 until his death in 1924, Gompers fought off socialists, allied himself with whichever major party supported labor, stressed gradual, concrete gains, and transformed the AFL into the most powerful amalgamation of trade unions in the country. By 1901 it had over a million members, almost a third of all skilled workers in America.

Gompers was less interested in vertical integration: combining skilled and unskilled workers. For most of his career, he preserved the prerogatives of crafts-men and acceded to their prejudices against women, blacks, and immigrants. Only two locals—the Cigar Makers' Union and the Typographers' Union—accepted women, and most affiliates restricted black membership through high entrance fees, technical examinations, and other discriminatory practices.

Despite the success of the AFL, the laboring classes did not organize them-selves as systematically as the barons of industrial America. Union membership never included more than 2 percent of the whole labor force and less than 10 percent of all industrial workers. Skewed by different languages and nationalities, deeply divided over race and gender, raised to value self-reliance, working men and women resisted unionization during the nineteenth century. In fact, workers often regarded such collective activities as alien, subversive, and un-American.

The Limits of Industrial Systems

As managers sought to increase their control over the workplace, workers often found themselves at the mercy of the new industrial order. Few could count on full-time employment, even when the economy was booming. One out of every three workers could expect to be out of work for at least three or four months a year. Changes in markets and weather brought seasonal unemployment, New machines that replaced old human skills led to structural or technological unem-ployment. And regular tailspins in the economy—on average one every five or six years—brought cyclical unemployment. In such hard times the industrial system was driven to its limits, and workers bore the brunt of it. Managers sped up work to increase labor productivity, insisted on longer hours, laid off hundreds, and cut wages.

When a man's pay dropped and his anger and frustration rose, when his wife began working all night to make ends meet and fell asleep during the day while taking care of her children, when food prices suddenly jumped—violence might well erupt. "A mob of 1,000 people, with women in the lead, marched through the Jewish quarter of Williamsburg last evening," wrote the New York *Times* in 1902, "and wrecked half a dozen butcher shops. Men and women who were seen coming out of the shops with meat and chickens in their hands were attacked. In the throng of women leaders of the mob there were many who carried bottles of kerosene oil."

Workers' strikes served more often than mobs as an outlet for protest. Most strikes broke out spontaneously, organized by informal leaders in a factory. "Mal-vina Fourtune and her brother Henry Fourtune it was them who started the strike," confessed a company informer in Chicopee, Massachusetts. "They go from house to house and tells the people to keep up the strike." Nor were strikes limited to the years of depression. Thousands of rallies and strikes were staged on behalf of the eight-hour workday, in good times as well as bad, by union and nonunion workers alike.

In 1877 Americans received an early view of labor troubles to come. When the Baltimore and Ohio Railroad cut wages by 20 percent, a crew in Martinsburg, West Virginia, seized the local depot and refused to let the trains move. The spontaneous strike spread to other eastern lines and then west to California until two-thirds of the nation's tracks were shut down. As strikebreakers came in, railyard after railyard went up in flames. Local police, state militia, and federal troops, sometimes fighting pitched battles with mobs supporting strikers, finally

Labor strikes, some of them bloody, plagued the late nineteenth century. Most involved working conditions rather than wages. Here labor and management confront each other directly. One striker reaches for a stone while an anxious mother looks on.

restored order after 12 days. The first nationwide strike in American history left 100 people dead and $10 million worth of railroad property in rubble. "This may be the beginning of a great civil war in this country, between labor and capital," read one newspaper editorial. In the face of violence, middle- and upper-class Americans came to fear the "Sampson-like strength" of labor.

Strikes became epidemic in the late nineteenth century. Between 1880 and 1900, some 6.6 million workers staged over 23,000 strikes. In 1886 alone, a record 610,000 workers were out of jobs as a result of strikes, lockouts, and shutdowns. The most violent episode of that year started innocently enough, at a rally at Haymarket Square in Chicago. Anarchists were protesting the brutality of police who had earlier killed two workers during a lockout at the McCormick Harvester Company. The turnout—around 3000—was disappointingly low, the speeches long-winded, the crowd placid and bored. As rain drenched the gathering, police moved into the square and ordered everyone to disperse. Moments later a bomb exploded, instantly killing one officer and mortally wounding six others. The police opened fire, and the crowd fired back. In addition to the 7 policemen who died, 70 more were injured. At least four civilians were killed and uncounted numbers hurt.

Conservatives charged that organized labor had encouraged the violence and anarchy of the "Haymarket Massacre." Even though the identity of the bomb thrower was never established, the courts found eight anarchists guilty of conspiracy to murder. Four were hanged, one committed suicide, and three later were pardoned by Governor John P. Altgeld. Even ordinary citizens called for action against radicals in laborers' clothing. Cities enlarged their police forces and states built more National Guard armories on the borders of working-class neighborhoods.

During the troubled 1890s federal and state governments firmly sided with business. In 1892, in the remote Coeur d'Alene district of Idaho, striking silver miners and company guards fought a guerrilla war until federal troops quashed the strike. In July of that year the Amalgamated Iron and Steel Workers, a powerful AFL affiliate, struck the Homestead steel mill after Carnegie's managing partner, Henry Clay Frick, cut wages by 20 percent and refused to improve working conditions. Determined to destroy the union, Frick imported 300 Pinkerton detectives to drive off picketing workers. The hired thugs arriving by barge under cover of darkness were suddenly engaged in a furious gun battle and beaten savagely as they marched to the main gate. When the melee ended, 10 strikers and 3 Pinkertons lay dead. Within days the governor had called out 8000 state militia; on July 15 the mill reopened under military guard. "I will never recognize the Union, never, never!" Frick insisted. By mid-November he had replaced most of the workers, broken the strike, and crippled the union for decades.

A broader confrontation between labor and capital took place just two years later. George Pullman, inventor of the plush Palace Car and owner of the company that built it, was a benevolent despot. He was determined to ensure efficiency on the job by controlling the lives of his workers. In the 1880s he built for his 5000 workers a model town south of Chicago on the shores of Lake Calumet. Pullman was a clean and pretty town, free of alcohol but never free from discontent. In addition to difficult working conditions, residents resented Pullman's relentless control over this compulsory heaven. "We are born in a Pullman house," one of them complained, "fed from the Pullman shop, taught in the Pullman school, catechized in the Pullman church, and when we die, we shall be buried in the Pullman cemetery and go to the Pullman hell."

As the depression of 1893 deepened, Pullman laid off workers, cut wages five times in one year, and refused to reduce the high rents charged for company houses. In 1894 frustrated workers struck. They managed to convince Eugene V. Debs' American Railway Union to support them by boycotting all trains that used Pullman cars. The General Managers Association, an organization of 24 midwestern railroads, appealed to President Grover Cleveland for federal help. On the slim pretext that the strike obstructed delivery of the United States mail (strikers had actually been willing to handle mail trains so long as they contained no Pullman cars), Cleveland secured an injunction halting the strike and ordered several thousand special deputies into Chicago to enforce it. In the rioting and looting that followed, 12 people died and scores were arrested. Debs and other union leaders were eventually sent to jail for defying the injunction. After his release, a bitter Debs became the foremost socialist leader in America.

At Pullman and in other labor disputes the central question, whatever the public issues, was power. Employers always enjoyed the advantage. They hired and fired workers, set the terms of employment, and controlled the workplace. To most of them, unions were a curse they fought to destroy with a formidable arsenal. "Yellow dog" contracts forced workers to forswear union membership. "Black-lists" circulated the names of labor agitators. Lockouts kept protesting workers from plants, and labor spies infiltrated their organizations. Workers were paid with "scrip," company money redeemable only at company stores charging inflated prices. With abundant migrant and immigrant labor, employers could replace strikers and so break their strikes. "I can hire one half the working class to kill the other half," Jay Gould once remarked.

When strikes spread, the government aided management not only with troops but also with powerful new legal weapons. The injunction had been used with devastating effect in the Pullman strike to stop workers from interfering with their employer's business. When the Supreme Court upheld Debs' sentence in *In re Debs* (1895), it legalized the federal injunction against the railway strikers. As the Court saw it, the strike hindered interstate commerce, an action deemed illegal under the Sherman Antitrust Act. The Sherman Act, intended to control monopolies, was thereby turned against labor. By the end of the century employers had weathered the protests of workers and emerged as masters of the mightiest industrial economy on earth.

The new industrial order was hard won, and its benefits were unevenly apportioned. The exploitative power of business grew as the number of those in control shrank. The gulf between the rich and the poor, always present, became more apparent. Laborers found themselves with fatter pay checks but less independence and satisfaction from their jobs. Yet the overall gain for the American economy was undeniable. On average, real wages rose for laborers, and Samuel Gompers agreed that "the social conditions of the working people have improved very materially within the past 35 years." At the end of the Civil War the United States had been fourth in the world in industrial production. By the mid-1890s the value of American manufactured goods nearly totaled those of France, Britain, and Germany combined, and by 1900 America ranked first among all industrial nations.

Whether rich or poor, worker, entrepreneur, or industrial baron, Americans were linked by new industrial systems, drawn closer to one another than ever before. Ore scooped from Mesabi might end up in a steel girder on James Eads' Mississippi bridge or in a steel pin bought by a California housewife or in a McCormick reaper slicing across the Nebraska plains. When a textile worker in Massachusetts struck, a family in Alabama might well pay more for clothes. A man in Cleveland now set his watch to agree with the time of a man in New York and vice versa, regardless of the sun. Such changes might seem effortless to someone like T. S. Hudson, scampering across the rails of America in 1882. But as the nineteenth century drew to a close, material progress seemed to go hand in hand with social upheaval. Americans had not yet adjusted to either.

SIGNIFICANT EVENTS

1859 — First oil well drilled near Titusville, Pennsylvania

1866 — Transatlantic cable links United States and Great Britain; National Labor Union founded

1868 — Philip Armour opens meat-packing factory in Chicago

1869 — Knights of Labor created

1870 — John D. Rockefeller incorporates Standard Oil Company of Ohio

1872 — George Westinghouse perfects air brakes; Crédit Mobilier scandal

1873 — Cable cars first used (in San Francisco); E. Remington and Sons begins making typewriters; Carnegie Steel Company founded; Panic of 1873

1874 — Massachusetts enacts first ten-hour workday law for women

1876 — Alexander Graham Bell invents telephone

1877 — Railroad wage cuts lead to violent strikes; Thomas Edison invents phonograph

1879 — Edison develops the incandescent light bulb; Henry George's *Progress and Poverty* published

1882 — Rockefeller's Standard Oil Company becomes the nation's first trust; Thomas Edison's electric company begins lighting New York City

1883 — Railroads establish standard time zones

1886 — American Federation of Labor organized; Haymarket Square bombing

1891 — Edison's motion picture camera patented

1892 — Homestead Steel strike

1893 — Panic of 1893

1894 — Pullman strike

1901 — U.S. Steel Corporation becomes the nation's first billion-dollar company

19

The Rise of an Urban Order

raziano's bootblack stand in the old County Court House off Foley Square was jammed with people. Almost everybody needed a shine, but practically nobody had come to get one. They were there to see George Washington Plunkitt, ward boss of Manhattan's Fifteenth Assembly district. Plunkitt sat above the din like an Irish king, dispensing favors and philosophy to loyal constituents. His crown was a top hat, his throne a chair perched atop the unassuming stand. On the wall behind him hung his coat of arms—crossed American flags cradling photographs of other party leaders. Doing whatever he could to help his people, he asked nothing in return except their votes on election day.

As one of the powers of Tammany Hall, the Democratic party organization that dominated New York City politics from 1850 to 1930, Plunkitt knew how to get those votes. On one typical day a bartender from his district woke him at two in the morning to bail a fellow saloonkeeper out of jail. Plunkitt didn't get back to sleep until after three, only to be roused by fire engines at six. He rushed to the fire to help burned-out tenants find food, clothing, and shelter at a nearby hotel.

After squeezing in breakfast, he visited the police court and secured the release of four drunken constituents "by a timely word with the judge." Half an hour later, at the Municipal Court, he directed one of his district captains to act as counsel for a widow in an eviction case and paid the rent of a poor family about to be dispossessed. As he left he handed the father a dollar for food. By eleven he was home again, where four men awaited him in search of jobs. It took him three hours, but he found work for all of them.

With barely enough time to eat lunch, he rushed to two funerals—one Italian over by the ferry, and one Jewish and closer to home. At both rites he stood conspicuously in front of the houses of worship to make certain he was seen. Then he dashed to a "Hebrew confirmation" at a local synagogue. By seven in the evening he was at district headquarters presiding over a meeting of his election captains. Each reported on the voters in his district: their attitudes toward Tammany, their needs and troubles, and the "best way to reach them."

The business of "the organization" thus cared for, Plunkitt went to a church fair at eight. He bought chances on everything, treated the children to ice cream,

Theodore Groll captures Washington Street, Indianapolis, at dusk in this detail from a painting done in the 1890s. The trolley cars are still horse-drawn (not electrified), but the telephone pole gives proof of the new urban era at hand.

kissed the little ones, flattered the mothers, and took the fathers around the corner for a quick drink. Then it was back to the clubhouse, where he promised some constituents a subscription for a new church bell. He bought tickets for an excursion of parishioners and a baseball game between two teams in his district. Before leaving, he told two dozen pushcart peddlers he would visit the precinct station in the morning to register their complaints of police harassment. He arrived at a Jewish wedding reception at half past ten (having already sent the bride "a handsome wedding present") and finally got to bed at midnight.

Such relentless exertion helped to make Plunkitt a fortune. Born to Irish immigrant parents in a shantytown called "Nanny Goat Hill" on Manhattan's Upper West Side, he died a millionaire in 1924 at the age of 82. His pluck and practicality would have made him the envy of the most successful industrialists. Like the Carnegies and Rockefellers, his rise from butcher boy to political boss was fueled by fierce ambition. City politics was his way out of the slums in a world that otherwise favored the rich, the educated, and the well established.

In the late nineteenth century the needs of rapidly growing cities and the people who lived in them gave political bosses like George Washington Plunkitt their chance. "I seen my opportunities and I took 'em," Plunkitt used to say. Every city building contract, every tax assessment, municipal bond issue, and rental on city property, every franchise and charter for a new business offered Plunkitt and his cronies an opportunity for lining their pockets with kickbacks, payoffs, and profits made from inside knowledge of city projects. This was "boodle," or honest graft (not to be confused with "black" graft, which came from vice and extortion). In Plunkitt's world boodle was the just reward for public service that normally paid so little.

How much boodle bosses collected depended on how successfully their organization controlled municipal politics. Control, in turn, hinged on electing the right officials, or as Plunkitt would have said, "turning out the vote." In the end, this whole system hung on the personal loyalty of bosses to immigrants and immigrants to bosses. That explains why Plunkitt spent so much time catering to his constituents. "When a poor man comes . . . for help," said one city boss, "we don't make one of those damned fool investigations like these city charities. No, by God, we fill his belly and warm his back and vote him our way."

Plunkitt's New York was the first great city in history to be ruled by men of the people in an organized and continuing fashion. Bosses and their henchmen came from the streets and saloons, the slums and tenements, the firehouses and funeral homes. More remarkable still, their families had only recently arrived in America. Usually bosses were immigrants or their children. Most remarkable of all, other great cities were ruled by them too. While the Irish of Tammany Hall ran New York, Germans governed in St. Louis, Scandinavians in Minneapolis, and Jews in San Francisco. In the late nineteenth century, the golden door of opportunity opened onto the city.

THE RISE OF CITIES

The modern city was the product of industrialization. The vast systems of communication and transportation, of manufacturing, marketing, and finance, of labor and management converged in the industrial city. Cities contained the great investment banks, the smoky mills and dingy sweatshops, the spreading railroad yards, the tenements and mansions, the new department stores and skyscrapers. They drew people like magnets from places as far away as Lincoln, Nebraska, and Minsk in Russia. By the end of the nineteenth century industrial cities had come of age. America—once an agrarian republic—was becoming urban, with tens of millions of "urbanites," an urban landscape, and a growing urban culture.

The Urban Explosion

"We cannot all live in cities," reformer Horace Greeley lamented just after the Civil War, "yet nearly all seemed determined to do so. . . . 'Hot and cold water,' baker's bread, gas, the theater, and the streetcars . . . indicate the tendency of modern taste." The city had all the household conveniences, temples of entertainment, and newfangled transports imaginable—and more: the best stores, the best restaurants, the best schools, the best newspapers, and virtually every museum, library, art gallery, bookshop, and orchestra. The city housed the delights of the age and most of the opportunity. Promising wages high enough to buy this good life, cities beckoned native-born Americans and a generation of immigrants to realize their dreams of success.

During the 50 years after the Civil War, world population rose by about 50 percent. The population of the United States quadrupled—from 23 million to 92

Realist painters like George Bellows, scorned by their critics as the "Ashcan School," captured the grittiness and vibrancy of teeming cities. Here Bellows evokes the cliff-dwelling ancestors of the Pueblo Indians with a turn-of-the-century scene of urban life. Like all his work, *Cliff Dwellers* makes dramatic use of light and dark, relying heavily on line, mass, and color to achieve naturalism.

million. Yet the number of people living in American cities increased nearly sevenfold. The census of 1870 defined a city as containing 8000 people or more. Ten years earlier, only one American in six qualified as a city dweller; in 1870 one in four did; in 1900, one in three. By 1910 nearly half the nation was urban.

Densely populated Europe and Asia boasted only a few cities of a million or more. In America giants sprouted overnight. Chicago (which rose from a swamp) had only 30,000 people in 1850, but it approached the million mark by 1890, making it the fastest growing metropolis in the world. So confident were city fathers of continued expansion that they laid new streetcar lines far into open cornfields. Just two American cities contained populations of over 500,000 at the outbreak of the Civil War. There were six when the century turned. Three—New York, Chicago, and Philadelphia—had more than a million each.

Cities grew in every region of the country, some faster than others. The Northeast and upper Midwest, where industrialization took hold earliest, were far more urban than the West and the South, although big cities could be found in those regions as well. Atlanta and Nashville (later Louisville, Memphis, Dallas, and Houston) boomed under the influence of railroads. In Birmingham, a steel town founded in Alabama in 1871, one early resident recalled that "property changed hands four or five times a day" during the real estate craze of the 1880s. Los Angeles had barely 6000 people in 1870. By 1900 it was the second largest city on the Pacific coast with a population of 100,000 and a set of nearby "satellite" towns, including Azusa (named, said its founders, "from A to Z in the USA!").

Size alone does not make a modern city. Without efficient ways of moving people and tying diverse functions together, without the means to control resources and capital, no settlement, however large, can perform as an organic, integrated unit, the mark of a modern metropolis. In the United States, the dynamic instruments of industry and commerce, along with striking advances in urban technology, helped to transform swelling towns into modern metropolises. Some cities became famous for their main product: Milwaukee for beer, Tulsa for oil, Houston for railroad cars, and Hershey, Pennsylvania, for chocolate. The giants continued to diversify. New York, the nation's banker, printer, and commercial center, also produced clothing and cigars. Chicago became the leading butcher, packer, and granary and by 1870 began to move into steelmaking.

The Great Global Migration

In the nineteenth century the world was moving to town. By some estimates 60 million people left farms and villages for cities between 1820 and 1920. Everywhere in Europe the forces of change pushed people off the land. After the mid-1820s and the end of the destructive Napoleonic Wars a cycle of baby booms continued at 20-year intervals for the rest of the century. Improved diet and sanitation, abetted by Louis Pasteur's pathbreaking discovery that bacteria cause infection and disease, reduced deaths. The population of Europe doubled between 1750 and 1850. Meanwhile the use of machinery enhanced productivity but cut the need for agricultural labor. In 1896 it took one man in a wheat field to do the work 18 had done just 60 years earlier.

Surplus farm workers became a ragtag army of rural migrants. Pushed from the land by machines, they were pulled by machines into the great industrial cities of Europe. The prospect of good pay and shorter hours drew them to urban factories. The young especially saw their fortunes in the city. In America those who stayed behind agonized as they watched their towns being robbed of the future.

*Includes immigrants from Great Britain, Ireland, Germany, and the Scandinavian countries.
**Includes immigrants from Poland, Russia, Italy, and other Baltic and East European countries.

IMMIGRATION AND POPULATION, 1860–1920

Frightened and envious, they shared Thomas Jefferson's view of cities as "ulcers on the body politic." The result was a voluminous literature of urban fear with sensational titles like *The Spider and the Fly; or, Tricks, Traps, and Pitfalls of City Life by One Who Knows* (1873) and *Metropolitan Life Unveiled; or the Mysteries and Miseries of America's Great Cities* (1882). No doubt their vivid pictures and splashy accounts seduced as many breathless readers as they repelled. By 1910 a third of all city dwellers had come from the American countryside.

Another quarter came from overseas, the crest of a tidal wave of immigration that began to hit American shores in the mid-1880s. Until then most immigrants had come from northern and western Europe—first the English, Scotch, Dutch, and French in the eighteenth century, then Germans, Scandinavians, and Irish in the mid-nineteenth century. Beginning in the 1880s "new" immigrants with swarthier faces appeared from southern and eastern Europe. Some were fleeing political and religious persecution. The assassination of Czar Alexander II in 1881 brought a resurgence of anti-Semitic pogroms in Russia. Polish and Russian Jews escaped by the tens of thousands from their "shtetls," or villages, into crowded European cities and then on to the new "Promised Land" across the Atlantic. Others left to evade diseases like cholera, which swept across southern Italy in 1887. But most came for the same reasons as migrants from the American countryside—a job, more money, a fresh start.

Ambitious, hardy, and resourceful, immigrants found themselves tested at every step of their journey. They were uprooted from old ways and old friends. Most left mothers and fathers, brothers and sisters, wives and children behind. In many cases it was too expensive to bring relatives along, at least on the first trip (the price one-way was about $50 in 1904). Wayfarers often stole across heavily guarded borders, sometimes on foot, sometimes by train. They traveled for weeks to reach a port like Le Havre in France or Bremen in Germany. If they could find no lodgings, they slept in the streets. At dockside, shipping lines vaccinated, disinfected, and examined them to ensure against their being returned at company expense (by 1907, some 40,000 emigrants had been rejected at Liverpool alone).

It took from one to two weeks to cross the Atlantic. Immigrants spent most of that time below decks in "steerage" compartments one passenger described as "a kind of hell that cleanses a man of his sins before coming to the land of Columbus." When they finally reached America (the main receiving station opened in 1892 on Ellis Island in New York's harbor), they still had to pass a dreaded medical examination that weeded out the physically and mentally unfit. No wonder the immigrant's arrival was, in the words of the hero of an immigrant novel, *The Rise of David Levinsky* (1917), "like a second birth to him. Imagine a new-born babe in possession of a fully developed intellect. Would it ever forget its entry into the world? Neither does the immigrant forget his entry into a country which is, to him, a new world in the profoundest sense."

Immigrants arrived in staggering numbers—over 6.3 million between 1877 and 1890, some 30 million by 1920. In 1907 alone, 1.2 million landed. By the turn of the century immigrants made up nearly 15 percent of the population. Most newcomers were young, between the ages of 15 and 40. They usually came from farms and tiny hamlets. Few spoke English, had skills, or had much education. They worshiped mainly in Catholic, Greek, or Russian Orthodox churches and Jewish synagogues. Almost two-thirds were men, a large number of whom came solely to make money for buying land or starting businesses back home. Some changed their minds and sent for relatives to join them, but returnees were common enough to have a name—"birds of passage." For every 100 eastern and southern Europeans who arrived between 1908 and 1910, 44 went back.

Jews were the singular exception. Over half came from cities and had been tailors, merchants, and artisans in Europe. Almost all stayed and brought their families with them. There was little else they could do. As one Jewish immigrant wrote of his Russian homeland, "Am I not despised? Am I not urged to leave? . . . Do I not rise daily with the fear lest the hungry mob attack me?"

The Immigrant in the City

When they put into port, the first thing newcomers were likely to see was a city—perhaps Boston, New York, or later Galveston, Texas. Enough of them traveled inland so that by the turn of the century three-quarters of the residents of Minnesota and Wisconsin and nearly two-thirds of Utah had at least one foreign-born parent.* Most immigrants, worn by physical and financial exhaustion, settled in cities, no matter where they came from. Even Italians, Slavs, and Greeks whose families had farmed for generations looked to cities for quick money.

Friends or labor contractors or just the drift of people speaking familiar tongues drew them to specific neighborhoods. Immigrants usually clustered together on the basis of their villages or provinces, reflecting old world habits and prejudices. In America Greeks from Athens still considered Spartans ignorant and belligerent, while Spartans found Athenians effete and decadent. Sometimes it seemed that only mutual mistrust of Sicilians united northern Italians with those from the central provinces. New York contained no "Little Italy" but distinct groups of Italians—Neapolitans and Calabrians in the Mulberry Bend district,

*Mormons serving as missionaries in Europe and Great Britain especially swelled Utah's population with converts.

Genoese on Baxter Street, northerners west of Broadway and on Sixty-ninth Street. Wherever they ended up, Jews tended to settle according to the regions in which they had lived in Europe.

Cities developed a well-defined mosaic of ethnic communities, but these neighborhoods were constantly in flux. As many as half the residents moved every 10 years, often to better quarters. More recent arrivals from Italy, Russia, and the Balkans replaced earlier ones from Ireland and Germany. Despite popular perceptions, no other group of immigrants lived like the Chinese in urban ghettos composed exclusively of one nationality. Racial prejudice forced the Chinese together, and local ordinances kept them from buying their way out. Though one nationality usually dominated a neighborhood, there was always a sprinkling of Poles, Slavs, or Greeks in Italian and Jewish areas and vice versa.

Ethnic communities served both as refuges from the strangeness of American society and springboards to a new life. In their neighborhoods immigrants could find comrades who spoke their native tongue and theaters that performed national plays and music, even as they were assaulted everywhere by a new language and culture. Familiar foods, sometimes prepared at ethnic restaurants like the German Luchow's or the Italian Mamma Leone's, competed with expensive American fare whose consumption was a sign of status and acceptance. The *Jewish Daily Forward* and scores of other foreign-language newspapers reported events from the homeland but also gave eager readers profiles of local leaders, advice on voting, and tips on adjusting to life in America. Organizations such as the Hebrew Immigrant Aid Society, the Polish National Alliance, and the Society for the Protection of Italian Immigrants furnished fellowship and assistance, usually in the newcomers' native languages. They also fostered assimilation by sponsoring baseball teams, insurance programs, libraries, and English classes.

Houses of worship were always at the center of immigrant life. They often catered to the practices of individual towns or provinces; yet occasionally they cast off orthodoxy under the cultural pressure of American experience. With Irish priests dominating the American Catholic church many immigrants formed new churches with priests from their homelands. Eastern European Jews began to break the old proscription against sitting next to their wives and daughters in synagogues, and the Orthodox churches of Armenians, Syrians, Rumanians, and Serbians gradually lost their national identifications.

Immigrants worked in factories, in the construction and needle trades, or as common laborers on the street. Their backgrounds and cultural values influenced the kinds of jobs they took. Italians, for example, were committed to family above individual success and were wary of children who did better than their parents. All but one of the nearly 500 bootblacks in New York in 1894 were Italian. Because Chinese men did not feel washing or ironing was women's work, more than 7500 of them could be found in San Francisco laundries by 1880. Sewing ladies' garments seemed unmanly to many native-born Americans but not to Russian and Italian tailors. Slavs tended to be the most physically robust of the new immigrants and valued steady income over education. They pulled their children out of school, sent them to work, and worked themselves in the mines for better pay than in factories.

On the whole, immigrants married later and had more children than the native-born. Greeks and eastern European Jews prearranged marriages according to tradition. They imported "picture brides," betrothed by mail and often from the same village as their prospective husbands. After marriage men ruled the household, but women managed it. Although child-rearing practices varied, immigrants resisted the relative permissiveness of American parents. Youngsters were expected to contribute, like little adults, to the welfare of the family. Caught between the past and the present, immigrants clung to tradition and assimilated slowly. Children adjusted more quickly, despite heart-rending clashes with their elders. They soon spoke English like natives, married whomever they pleased, and worked their way out of old neighborhoods.

The Shape of Cities

Cities of the late nineteenth century still exhibited the ringed residential pattern that had emerged in the old "walking cities" earlier in the century. In those days the professional and upper classes had lived within walking distance of their offices and shops in the city center. As the middle and upper classes moved outward from an increasingly industrial core, the poor, some immigrants, blacks, and lower-class laborers filled the inner void. They took over old factories and brownstones, shanties and cellars; they crammed themselves into dank tenements; and by sheer weight of numbers they transformed these areas into the slums of the central city.

Curled around the slums was the "zone of emergence," an income-graded band of those on their way up—second-generation city dwellers, factory workers, skilled laborers, and professional mechanics—living in progressively better tenements and neater row houses. Their residents had escaped poverty but could still slip back in hard times. Farther out was the suburban fringe, home to the white-collar managers and executives, who lived in larger houses on individual lots. With income determining residence, cities developed a concentric and fragmented look. Yet for all their differences, the circles of settlement held together as a part of a massive and interdependent whole.

Urban Transport

One reason cities remained whole was urban transportation. In the middle of the nineteenth century the horse-drawn railway had begun conveying people, some 35 million people a year in New York and 6.5 million in Boston. The railways' problems were legendary: so slow, a person could walk faster; so crowded (according to Mark Twain), you "had to hang on by your eyelashes and your toenails"; so dirty, thousands of tons of smelly horse manure were left in their wake every day.

Civic leaders came to understand that the modern city could not grow, much less survive, without improved transportation. One far-fetched scheme—trolley cars pulled by steam-driven cables up the steep hills of San Francisco—worked well enough so that Chicago, Seattle, and several other cities installed similar systems in the 1880s. Cable lines and steam locomotives were elevated on trestles high above crowded streets in New York and Chicago. New York completed the first elevated line in 1870. By the early 1880s its lines were hauling 175,000 passengers a day. The system spread to Kansas City, Chicago, and other large cities that could afford it. None of the breakthroughs quite did the trick. Cables remained slow and unreliable; "els" were dirty, ugly, and noisy.

It took electricity to rescue city travelers. In 1888 Frank Julian Sprague, a naval engineer who had once worked for Edison, installed the first electric trolley line, a 12-mile stretch of track in Richmond, Virginia, with overhead wires to power 40 cars. The ingenious Sprague also designed a multiple-unit system of control that permitted individual cars to be powered, lighted, and braked inde-

GROWTH OF NEW ORLEANS

Streetcars helped cities to spread beyond business districts while still functioning as organic wholes. By 1900, lines in New Orleans reached all the way to Audubon Park and Tulane University, bringing these once distant points within the reach of city dwellers and creating "streetcar suburbs."

pendently or together by a master switch located in any one of them. Streetcars moved along at the daunting speed of 12 miles an hour, twice as fast as horses traveled. By 1902 electricity drove nearly all city railways.

Sprague's innovations prompted the electrification of els and made possible the most dramatic advance in urban transport, "subways." The smoke and soot of the steam locomotives made the air of tunnels barely breathable in the first underground lines in London. Between 1895 and 1897 Boston built the first underground electric line, a mile and a half long, under Tremont Avenue. New York followed quickly in 1904 with a subway that ran from City Hall on the southern end of Manhattan north to 145th Street.

The rich had long been able to keep homes outside city limits, traveling to and fro in private carriages. New systems of mass transit freed the middle class and even the poor to live miles from work. Now for a nickel or two (the fare included a free transfer), anybody could ride from central shopping and business districts to the suburban fringes and back again. The segmented and sprawling city, held together by a network of moving vehicles, widened its reach out into suburbs.

Bridges and Skyscrapers

Since cities often grew along rivers and natural harbors, their separate parts sometimes had to be joined over water. The principles and techniques of river bridges had already been worked out by the railroads, most notably in Octave Chanute's bridge across the Missouri by Kansas City (1869) and James B. Eads' bridge across the Mississippi at St. Louis (1874). It remained for a German immigrant and his son, John and Washington Roebling, to make the bridge a symbol of urban growth.

The Roeblings built one of the wonders of the day: the Brooklyn Bridge. Begun in 1870, it took 13 years to complete, cost $15 million, and killed 20 men (including designer John Roebling). President Chester A. Arthur, his cabinet, and several governors attended the opening in 1883. Before them stood the longest suspension bridge in the world—over a mile across the East River with a passageway wide enough for a footpath, two double carriage lanes, and two railroad lines. Its arches were cut like the windows of a giant cathedral and its supporting cables hung, said one awe-struck observer, "like divine messages from above." Soon other suspension bridges spanned the railroad yards in St. Louis and the bay at Galveston, Texas. By 1909 there were over 350 new bridges of more than 500 feet in length.

Even as late as 1880 church steeples still dominated the urban landscape, towering over squat factories and office buildings. The increasing value of urban land put a premium on using available space to its limits. Congestion, which forced railways up on trestles over streets or underground, pushed buildings ever higher. Most large structures were built of masonry, with huge load-bearing walls that restricted floor space and supported no more than a dozen or so stories. The use of cast iron columns in factories and warehouses left more room to house large machines and stores of merchandise. Strong, durable, and fire-resistant "cloudscrapers" made of all cast iron were soon serving as office buildings and department stores too.

Steel, tougher in tension and compression, turned cloudscrapers into skyscrapers. First used in Chicago in William LeBaron Jenney's 10-story Home Insurance Building (1885), steel frames and girders raised buildings to heights of 30 stories by

the end of the century. "Instead of the building's being a shell," wrote architectural historian Lewis Mumford, "it became essentially a skeleton . . . with a tough
external skin." Studded with plate glass windows, Daniel Burnham's Reliance
Building (1894) in Chicago looked to contemporaries like "a glass tower fifteen
stories high."

It was no accident that many of the most stunning new skyscrapers arose in
Chicago, for the city had burned nearly to the ground in 1871. The "Chicago
School" of architects helped to rebuild it. A young maverick of the crowd,
Louis H. Sullivan, promised a new urban profile in which the skyscraper would be
"every inch a proud and soaring thing, rising in sheer exaltation that from top to
bottom is a unit without a single dissenting line." In the Wainwright Building
(1890) in St. Louis, the Prudential Building (1895) in Buffalo, and the Carson,
Pirie, and Scott department store (1889–1904) in Chicago, Sullivan produced towering structures that symbolized the modern industrial city.

For a building to be a "soaring thing" and still habitable required solutions for
some practical problems. Heating with a fireplace in each of hundreds of rooms
would have been too costly. A more efficient system of steam or hot water circulat-
ing through pipes came into use in the 1870s. When William Baldwin finally
perfected the "radiator" in 1874, high-rise buildings became year-round dwellings. To move people from the bottom to the top of tall buildings quickly and
safely, Elisha Graves Otis developed a trustworthy, fast elevator in 1861. By the
1890s faster electric elevators made "the passenger seem to feel his stomach pass
into his shoes," reported one visitor to Chicago.

Slum and Tenement

Far below the skyscrapers, jammed into block after block, lay the slums and
tenements of the inner city. In cramped rooms and sunless hallways, along narrow
alleys and in basements (some flooded every day by tidewaters) lived the city
poor. Some worked there, too, in "sweaters' shops" where as many as a dozen and
a half people labored and slept in dingy two-room flats. Writing in vivid detail in
How the Other Half Lives (1890), reporter and photographer Jacob Riis brought
his readers into the teeming tenement:

> Come over here. Step over this baby—it is a baby, spite of its rags and dirt—
> under these iron bridges called fire-escapes, but loaded down, despite the inno-
> cent watchfulness of the firemen, with broken household goods, with washtubs
> and barrels, over which no man could climb from a fire. This gap between dingy
> brick walls is the yard. That strip of smoke-colored sky up there is the heaven of
> these people.

By the late nineteenth century all cities had such slums and tenements. The
worst ones were in New York, where land rentals were highest and the pressure of
incoming immigrants was greatest. Crime flourished in places called "Bandit's
Roost," "Bottle Alley," "Hell's Kitchen," and "Kerosene Row." Bands of young
toughs (with names like the "Alley Gang," the "Sewer Rats," and the "Rock
Gang") stalked the streets in search of thrills and easy money. The darker forms of
vice—gambling, prostitution, and alcoholism—claimed their victims most readily
in the slums. The poor usually turned to crime when all else had failed. "Let God
Almighty judge who's to blame most," said a 20-year-old prostitute supporting a
sickly mother and four younger brothers and sisters, "I that was driven, or them
that drove me to the pass I'm in."

Disease was a constant and killing companion. Practices that had been safe in the open air of small villages helped turned crowded cities into hellholes. Until the late 1860s pigs and other animals roamed freely in the streets of New York. Visitors to one slum in the Midwest were shocked to discover a group of Greeks slaughtering sheep in a filthy basement and Italian ragpickers sorting their latest finds from the city dump in a courtyard filled with children. Tightly packed tenements and streets piled high with refuse were breeding grounds for deadly microbes. On the Lower East Side of New York nearly 1000 people dwelled on every acre of land in 1894, each of them a powerful transmitter of disease to family and neighbors.

Slum dwellers, often living on subsistence diets, were especially susceptible to epidemics. Cholera, typhoid, and a nasty outbreak of yellow fever in Memphis at the end of the 1870s killed tens of thousands. Tuberculosis was even deadlier. As late as 1900, among infectious diseases it ranked behind only influenza and pneumonia *combined* as a killer. Slum children—in fact all city children—as well as migrants from American farms who had little previous exposure to diseases were the most vulnerable. Infant mortality in cities was twice that of rural areas. In 1882 only half of the children born in Chicago could expect to reach the age of five, and almost a quarter of all children born in American cities in 1890 died before their first birthday.

The installation of new sewage and water purification systems helped. The modern flush toilet came into common use after the turn of the century. Until then water closets and communal privies, some catering to as many as 800 people, served the purpose. All too often cities dumped waste into old private vaults or, worse, into local rivers used for drinking water. In 1881 an exasperated mayor of Cleveland called the Cuyahoga River "an open sewer through the center of the city." The stench rising from open privies, from alleys filled with garbage, and from stagnant water, said a resident of one city, was "enough to knock you down."

Slum housing was often as dangerous as the water. An early tenement like New York's Gotham Court, built in 1850, was little more than a five-story barracks, 234 feet long and 34 feet wide, wedged between two alleys. Half the rooms of this "unventilated and fever breeding structure," as one observer called it, had no windows at all. The tubercle bacillus flourished. In 1879 New York enacted a new housing law, which required a window in all bedrooms of new tenements. Architect James E. Ware won a competition with an innovative design that contained an indentation at the middle of each side of the building. When the indentations of two tenements abutted each other, a shaft about five feet wide was formed. It furnished a small measure of air and light for interior rooms and made each building look like a giant dumbbell from above.

Originally hailed by reformers as a major improvement, Ware's dumbbell tenement spread over such cities as Cleveland, Cincinnati, and Boston "like a scab," said one disgruntled city dweller. Squeezed onto lots barely 25 by 100 feet, the dumbbell had as many as eight stories. Each contained 14 rooms divided into four apartments. Up to 16 families lived on a floor, which had but two toilets in the hall. With 10 tenements to a block, ordinary streets housed as many as 4000 people.

— SECOND STORY. —

"Dumbbell" tenements were designed to use every inch of available space in the standard 25 by 200 foot city lot while providing ventilation and reducing the spread of disease.

Overcrowding soon turned the reform into a dangerous blight. The much-vaunted airshafts became giant silos for trash, which blocked what little light had formerly entered, and carried fires from one story to the next. In 1890 Jacob Riis estimated that three-fourths of his poverty-stricken "Other Half" lived in tenements. When the New York housing commission met in 1900, after 33 years of tenement legislation, it concluded conditions were worse than when reformers started.

RUNNING AND REFORMING THE CITY

Those running the new industrial cities struggled to develop a more efficient way to govern their diverse populations. Many city charters dating from the eighteenth century included a cumbersome system of checks and balances. Mayors, city councils, and state legislatures checked each other so often that it was difficult to get anything done. The mayor vetoed the council; the council ignored the mayor. Jealous state legislatures allowed cities only the most limited and unpopular taxes, such as those on property. But to the cities more than the states fell the responsibility for providing services. Municipal government grew into a tangle of little governments—fragmented, dispersed, often at odds with one another. By 1890, Chicago had 11 branches of government, each a powerful fiefdom with its own hierarchy, regulations, and taxing authority. By the early twentieth century New York City had 1400 separate agencies.

At the very moment when such decentralization increasingly paralyzed cities, schools had to built, streets paved, garbage collected, sewers dug, fires fought, utility lines laid. The middle and upper classes, sources of political leadership for generations, were being drawn into business and moving to the suburban fringes, where they lost interest in governing the city (though not in how the city was governed). Meanwhile the dizzying pace of change left residents little time for planning. "Even the present," wrote Theodore S. Case in his 1888 history of Kansas City, "is more than they can keep up with."

Boss Rule

"Why must there be a boss," journalist Lincoln Steffens asked Boss Richard Croker of New York, "when we've got a mayor—and a city council?" "That's why," Croker broke in. "It's because we've got a mayor and a council and judges—and— a hundred other men to deal with." In other words, the boss and his system furnished cities with the centralization, authority, and services they so sorely needed.

Bosses ruled through the political machine. Often, like New York's Tammany Hall, the machines dated back to the late eighteenth and early nineteenth centuries as fraternal and charitable organizations. Over the years they became centers of political power, shifting their concern from the voting rights of the propertyless to the voting habits of immigrants. In New York the machine was Democratic; in Philadelphia, Republican. Some were less centralized, as in Chicago; some less ethnically mixed, as in Detroit. But wherever they appeared they both served and exploited the community.

The political machine bore a striking resemblance to the corporation. Like a corporate executive, the boss looked on politics as a profession and treated it as a business. His office might be a saloon, a funeral home, or, as in the case of George Washington Plunkitt, a shoeshine stand. His managers were party activists, arranged in a hierarchy with local committeemen reporting to district captains, captains to district leaders, and district leaders to the boss or bosses who ran the machine. Like a businessman, the boss sought to harmonize the competition or destroy it. His machinery was power and money; his workers, the party hacks; his consumers, the voting public.

The stock and trade of the machine was simple: a Christmas turkey, a load of coal for the winter, flowers for the sick, legal assistance and help with the authorities. "I think that there's got to be in every ward somebody that any bloke can come to—no matter what he's done—and get help," said Boston ward leader Martin Lomasney. *"Help, you understand; none of your law and justice, but help."* Bosses sponsored fun too—ball teams, glee clubs, torchlight parades, ward balls, and joy rides up the river with bands playing and drink flowing, even nursing bottles for the tiny ones. "You can't do nothin' with the people," said William Devery after organizing a joyride up the Hudson River for 10,000 of his New York constituents, "unless you do somethin' for 'em."

This crude welfare system not only won votes for machine-sponsored candidates; it also served as a form of public philanthropy. Private charities proved unable to cope with the crush of urban despair. By helping people, bosses also offered a path for advancement to the least privileged and a method of Americanization for the most foreign. To the unskilled, the boss doled out jobs in public construction. For bright, ambitious young men, he had places in city offices or in the party itself. These represented the first steps into the middle class. Help came in more basic forms too—English-language classes, guidance at the polls, speedy naturalization—which began to turn foreigners into grateful citizens.

It was votes that bosses really wanted. They went to almost any lengths to get them. William Tweed, whose ring ruled New York briefly in the 1860s and 1870s, streamlined the process of naturalization. His ward leaders filled out applications for citizenship, then had judges running for reelection sign them—up to 1000 a day. Every day 1000 new Americans became 1000 new supporters of Boss Tweed. "Little Bob" Davies of Jersey City was adept at mobilizing the "graveyard vote." He drew names from tombstones to pad lists of registered voters and hired "repeaters" to vote under the phony names. Democratic boss "Hinky Dink" Kenna of Chicago's First Ward liked to get his fraudulent names from the Hospital for the Insane at Dunning. Dunning inmates, he said, were more astute than Republican voters.

When reformers introduced the Australian (secret) ballot in the late 1880s to prevent fraud, bosses pulled the "Tasmanian dodge," premarking the election ticket to assure the vote went their way. Failing that, they dumped whole ballot boxes into the river or drove unpersuaded voters from the polls with gangs of barroom thugs. In an age when men alone had the right to vote, the most fearsome election day terrorists were women hired to intimidate opponents' voters: Euchre Kate Burns, the champion female heavyweight brick hurler of New York; Battle Annie, the ferocious leader of the Battle Row Ladies Social and Athletic Club; and Hell-Cat Maggie, who filed her front teeth to points and wore long artificial nails of brass. When she went tearing through the polls, nails clawing and teeth flashing, even the bravest citizen fled.

Why did bosses go to such lengths? Some, like "Honest" Ed Flynn of the Bronx, simply loved the game of politics. More often bosses loved money. Their ability to get it was limited only by their ingenuity or the occasional success of an outraged reformer. The record for brassiness must go to Boss Tweed. During a reign of barely a dozen years, Tweed bilked New York City out of millions of dollars. His masterpiece of graft was a chunky three-story courthouse in lower Manhattan originally budgeted at $250,000. When Tweed was through, the city had spent over $13 million—and the building was still not finished. Each window, consisting of a wooden frame, glass, and a small awning, was worth $12.50; each cost the city $8000. For carpeting valued at $13,000, the bill came to $350,000. The New York *Times* estimated that 65 percent of the total went back to the Tweed Ring. Tweed died in prison, but with such profits to be made, it is no wonder that bosses rivaled the pharaohs of ancient Egypt as builders.

In their fashion bosses played a vital role in the industrial city. Rising from the ranks of those they governed, they guided immigrants into American life and helped some of the underprivileged escape poverty. They forged a massive construction program that changed the urban landscape. Most of all they modernized city government by uniting it and making it perform. Choosing the aldermen, municipal judges, mayors, and administrative officials, bosses exerted new control that allowed them to provide the contracts and franchises needed to run cities.

The price was often outrageous. Inflated taxes, extorted revenue, unpunished vice and crime were only the obvious costs. A woman whose family enjoyed Plunkitt's Christmas turkey might be widowed by an accident to her husband in a sweatshop kept open by timely bribes. Filthy buildings might claim her children, as corrupt inspectors ignored flagrant violations. Buying votes and selling favors, bosses turned democracy into a petty business—as much a "business," said Plunkitt, "as the grocery or dry-goods or the drug business."

The Social Conscience of the City

Urban blight and the condition of the poor, particularly the immigrant poor, inspired social as well as political activism, especially within the churches. Some ministers told their middle class flocks that poverty resulted from weak character and a lack of morality. Others, like the popular Congregationalist minister Josiah Strong, simply concluded the city was "a menace to society." Along with a host of anxious economists and social workers, these church leaders blamed the trouble on new immigrants and urged restrictions on their entry. In the 1880s and 1890s nativist organizations like the American Protective Association and the Immigration Restriction League attacked Catholics and other non-Protestant newcomers. In 1897 the first bill requiring literacy tests to reduce immigration passed Congress, but President Grover Cleveland vetoed it.

Other clergymen took their missions to the slums, bridging the distance between the middle class and the poor. They became the social conscience of the city. Beginning in 1870 Dwight Lyman Moody, 300-pound former shoe salesman, joined gospel singer and organist Ira David Sankey to win armies of lowly converts with revivals in Boston, Chicago, and other cities. Evangelists helped to found American branches of the British Young Men's Christian Association and the Salvation Army. By the end of the century the Salvation Army had grown to 700 corps staffed by some 3000 officers. They ministered to the needy with food, music, shelter, and simple camaraderie.

A small group of ministers rejected the old ethos that personal guilt explained sin and turned to a new "Social Gospel." They believed individual salvation would come through the betterment of society, not the other way around. The influential Congregationalist minister Washington Gladden in *Applied Christianity* (1886) and other books spread the word that the church was responsible for performing good social works. Souls could be saved only if the bodies that contained them were first well fed, housed, and clothed. Charles L. Sheldon, a minister from Topeka, Kansas, asked readers of his best seller *In His Steps* (1896) to follow the lead of the charitable citizens of the fictitious town of Raymond. When confronted with the social ills of poverty, drunkenness, and slum life they asked themselves, "What would Jesus do?" Houses of worship, such as William Rainford's St. George's Episcopal Church in New York, became centers of social activity with boys' clubs and gymnasiums, libraries, glee clubs, and industrial training programs.

Church-sponsored programs often repelled the immigrant poor, who saw them as thinly disguised missionary efforts. Immigrants and other slum dwellers were more receptive to a bold new experiment called the settlement house. An agency of social reform imported from Great Britain (which had begun to grapple with the problems of the industrial city earlier in the century), the American settlement house first appeared on the Lower East Side of New York in 1886. Situated in the worst slums, these early community centers were run by middle-class women and men to help the poor and foreign-born. At the turn of the century there were over 100 of them, the most famous being Jane Addams' Hull House in Chicago (1889). In 1898 the Catholic church sponsored its first settlement house in New York, and in 1900 Bronson House opened in Los Angeles to aid the Hispanic community.

High purposes moved settlement workers. Leaving comfortable middle-class homes, they moved into the settlement houses. They dedicated themselves (like the "early Christians," said one) to service and sacrifice. They sought to teach new immigrants American ways and to create a community spirit that would foster "right living through social relations." Like political bosses, they helped, providing everything from day nurseries to playgrounds and libraries. Armed with statistics and personal experiences, they also entered the world of politics, lobbying for social legislation to regulate tenement housing, the working conditions of women, and the improvement of schools.

As they set about their work, settlement workers never lost sight of practicality or the humanity of their clients. Immigrants were to be made American, but they were also to be encouraged to preserve their heritages through festivals, parades, and museums. If the blight of the cities could be ended, decency, creativity, and wholesomeness would go a long way. "The delicious sensation to be found in a swimming pool," Jane Addams wrote, would doubtless outweigh the temptation "to play craps in a foul and stuffy alley."

CITY LIFE AND CULTURE

Settlement workers and other middle-class reformers offered Americans a startling look at the underside of the city, but a grand view of life at the top was available to anybody who strolled along Nob Hill in San Francisco, the North Shore of Lake Michigan near Chicago, or the Main Line outside Philadelphia. In New York, architect Richard Morris Hunt and the firm of McKim, Mead & White transformed Fifth Avenue into the most spectacular residential showplace in the country. William H. Vanderbilt's $11 million mansion on the corner of Fifty-First Street was actually three palaces under one roof. Just down Fifth Avenue was his grandfather's mansion, a limestone replica of a French château.

Few saw the insides with their gold walls, carvings, and Renaissance tapestries, their staircases and ceilings (in some cases ripped from medieval castles and shipped across the Atlantic). No matter—new, mass circulation newspapers gave anybody who wanted it a peek at the socially prominent. Before the Civil War, James Gordon Bennett, publisher of the New York *Herald,* pioneered journalistic voyeurism with lurid tales of what went on behind the potted palms at fancy dress balls. By the 1880s most newspapers had society pages. The upper crust of New York was a prime topic even in small cities like Mobile, Alabama. In 1889 its local paper devoted almost an entire issue to the 282 marriageable ladies of the Social Register, complete with their personal and financial assets. Under the guise of "news," high-toned city life invaded even the provinces of America.

The Urban Middle Class at Home

Between the top and the bottom stretched the vast and ill-defined middle of urban society—educated professionals, white-collar clerks and salesmen, shopkeepers,

Daily Lives

CLOTHING AND FASHION

Gender Roles and Fashions in the 1890s

At Chicago's vast Columbian Exposition of 1893, the Women's Building displayed the latest fashions of an industrial nation. A stunning new simplicity ruled, and the audience liked it. Dresses had less bulk. Skirts were shorter, waists wider and less confining. Shoes tipped at gentler angles on shrunken heels. As the models glided through the hall, women expressed "their great desire to be free from the bondage of skirts," one surprised journalist reported; "—women, too, who would, one would suppose, rather die in long skirts than let the world know they had legs." That same year the *Ladies Home Journal,* a respected women's magazine, proclaimed the female right to choose clothing for comfort. This was not quite a revolution in fashion, but it did signal a significant change, not only in what women were wearing but also in the roles they were playing in American society.

Through most of the nineteenth century Victorian convention dictated middle-class standards in women's dress. Strenuously laced steel-and-bone corsets pushed breasts up, stomachs in, and derrières out. The "Good Sense" corset waist even came in sizes to fit children. The resulting wasplike figure accentuated the image of women as procreators. So did outward apparel. Ankle-length skirts were draped over bustles, hoops, and petticoats—all of which made hips look larger, to suggest fertility. Wide-brimmed hats and high-heeled shoes stressed a delicate femininity. This complicated style bespoke wealth, status, and proper modesty, setting off middle- and upper-class women from those below, whose often shapeless

figures and plain clothes signaled drudgery and poverty.

Such elegance was cumbersome and sometimes debilitating. Corsets ("an instrument of human torture," one woman called them) constricted movement, circulation, and breathing. Internal organs pressed unnaturally against each other. Ribs occasionally cracked; uteruses sagged. Fainting spells and headaches were all too common. High collars, whether of satin or linen, chafed and choked. Yards of pleats could cake with ice in winter or overheat the wearer in summer. The sheer size of a full skirt, observed one women, meant "the wearer had to bunch it in great folds and devote

Daily Lives

one hand to nothing else but the carrying of it." With petticoats the costume weighed as much as 30 pounds. These clothes were designed for little except restricting the women who wore them.

Victorian morality gave men greater leeway in fashion as in conduct. At home they were figures of authority; outside they were free to make their way with few social encumbrances. Clothes, with the exception of stiff paper collars on shirts, expressed male independence. The dark suit coats and full, cuffless trousers afforded ample comfort. A paunchy waist, prominently displayed, signified success. For "dandies," there were checkered pants, floral waistcoats, and heavy gold watch chains.

In the 1840s health reformers and liberal educators had begun to attack women's dress. Feminists like Susan B. Anthony and Elizabeth Cady Stanton abandoned their corsets and donned "bloomers"—long-sleeved, high-necked, loose tunics worn over baggy trousers. Few women followed their lead, but by the 1890s new social and economic forces made simpler styles more acceptable. Health reformers continued to press their case, adding a new emphasis on the need for women to exercise more. New sports that included women became popular: ice-skating in the 1850s; croquet in the 1860s; and bicycling, the most vigorous of all, in the 1880s. Tennis and golf caught the fancy first of the wealthy and, after the turn of the century, of the middle class. All demanded greater movement and the clothes to make it possible.

As more women entered college and went to work, they grew impatient with convention. Women began to associate plainer dress not with the poor or with radical feminists but with new and appealing role models like college students, office clerks, and sports enthusiasts. Fashion became more sensible, reflecting the needs of these new women. Looser and lighter undergarments replaced corsets and bustles. "Shirtwaist" blouses (styled after men's shirts), skirts to the ankle, tailored suits, and lower heeled oxfords made getting to and from the office easier and work once there more efficient.

Meanwhile a revolution in the manufacture of clothing was quietly taking place. Before the Civil War, most garments were made at home. A ready-made–clothing industry had already begun to develop, but it specialized in refinishing castoffs and making only the cheapest grades of new clothes for sailors, slaves, and miners. Steady improvements on the sewing machine, along with the army's demand for uniforms during the Civil War, boosted sales and led to a new science of sizing. The development of cutting machines, pressers, and buttonholers allowed "ready-made" clothes to increase the range of styles offered in volume. In 1890 the value of factory-made clothing for women was under a third that of men's wear. But by 1914 it had soared to half a billion dollars, $20 million more than men's.

Ready to wear or not, newer styles failed to catch on immediately. Novelist Edna Ferber remembered that neighbors in her hometown of Appleton, Wisconsin, disapproved of her mother wearing shirtwaists and shorter skirts in the 1890s. Skirts generally remained long until World War I, and most women put on some kind of corset until the 1920s. Yet greater comfort was here to stay, and so were new roles for women.

corporate managers and executives, public employees, and their families. The earnings of the middle class had risen nearly 30 percent between the Civil War and the 1890s. By the turn of the century just over a third owned their homes. Often two or three stories in height, made of brick or brownstone, these suburban row houses stood within easy reach of new streetcars that could whisk residents to downtown business and shopping districts.

Houses of the nineteenth century served a variety of functions. The top floor of bigger homes contained a modest ballroom that doubled as a family room; in smaller homes it became a sewing room or a guest room for boarders. On the story below were the bedrooms and on the bottom floor, the living room, dining room, pantry, and kitchen. The most notable innovation of the household was the bathroom. Usually there was only one, so bedrooms still contained old-fashioned washstands. But new central heat gave urban bathers the luxury of no longer having to break through the ice that once covered washbowls on wintery mornings.

Technology had its greatest impact on the kitchen. More than any other room, it was a blend of tradition and progress. A "combination" stove (which could be fired by wood or coal if the gas failed) dominated the room. The "refrigerator," a newer and larger version of the old icebox, stood in the pantry, a telltale drip pan betraying its continued reliance on ice. Despite the likely presence of gas jets or electric lighting by the end of the century, a row of candles and kerosene lamps stood ready for use. Many middle-class homes had servants to do the cooking, laundry, and cleaning. According to one estimate about 25 percent of urban households had live-in servants. On call about 100 hours a week, off but one evening and part of Sunday, the average maid received room, board, and $2 to $5 a week in salary.

A woman was measured by the state of her home, which experts said shaped her family. "A clean, fresh, and well-ordered house," stipulated domestic adviser Shirley Murphy in 1883, "exercises over its inmates a moral, no less than physical influence, and has a direct tendency to make members of the family sober, peaceable, and considerate of the feelings and happiness of each other." The woman of the house was expected to prepare elaborate meals, clean, launder, and sew. Each took considerable time. Baking bread, for example, required nearly 24 hours from start to finish. In 1890, when bread was widely available at bakeries and grocery stores, four of five loaves were still made at home.

By the 1890s a cornucopia of commercially prepared foods eased some of the burdens of housework. Brand names began to appear, trumpeting a new age of convenience through consumerism—Campbell's soup, Quaker oats, Pillsbury flour, Jell-O, Canada Dry ginger ale, and Cracker Jacks, just to name a few. New appliances such as "self-working" washers and hand-pumped "vacuum" cleaners offered mechanical assistance, but shredded shirts and aching arms testified that mechanization was sometimes more trouble than it was worth.

The day had already begun to assume its modern form. Families rose early, and to the sound of a mechanical alarm rather than the crow of a rooster. City breakfasts were less hearty but more varied than country fare. Oatmeal and farina supplemented eggs, chops, and other meats. After breakfast the household dispersed. Children walked to grammar school or rode trolleys to high school. Fathers

Processed food labels for tin cans, ca. 1880.

commuted on streetcars to their places of business downtown. Mothers oversaw the domestic routine. The greatest boon to their mornings was the demise of the big noonday dinner. Husbands took their lunches at restaurants or saloons, and children ate at school. A quick cold meal of sandwiches, chicken, or leftovers sufficed for mother, maid, and any preschoolers at home.

Married women of the middle class were supposed to use their free time "to keep up intellectually, to look young and well and be fresh and bright." Lollie Osborn, a homemaker who lived near New York City, spent the winter of 1895 improving her mind "at Literature class," "at reading class at Lizzie Simonds," and "at Astronomy." Outside of literary clubs some women read uplifting religious novels like Lew Wallace's *Ben Hur* (1880) or popular "romances," frowned upon because of their titillating themes. Mrs. E. D. E. N. Southworth, the best-selling woman novelist of the nineteenth century, had heroines who were invariably strong, manipulative, and sensual. They defied contemporary mores through affairs of the heart and an occasional murder of passion.

A middle-class homemaker could also "go downtown" to shop or lunch with a friend. She might spend her afternoons doing needlepoint, an acceptable diversion because it combined the old virtues of housewifery with the new interest in arts and crafts. Or she could curl up with one of the new women's magazines such as the *Ladies Home Journal* for hints on dress, cooking, and home decorating and advice on health and manners.

The family reassembled at the end of the day for supper, a full meal of fish or roast meats, potatoes, canned and fresh vegetables, and breads, followed by a new treat from the refrigerator for dessert—ice cream. Nobody stayed long at the table to chat. Young girls raced to the porch steps to visit friends; boys went off for a game of baseball or "leap-frog"; fathers hurried to lodge meetings or sat smoking cigars and reading newspapers in the den or living room (either of which they could have completely to themselves); mothers cleaned up, then perhaps played the piano or looked at new three-dimensional slides through "magic lanterns." Increasingly, family members found themselves separated from each other and in the company of people their own age. Only on weekends did the routine vary. Toward the end of the nineteenth century, Saturday became less of a workday and more of a family day. Sunday mornings remained a time for dressing up and going to church, still an important center of family life. Afternoons had a more secular flavor with shopping trips (city stores often stayed open) and visits to lakes, zoos, and amusement parks (usually built at the end of trolley lines to attract more riders). In towns and villages, where the pace was slower and living less diversified, Sunday afternoons might offer only dinner and naps or reading, followed by another church service in the evening. In one form or another, outside institutions—fraternal organizations, uplift groups, athletic teams, and church groups—began to intrude on middle-class urban family life.

Victorian Mores

Taking its name from from the long-reigning British queen, Victorianism—a disciplined and prudish code of personal conduct—dictated middle-class behavior. It stressed sobriety, industriousness, self-control, and modesty, all designed to tame a turbulent urban-industrial society. When working-class Americans failed to follow middle-class cues, cultural reformers preached directly to them. In 1874

Frances Willard, fearing the corrosive effects of alcohol on the family, founded the Women's Christian Temperance Union. Under her leadership the WCTU worked relentlessly against the consumption of alcohol and for sexual purity and other middle-class virtues. At the turn of the century it had enlisted 500,000 members and was the largest women's organization in the country.

Anthony Comstock crusaded with equal vigor. A self-appointed custodian of public virtue, Comstock began in 1871 a 41-year campaign against obscenity that led to some 3600 arrests. His targets varied from the despicable to the harmless. In one two-year period he reported seizing 130,000 pounds of vice-ridden books, 194,000 pictures and photos, and precisely 60,300 "articles made of rubber for immoral purposes and used by both sexes." In 1873 President Ulysses S. Grant signed the so-called Comstock Law, a statute suppressing trade and circulation of "obscene literature and articles of immoral use." Two days later Comstock went to work as a special agent for the Post Office.

Crusaders like Comstock were not simply missionaries of a stuffy morality. They were apostles of a middle-class creed of social control and discipline. Inspired by their fear of disorder in an interdependent urban society they believed that the road to ruin lay behind the door of every saloon, dance hall, gambling parlor, or bedroom. And given the increasing incidence of alcoholism, venereal disease, gambling debts, unwanted pregnancies, divorce, industrial accidents, and other ills, moralists had cause for alarm. If taken to extremes either by individuals or society at large, such social pathologies could easily produce chaos and violence in the teeming cities of the late nineteenth century.

The insistence with which moralists warned against impropriety suggests that many people did not take their message to heart. Three-quarters of women surveyed toward the turn of the century reported that they desired and enjoyed sex. If some women did not, said physician Elizabeth Blackwell, they probably feared pain, injury from childbirth, or awkward sexual encounters.

Bold women challenged convention openly. Victoria Woodhull, publisher of *Woodhull & Claflin's Weekly*, divorced her husband, ran for president in 1872 on the Equal Rights party ticket, and pressed the case for sexual freedom. "I am a free lover!" she shouted to a riotous audience in New York's Steinway Hall. "I have the inalienable, constitutional, and natural right to love whom I may, to love as long or as short a period as I can, to change that love every day if I please!" While she made a public case for freedom of sexual choice, in private she followed convention. Like other social radicals, Woodhull believed in strict monogamy and romantic love for herself, just as middle-class readers of romance novels did.

Feminist writer Charlotte Perkins Gilman, author of *Women and Economics* (1898), disputed the ideals of womanly purity, domesticity, and idleness. After suffering a crippling depression in 1885 she wrote *The Yellow Wall Paper*, a fictionalized account of her illness that compared the confinement of a mental patient with the lot of a wife. For Susan B. Anthony sexual politics boiled down to female disfranchisement. She rallied women to demand the vote through the National American Woman Suffrage Association (1890). Despite such telling attacks on conventional behavior, most Americans heeded the message of the traditional moralists in spirit, if not in deed.

School Days

Public education was another powerful tool for imposing order and control on the city. The campaign for public education begun in the Jacksonian era did not have a serious impact until after the Civil War. As late as 1870 half the children in the country received no formal education at all. The average citizen had taken only four years of classes, and one in five Americans could not read. Then a great educational awakening occurred, as business required better educated workers and the number of compulsory state-supported school systems grew.

Attendance in public schools more than doubled between 1870 and 1900. The length of the school term rose from 132 to 144 days. Illiteracy fell by half. At the turn of the century, nearly all the states outside the South had enacted compulsory education laws. Almost three out of every four school-age children were enrolled. Yet an ordinary adult still had attended for only about five years, and less than 10 percent of those eligible ever went to high school.

The average school day started early, but by noon most girls were released (the assumption being they required less formal education than boys). Curricula stressed fundamentals—reading, writing, and arithmetic—but courses in manual training, science, and physical education were added as the demand for technical knowledge grew and opportunities to exercise shrank. In the classroom teachers had absolute control. Students learned by rote, sitting in silent study with hands clasped or standing erect while they recited phrases and sums. "Don't stop to think," barked a Chicago teacher to a class of terrified youngsters in the 1890s, "tell me what you know!"

A rigid social philosophy underlay the harsh discipline. In an age of industrialization, massive immigration, and rapid change, school curricula taught conformity and values as much as simple facts and figures. Teachers were supposed to be drillmasters, hammering their charges into shape for the sake of society. "Teachers and books," wrote New Jersey College Professor John L. Hart in 1879, "are better security than handcuffs and policemen." In *McGuffey's Reader*, a standard textbook used in grammar schools throughout the nineteenth century, students learned not only how to read but also how to behave. Hard work, Christian ethics, and obedience to authority would lead boys to heroic command, girls to blissful motherhood, and society to harmonious progress.

African-American students had to deal with the special problems of discrimination and segregation. As the federal commitment to Reconstruction faded, so did the impressive start made in public education for blacks. Yet they were so eager for education that by the end of the century nearly half of black America could read. It was a remarkable achievement, for most of the first generation of former slaves had been illiterate. Worse still, for nearly 100 years after the Civil War, the doctrine of "separate but equal," finally upheld by the Supreme Court in *Plessy v. Ferguson* (1896), kept black and white students apart but scarcely equal. By 1882 public schools in a half dozen southern states were segregated by law, the rest by practice. Underfunded and ill-equipped, serving dirt-poor families whose every member had to work, all-black schools drew only about a third of the South's black children.

Like African-Americans, many immigrants saw education as a way of getting ahead, while some educators saw it as a means of Americanizing immigrants. "Education," declared a New York principal, "will solve every problem of our national life, including that of assimilating our foreign element." Few public schools paid special attention to immigrants. Educators assumed that immigrant and native-born children would learn the same lessons and turn out the same way. But toward the end of the century, as immigration mounted, eastern cities began to offer night classes in English and civics for foreigners. When public education proved inadequate or failed to address their needs, immigrants established their own schools. Catholics, for example, started an elaborate expansion of their parochial schools in 1884. Public or private, the education of immigrants served the same purpose: teaching fundamentals while promoting citizenship through wholesome values. "The first step in civilization," wrote Father Paul Tymkevich of the Greek Catholic church, "is to acquire good habits, and where can they acquire them? On the streets? In the saloons?"

School was obviously the place, and by the 1880s educational reforms were already promoting "good habits" and marketable skills. A number of reforms came from Germany, already a center of innovation. Opened first in St. Louis in 1873, American versions of "kindergartens" put four- to six-year-olds in orderly classrooms while parents went off to work. "Normal" or teacher-training schools multiplied, so that in 1900 almost one teacher in five had a professional degree. Science and manual training supplemented more conventional curricula. Such vocational studies supplied industry with better educated workers and also helped to control them by reducing union influence over apprenticeship. By 1890, 36 cities had vocational high schools.

College Years

Increasingly colleges served the urban industrial society, not by controlling mass habits but by providing a corps of leaders and managers. Early in the nineteenth century, most Americans had regarded higher learning as effete and irrelevant. Of the few who sought higher education, many preferred the superior universities of Europe to those in the United States. As American society became more organized, mechanized, and complex, the need for professional, technical, and literary skills brought greater respect for what colleges could teach. The Morrill Act of 1862 generated a dozen new state colleges and universities, eight mechanical and agricultural colleges, and six black colleges.

Private philanthropy added more. In 1873 Johns Hopkins, who had acquired part of his fortune from ownership of the Baltimore and Ohio Railroad, bequeathed $7 million to found the university that bore his name. John D. Rockefeller reestablished the University of Chicago (1890), while railroad baron Leland Stanford endowed Stanford University (1891) with $24 million. The number of colleges and universities nearly doubled between 1870 and 1910. Their enrollments swelled to a third of a million. At that time the 16 universities of France had 40,000 students, a figure that roughly equaled the number of faculty of American institutions.

The "college man" enjoyed new respect as universities flourished. Small-town boys and girls admired him and children's novels like *Frank Merriwell at Yale* celebrated his exploits. No longer depicted as a wastrel or bookworm, he was now informed and virile. The upper middle class had a new ideal—the educated rogue in a ribbed turtleneck sweater. At his side, the envy of all to see, was a new phenomenon—the "co-ed." Before the Civil War women could attend only three private colleges. After the war they had new ones for themselves, among them Smith (1871), Wellesley (1875), and Bryn Mawr (1885). Many land-grant colleges, chartered to serve all people, admitted women from the start. By 1910 some 40 percent of college students were women, almost double the 1870 figure. Only one college in five refused to accept them.

Potent myths continued to make college life hard for women. As Dr. Edward Clarke of the Harvard Medical School told thousands of students in *Sex in Educa-*

tion (1873), the rigors of a college education could lead the "weaker sex" to physical or mental collapse, infertility, and early death. Women's colleges therefore included a stringent program of physical activity to keep students healthy. In addition to an academic curriculum similar to that of the best men's schools, women found an array of conventional courses in "domestic science" available to them. Pioneered in the 1870s by coeducational schools, they were developed to counter the claim that higher education would be of no value to most women. The first of these "Ladies Courses" had been a series of lectures on cooking offered by the wife of the president of Iowa State College. Eventually they included sewing and the application of chemistry to foods. Some women's colleges such as Bryn Mawr resisted, but 18 land-grant colleges, mostly in the West, had organized departments of home economics by 1905.

The practical impulse in higher education inspired several new black colleges. In the late nineteenth century, few institutions mixed races and most refused the rare African-American applicant who sought admission. Church groups and private foundations, such as the Peabody and Slater funds (supported by white philanthropists from the North), underwrote black schools after Reconstruction. By 1900, when a total of 700 black students were enrolled, about 2000 had graduated from college. Some, through hard work and persistence, had even graduated from institutions generally considered reserved for whites.

By the turn of the century, higher learning, though pursued by less than 5 percent of college-age Americans, extended more and more beyond college. In keeping with the new emphasis on practical training, professional schools multiplied. American universities adopted the German model requiring young faculty members to perform scholarly research as part of their training. The number of medical schools more than doubled between 1870 and 1900; the number of medical students almost tripled. Ten percent of medical students were women (a peak enrollment that soon shrank as the medical profession became more organized and exclusive). The number of law schools (a uniquely American development) jumped from 51 in 1880 to 102 in 1900, while schools of nursing grew by 300 percent. New professionals swelled the ranks of the middle class. Slowly the professional was becoming a new force in the society of urban America, replacing the ministers and gentlemen freeholders of an earlier day as community leaders.

Palaces of Consumption

In the city, middle- and working-class urbanites had access to a new material culture that was leveling and homogenizing American society. In the eighteenth century clothes signaled status. As sewing machines became household items in the nineteenth century, common people began wearing garments that fit them and made them look more like the well-to-do. The demand for hundreds of thousands of uniforms during the Civil War encouraged mass manufacturing, and new immigrants skilled at the needle trades supplied the labor. A revolution in clothing substituted store-bought "ready-made" garments for those manufactured at home or consigned to high-priced tailors. By 1890 millions of boys and men dressed in "ready-to-wear." Similar shifts affected the food people ate and the furnishings in their homes.

Young girl selling newspapers in New York, ca. 1895.

Well-made, inexpensive merchandise in standard sizes and shapes found outlets in new palaces of consumption called "department stores" (so named because they displayed their goods in separate sections or departments). The idea was imported from France, where shopping arcades had been built as early as the 1860s. Unlike the small exclusive shops of Europe, department stores were palatial, public, and inviting. Rising several stories, like the Cast Iron Palace of A. T. Stewart in New York, they were usually found in central business districts, where they were easily accessible by streetcars and other public conveyances.

A trip to the department store offered a day's entertainment. In addition to shopping, patrons found restaurants, dance floors, and beauty salons. Most of the new stores had intricate facades that sometimes duplicated Venetian palazzos. There were large plate glass windows filled with enticing merchandise that invited strollers to participate in the new pastime of "window shopping." The wide, unbroken interiors, painted in soft colors, imparted a dreamlike quality to rooms with appealing displays of furniture, housewares, and clothing.

Retailers did not rely on their stores alone to woo customers. From the start they publicized their wares in daily newspapers. Under the impact of new printing techniques and aggressive publishers such as Joseph Pulitzer, newspapers broadened their coverage, sought out sensational "news" stories, and increased their circulation. The advertisements of department stores contributed to their success and also helped to keep them free of the political subsidies that prejudiced newspapers in France and Italy. Between 1870 and 1900 the amount of money spent on advertising quadrupled.

Emile Zola, the French novelist and crusading journalist, observed that department stores "democratized luxury." Anyone could enter free of charge, handle the most elegant and expensive goods, and buy whatever was affordable. When consumers found goods too pricey, department stores pioneered "lay-away" plans, which allowed for deferred payments. Free delivery and free return or exchange of purchases helped to make buying and selling a public affair built on policies offered to all, not just the favored customers of exclusive fashion makers. The department store also educated people. It showed them models of what proper families owned and taught them the correct names for things like "women's wear" and "parlor furniture." Mass production, along with massive advertising campaigns, was beginning to produce a mass culture.

Slowly popping up in city after city, "chain stores" (a term coined in America) served a similar function but without frills. They catered to the working class, who could not afford department stores, and operated on a "cash-and-carry" basis. Owners kept their costs down by buying large quantities to fill the small stores in their long neighborhood chains. The Great Atlantic and Pacific Tea Company, founded in 1859, was the first. It gradually added other groceries to its list of teas. By 1876 there were 76 A & P branches, all featuring the distinctive red-and-gold facade. F. W. Woolworth opened his first "5-and-10-cent" store in 1879. In the twentieth century such centrally operated chains would drive local merchants out of business.

Rural Americans, far from department and chain stores, joined the community of consumers by mail. From a loft over a livery stable in Chicago, Aaron Montgomery Ward started sending a price sheet to farmers in 1872. By cutting out the middleman Ward promised savings of 40 percent on fans, parasols, needles, trunks, harnesses, cutlery, and scores of other goods. In 1884 his catalogues boasted 10,000 items, each illustrated by a lavish woodcut. Country folk came to rely on Ward for almost all their needs, even things he could not possibly supply. "As you advertise everything for sale that a person wants," one faithful customer reasoned, "I thought I would write you, as I am in need of a wife, and see what you could do for me."

Similarly, Richard W. Sears and Alvah C. Roebuck built a $500 million mail order business by 1907. In the early 1900s Sears, Roebuck was distributing 6 million catalogues every year. Schoolrooms that had no encyclopedia used a Ward's or Sears' catalogue instead. Children were drilled in reading and spelling from it. They learned arithmetic by adding up orders and geography by studying the postal zone maps. When asked where the Ten Commandments came from, one farm boy replied without hesitation that they came from Sears, Roebuck.

Americans were already beginning to think of themselves as consumers, even as machines and factories weakened the old work ethic of individual productivity. Reaching out from city to countryside, a vast community of consumption was growing. Rural free delivery of mail, standardized by the Post Office in 1898, and the inauguration of parcel post in 1913 made everyone's home a potential marketplace. Increasingly city businesses sold the same goods to farmer and clerk, rich and poor, native-born and immigrant. Common patterns and articles of consumption bound up the nation as never before.

Arts and Entertainment

People in cities turned leisure into a consumer item, spending time and money in new ways. While churchgoing remained a primary leisure activity, hundreds of new fraternal, business, civic, and patriotic organizations sprang up. Members paid annual dues to a special fellowship that reduced the anonymity and isolation of urban life and furnished important contacts in the community. Sports, traditionally the province of the rich, slowly broadened their appeal. The recently imported English game of tennis attracted new players at country clubs but few in public parks. Most people regarded it as a game for women and frail men. Polo and golf, which required expensive equipment, considerable space, and some training, were also limited to the country-club set.

Croquet had wider appeal, since it required less skill and special equipment. Perhaps as important, it could be enjoyed in mixed company, like the new national craze of bicycling. Bicycles evolved from the unstable "ordinary" with its large front wheel to the "safety" bike, which had equal-sized wheels, a dropped middle bar, pneumatic tires, and coaster brakes. By the early 1890s, Americans owned more than a million bicycles (a good one cost about $100, far beyond the reach of a factory worker). On Sunday afternoons city parks became crowded with cyclers, and cycling clubs such as the League of American Wheelmen began lobbying for better roads.

More and more women rode the new safety bikes along with the earlier tricycles. Their participation was governed by elaborate rules, including a strict proscription against riding alone. But cycling broke down conventions too. Inevitably it required looser garments, freeing women from corsets. Lady cyclists demonstrated that they were hardly too fragile for physical exertion. Tandem bikes encouraged couples to ride together. In 1896, at the height of the fad, one enterprising manufacturer even brought out an unadorned black bicycle for widows in mourning.

Mannered sports of the wealthy and middle class had their counterparts in organized spectator sports that attracted crowds from every walk of life. Baseball overshadowed all others. For city dwellers with dull work, cramped quarters, and isolated lives, baseball offered the chance to join thousands of people for an exciting outdoor spectacle. In the 1890s it was attracting crowds of 60,000. Like roller skating, baseball began as a fashionable exercise played in natty blue trousers and straw hats, attended by ladies and gentlemen in stylish coaches, and followed by a formal dinner. Boston teamsters soon confirmed its status as a "democratic" sport of amateurs by scheduling games on the Common before work.

Slowly the game took its modern form: in 1869 the first professional team, the Cincinnati Red Stockings, appeared; umpires called balls and strikes; the overhand replaced the underhand pitch; fielders put on gloves and catchers, protective gear; lively experimental balls that produced scores of 201 to 11 were abandoned. Newspapers began covering baseball in specialized sports sections with detailed statistics for fans. Teams from eight cities formed the National League of Professional Baseball Clubs in 1876, followed by the American League in 1901. In 1903 the Boston Red Sox beat the Pittsburgh Pirates in the first World Series. League players were distinctly working class, with few of the high salaries of today's professionals. When the players tried to unionize and form their own league, owners beat them back.

Horse racing, bicycle tournaments, and other sports of speed and violence helped to break the dullness, frustration, and routine of the industrial city. In 1869, without pads or helmets, Rutgers beat Princeton in the first intercollegiate football match. By the 1890s the service academies and state universities fielded teams. But not everyone cheered. Cornell University forbade its team from playing the University of Michigan. "I will not permit 30 men to travel 400 miles, " said President White in 1873, "to agitate a bag of wind." Despite protests against rising death tolls (18 players died in 1905), football soon attracted crowds of 50,000 or more. Then, beginning in 1891 when Dr. James Naismith nailed a peach basket to the gymnasium wall at the Y.M.C.A. Training School in Springfield, Massachusetts, "basketball" became the indoor interlude between the outdoor sports of spring and fall.

Variety also marked social life in the city. Workingmen took their dates to dance halls and boxing exhibitions, staged in small rings used for variety acts between fights. Wealthier couples went to theaters and symphonies. A "star system," developed long in advance of Hollywood, promised audiences their favorite actors. Popular melodramas gave theatergoers a chance to escape the ambiguities of modern life. The audience booed villains, cheered heroes, shuddered for heroines, and marveled at tricky stage mechanics that made ice floes move and players float upward to heaven. Whatever was happening on the street, virtue and honor triumphed at every performance of Harriet Beecher Stowe's *Uncle Tom's Cabin* and Augustin Daley's *Under the Gaslight*, the two biggest attractions at the end of the century. Even "serious" theater, such as the tragedies of Shakespeare, furnished excitement—swordplay, gasping deaths, and gloriously anguished monologues.

Cities put together symphony orchestras, expert ones in New York and Chicago, half-professional and half-amateur ones in smaller cities. To appeal to broad audience tastes, the orchestras played a mixture of popular tunes, John Philip Sousa marches, and the music of classical European composers. Theatergoers with lighter tastes relished weak American imitations of operettas by Gilbert and Sullivan and home-grown vaudeville revues. Touring companies bringing city culture

The catcher wears no mitt in this 1875 painting of two baseball players, by Thomas Eakins. Eakins, a master of realism, shocked his staid faculty colleagues at Philadelphia's Pennsylvania Academy of Fine Arts by working from live nude models and by painting scenes and portraits that, while insightful and penetrating, did not always flatter their subjects.

to small towns caused such excitement that crowds gathered at the train station to greet them.

In towns and cities a stunning assortment of music filled the air. Organ grinders churned out Italian airs on street corners; steam-powered calliopes tooted spirited waltzes from amusement parks and riverboat decks; in bandstands brass ensembles played German-style concerts of the latest compositions of Patrick Gilmore. By 1900 the sale of phonograph records had reached 3 million, helping to make popular music a big business. Ballads like "My Mother Was a Lady" ran to nostalgia, moralism, and sentimentality. Topical songs celebrated the discovery of oil, the launching of baseball's National League, and the changing styles of women's clothing. In Scott Joplin's "Maple Leaf Rag" (1899) the lively syncopation of ragtime heralded the coming of jazz.

As the nineteenth century drew to a close the city was reshaping the country, just as the industrial system was creating a more specialized, diversified, and interlocking national and even international economy. Most Americans were ambivalent about this process. The old Jeffersonian bias against cities warred with the gospel of material progress and wealth that cities so dramatically embodied. Cities beckoned migrants and immigrants with unparalleled opportunities for work and pleasure. The playwright Israel Zangwill celebrated the city's transforming power in his 1908 Broadway hit *The Melting Pot.* "The real American," one of his characters explained, "is only in the Crucible, I tell you—he will be the fusion of all the races, the coming superman."

Where Zangwill saw a melting pot with all its promise for a new super race, champions of traditional American values like the widely read Protestant minister Josiah Strong saw "a commingled mass of venomous filth and seething sin, of lust, of drunkenness, of pauperism, and crime of every sort." Economist David A. Wells, alarmed at rising rates of heart disease and mental illness, bemoaned what he called these "diseases of civilization." "Never was there, perhaps, more hollowness of heart than at present, and here in the United States," wrote poet Walt Whitman. The gap between rich and poor yawned most widely in cities. Progress and poverty, as Henry George observed, seemed to go hand in hand.

Both the champions and critics of the late nineteenth century had a point. Corruption, crudeness, and immorality were no more or less a part of the cities than the vibrancy, energy, and opportunities that drew people to them. In the end moral judgments, whether pro or con, missed the point. Forces much deeper than individual vices and virtues gave cities their new form. Integrated systems of transportation, manufacturing, communications, capital accumulation, and the mass distribution of goods and culture had cities as their indispensable nodes. Those cities grew so rapidly, and in such an unplanned, helter-skelter fashion, that their disorderliness threatened the operation of the very systems that helped to bring them into being.

Somehow the political system had to find within the traditions of a democratic republic a way to bring order out of this seeming chaos. More would be needed than Jacob Riis' moralistic warnings to the privileged few to observe the desperate plight of "the Other Half." People divided by wealth, race, ethnicity, religion, region, social class, age, cultural habits, and gender had somehow to be shaped into a coherent whole. The arbitrary rule of the bosses would have to give way to government that met the industrial order's need for efficiency, the public's need for services, and the need of the poor for compassion, all at a price society could afford. Since Americans could not agree that modern urban life was desirable in the first place, they would have great difficulty finding any way to make their cities work.

SIGNIFICANT EVENTS

1869 — Cincinnati Red Stockings become first professional baseball team; Rutgers beats Princeton in first intercollegiate football game

1870 — Elevated railroad begins operation in New York City

1871 — Fire destroys most of Chicago

1872 — William "Boss" Tweed convicted of defrauding city of New York

1873 — Comstock Law enacted

1874 — Women's Christian Temperance Union founded

1875 — Dwight Moody begins urban evangelical revivals

1876 — First National League baseball game; Central Park completed in New York City; Johns Hopkins University opens nation's first graduate school

1879 — F. W. Woolworth opens first "5-and-10-cents" store

1882 — Chinese Exclusion Act

1883 — Brooklyn Bridge opens

1885 — Home Life Insurance Building, world's first skyscraper, built in Chicago

1886 — Statue of Liberty dedicated

1887 — Edward Bellamy's *Looking Backward, 2000–1887* published; free mail delivery in all communities with 10,000 or more people

1888 — Nation's first electric trolley line begins operation in Richmond, Virginia

1889 — Hull House opens in Chicago

1890 — Jacob Riis' *How the Other Half Lives* published

1891 — Basketball invented

1892 — Ellis Island opens as receiving station for immigrants

1893 — World's Columbian Exposition in Chicago

1894 — Immigration Restriction League organized

1896 — *Plessy v. Ferguson*

1897 — Boston opens nation's first subway station

Generations of the Republic

The Family in an Urbanizing Culture (1860–1920)

The generation born after 1860 lived in an America suspended between two worlds, one urban and the other rural. By the end of the nineteenth century, nearly half of all Americans dwelled in cities, contrasted with only 20 percent in 1860. The urban middle class became firmly established, and for the first time in American history agricultural workers made up less than half of the labor force.

Following a pattern set earlier in the century, the rate of population growth continued to decline. Traditionally birth rates had been highest along the frontier, where abundant land represented opportunity for succeeding generations and so encouraged fertility. As the frontier slowly receded, birth rates fell: the average number of children born to a white woman was 5.2 in 1860; by 1890 it was 3.9. High infant mortality kept most families even smaller, usually to about 3 children.

This decline was widespread: it not only affected virtually all classes, races, and ethnic groups but touched other Western nations as well. Historians speculate that the change reflected the impact of a rising urban middle class, maturing industrial economies, and changing ideals of the family. For middle-class families, re-

ducing family size made sense, given the premium on urban dwelling space and the opportunity to improve their own material lives by raising fewer children. Higher birth rates among immigrants and working-class urbanites remained common, but in time even these families began to shrink as they improved their status, spent more money on educating their children, and sent fewer of them to work at a young age. Despite declining birth rates, the nation as a whole remained young. The population pyramid retained its classic shape—wide at the youthful base and narrower toward the elderly top.

The experiences of those growing up in the new urban environment differed widely, in large measure depending on class and economic status. The parents of the new urban middle class viewed families as havens, away from the bustle of the city's business district, its sooty factories, and the threat of strikes and labor violence. Chaos might reign in the industrial city, but orderliness, tranquillity, and hierarchy ruled the Victorian home. Seventeenth-century notions of children as inherently sinful had given way to greater optimism about their capacity to be shaped. By the late nineteenth century

1870

Birth Year	Males	Females	Age
Before 1796			75 +
1796–1800			70–74
1801–05			65–69
1806–10			60–64
1811–15			55–59
1816–20			50–54
1821–25			45–49
1826–30			40–44
1831–35			35–39
1836–40			30–34
1841–45			25–29
1846–50			20–24
1851–55			15–19
1856–60			10–14
1861–65			5–9
1866–70			0–4

3 2 1 0 1 2 3

As middle- and upper-class youngsters reached the age of courtship, they faced increasingly elaborate rituals. Sixteen was the recommended age for young women to start "keeping company" with men, though they could begin as early as fourteen. Flirting was an accepted means for women to seize the romantic initiative normally reserved for men. New leisure activities such as roller skating and bicycle riding gave couples acceptable ways to hold hands in public or be alone together. The new urban culture also offered women greater opportunity to be self-supporting than their mothers and grandmothers had. As a result, more than one woman in ten never married, the highest proportion in American history. (Among college-educated women the percentage was even higher.) "I don't want to be married," a young schoolteacher told her beau. "I can take care of myself."

Men had responsibility for proposing marriage and, once accepted, an obligation to seek the approval of their fiancées' father. Since the prospective husband was expected to support his wife and children, he had to outline his financial prospects. Women remained subordinate, and once engaged they were expected to obey their betrothed as they had their father. They also were to remain pure and innocent until marriage, whereupon they were advised to control the "lower natures" of their husbands by cultivating their own supposed indifference to sex. Despite this

clergy and child experts were advising parents that "bad habits" resulted from improper training, not innate depravity.

Thus children required gentle nurturing, usually at the hands of the mother. It began in infancy with a new emphasis on breast-feeding. As children grew, "reason and affection" were the favored tools for training. Parental advisers now condemned the practice of wrapping babies tightly, viewing swaddling clothes as "so many bonds by which [the baby] is restrained of the natural freedom of its body."

advice, so often tendered by marriage manuals of the day, middle-class Americans became more conscious of sexuality as an emotional dimension of a satisfying union, not merely a function to be performed for the purposes of procreation. The stereotype of the frigid, repressed Victorian marriage is at best overdrawn.

Middle-class weddings were often lavish affairs, with printed invitations for the larger ones. Gifts were often displayed on the day of the marriage and enviously inspected by the guests. Around 1870, when the cost of photography dropped, wedding portraits became popular. Taken well after the ceremony, they usually commemorated the bride alone. Also by the 1870s, a growing railroad network helped spawn a new institution—the honeymoon resort. Hotels at Saratoga and Niagara Falls, New York, greeted new couples with band music and offered special honeymoon suites to make memorable the interlude between courtship and married life.

The gritty realities that confronted urban working classes made any talk of family "havens" or elaborate weddings somewhat fanciful. Most families moved frequently, in search of work, and lived in cramped quarters. To supplement family incomes as many as 30 percent took in boarders, usually unmarried men and women between the ages of 20 and 35. (In some cities, nearly half the immigrants who arrived toward the end of the century had boarders in their homes.) In such households mothers took responsibility for child rearing, often working outside the home as well to help support the family. The consequence of such pressures could be grim. Gertrude Moselle, a black journalist in New York writing a column of advice to women, warned working mothers against the practice of drugging their children or locking them in closets to keep them out of mischief while the mothers were absent.

In the "family economies" of the working classes, key decisions—over whether and whom to marry, over work and education, over when to leave home—tended to be made on the basis of collective rather than individual needs. Though boys were more likely to work than girls, daughters in immigrant families often went to work at an early age so sons could continue their education. It was customary for one daughter to remain unmarried so she could care for younger siblings or aged parents. Young men and women generally worked for seven years before marrying and often did not establish their own households until their early thirties.

The rise of urban centers even affected family lives in rural areas, as a larger proportion of young farm men were drawn to the opportunities in the city. By the second or third generation of settlement many farming communities consisted of close networks of female kin, since daughters often married neighbors and set up house near their parents. The bonds of family and kinship were equally strong among African-Americans, the vast majority of whom lived in the southern countryside. Black families had existed in slavery, though with restrictions on visitation for slave couples belonging to different masters and with constant threats of separation by sale. The strength of such attachments became clear after the Civil War when thousands of former slaves wandered the South in search of spouses, siblings, and children separated by sale or war. As late as 1900, so many ex-slaves were seeking relatives that one Virginia newspaper created a special section—"Do You Know Them?"—to satisfy the demand for information.

Beginning in the 1880s, in both rural and urban settings, American mortality rates began gradually declining. (There were notable exceptions among African-Americans; see page 938.) In cities, the decline resulted from a host of factors: the coming of purer water, better access to medical care, pasteurized milk, and—by the early twentieth century—improvements in sewage systems. As a result of the drop in mortality, the population grew steadily older. By 1900 about 6.5 percent of all Americans were 60 or older, compared to 4 percent in 1860. Still, with so few members of society reaching old age, no fixed policy toward retirement existed in most businesses. Voluntary retirement did increase. In 1920 some 60 percent of

men 65 and older continued to work, down from the 75 percent who had worked in 1870. The growth of the factory system helped to account for the decline by accelerating retirement among workers who could not keep pace. Those who continued to work often found themselves moved from assembly lines to lower-paying janitorial jobs.

Poverty among the aged increased. As late as 1922 no state had enacted a workable old-age pension system, despite recognition (dating from around 1910) that old age was becoming a social problem. By 1930 one elderly American in four was dependent on some form of assistance. Most relied on savings or help from families, but many found themselves in asylums and state poorhouses, the majority of whose populations were 65 or older. Not until 1935 did Congress enact a national pension program in the Social Security Act, at least 50 years later than most European countries. Even then its provisions and support were limited. Society still held that individuals were responsible for themselves, whatever their age.

In their declining years this generation saw America assuming its characteristic twentieth-century shape, in which the urban middle classes achieved a dominant social position. Births were becoming less frequent, and the population was steadily growing older and more diverse. Modern America was coming of age with the passing of this generation.

20

Agrarian Domains: The South and the West

The news spread across the South during the late 1870s in a variety of ways: sometimes merely as rumors, passed by word of mouth in the cotton fields. Perhaps a man came around with a handbill, telling about cheap land to be had. Or it might be in a letter from friends or relatives, read aloud to the congregation at church. The news spread in different ways, but in the end, the talk always spelled *Kansas*.

Few black farmers had been to Kansas themselves, of course. But more than a few knew that Old John Brown had lived there before coming east to launch his famous raid on Harpers Ferry. Kansas was a state where it seemed black folk might be able to live more freely. "You can buy land at from a dollar and a half to two dollars an acre," wrote one settler to his friend in Louisiana, also noting another distinct advantage. "They do not kill Negroes here for voting." *The Colored Citizen*, a newspaper in Topeka, received so many inquiries that it printed advice on how to travel and where to settle, concluding, "COME WEST. COME TO KANSAS." Even more enticing were the chromoliths—colored promotional handbills showing "freedman's homes" with floor-length French windows, living rooms with young children playing the piano, black mothers directing a host of servants in the kitchen and fathers hauling home turkeys and deer from the verdant prairies.

In 1878 such prospects excited hundreds of black families already stretched to their limits by economic hardship and political violence. With Rutherford Hayes president and Reconstruction officially superseded by white "redemption," the future in the South seemed uncertain indeed. Henry Adams, founder of the Negro Union Co-operative Aid Association in Louisiana, sent 150 members of his organization across the South to study the plight of ordinary blacks. By 1877 he had concluded that migration out of the South was the best solution available. But there were individuals aplenty who needed no committee to come to that conclusion. "Colored people are looked upon by the white people with disdain and scum," one black farmer from Texas complained. "I have suffered the bukes and scums long enough down South here."

St. Louis first learned of these rumblings in the first raw days of March 1879, as steamers from downriver began unloading unusual numbers of freedmen. Some came with belongings and money; others had little more than the clothes on their

Blasting away with pressurized water jets, miners loosen gold-bearing gravel. Such techniques damaged the environment in the rush to exploit western resources. The artist, Mrs. Jonas Brown, lived in Idaho City during the height of its gold rush.

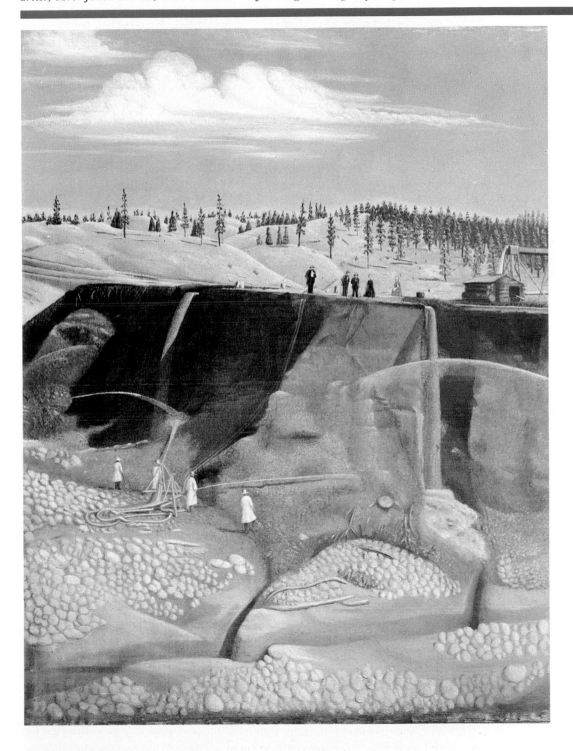

backs. While the weather was still cold, they sought shelter beneath tarpaulins along the river levee, built fires by the shore and got out frying pans to cook their meals while their children jumped rope nearby. By the end of April over 6,000 had arrived; by the end of 1879, over 20,000. When the crowds became too much for the wharves and temporary shelters, the city's black churches banded together to shelter the "refugees," feed them, and help them continue toward Kansas. The news that rail passage would not be free, as many rumors had it, did not shake their almost millennial faith in their mission. "We's like de chilun ob Israel when dey was led from out o' bondage by Moses," one explained, referring to the exodus from Egypt across the Red Sea. "Dis is our Red Sea, right hyah in St. Louis, atween home an' Kansas, an' if we sticks togeder an' keeps up our faith we'll git to Kansas and be out o' bondage for shuah." So the "Exodusters," as they became known, pressed onward.

Adjusting to the new land was often not easy, any more for black emigrants than for whites. Both northerners and southerners were accustomed to forested country, where lumber was plentiful for building houses and for cooking. The Exodusters were not prepared for the harsh Kansas winters either. "Kansas has the roughest wind you ever run across in *your* life," commented one; another was dismayed to find that cotton did not flourish in prairie soil. "If I were back home I might get in a crop of cotton; but I cannot make enough here." Those who did manage to settle on farms met with the hatred of cattlemen whose herds grazed the prairies. One settler from Nicodemus, an early black colony, wrote the governor of Kansas, begging him to "please get rede of the Catel we are so rounded with the hured [herders] do not care for us."

In the end, more black emigrants settled in the growing towns like Topeka, Lincoln, or Kansas City. Men might get jobs as hired hands, while the women worked as washerwomen. With luck, couples made $350 a year, saved a bit of it for a home, and put down roots. Bill Sims, an emigrant who settled in Ottawa, Kansas, put down roots literally—working at tree husbandry for a living. When his wife died, he promised her on her deathbed that he would educate their two daughters. By the 1930s, when he was in his nineties, he could boast that his oldest had been the "first colored girl to ever graduate" from Ottawa University; his other daughter had become a schoolteacher. And on the courthouse grounds at the center of town, the trees he had planted years before were still standing.

Sims and the host of Exodusters who poured into Kansas were part of a more general flood westward. In 1879, as blacks traveled up the Mississippi to St. Louis, a thousand white emigrants arrived in Kansas every week. Special trains brought settlers to the plains, all eager to start anew, whether they were farmers from Pennsylvania or Russian Mennonites newly emigrated. During the 1870s, Nebraska's population increased from 123,000 to over 450,000; during the 1880s the number of Kansans jumped from a million to a million and a half. "We have plenty of room for all creation," boasted a newspaper in Olathe, Kansas.

Yet the spirit of boosterism and hope could not mask serious strains in the rapidly expanding nation, especially in the South and West. The boom economies of cotton, cattle, and grain all depended on urban markets. The market for cotton lay with the textile mills of New England (and, increasingly, the "New South"), while the demand for beef and western grains came from metropolitan centers. Especially during hard times, westerners and southerners saw themselves as the victims of a colonial economic system, in which their fortunes were controlled by the industries of the Northeast. Like colonial subjects of European imperialists, the West and South exported inexpensive raw materials and imported more expensive manufactured goods. And as rural people, they found themselves alienated from a culture that was increasingly urban.

The more rural South and West were also marked by the conflicts of race and ethnicity, just as the centers of industry had been. The racism of these regions provided the rationale for creating a society based on caste; violence offered one means to establish and sustain it. The Exodusters of 1879 had left the South in large part because of the increasing violence of white "Redeemers." On the western ranges racism took the form of open warfare between whites and Indians, whose cultures clashed directly. (The cowboys, after all, could not have expanded their rangeland farther west so long as the Indians' wild cattle—the buffalo— dominated the grazing lands of the Plains.) Against Hispanics, Asians, and African-Americans, whites adopted a mixture of physical intimidation, segregation, and other legal mechanisms that denied minorities the rights of citizens.

As the two regions became tied more closely to the industrial Northeast, the tensions and imbalances between the regions subjected the national political system to stresses even in boom times. Drought, exhausted mines, overcut timberlands, and overproduction in cattle and grain demonstrated the limits of the regions' economies. The inevitable adjustments were often wrenching.

THE SOUTHERN BURDEN

In the era following Reconstruction a faith in economic progress flourished in the South. Propagandists for this ideal, led by Henry Grady of the Atlanta *Constitution*, envisioned a "New South" based on bustling industry, cities, and commerce. The business class and its values would displace the old planter class as southerners raced "to out-Yankee the Yankee." Yet while Grady spread the gospel of laissez-faire capitalism and economic diversity, no amount of hopeful rhetoric could change the economic structure of the South as an agrarian society. As late as 1890 the census counted less than 10 percent of all southerners as urban dwellers, compared to more than 50 percent in the North Atlantic states. The South had not only fewer large cities but also fewer small towns, which had become an important source of economic diversification in the Midwest.

Even more relevant to the South's problems, its antebellum economy had depended largely on slave labor. In 1860 the value of slaves in the five cotton states—Alabama, Louisiana, South Carolina, Georgia, and Mississippi—had amounted to 60 percent of all agricultural wealth, whereas the value of farmlands and buildings amounted to less than a third. In Harrison County, Texas, for example, a typical slaveholding family owned $10,000 worth of property in slaves, three times the value of their land and buildings. This fundamental fact ensured that slaveholders tried to concentrate their wealth in slaves, not land, which often seemed almost disposable. Planters would clear new fields, plow them, exhaust them in a few years, and move on in search of new profits rather than settling down, as prosperous northern farmers did. Not only the larger "cotton lords" but smaller operators too carried their wealth in slaves. A farmer who owned only three slaves had a greater investment in his human property than the average nonslaveholding farmer had in all his assets combined.

Thus while northern society in the 1840s and 1850s was building canals and rail links, developing towns that would serve surrounding farms and drive up land values, southerners were accumulating comparatively little wealth in land, factories, buildings, or transportation facilities. The railroads and canals that did exist tied staple crop areas to ports rather than opening the back country to economic development. The southern economy that emerged from the Civil War was therefore decentralized, isolated, and agricultural.

Certainly publicists like Henry Grady were right about the South's potential. The region extending from Delaware south to Florida and west to Texas and Oklahoma took in a third of the nation's total area, a third of its arable farm lands, two-thirds of the land with over 40 inches of rainfall each year, vast tracts of lumber, and rich deposits of coal, iron, oil, and fertilizers. But to overcome the devastation inflicted by the war and the loss of wealth based on slaveholding, southern entrepreneurs needed to wage a major campaign to catch up with the rest of the nation. Indeed, they did better than popular myth would suggest. In rates of growth for urban areas, as well as for mining, textiles, lumber, and railroad building, the postwar South equaled or surpassed other regions of the country.

Still, the South lagged far behind. The war had abolished slavery, but it had not wiped out the inferior status of blacks, who continued to receive distinctly lower wages for their labor than did northern or western workers. This economic hardship not only worked a disservice to blacks, but it depressed the wage scale for the region as a whole. Despite all its natural and human resources, the South remained the poorest section of the United States well into the twentieth century. It was the low-wage market that unified the experience of blacks and whites who were otherwise separated by caste and culture.

Cotton in the New South

One barrier to economic development arose from continued reliance on agricultural staples like tobacco, rice, sugar, and especially cotton. Although southerners had boasted that cotton was king in the region and nation during the 1850s, between 1870 and 1900 the number of acres planted in cotton more than doubled. In a turnabout, as the use of fertilizers increased, the crop spread eastward into areas that had once been considered marginal for cotton.

In good years, southern farms were more profitable than those in other regions. But from 1880 to 1900 the world demand for cotton grew at only about 2.7 percent per year, so prices fell. Even as cotton farmers worked to increase their productivity, they lost ground. While farms in other parts of the country were becoming larger, more efficient, and tended by fewer workers per acre, the average size of a southern farm fell. This partly reflected the breakup of large plantations before the war, but it also was caused by a continued high birth rate in the South. In other regions of the country, the number of children born per mother was dropping, but in the South, the continuing large family size meant that fewer acres of land were available for each person to cultivate. Thus even though the southern economy kept pace with national growth, per capita income fell behind. Before 1900, the South prospered in only a few pockets, such as South Carolina's fertilizer regions, Birmingham's steel industry, and areas of Kentucky, North Carolina, and Virginia that benefited from a rise in tobacco prices.

Some southern farmers sought roads to prosperity other than cotton. George Washington Carver, of Alabama's Tuskegee Institute for blacks (page 786), persuaded many poor farmers to plant peanuts. But most southern soils were too acidic and the rains too heavy in the spring for grains and legumes to flourish. Corn and other food crops offered a hedge against poor cotton prices, but they brought in no cash. Parasites and diseases plagued cattle herds, reducing weight and milk yields. Work animals like mules were raised more cheaply in other regions. As much as southerners might seek alternative sources of income, cotton still dominated the region's economic life. "When southern cotton prices drop, every man feels the blow," one observer commented; "when cotton prices advance, every industry thrives with vigor."

Sharecropping

Emancipation during the Civil War had brought to John Solomon Lewis and other former slaves not only freedom from servitude, but hopes of economic independence. In the era after the war Lewis rented land to grow cotton in Tensas Parish, Louisiana. The devastations of war followed by the severe depression of the 1870s dashed his hopes. "I was in debt," Lewis explained, "and the man I rented land from said every year I must rent again to pay the other year, and so I rents and rents and each year I gets deeper and deeper in debt."

Lewis' lament expressed the plight of small farmers both black and white in the cotton South. The South's best lands remained in the hands of large plantation

---

"Forty acres and a mule" had been the dream of newly freed slave families at the end of the Civil War; sharecropping or tenant farming was more often their lot. At least 'croppers had the advantage of living in cabins much closer to the fields they worked. This scene was sketched in 1901 by H. T. West.

The Geography of the Postwar South

In 1860 slaves accounted for nearly 60 percent of the agricultural wealth in the cotton states stretching from South Carolina to Louisiana. The value of farm lands and buildings amounted to less than a third. Emancipation changed all that. With slaves no longer "property" that could be controlled or moved at will, land itself became an important measure of worth. Southern planters and farmers who had once been "labor lords" became landlords to whom property now meant land. This shift was reflected in the geography of the postwar South.

Railroads increased the value of land by opening up interior markets; after the Civil War, southerners eagerly participated in the nationwide railroad boom, in marked contrast with the pre-war years. By 1890 (see maps at left) an enlarged rail network was well established. Cotton production also rose sharply. In southeastern regions, where soils had been thought "exhausted," fertilizers increased output. Farther west, more intensive use of labor increased per acre yields. In both cases, greater crop volume enhanced the value of land, to the advantage of farmers and planters alike.

As the new agricultural system stabilized after 1880, large landowners divided their holdings into plots that they worked for themselves, bringing in wage laborers who lived in quarters the owners provided (see map at left) and land that they rented to tenants or sharecroppers. On the one hand, wage laborers allowed landowners the flexibility of bringing in workers for peak harvesting seasons, then laying them off later; on the other hand, sharecroppers and tenants, having signed a yearly contract, provided the security of knowing someone would be there to work the land. Because wage laborers had to travel from farm to farm in order to continue working, they tended to be young, single males. Sharecroppers and tenants were usually families who preferred to stay in one place.

Shortages of capital needed to establish independent farms made tenantry the dominant pattern in southern agriculture after the war (see map below). But notice that by 1900 tenantry accounted for much of the farm labor in areas of the trans-Mississippi West settled under the generous terms of the Homestead Act of 1862. There, too, low crop prices, the heavy cost of land and equipment, and severe environmental conditions forced independent farmers into tenantry.

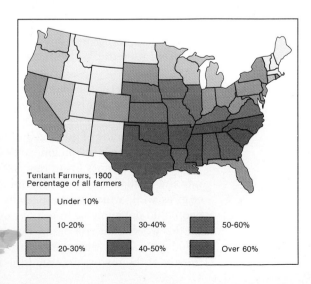

Tenant Farmers, 1900
Percentage of all farmers

Under 10%
10-20%
20-30%
30-40%
40-50%
50-60%
Over 60%

owners. Those owners had little cash to pay wages for farm labor. And only a few among the land-hungry freedmen or poor whites had the wherewithal to acquire land of their own. So, like Lewis they rented, and like Lewis they saw their debts pile up. The average tenant in the Deep South from Alabama to Texas seldom had more than 15 to 20 acres. Since cotton was king and money scarce, rents were generally set in pounds of cotton rather than in dollars. Usually the amount added up to about one-quarter to one-half the value of a farmer's annual crop. If a tenant was lucky enough to find a generous planter, or if an area had a shortage of tenant farmers, or if the tenant had tools and farm animals of his own, then the terms of the rent might be less burdensome.

This system of farming on shares, or sharecropping, would not have proven so ruinous if the South had possessed a more equitable system of credit. But before they could sell their crop in the fall, farmers without cash had to borrow money in the spring to buy their seeds, tools, and other necessities. The only source for those supplies in most areas of the South was the local store. When John Solomon Lewis and other tenants entered the store they saw two prices, one for cash and one for credit. The credit price might be as much as 60 percent higher, in effect a 60 percent interest charge. By contrast, merchants in New York City seldom charged their customers more than 6 percent to buy on credit. The only asset most sharecroppers could offer as security was a mortgage or lien on their crops. This meant in turn that the shopkeeper rather than the sharecropper had first claim on the crop until the debt was paid off, a practice that was known as the crop–lien system.

Many planters recognized that running a store was a way to increase profits. They would rent the land and then sell the goods needed to farm. At the same time storeowners without land often held mortgages on nearby farms. As farms failed, the merchants took them through foreclosure, thereby becoming large landholders themselves. Most tenants found they were twice indebted: they owed part of the crop to the landlord and the remainder to the shopkeeper—more often than not the same person.

The combination of sharecropping and crop liens led to debt peonage. Economic dependence robbed the small farmers of their freedom. The landlord–shopkeeper could insist that sharecroppers devote their efforts solely to producing profitable crops rather than foodstuffs. In the post–Civil War South that almost always meant cotton, which yielded more value per acre than any other crop. Instead of raising corn and hogs, sharecroppers had to use credit to buy food imported from the Midwest. One observer noted that Louisiana farmers "had not as much as twenty-five to fifty dollars cash money (about the value of one 400- to 450-pound bale) at the end of any one year. That they always, at the owner's mode of settling, was in his debt. Yet, they did not even have half enough to eat or scarcely anything to wear."

The problems of ginning and marketing made matters worse. Few areas had more than a single cotton gin, so that no price competition existed. Most landlords insisted that tenants bring raw cotton to their mills to be ginned and baled, at a rate the landlord set himself. And most landlords claimed the right to market the crop as well, which was especially onerous to black sharecroppers. "The white people do not allow us to sell our own crops," blacks regularly remarked. "When we do, we do it at risk of our lives, getting whipped, shot at, and often some get killed." Or as one disgruntled farmer complained, "We had to carry the cotton to the gin of the man who owned the land we rented, and he would take it all from us." Though statistics show that blacks were economically better off in freedom than in slavery, sharecropping, crop liens, and monopolies on ginning and marketing added up to inequality and crushing poverty for the South's small farmers.

Southern Industry

By the 1880s many southerners came to believe that industrialization was the only way the South could shed its yoke of poverty. The gospel of the New South swept some localities with the fervor of a religious camp meeting. By soaking up unemployed agricultural labor, new industries would become as much social as business enterprises. "People were urged to take stock . . . for the town's sake, for the poor people's sake, literally for God's sake," one writer explained.

In many ways the crusade for a New South was crowned with success. Southern industrial production from 1869 to 1909 grew faster than the national rate. So did productivity for southern workers. A boom in railroad building after 1879 furnished the region with a good transportation network. The number of industrial workers tripled (209,000 to 600,000), as did the value of manufactures.

In two areas, cotton textiles and tobacco, southern advances were especially striking. Aided by easy access to cotton fiber and abundant cheap labor, 161 cotton mills were in operation by 1880. That number jumped to 400 by 1900, with the mills employing almost 100,000 workers. Local custom dictated that most textile workers be whites, drawn from the ranks of poorly paid agricultural wage earners escaping the competition of blacks, or mountain folk escaping the poverty of poor soils. Many mills employed entire families, though it soon became clear that older men used to working outdoors in a rhythm dictated by the sun and seasons lacked the temperament demanded to tend spindles and looms. But over time, as southern farm folk were socialized to the monotonous rhythms of indoor factory work for wages, they became competitive with workers from other regions of the United States and western Europe.

The tobacco industry also thrived in the New South. Before the Civil War American taste in tobacco had run to cigars, snuff, and chewing tobacco. By the 1880s popular taste in the North shifted to a new product, cigarettes. (Southern men tended to consider them effeminate.) James Bonsack had coincidentally in-

Textile production was critical to the industrial expansion of the New South. Most mill towns attracted entire families, almost all of them white. Conditions were generally cramped, noisy, and unsafe. These women at the White Oaks Mills in Greensboro, North Carolina, are measuring and sewing denim.

vented in 1880 a machine that made it possible to roll vast numbers of cigarettes at low cost. The growing popularity of smoking was reflected in the rate of annual tobacco consumption, which soared from 1.5 pounds per person in 1860 to 5.5 pounds in 1900. Americans spent more money on tobacco than on clothes or shoes. The health consequences of the new fad would not become evident until nearly a hundred years later.

The sudden taste for smoking offered southerners a rare opportunity to control a major national market. But the factories were so hot, the smells so strong, and the work so unskilled that whites generally refused the jobs. James Buchanan Duke solved the labor problem by hiring Russian Jewish immigrants to train local blacks in the techniques of tobacco work. Then he adopted the Bonsack machine to mechanize cigarette rolling. A vigorous national advertising campaign and ruthless use of promotional gimmicks allowed Duke to destroy or buy out his competitors. By 1890 he had built his American Tobacco Company into a major trust that dominated the industry.

The Colonial South

Jobs in textiles and tobacco paid better wages than agricultural labor and thus formed the basis of industrial growth. These industries also encouraged urbanization and investment of capital for regional development, but they could not by themselves lift the region from poverty. Both reflected the prevailing low-wage pattern of southern agriculture rather than the higher wage patterns of the industrial Northeast and upper Midwest. During the same period when the heavy flood of immigrants was expanding both work forces and markets in other sections of the nation, low wages discouraged immigrants from settling in the South. Isolated from the international labor pool, the southern labor force grew almost exclusively from natural increase.

The realities of southern economic life were more accurately reflected in lumber and steel than in tobacco and textiles. In the postwar era, the South possessed over 60 percent of the nation's timber resources. With soaring demand to meet the needs of the nation's rapidly growing towns and cities, lumber became the South's leading industry and number one employer. If anything, however, aggressive lumbering left the South far poorer. Corrupt state governments and relaxed federal timber policy allowed northerners and foreigners to acquire huge forest tracts at prices far below their actual value. Most of the timber was sold as raw lumber rather than finished products such as cedar shingles or newsprint, though the manufacture of furniture did flourish in North Carolina.

Logging camps were set up as isolated and temporary settlements. Visitors described the predominantly black work force as "single, homeless, and possessionless." The ruthless overcutting and other bad lumbering practices typical in all regions during this exploitative era destroyed the southern forests' capacity for self-renewal and led to severe problems of soil erosion and flooding. Having devastated the forests around their camps, the loggers quickly moved on to repeat their acts of destruction elsewhere. The sawmills to which they sent the cut timber were scarcely more permanent. The workers, mostly single, young black men, had little time to forge bonds of common interest among themselves or roots in the local community. Most mills operated for only a few years in any one place before the owners followed the loggers to a new area. They generally left without having contributed significantly to local development.

The fact that most mill workers were black added to the industry's relative isolation from nearby towns. Logging and lumbering provided young southern blacks the single greatest source of employment. The work was unskilled, dirty, dangerous, and temporary. High turnover and low morale often led southerners to blame the workers, not the operators, for the industry's low standards. As one critic complained, "The sawmill negro is rather shiftless and is not inclined to stay in any one location and consequently there is little incentive on the part of the owner or operator to carry on welfare work in any extensive manner." In fact, most blacks left the mills in search of higher wages or to settle down to sharecropping in order to marry and support families.

Even more symptomatic of the South's economic woes was the failure of the iron and steel industry to meet the expectations of the New South's promoters. By burning coke as a fuel to produce pig iron, Chattanooga, Tennessee, and Birmingham, Alabama, became major centers for foundries. Birmingham had the special advantage of being located closer than any other industrial center to *both* iron and coal deposits. By the 1890s the Tennessee Coal, Iron, and Railway Company (TCI) had turned its Birmingham facilities into the major producer of iron pipe for use in the gas, water, and sewer lines vital to urban growth. Unfortunately for Birmingham, its iron deposits were ill suited to produce the kinds of steel in high demand. By 1907 TCI had become so financially strapped that it had to sell out to the giant U.S. Steel Corporation, controlled by northern interests.

The disappointing contribution of the lumber and iron industries to southern economic growth was paralleled by other leading industries such as mining, chemical fertilizers, cottonseed oil, and railroads. Though all these industries grew dramatically in employment and the value of their products, they failed to meet the rosy predictions of the apostles of the New South. The region remained largely rural, agricultural, and poor.

Southerners of the day as well as modern historians have argued that the South suffered from the exploitation of outside financial interests. The region was in short a colonial economy, they claimed, relying for its wealth on extractive products such as minerals and timber or staple crops whose value had not increased through processing into finished goods. Profits that might have been used to foster development in the South were siphoned off to other regions, as decisions affecting the region's economic health were made in New York or Pittsburgh, not in Atlanta or New Orleans.

More recent analysis, however, suggests that economic growth lagged due to three factors peculiar to the South, rather than any conspiracy of outside capitalists. First, the South began to industrialize later than the Northeast, so northern entrepreneurs and workers had a head start on learning the new manufacturing techniques. Northern workers could be more productive, not because they were more energetic or disciplined, but because they were more experienced. Once Southern workers overcame that differential, they competed equally. Second, the South commanded only a small technologically skilled community to guide its industrial development. Since northern engineers and mechanics seldom followed northern capital into the region, few people were available to adapt modern technology to southern conditions. Southerners who did want to remain in the region found it difficult. For example, George Gordon Crawford, a Georgian who eventually became director of Tennessee Coal and Iron's Alabama operations, had to travel to Germany to receive his graduate education and then spent 15 years mastering steel operations at the Carnegie plant in Pennsylvania before returning to his homeland. Thus the South found itself importing advanced technologies and machinery even when they were ill adapted to southern conditions. The Bessemer process, for instance, did not work well with the type of iron ore found near Birmingham.

Southerners might have overcome this problem by upgrading the region's work force through better education. But no region in the nation spent as little on schooling as the South. Even before the war southern leaders were hostile to government services in general, largely to keep taxes low. The elite cared little about educating ordinary whites and openly resisted educating blacks. Education, they contended, "spoiled" otherwise contented workers and led them to demand higher wages and improved conditions. More important, better educated workers often left the region in search of higher paying jobs. Nor did the region invest heavily in technical colleges and engineering schools like the ones northern capitalists funded at Cornell University (1865) and the Massachusetts Institute of Technology (1859).

The lack of education was a critical factor behind the third and most central source of southern poverty, the isolation of the southern labor market. In 1900 agriculture still dominated the southern economy, and it required an unskilled, low-paid work force of sharecroppers and wage laborers. Ever fearful of outside influences that might spread discontent among the industrial and agricultural poor, southerners perpetuated conditions that also discouraged much needed outside human and capital resources. The South remained poor because it received too little, not too much, outside investment.

THE RISE OF JIM CROW

When Reconstruction and Radical Republican rule ended in the South after 1876, northerners gave up any pretense of protecting black freedmen. To achieve sectional reconciliation, whites both North and South were willing to sacrifice the rights of blacks. Southerners were relieved that in the matter of race relations they would be "left alone" by the federal government. That laissez-faire approach suited northern former champions of black rights like *The Nation* magazine, which had come to doubt whether former slaves could participate in "a system of government for which you [northern readers] and I have much respect." The Compromise of 1877 (page 637) guaranteed that blacks would remain free but did not guarantee political equality.

Segregation

Whatever their politics before the war, the Redeemer politicians who came to power in southern states afterward adopted a probusiness posture. Mostly Democrats, they were eager to develop the New South and reap benefits from its economic expansion. To attract the business-oriented elements—bankers, railroad promoters, industrial leaders—the ruling Democrats sometimes referred to themselves as Conservatives or conservative Democrats. As their part of the bargain, the Redeemers assured anxious northerners that home rule would not mean the wholesale political disfranchisement of the freedmen. So long as freed blacks identified their interests with those of conservative whites, leading southerners like

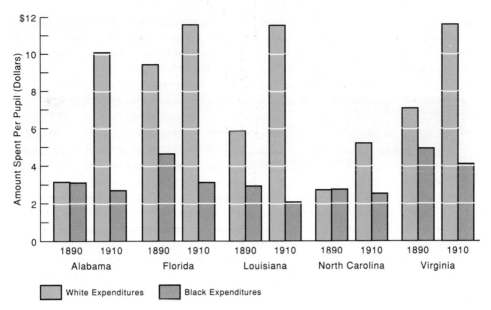

Source: Data from Robert A. Margo, *Disfranchisement, School Finance, and the Economics of Segregated Schools in the U.S. South, 1890-1910* (New York: Garland Press, 1985), table I-1.

SPENDING ON EDUCATION IN THE SOUTH
BEFORE AND AFTER DISFRANCHISEMENT
With disfranchisement and segregation, education was separate, but hardly equal for blacks and whites.

Alexander Stephens of Georgia, Wade Hampton of South Carolina, and L. Q. C. Lamar of Mississippi saw no reason to "take [blacks] out of politics as a factor or leading issue." And blacks did continue to entertain clear ideas about their political interests, to vote, and to hold some minor public offices, especially in states like South Carolina, where black majorities held the balance between rival political factions.

Whatever tolerance had existed began to disappear in the 1880s, as the new Redeemer governments moved to formalize a "Jim Crow" system of segregation.* As more blacks moved into southern towns and cities to compete for jobs with whites, and as their status as free laborers (and often voters) blurred the social line between them and poor whites, pressures increased to separate blacks as social inferiors. That was made somewhat difficult by the Civil Rights Act of 1875, in which Congress had guaranteed persons of every race the right to use public facilities such as hotels, theaters, and railroads. But when a number of blacks sued after being denied those rights, the Supreme Court ruled (in the *Civil Rights Cases*, 1883) that the 1875 law was invalid. Hotels and railroads were not "public" institutions, the Court argued narrowly; they were owned by private individuals. The Fourteenth Amendment was thus said to protect citizens from violations of their civil rights only by states, not by private individuals. The national policy of laissez faire in race relations could not have been made any clearer, and southern legislatures got the message.

*The term "Jim Crow," to denote a policy of segregation, originated in a song of the same name sung in minstrel shows of the day.

Within 20 years every southern state had enacted a legal system of racial separation. The earliest laws limited segregation largely to schools and trains, but soon a complex web of Jim Crow statutes had drawn a color line indelibly in prisons, parks, hotels, restaurants, hospitals, and virtually all public places except streets and stores. And again the Supreme Court accepted the new state of affairs in *Plessy v. Ferguson* (1896). That decision upheld a Louisiana law requiring segregated railroad facilities by arguing that segregation did not constitute discrimination under the equal protection clause of the Fourteenth Amendment, so long as accommodations for both races were equal. In reality, of course, the segregated facilities stigmatized blacks. Such facilities were always separate but seldom met the standard of equality.

By the turn of the century segregation was firmly in place. Jim Crow effectively stifled significant economic competition. Jobs such as those in textile mills were restricted largely to whites, while skilled and professional blacks were generally allowed to serve only a black clientele. Blacks could enter some white residential areas only as servants and hired help. They were barred from juries and generally received far stiffer penalties than whites who committed similar crimes. And as the law became entrenched, so did social custom. Blacks always called whites, even those of lower status, Mister, Miss, and Ma'am, but to whites, no matter what age or profession blacks might be, they were called by first name or more simply Sister or Boy. If any black crossed the lines drawn by whites, the consequences were often violent. A rapid increase in lynchings accompanied the rise of Jim Crow. Of the 187 lynchings averaged in each year of the 1890s, some 80 percent occurred in the South, where the large majority of victims were black.

Disfranchisement

"The best friends of the colored men are the old slaveholders," politician Wade Hampton told a group of black voters in 1878. " . . . They will defend your right to vote because it gives to the South infinitely more power than we ever had before." Hampton and other conservative Democrats espoused this policy so long as black voters marched to the polls to vote their way. But if wooing failed, whites resorted to various forms of coercion. Implicit on many occasions was the threat of violence if blacks did not vote according to instruction. One Mississippi newspaper observed in 1883 that should freedmen "not vote with the Democrats, it would be better for them and the county that they refuse to participate in the election. The weather might be warm that day and they might get sun-struck." Whether by persuasive appeal, bribery, fraud, or intimidation, the conservative Democrats did regularly manage to remain in power with the help of blacks.

Those who sought to reform either the political or economic system courted black votes too. The issues varied from state to state—"greenback" currency reforms, public school legislation, complaints about the laws that allowed convict labor (poor whites as well as blacks) to be hired out—but in each case, the threat of an alliance between poor whites and poor blacks was always there. Conservatives began to argue that it might be better if blacks were disfranchised, eliminating even their minimal influence in politics.

Mississippi, which during Reconstruction had led the move to "redeem" its state from Radical Republicans, in 1890 again took the lead in disfranchising black voters. In a constitutional convention, delegates required that voters henceforth would be required to pay a poll tax and pass a literacy test. Such tests made it possible to eliminate the great majority of black voters, especially if election officials interpreted the requirements strictly. Poll taxes were first adopted in the North and South to fund schools. Since many blacks were too poor to pay even a small amount, the new poll tax would keep them from voting. Then, too, Mississippi required that the tax be paid in advance and the receipt presented on the day of voting, a cumbersome and discouraging procedure. Conservative Democrats favored the plan because it reduced not only black voting but also that of poor whites, who were most likely to join opposition parties. Before Mississippi's new constitution went into effect, there were 257,305 eligible voters in the state; in 1892, after its adoption, that number plummeted to 76,742.[*]

Conservatives in other southern states were envious. "We would do well to imitate the wise politicians of Mississippi," noted one Alabama journal. "The poll tax gets rid of most of the negro votes there," wrote an enthusiastic Louisiana observer, "but it gets rid of a great many whites at the same time—in fact a majority of them." But for just that reason, the issue of voter disfranchisement remained explosive in many southern states. As more and more small farmers angrily challenged the corruption of conservative Democratic rule in the early 1890s, some held out for an alliance with black voters to change the system. Once that challenge failed, the move for disfranchisement swept the rest of the South by the end of the century, with devastating results for blacks.

THE TRANSFORMED WEST

The West, like the South, has been defined not so much as a particular place but as a distinctive culture shaped by an unusual set of conditions. For historian Frederick Jackson Turner, writing in the 1890s, the West was shaped by the frontier, an area of "free land" to be found beyond the point of white settlement. In the ethnocentric fashion of his age, Turner ignored the presence of rich and varied tribal cultures beyond the frontier, where Indians hardly considered their lands "free" for use by whites. By the time the Civil War broke out, the frontier of white settlement had moved beyond the Mississippi, but it had "jumped" across the Great Plains to the Pacific, as "Overlanders" settled the farmlands of California and Oregon. The frontier then pushed east from the Pacific coast, following miners into the Sierra Nevadas. At the same time, farmers and ranchers pushed west from the Mississippi into what had been popularly known as "the Great American desert."

Most areas of this Great Plains region, west of the 98th meridian, receive less than 20 inches of rainfall a year. In the Great Basin area of Utah, Nevada, and eastern California the climate is even drier. In extreme cases, the air becomes so dry that rain evaporates before hitting the ground. The infrequent stands of timber cluster along river bottoms, making wood for housing and fences scarce. To eastern farmers accustomed to ready access to water, timber, and tillable land, the region between the 98th meridian and the fertile valleys of the West Coast at first seemed suitable for neither man nor beast. Many Overlanders of the 1840s and 1850s compared its vast windy spaces to the oceans, a "sea of grass" stretching to the horizon crossed by "prairie schooners."

---

[*]It was perhaps doubly ironic that the convention, convinced that lower-class whites as well as blacks would oppose the changes, simply declared the new constitution adopted. They never allowed it to be ratified in a popular vote.

Native Americans and the Western Environment

Easterners who watched the wagons head west liked to conjure up the image of a "trackless wilderness," but in truth, even in the 1840s the Great Plains and mountain frontier comprised a region in which Spanish, Anglo-American, and Native American cultures were interacting with one another in unstable, swiftly changing ways. The horse, introduced into North America by the colonial Spanish, had spread by the eighteenth century across the plains. By the nineteenth century the Comanche, Cheyenne, Sioux, Kiowa, Blackfoot, Apache, and other tribes were among the great equestrians of the world. The mobility they attained on horseback significantly increased the area in which they could hunt the buffalo, and it transformed many of their cultures from a relatively settled, village-centered, horticultural way of life to a more aggressively nomadic existence.

Under the Indian Removal Act of 1830 the forced relocation of eastern tribes to lands west of the Mississippi also disturbed intertribal patterns. The dry climate of the western plains was an environment for which the woodland cultures of eastern tribes were ill-suited. Western tribes such as the Comanche, Pawnee, and Osage resented the intrusion of the newcomers, who raided their camps and drove off livestock. The Sioux, perhaps the most feared warriors of the Plains in the mid-nineteenth century, had emerged from the forests of the Great Lakes only a century earlier. They were able to expand partly because they began using firearms before other tribes and partly because they escaped the worst ravages of white diseases, which decimated many plains tribes.

Some whites—usually those who had the least contact with native Americans—viewed Indians as "noble savages," whose "natural" way of life remained in harmony with the elements, a myth still perpetuated by far too many scholars. To be sure, the population density of Indian settlement remained low enough so that their impact on the western environment was relatively small compared with later white settlement. And Indians could be remarkably inventive about making the most of the resources around them. The bark of the cottonwood proved good food for horses during the winter, while the buffalo supplied not only meat but also bones for tools, fat for cosmetics, and sinews for thread. But Indians had traditionally hunted bison by stampeding them over cliffs, which resulted in tremendous waste of food. They irrigated crops, set fires on the plains to improve the game and vegetation, and in other ways actively altered their environment.

By the mid-nineteenth century they had also become enmeshed in a web of white trade, supplying furs in return for firearms, cloth, metal tools, and jewelry. Since the environment could sustain only a finite amount of use, Indians suffered, just as white trappers did, when the fur trade led to overtrapping. And the Sioux nation expanded so aggressively because its increasing population forced the tribe to enlarge its base of resources. It would be misleading, then, to view native societies in the Great Plains as isolated from white cultures, living as they had from time out of mind. For more than a century, the West had been in dramatic flux, as white and Indian cultures borrowed and adapted from one another, often clashing in competition for the region's limited resources.

Whites and Indians found themselves in conflict because their values were so much at odds. Generalizations about Indians in the West are hard to sustain because their cultures were as varied as the western environment. Although big-game hunting was common among western Indians, the nomadic buffalo culture of the Great Plains was hardly representative. Along the Pacific Northwest coast the

The cultures of western Indians were remarkably varied, ranging from the nomadic Plains tribes to the more settled peoples of the northwest coast who lived off the sea. This Sioux woman gathers firewood; the photograph was taken by Edward Curtis, who spent many years recording the faces and lives of western tribes.

Yuroks, Coos, Umpqua, Chinook, and other tribes hunted the woods and mountains for bear, moose, elk, and deer. They also took from the ocean whales, seals, and a variety of fish. The Klamaths, Yakimas, and Walla Wallas moved into the river valleys for the great salmon runs. Where the land was less bountiful, Indian tribes lived close to starvation. Utes, Shoshones, Paiutes, and Pavistos scoured the hot, arid Great Basin deserts to eke out a diet of rabbits, snakes, insects, roots, berries, seeds, and nuts. The early Hohokams and later the Havasupais, Pima, and other tribes in New Mexico and Arizona developed irrigation to allow farming of beans, squash, and corn in the arid climate.

Despite such diversity, Indian tribes did share certain values. Most were small, extended kinship groups in which the well-being of the community outweighed the needs of the individual. While some tribes were materially better off than others, the gap between rich and poor within tribes was seldom large. Egalitarian material culture tended to promote egalitarian decision making. The Cheyenne, for example, employed a council of 44 to advise the chief.

What most separated white and Indian cultures were attitudes toward the land and all that was on it. Man, for the Indians, was not a transcendent being, but a single part of a complex web of animals, plants, and other natural elements—all with souls of their own. Whereas Europeans viewed nature as a resource to be exploited, the Indians saw it as sacred. The Taos of New Mexico, for example, believed that each spring the pregnant earth issued new life. To avoid disturbing "mother" earth, they removed the hard shoes from their horses and themselves walked in bare feet or soft moccasins. Whites were mystified by the attitude of Chief Somohalla of the Wanapaun tribe who explained why his people refused to farm: "You ask me to plow the ground! Shall I take a knife and tear my mother's bosom? . . . You ask me to cut grass and make hay and sell it, and be rich like white men! But how dare I cut off my mother's hair?"

Such reverence for the land gave Indians a religious loyalty to special places. The Taos centered their spiritual and economic life on Blue Lake in northwest New Mexico, the source of life and the revelations of the great spirit of the universe. The Shoshone in eastern California came to Coso Hot Springs for healing and worship. To white migrants from the East or from Europe, these places had no special meaning. Where the Sioux saw in the Black Hills the sacred home of Wakan Tanka, the burial place of the dead and the site of their "vision quests," whites saw the possibility of gold and grass for grazing their herds. From such misunderstandings came conflict. To some white Americans, the Indians seemed a hopelessly savage people whose just fate was extermination. To other whites, moved by Christian zeal or "enlightened" sympathy, the Indian was a child, an inferior being, who needed to be first protected and then assimilated into American society. To survive either killing or kindness, Indians had to find ways to resist both forms of attack.

Whites and the Western Environment

The balance of power between white and Indian cultures changed dramatically in the years following the Civil War. For Indians it was a time of transition and rebuilding as well as military defeat and despair. For white Americans the new industrial order created both the means and the motive to close the final western frontiers. Transcontinental rail lines, standardized rail gauges and freight systems, telegraph lines to coordinate communications, systems of large-scale finance and military power, and rapidly growing urban markets all made it easier to accelerate white settlement in the West, especially in the least settled areas of the Great Plains.

Even among whites, however, attitudes varied as to how Americans should take advantage of the frontier region. As repeated discoveries of gold and silver brought whites into Indian territory, many adopted the confident, booster outlook of Missouri politician William Gilpin. To Gilpin, the Indians seemed just one more impediment that would be pushed aside by the expansive force of the American people. Only the lack of vision among those in the East prevented the nation from opening the West for exploitation, he told an Independence, Missouri, audience in 1849. What was most needed were cheap lands and a railroad linking the two coasts "like ears on a human head."

By 1868 the dreams of western expansionists were becoming reality. A generous Congress had granted the West its two greatest wishes: free land, under the Homestead Act of 1862, and a transcontinental railroad. As the new governor of Colorado, Gilpin told a July Fourth audience that the resources of the region were so limitless that the land would one day support over a billion people. The limited rainfall and water resources did not daunt him, for in his eyes the West was a garden, not "the Great American desert" it had been called for so many years. If the rains did not come, farmers would find all the water they needed in artesian wells deep underground. Once the land had been planted, the rains would develop naturally, Gilpin assured his listeners, for he subscribed to the popular myth that "rain follows the plow."

Unlike the visionary Gilpinites, John Wesley Powell actually knew something about water and farming. After service in the Civil War that cost him his right arm, Major Powell, a geologist, had come west in 1869 to lead a scientific expedition down the Green and Colorado rivers through the Grand Canyon. No whites had

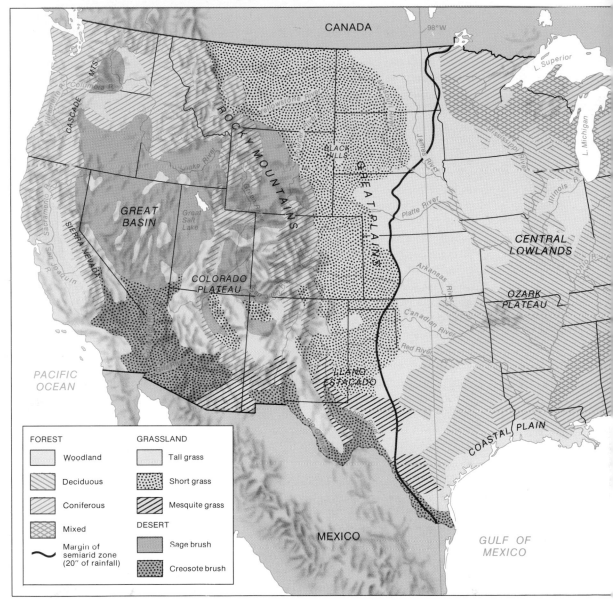

NATURAL ENVIRONMENT OF THE WEST

With the exception of the Pacific Northwest in Oregon and Washington, few areas west of the 20-inch rainfall line receive enough annual precipitation to support agriculture without irrigation. Consequently water has been the key to growth and development in the area west of the 98th meridian, encompassing over half the land area of the continental United States. The dominance of short grasses and coniferous (evergreen) trees reflects the rainfall patterns.

ever made that trip; indeed most people doubted it could be done. Powell not only survived, but he also repeated the feat in 1871, impelled as much by his fascination with Indian customs as with the remarkable terrain. Capitalizing on his success, he told Congress that the development of the West required more scientific planning. Much of the region had not yet even been mapped or its resources identified. In 1880 Powell was appointed director of the recently formed U.S. Geological Survey.

Powell too had a vision of the West, in his case based on the realities of the environment rather than the power of myth. In the East, where rainfall was adequate, a family could make a decent living farming a plot even half of the maximum 160 acres allotted settlers under the current policy for sale of federal land. But eastern land law had little relevance in a region whose arid climate rendered 1280 acres barely enough for farming, while grazing a small herd required at least 2560. And with no water at all, most land was useless.

For the West to grow in an orderly fashion, Powell believed that the laws had to be revised to suit the environment. The key was to treat water, not land, as a precious commodity. In the water-rich East, the English tradition of riparian rights prevailed. Those who owned the banks of a river or stream controlled as much water as they might take regardless of the consequence for others downstream. Such a practice in the West, Powell recognized, would enrich the few people with access to water while spelling ruin for the rest.

The alternative was to allow the community to distribute water to the benefit of the many rather than the powerful or privileged few. To that end the federal government would have to establish political boundaries defined by watershed areas rather than the grid pattern of settlement, which dated back to the Northwest Ordinances of the 1780s. Scientifically based planning would replace the laissez-faire custom under which the unregulated individual or corporation pursued narrow ends of profit with little regard for its environmental costs or the greater social good. But Powell's scientific realism could not overcome the vision of the West as the new American Eden. Development would proceed with the same enthusiasm for laissez faire and immediate results as captivated the East. And the first victims of this unrestrained expansion were Indians.

THE WAR FOR THE WEST

Since Andrew Jackson began moving eastern tribes beyond the Mississippi River, federal officials considered the Great Plains marginal land that could safely be given to the Indians. White estimates of the land began to change with a series of gold and silver discoveries beginning in 1848. By 1851 federal officials introduced a policy of "concentration," trying to get various tribes to sign treaties limiting the boundaries of their hunting grounds. Such treaties were often claimed to be settlements that would last "forever," but time after time, land-hungry pioneers squatted on Indian lands, then demanded protection from the government. The government, in turn, forced new, more restrictive agreements on the western tribes. In the Pacific Northwest, for example, many Indians had welcomed the first farmers, but by the 1850s the pressures on their land had become disruptive. Territorial governor Isaac Stevens, by often devious means, induced representatives of the Cayuse, Yakima, Walla Walla, and Nez Percé to cede millions of acres of land on which they had once freely hunted.

By 1862 the lands of the Santee Sioux had been similarly whittled down to a strip 10 miles wide and 150 miles long along the Minnesota River. Lashing out in frustration, the tribe attacked several undefended white settlements along the Minnesota frontier. The alarmed governor informed Washington that a full-scale war had broken out. In response, General John Pope came to St. Paul declaring his intention to wage a war of extermination. "They are to be treated as maniacs or wild beasts and by no means as people with whom treaties and compromises can be made," he instructed his officers. When Pope's forces under Colonel Henry Sibley captured 1800 Sioux braves, vindictive Minnesotans were outraged that President Lincoln would authorize the hanging of only 38.

War

The campaign under General Pope was the opening phase of a guerrilla war that raged intermittently between the U.S. Army and western Indians for some 30 years. The conflict gained momentum in November 1864, when a force of Colorado volunteers under Colonel John Chivington fell upon a band of friendly Cheyenne gathered at Sand Creek under the protection of the army. Black Kettle, the Cheyenne chief, raised an American flag to indicate friendship, but Chivington was having none of it. "Kill and scalp all, big and little," he told his men. When the massacre ended, all 80 Cheyenne, including women and children, lay dead. Settlers and soldiers alike felt the consequences of Chivington's unprovoked brutality, as virtually all the plains Indians joined the Sioux efforts to drive the whites from their lands.

The Sand Creek massacre was severely criticized by many eastern reformers, who understood the sources of Indian violence. The commission appointed to negotiate peace terms in 1867 observed that "when the progress of settlement reaches the Indian's home, the only question is, 'How best to get his land.' When they are obtained, the Indian is lost sight of " Fair-minded generals like George Crook and O. O. Howard honored treaty obligations and tried to inform insensitive politicians about the injustices that provoked Indian hostility. But the gap between the two cultures was so great that even reformers were largely unwilling to consider the possibility of allowing Indians to continue their traditional lives, protected from white encroachment. Instead they campaigned to turn nomadic Indians into farmers with 160-acre plots of land. General Pope, who went on to become commander of the Department of the Missouri, recognized the folly of this notion but proposed the equally unlikely solution of making Indians into stock raisers and cattlemen.

In the end, war was only one of several determining factors in the defeat of tribal cultures. Over the course of centuries only an estimated 4000 Indians (and about 7000 whites) were killed in direct warfare—a paltry few compared to the casualty lists of the Civil War. Far more devastating were white diseases, which continued to take their toll, and the debilitating influence of liquor. On the Great Plains the railroad disrupted the migratory patterns of the buffalo and in turn the patterns of the hunt. Tourist parties came west on the trains to bag the buffalo from railside; and when hides became popular back east, commercial companies hired hunters who could mow down over 100 bison an hour. In three short years, from 1872 to 1874, approximately 9 million of the herd were killed. By 1883 bison were nearly extinct on the plains. In other areas mining, farming, grazing herds, and fencing disrupted the Indians' traditional hunting and farming lands.

Last Stands

Among those who joined in Cheyenne raids on white settlements after Sand Creek
was a young Sioux named Crazy Horse. His western band had always worried that
too much contact with whites would destroy the Indian way of life. As the Civil
War ended, veteran troops swelled the ranks of the western army assigned to
protect the Northern Pacific Railroad and to open a trail from the gold fields of
western Montana through Sioux country along the South Platte River. Crazy
Horse led regular raiding parties that made that trail unsafe for soldiers and civilians. In December 1866 Captain William Fetterman, a brash commander who
believed his 80 men could make short work of any Sioux war party, rode straight
into an ambush Crazy Horse had helped set. There were no survivors.

This campaign was effective enough to cause federal negotiators to sign a
treaty in 1868 promising to abandon the trail to the gold fields, as well as three
military posts. It agreed also to the establishment of two large Indian reservations,
one in Oklahoma and the other in the western Dakotas. But many of the Sioux did
not understand that the terms restricted them to hunting in the area of the Powder
River and Bighorn country and to living in a reservation area of South Dakota west
of the Missouri. To protect the transcontinental route and the trail to Montana, the
treaty banned all trade between whites and Indians along the Platte. Thus the
tribes could not replenish their supplies of guns, ammunition, and blankets. Much
to the Indians' dismay, the army began to harass bands that traveled outside the
reservation area.

Only Chief Sitting Bull's northern Tetons and their Cheyenne allies had refused to sign the treaty, and Crazy Horse joined them, determined to draw a firm
line. But in the summer of 1874 Colonel George Armstrong Custer flagrantly
disregarded the 1868 treaty by leading an expedition into *Pa Sapa*, the sacred
Black Hills of the Sioux. Custer, a Civil War veteran, had gained fame among the
plains tribes as a "squaw killer" for his cruel warfare against the Indians of western
Kansas. Among white critics he was known for his monumental vanity and pub-
licity-seeking ways. When his expedition returned, its members spread rumors
that the Black Hills were rich with gold "from the grass roots down." As prospectors poured into Indian country, the army made little effort to keep them out.
Once again, federal negotiators tried to force another treaty to gain control of the
Black Hills, but when that failed, President Grant ordered all "hostiles" in the
area rounded up and driven onto the reservations.

The stage was set for a showdown, as the Cheyenne allied with the Sioux for
the first time under the leadership of Crazy Horse. Against them marched several
army columns, including Custer's 7th Cavalry, a force of over 600 troops. Custer,
ever eager to win fame, arrived at the Little Big Horn River a day earlier than the
other columns. Hearing a rumor of a native village nearby, he impulsively attacked, only to discover that he had stumbled onto an encampment of over 12,000
Sioux and Cheyenne, extending for almost three miles. From a deep ravine Crazy
Horse charged Custer, killing him and some 250 soldiers.

"It is a good day to die!" Crazy Horse cried—the traditional war cry. Even in
the midst of victory he spoke truly. For while Custer had been conquered, the
railroads still stood ready to continue their work, the prospectors remained eager
to make fortunes, and soldiers continued to come from the East. By late summer
the Sioux were forced to split into small bands to evade the army sent to punish

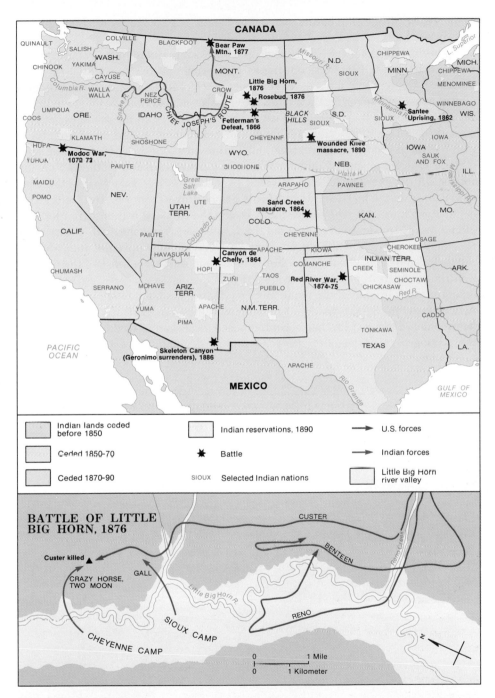

THE INDIAN FRONTIER

As conflict erupted between Indian and white cultures in the West, the government sought increasingly to concentrate tribes on reservations. Resistance to the reservation concept helped unite the Sioux and Cheyenne, traditionally enemies, in the Dakotas during the 1870s. Along the Little Big Horn River, the impetuous Custer underestimated the strength of his Indian opponents and attacked before the supporting troops of Reno and Benteen were in a position to aid him.

them. While Sitting Bull barely escaped to Canada, Crazy Horse and 800 with him surrendered after a winter of suffering and starvation.

The battles along the Platte and upper Missouri rivers did not end the war between whites and Indians, but never again would such a substantial threat be mounted. Even peaceful tribes like the Nez Percé of Idaho found no security once whites began to hunger for their land. The Nez Percé had become effective breeders of livestock, rich in horses and cattle that they grazed in the meadows of grass west of the Snake River canyon. That did not prevent the government from trying to force them onto a small reservation. Rather than see his people humiliated, Chief Joseph led a band of almost 600 toward Canada, pursued by the U.S. Army. In just 75 days the Nez Percé traveled over 1300 miles. Every time the army closed to attack, Chief Joseph and his warriors drove them off. But before they could reach the border they were trapped, and the chief's words of surrender were eloquent: "Hear me, my chiefs, I am tired; my heart is sick and sad. From where the sun now stands I will fight no more forever." The government then shipped the defeated tribe to Oklahoma, where disease and starvation finished the destruction the army had begun.

Almost as mythic as the name of Crazy Horse was Geronimo, whose band of Apaches was the last to succumb to white conquest. In 1872 Cochise, the great battle chief of the Apache, had accepted peace terms and moved his people onto a reservation in the Arizona territory. Geronimo decided to keep up the fight, re-

More than warfare, acculturation threatened the survival of traditional Indian ways. By 1905, some 20 years after his surrender, Geronimo had adopted Christianity and other white ways (including this top hat). He rode as a celebrity that year in Theodore Roosevelt's inaugural parade.

treating across the Mexican border into a mountain camp and from there leading sporadic raids on settlements and ranches across the territories. Terrified whites begged Washington for protection, but not until 1886 did the army finally capture Geronimo and send him to an exile in Florida.

By 1887 reformers recognized that the policy of concentrating Indians on reservations was a failure. Deprived of their traditional lands and culture, the reservation tribes became dependent on the government. And whites who coveted the resources of reservation lands were quick to violate treaty terms. Railroad barons like Collis P. Huntington and Jay Gould had ignored Apache rights as they ran tracks across the reservation. In a spirit that mingled good intentions and unbridled greed, Congress adopted the Dawes Severalty Act of 1887 to end reservation policy and bring once-nomadic Indians into white society as farmers and small landowners.

In practice, the Dawes Act was more destructive than any blow struck by the army, because it attacked the communal tribal structure upon which Indian life was based. Lands held in common would now be allotted to individuals: 160 acres to the head of a family and 80 acres to single adults or orphans. But as John Wesley Powell had warned, small homestead farms in the West would not support a family—white or Indian—unless they were irrigated. And most Indians of the region had no experience with farming, managing money, or other white ways. The sponsors of the Dawes Act, knowing that whites might swindle Indians out of their private holdings, arranged for the government to hold title to the land for 25 years, but that did not stop unscrupulous speculators from "leasing" lands. Furthermore, all reservation lands not allocated to Indians were opened to non-Indian homesteaders. Few Indians were able to assimilate into white society as the Dawes Act intended.

Against such a bleak future, many Indians sought solace in dreams of the past. In 1890 a religious revival spread when word came from the Nevada desert that a humble Paiute named Wovoka had received revelations from the Great Spirit. Wovoka told the pilgrims that God wanted them "to be good and love one another, and not fight, or steal, or lie." With that message God also sent a dance. Wovoka preached that if they adopted his message and mystical rituals, the dead Indians would come back, whites would be driven out of the land, and game would be thick again. As the rituals spread from tribe to tribe, alarmed settlers called the strange shuffling and chanting the "Ghost Dance." The army moved to stop the proceedings among the Sioux, for fear of another uprising. The great Sitting Bull himself was killed in one scuffle, while the 7th Cavalry, Custer's old unit, set out to track down other members of the tribe. At Wounded Knee the cavalry fell upon one band and with devastating machine-gun fire killed at least 200 men, women, and children.

Wounded Knee was a last symbolic act of violence against an independent Indian way of life. After 1890 the real battle was over assimilation, not extinction. The system of markets, rail and freight networks, and extractive industries was linking the Far West with the rest of the nation, replacing free-roaming bison with herded cattle and sheep, nomadic tribes with prairie sodbusters, and sacred hunting grounds like the Sioux's *Pa Sapa* with gold fields. Armed with the Dawes Act and often pressed by those with designs on Indian lands, reformers sought to use a combination of education, citizenship, and allotments to draw Indians from their communal lives into white society. Most Indians were equally determined to preserve their tribal ways and a sense of themselves as a separate people.

THE WESTERN BOOM

Though opportunity in the West lay in the land and its resources, wealth also accumulated in the towns. Each time a speculative fever hit the region, new communities sprouted to serve those who rushed in to strike it rich. The boom began with the "forty-niners" of 1849 and San Francisco; in the next few decades new hordes threw up towns in Park City, Utah; Tombstone, Arizona; Deadwood in the Dakota Territories; and other promising sites. Then in the 1860s came the railroads, which created cities like Denver and would awaken sleepy communities like Los Angeles. Railroads opened the Great Plains to the cattle drives that in the 1870s brought the great herds to "cowtowns" like Sedalia, Missouri; Dodge City, Wichita; and Abilene, Kansas; and Cheyenne, Wyoming. Fast behind the cattle boom came the sodbusters by the late 1870s to turn the thick prairie soils left open by the destruction of the buffalo herds. By the 1890s the once unsettled Great Plains were dotted with towns, crisscrossed by rails, and divided into farms, ranches, and Indian reservations. Historian Frederick Jackson Turner could announce by 1893 that the frontier had closed.

The gold and silver strikes established a pattern the other booms would follow. Stories of easy riches would attract small entrepreneurs. The populations of boom towns were largely male (as much as 90 percent) and almost half foreign-born. Someone entering the local saloon could expect to hear English, the Irish brogue, German, French, Spanish, Chinese, Italian, Hawaiian, and various Indian dialects. Once the quick profits were gone, a period of consolidation brought more order to towns and larger scale to enterprise. In the mine fields, that meant corporations with the capital to invest in high-pressure hydraulic water jets to blast ore loose and other heavy equipment to crush rock and extract silver and gold from deeper veins. In their concern to secure quick profits, such operations often led to environmental disaster as floods, mud slides, and dirty streams threatened the livelihood of farmers in the valleys below. In state and territorial governments bitter disputes erupted between agricultural and mining interests.

Conflict erupted, too, between the corporations and the paid labor force that replaced the prospectors. Struggles between the companies and miners seeking union recognition, better wages and hours, and improved working conditions sometimes turned into pitched battles. In Coeur d'Alene, Idaho, in 1892, troops seeking to break a strike killed seven miners. The miners, refusing to knuckle under, created the Western Federation of Miners, which in the decade after 1893 attracted some 50,000 members and a reputation as one of the nation's most militant unions. In short, the mining frontier, which had begun as a rowdy and individualistic collection of small-scale prospectors, had been integrated into the industrial system of wage labor, large-scale resource extraction, and high-finance capital.

Rail Towns and Cattle Drives

As William Gilpin had predicted in 1849, the development of the West awaited the coming of the railroads. Before the gold spike joined the Central and Union Pacific at Promontory Point, Utah, in 1869, travel across the West was slow and dusty. Mail, cargo, and people moved on stagecoaches, wagons, horseback, and

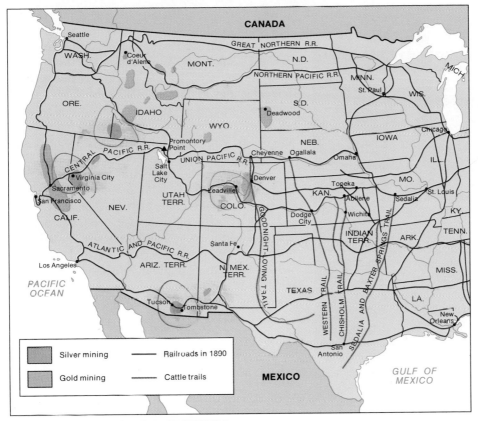

THE MINING AND CATTLE FRONTIERS

In the vast spaces of the West, railroads, cattle trails, and gold mining usually preceded the arrival of settlers in large enough numbers to establish towns and cities. The railroads forged a crucial link between the region's natural resources and urban markets in the East and in Europe, but by transecting the plains they also disrupted the migratory patterns of the buffalo herds, undermining Plains Indian cultures while opening the land to cattle grazing and farming.

foot. Given the vast distances and sparse population, entrepreneurs had little opportunity to follow the eastern practice of building local railroads from city to city.

But such difficulties put no end to dreaming, especially for the likes of Collis P. Huntington. A transplanted New Yorker, Huntington soon discovered that the way to make a fortune was not in the hunt for gold but by supplying the boom society that came with the rush for mineral wealth. Setting up a hardware business in Sacramento, he often strapped bags of gold to his waist and rowed out into San Francisco harbor to meet incoming supply ships. Before they could land, he had bought up the entire cargo, which he then sold at highly inflated prices. Huntington understood all too well the credo of the West in those early days: "It pays to be shifty in a new land." He and three other Sacramento business leaders, Mark Hopkins, Leland Stanford, and Charles Crocker—the "Big Four" (all happened to be ample in girth as well as in wealth)—incorporated the Central Pacific Railroad.

In 1862 the Central Pacific won from Congress the opportunity to build the western link of the transcontinental railroad eastward from San Francisco. To the Union Pacific Corporation fell the right to construct the section from Omaha westward. But the real money in this and other ventures lay not so much in the revenues from passengers and freight, but from generous loans and gifts of federal and state lands. For every mile of track completed, the rail companies received twenty sections of land in the states along the route and forty sections per mile in the territories. (One section equaled 6,400 acres or ten square miles.) By the time the Central and Union Pacific railroads were completed, they had received some 45 million acres. Fraudulent stock practices, corrupt accounting, and wholesale bribery (with the complicity of the vice-president and at least two members of Congress) enabled the promoters to earn large profits.

General Grenville Dodge, an army engineer on leave to the Union Pacific, recognized that the immense labor force needed to build the railroad might be recruited cheaply from the mass of Irish and other European immigrants. He drove his workers with ruthless army discipline, completing as much as ten miles of track in a single day. Charles Crocker had no similar source of cheap labor in California for the Central Pacific, since the gold rush era had passed. Worse yet, he faced the formidable task of forging a route through the Sierra Nevadas. When his partner Leland Stanford suggested imported Chinese labor, Crocker dismissed him with a laugh—at first. But it was some 10,000 Chinese laborers ("the Asiatic Contingent of the the Grand Army of Civilization," one observer dubbed them) who accomplished the daunting task. With wheelbarrows, picks, shovels, and baskets they advanced eastward, building trestles like the one at Secrettown (left) and chipping away at the steep Sierras' looming granite walls. On the worst stretches they averaged only eight inches a day.

Once the Chinese crews had broken into the flat country of the desert basin, the two railroads raced to claim as much federal land as possible. Labor bosses pushed their men with blatant appeals to racism. In the resulting scramble, the two sides passed each other, laying over two hundred miles of parallel track before the government ordered them to join at Promontory Point, Utah, in the spring of 1869. The headlong rush had involved waste and the cutting of corners: many sections of the first track had been thrown up on narrow embankments and over flimsy bridges. Still, East and West were finally linked across the American continent. Writer Bret Harte described the Central and Union Pacific engines as

> Facing on a single track
> Half a world behind each back.

Over 75 western railroads benefited from similar government generosity. The Northern Pacific line, from Minnesota to Seattle, received almost twice as much land as the Central Pacific and the Union Pacific. The Atchison, Topeka, and Santa Fe, which followed the old Santa Fe Trail, acquired some 3 million acres. Only the Great Northern, the last of the major transcontinental lines, built its track without federal aid.

The rail companies recognized the strategic value of their enterprise. If the key to getting rich off the gold rush was supplying miners, the key to prospering in the developing West was control of the means of transport. Just by threatening to bypass a town, a powerful railroad could extract important concessions on rights of way, taxes, and loans. No one topped Collis Huntington for ruthlessness and audacity. "If the Great Wall of China were put in his path, he would attack it with his nails," an acquaintance remarked. To Huntington the Big Four assigned the task of managing Congress, judges, and local officials. "If a man has the power to do great evil and won't do right unless he is bribed to do it, I think . . . it is a man's duty to go up and bribe the judge," he admitted with characteristic bluntness.

When Los Angeles resisted Charles Crocker's demands for major concessions, the Big Four threatened to ruin the town by leaving it off their route. As an example to Angelenos they bypassed nearby San Bernardino and simply built another town, Colton. After acquiring waterfront land in Oakland, the Central Pacific eventually gained control of all the railroad, ferry, and dock land around the rim of San Francisco Bay. And as huge landowners with control of transportation, the railroads had an enormous influence on the development of farming and cattle grazing.

Westerners developed a peculiar ambivalence toward government and the railroads. Both were necessary for growth and development of the region. Yet, in the words of the Sacramento *Union*, miners, small ranchers, farmers, and the newly settled towns found their lives hinging on decisions made by "coldhearted, selfish, sordid" robber barons and officials in Washington, over whom they had little direct control. Such antagonism helps explain the legends that abounded concerning the exploits of train robbers like the James brothers, Jesse and Frank, and the Hole-in-the-Wall Gang, led by Butch Cassidy and the Sundance Kid. If the railroads could, with government support, rob the people, then the train robbers were latter-day "Robin Hoods," giving the railroads a little of their own medicine.

So the railroads sparked urban growth in coastal cities like Seattle, San Francisco, and Los Angeles, where sea and land transportation routes met. Los Angeles, a sleepy town of 6000 people in the 1870s, jumped to over 50,000 with the coming of the Southern Pacific and the Santa Fe. San Francisco and Oakland prospered as major transportation centers after the gold rush ended. For western cities of the interior like Denver, Cheyenne, Abilene, and Wichita, growth came with the joining of the railroads to the great cattle trails.

In many ways Wichita, Kansas, typified the scattered towns and cities that sprouted as the West opened to speculative fever. Wichita, on the Arkansas River, first served as a campsite for Indians and fur traders. After the Civil War, land speculators recognized that the proximity to the Chisholm Trail would bring the cattle herds and the hungry and thirsty cowpokes who drove them to Abilene. When the railroad came through in 1872 the boom began in earnest. Area farmers now had far wider access to distant markets. And towns like Wichita offered farmers and cowhands alike an escape from the isolation that was their common lot. In the five years after 1869 the town's population grew from 300 to 2500 people.

Cattle Kingdom

The towns thrived, of course, on the business of ranchers, whose longhorn steers were driven to market beginning in 1866. Mexican ranchers had introduced not only the cattle but the basic techniques for their management with a minimum of cost and labor. The ranchers allowed their herds to roam the range freely, identified only by a distinctive mark or brand. Each spring the cowboys rounded up the herds, branded the calves, and selected the steers to send to market. Anglo-Americans who came to Texas readily adopted the Mexican equipment: the tough mustangs and broncos (horses suited to managing the mean longhorns), the branding iron for marking the herds, the corral for holding cattle, and the lariat for roping. So too the cowboys donned the distinctive Mexican outfits—chaps, spurs, and a broad-brimmed hat.

Clara Williamson painted this herd on the long drive north from Texas. Cowboys normally worked in pairs, opposite each other, as shown here; the chuck wagon can be seen at the rear of the train. So strenuous was the work that each cowboy brought with him about eight horses, so fresh mounts would always be available.

When the early routes to Sedalia, Missouri, proved unfriendly, a more direct route through easier country along the Chisholm Trail, running from San Antonio to Abilene and Ellsworth, made the cattle drive practical. But the railroads that carried cattle east also brought farmers determined to close the open ranges of western Kansas. The resourceful Texans had soon blazed new trails, the Western to Dodge City and the Goodnight-Loving to Pueblo, Denver, and Cheyenne.

Since cattle grazed on the open range, early ranches were relatively small. Most had a house for the rancher and his family, a bunk house for the cowboys and other hired hands, and some grazing lands. Ranchers either owned the lands and herds or managed them for corporations and investors. Women were rare in the masculine world of cattle and cowboys. Most were ranchers' wives, who cooked, nursed the sick, and helped run the ranch. By necessity these women were strong and resourceful. When Helen Wiser Stewart of Nevada learned in July 1884 that her husband had been murdered, she took over operation of the ranch. Her life was an endless round of buying and selling cattle, managing the hands, and tending to her family. She did heavy physical labor as well, gathering crops, racking wine, grubbing mesquite, slaughtering hogs, and tending her garden.

After the Civil War veterans of the Confederate army made up the majority of the cowhands who tended the herds in Texas. But at least a third of all cowboys were black freedmen and Mexicans. Some cowhands dreamed of setting aside enough wages to start a herd of their own. A few took the easier route of cattle rustling. But in the end, most became wage laborers employed by the large corporate enterprises that came to dominate the industry. When Richard King, founder of the huge King Ranch of Texas, made $50,000 on the drive of 1875, he paid his 43 hands (over half of them Hispanic) anywhere from $43.20 a month for the most experienced to $25 for ordinary horse wranglers. Once again, the eastern pattern of economic concentration and labor specialization was being applied in the West.

Life in the saddle was far from romantic. For his labors, a cowboy was fed, housed, and paid a wage of about a dollar a day. No more than 12 hands tended from 2000 to 5000 head along the trail. During the drives of some 800 miles, lasting several months, the hands spent long hours chasing strays, guarding against human and animal predators, and heading off stampedes. Heavy dust clung to the skin and a cough brought up black phlegm from the lungs. There were days when the sun shone and the spectacle of the herd elevated spirits. More often, though, the cowboy reached the end of the day gloomy and heartsick, his stomach hurting from hunger, his body aching with fatigue. His only relief came in the raucous cattle towns where saloonkeepers, card sharps, and dance hall madams waited to separate him from his hard-earned wages.

The cattle boom that began with the first long drive of 1866 reached its peak from 1880 to 1885. Ranchers came to expect profits of 25 to 40 percent a year. Millions of dollars poured into the west from eastern and foreign interests eager to cash in on soaring cattle prices. Ranching corporations extended the open range from Texas into Wyoming and Montana. But as in all booms, forces were at work bringing the inevitable bust. High profits swelled the size of the herds and led to overproduction, increased foreign competition, and sagging beef prices. The big ranchers sometimes banded together to squeeze out the cowhands and farmers who sought to start herds of their own. In 1892 a range war broke out between the hired guns of the Wyoming Stockgrowers' Association and the small independent ranchers. The same forces that led to consolidation of industrial firms began to drive the small operators out of the cattle business.

Cattle ranchers were not the only entrepreneurs with an eye on the public domain. Rising food prices and cheap lands brought farmers into the Great Plains too. The "nesters," as ranchers disdainfully called them, fenced off their lands, resulting in a continually shrinking open range. Vast grants to the railroads limited the area of free land, while ranchers intent on breeding heavier cattle with more tender beef began to fence in their stock to prevent them from mixing with inferior strays. Even after Congress declared it illegal to fence the public domain, nesters and cattlemen fought an intermittent guerrilla war to establish their conflicting claims.

And cows were not the only grazing animals the Mexicans had introduced to the West. Cattlemen had particular contempt for the sheep raiser and his "woolies." Sheep tended to crop grasses so short that they ruined land for cattle grazing. To protect the range they saw as their own from the "hooved locust," cattlemen attacked shepherds and their flocks. On one occasion raiders along the Green River in Wyoming clubbed 8000 sheep to death. The sheep raiser–cattle rancher feuds produced violence often more severe than that between the farmers and ranchers.

In the end it was nature that imposed its own limits on the boom. There was simply not enough grass along the trails to support the millions of head on their way to market. The need to buy feed and land to raise hay drove costs up. Diseases like "Texas fever" sometimes wiped out entire herds. Then in 1886 and 1887 came two of the coldest winters in recorded history. The winds brought blizzards that drove wandering herds up against fences, where they either froze or starved to death. Exhaled breath congealed into sheets of ice so heavy a cow could not raise its head. Summer brought no relief, as severe heat and drought dried up waterholes and scorched the grasslands. In the Dakotas, Montana, Colorado, and Wyoming, losses ran as high as 90 percent. Future president Theodore Roosevelt was among the easterners who lost investments.

By the 1890s the open range and the long drives had disappeared. What prevailed were the cattle corporations like the King Ranch of Texas, with sufficient capital to acquire and fence vast grazing lands, hire ranchers to manage the herds, and pay for feed during winter months. The free and independent cowboy sitting tall in the saddle lived on mostly in the mythology of western writers and Hollywood movies.

THE FINAL FRONTIER

In the 1860s they had come in a trickle; in the 1870s they became a torrent. They were farmers from the East and Midwest, black freedmen from the South, and immigrants from Europe. What bound them together was a hunger for land based on their rural and peasant backgrounds. They had read railroad and steamship advertisements and heard stories from friends about millions of acres of fertile lands in the plains west of the 98th meridian. New, hardier strands of wheat like the "Turkey Red" imported from Russia, improved farm machinery, and techniques like dry farming made it possible to raise crops under harsh climatic conditions. The number of farms in the United States increased from around 2 million on the eve of the Civil War to almost 6 million in 1900.

The Land Rush

So intense was the craving for land that in March and April of 1889 some 100,000 people traveled by wagon, horseback, carriage, buckboard, mule, and on foot to a line across the Oklahoma panhandle. These were "Boomers," gathered for the greatest land rush in history. On April 22, 1889, with a signal from the U.S. cavalry, the Boomers raced across the line to claim some 2 million acres of Indian territory opened for settlement. And beyond the line lay the "Sooners"—those who had jumped the gun and hidden in gullies and thickets, ready to leap out one minute after noon to claim a stake in prosperity.

Even though more land would be settled after 1900 than before, the Oklahoma land rush marked the end of the opening of the West. No longer would geographers be able to mark a line on a map demarcating the point where settlement ended. Even before then the myth of the garden had foundered on the realities of weather and uncertain markets. Overproduction, combined with competition from newly opened lands in Canada, Argentina, Russia, and Australia, steadily drove down prices from the 1870s to the early twentieth century. Wheat, which sold for as much as $1.60 a bushel during the Civil War, fell as low as 49 cents during the 1890s and would not rise over a dollar until the demands of World War I drove prices up. Periods of above-average rain inevitably gave way to dry cycles. Farmers, like cattle ranchers, suffered through the drought and fierce winter cold of 1886 and 1887. They, especially, had to confront the harsh realities of a dry, treeless land that left families isolated in the vast loneliness of its boundless horizons. So even as the hopeful crowds lined up in Oklahoma, thousands of others abandoned their farms to escape mounting debts. Some returned east while others headed farther west, pursuing what one historian described as "the mirage of an infinity of second chances."

The West never conformed to the myth popular in the East that a poor farmer, with fortitude, self-reliance, and luck, could prosper on free and fertile land. For one thing, most of the desirable land in the West was not free. For every acre the government granted under the Homestead Act (80 million by 1900) farmers bought six. Land that the government had granted to Indians, the states, or the railroads had to be purchased. And the best lands were those near the railroad tracks that gave access to eastern markets. By the 1890s railroad land sold for around $25 an acre, compared to $1.25 if bought under the Homestead Act.

Speculators managed to control much of the choicest land, purchasing large blocks from states eager to raise revenues. Or they employed shills willing to establish a "dummy entry" on a quarter section and then turn it over to the speculator for a modest fee. Some even built cabins on wheels, which they could move from section to section to comply with the law's requirement for a building on the land. Others dropped a cup of water on the ground to meet the terms of the Desert Land Act of 1877, which entitled a farmer to 640 acres if the land was irrigated within three years.

Land was not the only expense for newly settled farmers. Farming the plains required substantial investment in equipment. Only a steel plow could cut the dense root systems of prairie grasses. The threat of cattle trampling the fields forced farmers to erect fences. Lacking wood, they found the answer in barbed wire, first marketed by an Illinois farmer, Joseph Glidden, in 1874. Between 1880 and 1900 the sale of barbed wire imported from the East grew from 80 million to 297 million pounds per year. And with little rain, many farmers had to install windmills and pumping equipment to draw water from deep underground.

On the vast open prairies, successful farming in export staples, especially wheat and oats, demanded heavy investment in machinery: special plows and harrows (which turned the heavy sod before spring rains and harrowed quickly to capture moisture once it fell) to permit dry farming; threshers, combines, and harvesters to bring in the crop; and powerful steam tractors to pull the heavy equipment. The average farmer spent what was for the poor a small fortune, about $785 on machinery alone and another $500 for land. The bigger operators often invested 10 or 20 times as much. Farms of over 1000 acres, known as bonanza farms, were most common in the wheatlands of the northern plains. The resulting efficiencies made a great difference. A steam tractor working one of the huge bonanza farms could simultaneously plow, harrow, and seed up to 50 acres a day—about 20 times more than a single person could do without machinery. Against such competition, small-scale farmers could scarcely compete. Like small farmers in the South, many westerners became tenants on land owned by others. Bonanza farmers hired as many as 250 laborers to work each 10,000 acres in return for room, board, and as little as 50 cents a day in wages.

A Plains Existence

For poor farm families, life on the plains meant a sod house or a dugout carved out of the hillside for protection from the winds. Tough, root-bound sod was cut into bricks about a foot wide and three feet long and laid edgewise to create walls three feet thick; sod bricks were laid over rafters for a roof. The average house was seldom more than 18 by 24 feet, and in severe weather it had to accommodate animals as well as people. One door and usually no more than a single window provided light and air. A sod house had the advantage of being cheap, too heavy to blow away in the wind, and too wet to catch fire. The thick walls kept the house warm in winter and cool in summer. In the spring, wildflowers and grass turned the roof into a small garden.

But bad weather made the disadvantages all too apparent. A heavy, soaking rain or snow could bring the roof down, or at the least allow mud and water to seep into the living area, where wooden floors were an uncommon luxury. Katherine Gibson of the Dakota territories recalled that no sooner had she lighted the stove one cold fall morning than she was beset by a rattlesnake and its offspring. She escaped through the window. As soon as a home was established, armies of flies, gnats, mosquitoes, and fleas moved in. Privacy was nearly impossible for families of six or more. Whenever they could afford to do so, farm families erected a wood frame house and turned the sod hut over to the livestock.

The heaviest burdens of farm life fell on the women, who faced a seemingly infinite variety of chores and deprivations. Stores were scarce and money for supplies even scarcer. Matches, window glass, kerosene for light and heat, and soap for laundry were generally unavailable. That meant long days over hot tubs preparing tallow wax for candles or soaking ashes and boiling lye with grease and pork rinds to make soap. Equally time-consuming was the sewing of clothing. Some families brought carding brushes and spinning wheels, but wool in the first years of settlement was often in such short supply that resourceful women used hair from wolves and other wild animals. Wagon covers and tents were often the only other cloth available. Buttons had to be fashioned from old spoons.

Even worse than disease and the shortage of basic necessities were the hard-

Sod houses built on the treeless plains were limited in size by a shortage of wood needed to support the roof, which often was over a foot thick. Having to haul possessions over long distances obviously restricted what a family could carry.

ships imposed by the natural elements. Women in the Southwest lived in dread of the stinging centipedes and scorpions that inhabited wall cracks. For the farmers from Missouri to Oregon, nothing spelled disaster like the locusts that periodically descended without warning. Swarms were sometimes more than 100 miles long, beating against the houses like hailstones. Though they seldom bothered people, they stripped all vegetation in their paths, including the bark of trees. They even devoured the laundry on the line and curtains in the windows. Many a farm family survived the harsh weather only to see an entire year's labor destroyed in a day. "I saw heaps of grasshoppers as large as a washtub," Elizabeth Roe recalled. "They commenced on a forty acre field of corn at 10 o'clock and before night there was not an ear of corn or green leaf to be seen."

The hot summers, disease, Indian wars, isolation, and material deprivation all taxed the courage of pioneer farm families, but winter had its special horrors. Blizzards could sweep the plains for days, piling snow to the rooftops and halting

Daily Lives

FOOD/DRINK/DRUGS

The Frontier Kitchen of the Plains

Out on the treeless plains the Indians had adjusted to scarcity of food, water, and other necessities by adopting a nomadic way of life. Their small kinship groups moved each season to wherever nature supplied the food they needed. Such mobility discouraged families from acquiring extensive material possessions. Tools and housing had to be light and portable. Even tribes that raised crops as part of their subsistence cycle often moved with the seasons.

White settlement was different. Farmers, ranchers, and townspeople rooted themselves to a single place. What the surrounding countryside could not supply had to be brought from afar, generally at great effort and expense. In areas distant from the railroad or other transportation links, families generally had to learn either to do without or to improvise from materials at hand. Keeping food on the table was nearly impossible some seasons of the year. Coffee and sugar were staples in such short supply that resourceful women invented a variety of substitutes. "Take a gallon of bran, two tablespoonsful of molasses, scald and parch in an oven until it is somewhat browned and charred," one women suggested. Something as simple as finding water suitable for drinking or cooking became a problem in many western areas, where the choice might be between "the strong alkaline water of the Rio Grande or the purchase of melted manufactured ice (shipped by rail) at its great cost." To prepare for the lean winter months, women stocked their cellars and made wild fruits into leathery

A box mill was essential for grinding the coffee beans and "stretchers"—rye, barley, and other grains used to extend coffee, which was often in short supply on pioneer farms.

cakes, eaten to ward off the scurvy that resulted from vitamin deficiency.

Gardening, generally a woman's responsibility, brought variety to the diet and color to the yard. The legume family of peas and beans, in particular, provided needed protein. Superstition had it that plants which grew above ground, like peas, beans, and squash, should be planted in the new moon, whereas root plants such as carrots, potatoes, radishes, and turnips went in as the moon waned. As the moon rose, the theory went, plants rose; as it dropped, so did the root plants. Flowers were much prized but seldom survived the winds, heat, and dry periods. Dishwater and laundry water helped keep them alive. One woman was so excited by the discovery of a hardy dandelion that she cultivated it with care and planted its seeds each spring.

Daily Lives

Until rail lines made shipment of goods cheap and Sears, Roebuck "wish-books" brought mail order to the frontier, a woman's kitchen was fairly modest. A cast iron stove, which sold for $25 in the East, was in such demand and so expensive to ship that it fetched $200 in some areas of the West. One miner's wife in Montana during the 1870s considered her kitchen "well-furnished" with two kettles, a cast iron skillet, and a coffeepot. A kitchen cupboard might be little more than a box nailed to a log. In sod houses cooking could be difficult after a cloudburst. One "soddie" recalled that her kitchen remained snug and dry during a rainstorm, but she discovered that the downpour had taken its toll as the water seeped slowly through the thick roof. After the sun came out, the still-waterlogged roof began to leak. She ended up frying pancakes on her stove under the protection of an umbrella while the sun shone brightly outside.

Without doctors, circumstances forced women to learn the rudiments of caring for the hurt and sick. Most folk remedies did little more than ease pain. Whiskey and patent medicines, often more dangerous than the disease, were used to treat a range of ills from frostbite to snake bite and from sore throats to burns and rheumatism. Settlers believed that onions and gunpowder had valuable medicinal properties. Cobwebs could bandage small wounds; turpentine served as a disinfectant. Mosquitoes were repelled with a paste of vinegar and salt. One woman in Wyoming prevented winter snow blindness by burning pitch pine until it was black and smudging the skin below the eyes with it to cut glare. Most parents thought the laxative castor oil could cure any childhood malady. And if a family member had a fever, one treatment was to bind the head with a cold rag, wrap the feet in cabbage leaves, and then force down large doses of sage tea, rhubarb, and soda. Some women adapted remedies used on their farm animals. Sarah Olds, a Nevada homesteader whose family was plagued by fleas and lice, recalled that "we all took baths with plenty of sheep dip in the water. . . . I had no disinfectant . . . so I boiled all our clothing in sheep dip and kerosene."

Gradually, as the market system penetrated the West, families had less need to improvise in matters of diet and medicine. Through catalogs one might order spices like white pepper or poultry seasoning and appliances such as grinders for real coffee. If a local stagecoach passed by the house, a woman might send her eggs and butter to town to be exchanged for needed store-bought goods like threads and needles. It took a complex commercial network to bring all that the good life required to a land that produced few foods and necessities in abundance.

all forms of travel. Stockade fences built to keep the blizzards out and the animals safe made many a farm house seem like a prison. After living through several severe Dakota winters, Mary Woodward was amused by an eastern poet's romantic view of a winter snowfall. "I doubt if there is a poet living who possesses enough vim to write a poem about a Dakota blizzard. I guess a blizzard would knock all the poetry out of a man."

In the face of such hardships many westerners found comfort in religion. Though Catholics and Jews came West, evangelical Protestants dominated along the frontier, in the mining towns, and in other western communities. Worship offered an emotional outlet, some intellectual stimulation, a means of preserving older values, and a source of hope. Circuit riders compensated for the shortage of preachers, while camp meetings offered an opportunity for socializing; both brought contact with a wider world. In many communities it was the churches that first instilled order on public life. Through church committees westerners could deal with local problems like the need for schools or charity for the poor.

The sense among westerners and southerners that they were outside the American mainstream came not so much from their isolation from the industrial Northeast or Midwest, but from their links to it. The struggle by promoters of a New South to out-Yankee the Yankee could not overcome the region's low wage structure and high fertility rates. And so by 1900 southerners earned half as much as the national average—$509 versus $1165. The promoters of a fertile West had greater success in adopting the techniques of large-scale industry and investment to mining, cattle ranching, and farming. But they too discovered limits to an arid land, whose mineral and timber resources were not endless and where rain, contrary to William Gilpin's hopes, did not follow the plow. Like easterners, ordinary citizens in the West found that large corporations with near-monopoly control over markets and transportation bred inequality, unfair business practices, and widespread resentment.

These regional upheavals could not help but affect the political system as conflicts of class and race and region spilled over into the national arena. By the late 1880s and early 1890s, an agrarian revolt had begun to sweep the South and West. In both sections disillusionment and despair turned to bitterness as more small farmers, both black and white, found themselves enslaved to debt and driven toward bankruptcy, tenantry, or wage labor. It was small wonder that the South and West gave rise to a "People's party," determined to end the "business as usual" approach of the Democratic and Republican parties.

SIGNIFICANT EVENTS

1849–1859	Gold and silver strikes open western mining frontier
1862	Homestead Act; Minnesota Sioux uprising begins Plains Indian wars
1864	Chivington massacre
1866	Drive to Sedalia, Missouri, launches cattle boom
1869	Completion of first transcontinental railroad; Powell explores the Grand Canyon
1872–1874	The great buffalo slaughter
1874	Black Hills gold rush; barbed wire patented
1876	Battle of Little Big Horn; Nez Percé resist relocation
1877	Compromise of 1877 ends Reconstruction; Crazy Horse surrenders; Desert Land Act
1879	Height of Exoduster migration to Kansas
1880	Bonsack cigarette-rolling machine invented
1883	*Civil Rights Cases*
1885–1887	Severe winter and drought cycle in the West
1887	Dawes Severalty Act
1889	Oklahoma opened to settlement
1890s	Tennessee Coal, Iron, and Railway Company makes Birmingham, Alabama, a major steel center
1890	Ghost Dance Indian religious revival; Wounded Knee
1892	Union violence at Coeur d'Alene, Idaho; Wyoming range wars
1893	Frederick Jackson Turner's "Frontier Thesis" presented
1896	*Plessy v. Ferguson* upholds separate but equal doctrine

21

The Failure of
Traditional Politics

he Democratic brass band gathered on a hot September day in Sparta, Georgia, to play a few patriotic numbers. Set up at one end of the grove, it launched tune after tune, each louder than the last. At the other end of the crowd, from a platform in the semiwooded countryside, Tom Watson addressed the assembled folks. On the surface, it was a scene reenacted all across America in that election season: brass bands, barbecues, and ballyhoo. But this was 1892—not an ordinary election year—and the assembly at Sparta was profoundly unsettling to many observers.

To begin with, the Democratic band that played so loudly at the far end of the grove did not belong to Tom Watson, the campaigner. Watson, a Congressman from northeast Georgia, had left the Democratic ticket in disgust and was running on behalf of a new third party, the Populists. His opponent's gathering was down the grove less than a mile away, and the band had come over to whoop it up and distract Watson's followers. What seemed especially unsettling to the rival Democrats was that the Watson crowd was largely black. Blacks still went to the polls in Georgia in 1892; and most of them knew, from the habits of the past decades, the way they were supposed to vote if they wanted to stay healthy. On Election Day the white owner they sharecropped for or some other local worthy would gather 25 or 50 blacks and march them off single file, down a dusty road to the polls. Blacks remembered well enough the nights in the 1870s when the Ku Klux Klan galloped through the countryside, and southern whites "redeemed" their states. Redeemer politicians treated blacks courteously enough during election season, so long as they voted the way they were meant to.

As the band continued playing, a Democrat on horseback pushed his way into Watson's Populist crowd shouting, "A free dinner for everybody; you are all invited down to the barbecue—white and colored!" Watson had no dinner plans but he had his lungs. "You may have the trees," he shouted to the rider, "but we have got the men; and these men are not going to be enticed away from free, fair discussion of these great public questions by any amount of barbecued beef!" Nor did the crowd move. They wanted to hear Watson out.

Thomas E. Watson was no ordinary farmer and no typical southern politician. He was, in fact, the single largest landowner in Georgia, with more tenants on his land than his grandfather had owned slaves. Yet like some other members of the

New York City's Democratic party machine grew out of the Tammany Society, an eighteenth-century fraternal order named for a Lenni Lenape chief who welcomed William Penn. Here, Tammany Hall is decorated for the Democratic Convention of 1868.

landed class, Watson identified with the poor farmers, tenants, small landholders, and impoverished industrial workers who rallied to the Populist party. During the past two decades, the price of cotton had fallen steadily at the same time that deflation had increased the value of money. For farmers in debt, these conditions meant that paying back loans had become even more expensive. Land in the South was so cheap that farmers could not mortgage it; merchants and banks would allow them only to take out "liens"—obligations to pay back their debts from the sale of future crops. If the crops fell short or prices dropped, they lost their land. Each year fewer farmers owned the land they tilled; a third had become tenants by the time the 1892 election rolled around. "Hundreds of farmers will be turned adrift, and thousands of acres of our best lands be allowed to grow up in weeds. . . . The roads are full of Negroes beggings homes," one newspaper editor warned. Urban workers were equally desperate. The mills that belched the smoke of Henry Grady's New South left their workers in "rooms wherein eight and ten members of one family are stricken down, where pneumonia and fever and measles are attacking their emaciated bodies; where there is no sanitation, no help or protection from the city, no medicine, no food, no fire, no nurses—nothing but torturing hunger and death."

Such folk acted "like victims of some horrid nightmare . . . powerless—oppressed—shackled," Watson observed. To him the agents of ruin were all too evident. They included the huge railroad companies, which charged exorbitant fees to ship cotton, and the industrialists and finance capitalists, who held a "monopoly of power, of place, of privilege, of wealth, of progress." Nor was Watson alone in his views, for many western as well as southern farmers were experiencing hard times. Watson and eight members of Congress from the West had organized a splinter party, called the Populists, or People's party. It ran its first major candidates in the 1892 elections.

Throughout the campaign Watson received continual threats against his life and later regarded it as something of a "miracle" that he hadn't been killed. The hatred resulted not so much from his social program (though proposals like nationalizing the railroads upset many conservatives) as from his decision to build a political alliance between poor whites and poor blacks, against the Republican industrialists of the Northeast and the conservative Democratic ruling class of the South. Watson told his racially mixed audiences that both Democrats and Republicans wanted to keep them divided from each other:

> You are kept apart that you may be separately fleeced of your earnings. You are made to hate each other because upon that hatred is rested the keystone of the arch of financial despotism which enslaves you both. You are deceived and blinded that you may not see how this race antagonism perpetuates a monetary system which beggars both.

As the campaign of 1892 heated up, white Populists found themselves barred from their churches by hostile fellow citizens, denied credit at local stores, even driven from their homes. Citizens of both races nevertheless worked eagerly for Watson. One young black preacher, the Reverend H. S. Doyle, made over 60 speeches in the candidate's behalf; when Doyle was threatened with a lynch mob, Watson gave him haven on his own lands and mobilized some 2000 Populists to protect him. They arrived on "buggies and horses foaming and tired with travel." "We are determined," said Watson, "in this free country that the humblest white or black man that wants to talk our doctrine shall do it, and the man doesn't live who shall touch a hair of his head, without fighting every man in the people's party."

Still, upright intentions could not outweigh fraud and outright violence. As many as 15 blacks died in the Democratic campaign of intimidation. Whiskey was

Georgia firebrand Tom Watson in 1904.

dispensed liberally to persuade citizens to vote Democratic; blacks were trucked in from across the South Carolina line to vote; many Democrats voted repeatedly as ballot boxes were stuffed. Even cash bribes routinely changed hands. After winning through such a convincing show of force, Watson's opponents expected that their adversary had learned his lesson—was so badly beaten that he would have to be laid out in state, like a corpse at a funeral. Watson was having none of it. "We decided not to die," he announced, on behalf of his party. "We unanimously decided to postpone the funeral."

The conditions breeding rebellion and resistance in the South and West would not go away. By the early 1890s the national system of politics as usual was not working. An economic and social revolution had been reshaping America, creating industrial and financial systems of remarkable size, cities whose social diversity and stratification had become much greater than the cities of prewar America, regional economies in the South and West whose raw materials had been drawn into national and international markets over which farmers and ordinary workers had little control.

The political system changed much more slowly. Real social and economic problems were allowed to simmer unattended. Pressures built in the 1890s as the business cycle plunged and a great depression worked its stringent discipline, throwing millions out of work and driving many to violent protest. Politicians were forced to change and adjust. Men and women like Watson ensured that politics could not go on as usual.

THE POLITICS OF PARALYSIS

As he traveled through the United States in the 1880s and 1890s, Moisci Ostrogorski, a Russian political scientist, observed that "the constituted authorities are unequal to their duty." Ostrogorski was part of an invasion of foreign visitors who had come to see the American democratic experiment in action. By the end of the century they were in agreement: the experiment was imperiled, the victim of private greed, middle-class indifference, and political mediocrity. In fact, there were deeper problems—the widening gulf between rich and poor, the growing power of corporate industry, the wretched poverty of city and farm, the endless cycle of boom and bust, the needs of blacks, women, Indians, and other Americans. They had scarcely been addressed, let alone resolved. Politics, the traditional medium of resolution, was grinding into paralysis as Republicans and Democrats fought to a dangerous stalemate.

The Party Stalemate

Another foreign visitor to America in the 1880s, the British historian and diplomat Lord James Bryce, concluded that "neither party has any clean-cut principles, any distinctive tenets. . . . All has been lost, except office or the hope of it." Bryce's judgment, echoed by generations of historians, is too harsh. That the two parties seemed so similar and produced so little were marks of the delicate balance of power on which partisan politics rested in the Gilded Age. From 1877 to 1897 Republicans inhabited the White House for 12 years, Democrats for 8. Margins of victory were paper thin. In 1880, for example, the Republicans won the presiden-

Daily Lives

POLITICAL CULTURE

The Bosses Throw a Party

Chicago's First Ward Ball was a lavish if chaotic affair held in the city's spacious Coliseum. Mounted by ward bosses "Bathhouse" John Coughlin and Michael "Hinky Dink" Kenna, the annual bash had something for everyone. With wine merchants pledged to spend $1500 each, waiters paying $5 just to work the floor, and ordinary tickets running $3 apiece, Hinky Dink and the Bath turned a $20,000 profit in 1907. That was enough to replenish their war chest for the 1908 elections. The 20,000 revelers had thoroughly enjoyed themselves, downing 10,000 quarts of champagne and 30,000 quarts of beer. "Enjoy" was perhaps too tame a judgment. Riotous, drunken carousers stripped unguarded young women naked, overran a lurid "circus act," and smashed a 35-foot bar. "If a great disaster had befallen the Coliseum last night," reported the unamused *Tribune*, "there would not have been a second story worker, a dip or plug ugly, porch climber, dope fiend or scarlet woman remaining in Chicago."

Reformers railed against the "vile orgy," but Hinky Dink and the Bath paid no heed. For 1908 the Coliseum was again rented and the liquor license—all neat and legal—renewed. When the *Tribune* threatened to publish the names of any "better grade" politicians or business leaders (the ball's biggest supporters) who attended, Hinky Dink himself took charge of promoting ticket sales. Any house of ill repute employing two more prostitutes than the year before received an additional 50 tickets to sell. A barber who had been allowed the privilege of placing his pole on the city sidewalk free of charge was encouraged to show his gratitude by purchasing tickets and giving them away. Every saloonkeeper and theater owner in the ward received an extra block to dispose of, and those who refused could be found cooling their heels in jail or suddenly deprived of their mortgages. A few could not be found at all.

When a bomb mysteriously shattered the back windows of the Coliseum two days before the party, Bathhouse John blamed reformers. Asked to compromise with them, the Bath winked: "All right. . . . We won't let parents bring their children." Still, he made a few concessions. Pickpockets were told they were no longer welcome at this year's event and warned that they would be driven from the city if anyone reported a theft. Two hundred burly ward heelers, collectors, and party thugs, each wearing a bright blue ribbon, were detailed as bouncers. (Trusted precinct captains and ward jobholders got red ribbons to identify them as clerks in the cloakroom.) A hundred extra policemen were put on duty to control the crowd.

As night fell on the appointed date, Bathhouse John hurried to the Coliseum from a meeting of the city council. As an alderman, he had just voted against a low bid from an unfriendly contractor to construct a new city hall. He arrived at the celebrations to find 15,000 people jammed along Wabash Avenue waiting to enter. Rushing inside, he spoke briefly to Hinky Dink, checked the preparations one last time, and cried, "O.K.! Let 'em in."

The crowd flooded the hall, knocking over tables and potted palms, crashing like a giant wave onto the bars, and spilling finally into the annex and basement. Some were already in their cups; others demanded beer so ferociously that bartenders had no time to ask for payment. Soon the empty champagne bottles were piled

Daily Lives

Michael "Hinky Dink" Kenna and "Bathhouse" John Coughlin, bosses of Chicago's notorious First Ward and "Lords of the Levee."

high atop tables, the better for Hinky Dink and the Bath to see how the party and the "take" were coming along. The hall became a madhouse, so tightly packed that "even those already drunk were forced to stand erect." High above the throng, in the royal boxes, sat a more dignified group of fun-lovers—the important lawyers, politicians, railroad executives, and businessmen, all wearing masks to avoid detection by reporters.

Then the ladies arrived—painted, daringly dressed, and ready for an evening of sport (despite already having put in half-shifts at the local brothels). At midnight sharp, a huge procession gathered at one end of the Coliseum and strutted, 25 abreast, across the floor. At the head of the Grand March stood Hinky Dink and the Bath, trailed by an army of card sharps and gamblers, prostitutes, pimps and madams, female impersonators, tramps, dive owners, and other assorted characters of unsavory reputation. Then Bathhouse John gave the nod, and the band struck up the evening's theme: "Hail! Hail! The Gang's All Here!"

Loyal voters continued dancing, brawling, and drinking until near dawn, when the Bath called for a final chorus or two of "Home, Sweet Home." A sleepy-eyed Coughlin tarried a bit longer to count receipts. With all the gate crashers and cheapskates, the take was less than $20,000, but no matter—there was always next year!

Chicago's First Ward Ball was not the only such party, only the most notorious. All across turn-of-the-century America similar scenes were enacted. Whether in Boss Cox's Cincinnati, Boss Behrman's New Orleans, or Boss Reuf's San Francisco, political machines were mounting barbecues, boatrides, and balls to raise funds and reward their followers. Reformers might fulminate, but bosses like Hinky Dink and the Bath continued to levy tribute and rule the wards for years to come.

tial race by only 7000 votes out of more than 9 million cast. No president had a majority of his party in both houses of Congress for his entire term. Democrats won control of the House in 1874, lost it in 1880, regained it in 1882, only to lose it in 1888 and win it again in 1890. Republicans held the Senate throughout the period (except for 1879–1881), but between 1876 and 1890 they enjoyed a margin of more than three for only two years.

With elections so tight, the parties orchestrated mass spectacles to bring out the vote. "For three months," reported a British observer, "processions, usually with brass bands, flags, badges, crowds of cheering spectators, are the order of the day and night from end to end of the country." In cities political machines turned out loyal followers on cue. Party workers distributed leaflets and pinned campaign buttons on passers-by, while local postmasters (party appointees) delivered campaign pamphlets with the mail. Picnics and rallies, highlighted by spellbinding speakers, drew people from miles away. Campaigns stressed entertainment and symbols, lest either party risk losing precious votes. "Political oratory," remarked still another foreign traveler, was "not directed towards instruction, but towards stimulation." When election day finally arrived, stores closed and businesses shut down. At political clubs and corner saloons men lined up to get voting orders (along with free drinks) from ward bosses. In the countryside, fields went untended as farmers took their families to town, cast their ballots, and bet on the outcome.

It is no wonder that an average of nearly 80 percent of those eligible cast their ballots in presidential elections between 1876 and 1900, a figure higher than any time since. Even so, the electorate was only a small percentage of the population. Between 1876 and 1892, less than one American in five voted in presidential elections. Other than white males, few citizens even met voting qualifications. Only in Wyoming, Utah, Idaho, and Colorado could women vote in national elections. In 1875 the Supreme Court ruled in *Minor v. Happersett* that states could deny women their franchise. The efforts of the National Woman Suffrage Association to enact a constitutional amendment granting women the right to vote failed miserably, and between 1870 and 1910 almost a dozen states defeated similar referenda.

Party loyalty was unwavering. In every election, 16 states could be counted on to vote Republican, 14 Democratic. Only in Connecticut, New Jersey, Illinois, New York, Indiana, and Ohio were the results ever in doubt. National victories often hung on their returns. Both parties courted them with money, time, and— most flattering of all—presidential candidacies. Between 1868 and 1900 these states produced five of six Republican and four of six Democratic candidates for president. Ohio alone supplied four Republican presidents, New York four Democratic candidates for president.

Republicans and Democrats did have similarities but also clear differences. Both parties supported business and condemned radicalism; neither offered embattled farmers and workers much help. Democrats believed in states' rights and a decentralized, limited government. They were often naysayers, especially to spending. Their regional center of power was the South, which embraced the party not only because Democrats had led the Old Confederacy and "redeemed" it from Reconstruction but also out of fear that federal authorities might try again to protect the rights of African-Americans.

Urban political machines and their immigrant constituents composed a second wing of the Democratic party. The cultural politics of religion and ethnicity

Even as a teenaged printer's apprentice around 1850, Samuel Clemens seemed a cocky "man of letters," displaying his name on a printer's stick. By 1873 his humorous essays and books, published under the pen name of Mark Twain, had made him famous. When he and Charles Dudley Warner published a satirical novel, its title, *The Gilded Age*, became synonymous with an era rife with political spoils and corruption. Twain's masterpiece, *The Adventures of Huckleberry Finn* (1884), combined a realistic ear for dialect with humor that, at bottom, reflected a somber view of human nature.

guided them. Often members of ritualistic religions such as Roman Catholicism, German Lutheranism, and Judaism, they saw salvation in following the rituals of their faith, not in dictating codes of conduct for all society. For an Italian Catholic or a Russian Jew, morality was an individual and family matter. They regarded the Democratic party as a protector of liberty because it opposed such moral and ethnic controls as prohibition of alcohol, Sunday-closing laws, and English-only public schools.

Whereas the Democrats were the party of localism and restraint, the Republicans had begun to develop a national vision and invoke modest federal activism. Drawing on their Whig heritage, they promoted economic growth through the Homestead Act (1862), subsidies to railroads, and protective tariffs. Business interests therefore formed the solid core of their support, around which a substantial portion of the middle class rallied. With memories of emancipation and Reconstruction, African-Americans too voted for the party of Lincoln. (Black voting power, of course, had dwindled as white Democrats "redeemed" the South.) By 1890 well over a million surviving veterans remained loyal to the Grand Old Party. Regionally Republicans could count on the Northeast and Midwest to offset Democratic control of the South. And ethnically they drew on Anglo-Saxon Protestant sects that put their faith in the value of good works to encourage pious behavior throughout society. In the Republican party, which had risen to power with moral condemnations of slavery, these pietistic groups found eager supporters of social controls such as prohibition.

Both parties suffered from deep divisions and personal feuds. The Republicans were split among various factions with colorful labels like "Stalwarts," "Half-Breeds," and "Mugwumps" (an Algonkian word meaning "chief"). Stalwarts looked for leadership to "Lord" Roscoe Conkling, the haughty and vain senator from New York. Tall, graceful, a former boxer, Conkling summed up his philosophy in one line: "I do not know how to belong to a party a little." He and his followers hewed to the old tenets of Republicanism, especially its commitments to Reconstruction and establishing the Republican party in the South. Most of all they believed in the time-honored political traditions of acquiring power and dispersing the "spoils" (federal, state, and local offices) to supporters and party workers.

No less a master of spoils was the charming, sharp-tongued senator from Maine, James G. Blaine, who led the Half-Breeds. These forward-looking party members embraced the new Republicanism of economic nationalism, tariff protection, and the development of an urban industrial society. Opposed to both factions were the Mugwumps. Elitist and socially prominent, out of touch with the mass of voters, they wanted to end corruption and replace the spoils system with a rational civil service that employed men of wealth, education, and standing. Essentially conservative, they favored a limited supply of money and laissez-faire government. For their part the Democrats, as ardent a collection of spoils-seekers as the Stalwarts and Half-Breeds, were split among southern white supremacists and family farmers, urban machine politicians, and business interests bent on lowering tariffs.

Impassioned reformers usually created their own political instruments. Some formed nonpartisan groups that aligned themselves behind issues rather than parties. Opponents of alcohol formed the Women's Christian Temperance Union (1874) and the Anti-Saloon League (1893). Champions of the rights of women joined the National Woman Suffrage Association (1890), a reunion of two branches of the women's suffrage movement that had split in 1869. Formal political parties sometimes crystallized around a single concern or a particular group. Advocates of prohibition rallied to the Prohibition party (1869). Those who sought inflation of the currency formed the Greenback party (1874). Disgruntled farmers in the West and South created the Populist, or People's, party (1892). All drew scores of supporters from both conventional parties, but as single-interest groups, they mobilized minorities, not majorities.

Congressional Politics

Congressional politics focused on the well-worn issues of regional conflict, patronage, tariffs, and money. With the presidency weakened by the impeachment of Andrew Johnson, the scandals of Ulysses S. Grant, and the contested victory of Rutherford B. Hayes in 1876, Congress enjoyed the initiative in making policy. Time after time, legislators squandered it amid electioneering and party infighting.

Some divisive issues were the bitter legacy of the Civil War. Well into the 1880s Republicans symbolically waved the "bloody shirt" by labeling Democrats the "party of treason," responsible for the war between the states and unworthy of governing. "Not every Democrat was a Rebel," they reminded voters, "but every rebel was a Democrat." South of the Mason–Dixon line, Democrats waved the bloody shirt too, only it was the Republicans who were called traitors.

The war's politics also surfaced in the lobbying efforts of veterans. The Grand Army of the Republic, an organization of over 400,000 former Union soldiers, petitioned the government for pensions to make up for poor wartime pay and to support the widows and orphans of their fallen comrades. By the turn of the century Union army veterans and their families were receiving $157 million annually, one of the largest programs of public assistance in American history. Veterans of the Confederacy, on the other hand, got nothing except small pensions from several southern states.

Less divisive but more relevant was the campaign for a new method of staffing federal offices. Since the early nineteenth century, government jobs had been awarded by political victors, who simply gave them away to loyal followers regardless of their qualifications. After elections, winners faced an army of office seekers, "lying in wait . . . like vultures for a wounded bison." President Hayes found that even his wife was hounded by applicants, and Benjamin Harrison despaired that he spent as many as six hours a day dealing with them during the first 18 months of his presidency.

The increasing size of the federal bureaucracy made the situation almost intolerable by the late 1880s. From barely 53,000 people on the payroll at the end of the Civil War, the federal government had grown to 166,000 by the early 1890s. In addition, far more government jobs required special skills. For example, the use of typewriters (20 of them were hammering away at the Justice Department by the mid-1880s) meant that literacy and intelligence alone no longer qualified someone for a clerkship. As government expanded, the need for scientists, engineers, and other well-trained professionals grew accordingly.

Dismantling the spoils system, whatever the need, stirred great controversy. American politics rested on patronage. Without it, politicians—from presidents to lowly ward captains—feared that they could attract neither the workers nor the money required to run their parties. Reacting to the scandals of the Grant administration, a group of young independents, generally well educated and well-to-do, banded together in 1881 to form the National Civil Service Reform League. The league promoted the British model of civil service based on examination and merit. Defenders of the spoils system called the reform "snivel service," with neither party in Congress willing to take action when it held power (and thus controlled patronage). Presidents, not nearly so dependent on appointees for influence, could more easily afford to advocate reform.

The assassination of President James A. Garfield in 1881 by Charles Guiteau, a demented and frustrated office seeker, finally produced a clamor for reform. In 1883 the Civil Service Act, or Pendleton Act, created a bipartisan civil service commission to administer competitive examinations for a select number of federal jobs. It also outlawed the assessments political leaders charged their appointees and established an orderly, nonpartisan method of promotion. While the new system applied to only 10 percent of all federal jobs, presidents could expand the list. By 1896 almost one federal worker in two came under civil service (though whether the new system actually improved the quality of bureaucrats was hotly debated).

As much as any issue, the protective tariff ignited popular emotions while baffling politicians. The tax on imports of manufactured goods and some agricultural products had been created early in the century to protect developing "infant industries." Since then the debate on whether to increase or lower tariffs had set regions and interest groups against one another. Northern and eastern industrialists supported high schedules to keep up the prices of their foreign competitors. So did laboring men and women, who wanted to protect their wages and jobs. Southerners saw the tariff as more unfair protection for the industrial Northeast and opposed it on all but the products made within their region. Farmers, while favoring protection for agriculture, wanted rates on manufactured goods reduced. Consumers maintained that high tariffs gouged them by keeping prices up, regardless of the jobs they preserved.

As promoters of economic growth, Republicans usually favored high tariffs.

Democrats generally sought reduction to encourage foreign trade and cut the federal surplus. In 1890, when Republicans controlled the House, Congress enacted the McKinley Tariff (1890), which raised schedules to an all-time high. The McKinley Tariff also contained a novel twist, a reciprocity clause to promote foreign trade. The president was given authority to lower rates if other countries did the same. In 1894 Democrats in the House, supported strongly by President Grover Cleveland, succeeded in reducing rates, only to be thwarted by some 600 Senate amendments restoring most cuts. In 1897 the Dingley Tariff raised rates still higher but soothed reductionists by broadening reciprocity.

Just as murky and emotional was the currency controversy. Until about the mid-1800s American money, like that of other nations, was coined from both gold and silver. In this policy of "bimetallism," the Treasury periodically adjusted the number of grains of each metal in the dollar according to the price of gold and silver bullion on the open market. The need for more money during the Civil War led Congress to issue "greenbacks"—currency printed on green paper that was not redeemable in gold or silver. For the next decade and a half Americans argued over whether to print more unsupported paper money or take it out of circulation entirely. In 1878 the "Greenback" party polled over a million votes and elected 14 representatives to Congress. Yet fear of inflation led Congress first to reduce the number of greenbacks in circulation, then in 1879 to make what remained convertible into gold on demand. The currency and the question faded from the scene.

Meanwhile a more heated battle was developing over silver-backed money. In a sense it pitted "have-nots" against "haves." The have-nots of business— aggressive entrepreneurs interested in starting new ventures—were hungry for capital to build factories, warehouses, or railroads. They wanted more silver coined to expand the money supply. Prices would rise and interest rates would fall, an ideal situation for eager new businessmen.

Farmers also looked to silver for salvation. Some had bought cheap land from railroads or from the government on credit. Others borrowed every year to purchase seed and equipment for planting and harvesting. As the prices of wheat, corn, and other agricultural products steadily slipped, these farmers found themselves unable to pay their debts. They blamed "the money power"—gold-oriented northeastern bankers and financiers—for keeping the supply of money low and interest rates high. Inflation, they believed, would increase farm prices and fatten farmers' profits. It would even cheapen their debts by permitting them to repay loans with dollars worth less than those originally borrowed. Western miners, who had just hit a mother lode of silver, also supported bimetallism.

Bankers, other creditors, and established businessmen—the haves—stood firmly for "sound money," a limited supply of currency that rested on the time-honored standard of gold. It was an article of their faith that dollars exchangeable for gold induced the business confidence required for prosperity by keeping the monetary system tight and stable. "Atheism is not worse in religion," declared the New York *Christian Advocate* in 1878, "than an unstable or irredeemable currency in political economy."

By the early 1870s the United States and Europe used so little silver that Congress stopped coining it. A silver mining boom in Nevada soon revived demands for coining the metal. In 1878 the Bland–Allison Act inaugurated a limited form of silver coinage. The Treasury was required to purchase between $2 million and $4 million worth of silver each month. Pressure for unlimited coinage of silver—coining of all silver presented at United States mints—mounted as silver production quadrupled between 1870 and 1890. Under the Bland–Allison Act, moreover, the money supply was growing too slowly for inflationists. Each year the government was able to buy all the silver it needed with fewer and fewer dollars because new discoveries reduced silver prices. The money supply grew too slowly. By 1890 the pressure to coin silver had reached such a level that President Harrison and Republican leaders in Congress adopted the Sherman Silver Purchase Act. The government was obligated to buy 4.5 million ounces of silver every month regardless of the price. Paper tender called "treasury notes," redeemable in either gold or silver, would pay for it. The compromise satisfied both sides only temporarily, and by the mid-1890s silver was again a hot issue.

The White House from Hayes to Harrison

From the 1870s through the 1890s a run of nearly anonymous presidents presided over the country. Not all were mere caretakers; some tried to revive the office, but Congress continued to reign supreme in Washington. Despite the criticism of modern historians, such legislative supremacy more closely reflected the intentions of the Founding Fathers. The dynamic presidency is more a product of twentieth-century circumstances and political values.

The first of the "Ohio dynasty" (three presidents from 1876 to 1900), Republican Rutherford B. Hayes was, in the opinion of one Democratic leader, "far better than four years of unrest which we should undoubtedly have had if Tilden had occupied the office of President." ("Rutherfraud" Hayes, as the angry losers called him, had reversed the popular election victory of Samuel Tilden in 1876 with secret deals for contested electoral votes.) A Harvard-trained lawyer, wounded veteran of the Civil War, and reform governor of Ohio, Hayes was moderate in his personal habits. When Rutherford and "Lemonade Lucy" Hayes threw a dinner party, said one guest, "the water flowed like champagne." As president, Hayes moved quickly to end Reconstruction and tried unsuccessfully to woo southern Democrats with promises of economic support. He pursued civil service reform so staunchly that one angry spoilsman called him "George Washington." Making few inroads against the spoils system, he left office after a single term, happy to be "out of a scrape."

Republican James Garfield succeeded Hayes, but not for long. Another former soldier from Ohio, Garfield won by a handful of votes and spent his first hundred days in the White House besieged by office hunters and indecisively trying to placate the rival Half-Breed and Stalwart sections of his party. On July 2, 1881, Garfield was shot while standing in a Washington railroad station, on route to a vacation in New England. "I am a Stalwart and Arthur is President now!" shouted Charles Guiteau, the crazed assassin who had failed to receive an appointment in the administration. Garfield lingered for 11 weeks before succumbing to his wounds. Chester A. Arthur, a "spoilsman's spoilsman" and protégé of party boss Roscoe Conkling, was president. "Chet Arthur, President of the United States," exclaimed a dismayed Republican. "Good God!"

"He isn't 'Chet' Arthur any more," concluded one former associate soon after the inauguration. To almost everyone's surprise, the fastidious Arthur turned out to be an honest president. He transformed the gloomy and dilapidated White House into an elegant social center. He broke with machine politicians, including his mentor Roscoe Conkling. He worked to lower the tariff, warmly endorsed the

Handsome and urbane, Chester A. Arthur was the era's most fashionable and least distinguished president.

new Civil Service Act, and reduced the federal surplus by beginning construction of a modern navy. Such even-handed administration left him little chance for renomination from party leaders. Half-Breeds regarded him as a Stalwart, Stalwarts as a renegade. Arthur could never have accepted anyway; he was dying and knew it.

The election of 1884 was, in the words of a contemporary, the "vilest" ever waged. It pitted Half-Breed Senator James Blaine, the beloved "Plumed Knight" from Maine, against Democrat Grover Cleveland, the former mayor of Buffalo and governor of New York. Despite superb talents as a leader and vote-getter, Blaine was haunted by renewed charges that he helped to secure illegal favors for the Little Rock and Fort Smith Railroad. "Grover the Good," on the other hand, had won a well-deserved reputation for honesty by fighting corruption and the spoils system in New York. The diligent and portly Cleveland, sighed a reporter, "remains within doors constantly, eats and works, eats and works, and works and eats." Unfortunately Cleveland, a bachelor, spent enough time away from work to father an illegitimate child. "Above all, tell the truth," he instructed his campaign managers, when the scandal broke, whereupon Republicans throughout the country broke into a chant of "Ma, ma, where's my pa?" In the last week of the tight race, Democrats circulated among the numerous Irish-Catholic voters of New York the statement of a local Protestant minister that labeled Democrats the party of "Rum, Romanism, and Rebellion" (alcohol, Catholicism, and the Civil War). Most of the Irish who had been tempted to support Blaine returned to the Democratic fold and New York swung to Cleveland. When Cleveland won the election (by a mere 25,000 out of 10 million votes), Democrats told Republicans where to find the bachelor father: "Gone to the White House, ha, ha, ha!"

A Chinese laborer, queue in hand, proudly displays patches in support of the 1888 Democratic presidential candidate Grover Cleveland and his running mate, Allen B. Thurman. Cleveland and Thurman lost to Benjamin Harrison and Levi P. Morton.

Cleveland was the first Democrat elected to the White House since James Buchanan in 1856. He pleased reformers, especially Mugwumps who had deserted the Republican party to support him, by expanding the civil service. Businessmen praised his conservative devotion to gold, economy, and efficiency. He endorsed the growth of federal power by supporting the Interstate Commerce Act (1887), new agricultural research, and federal arbitration of labor disputes.

Cleveland's presidential activism remained limited. He vetoed two of every three bills brought to him, more than twice the number of all his predecessors combined. Toward the end of his term, embarrassed by the large federal surplus, Cleveland finally exerted leadership by attacking the tariff as "the vicious, inequitable, illogical source of taxation" and pledging to lower it. The Republican-controlled Senate blocked this move, and in 1888 Republicans nominated a sturdy defender of protectionism, Benjamin Harrison, the grandson of President William Henry Harrison. Cleveland won a plurality of the popular vote but lost in the Electoral College. Since the Republicans also won both houses of Congress, 1888 marked the most sweeping victory for either party in nearly 20 years.

Benjamin Harrison (called by his colleagues the "human iceberg") worked hard, rarely delegated management, and turned the White House into a well-regulated office. Cautiously active, he began to bring the presidency back to life. As a former senator, he understood the value of executive advice and pressure; he offered both at informal dinners at the White House with leaders of the House and Senate, in trial balloons released to reporters, and in well-timed messages to Congress. He helped to shape the Sherman Silver Purchase Act (1890), kept up with the McKinley Tariff (1890), and accepted the Sherman Antitrust Act (1890), which limited the control exerted by business combinations over markets. At his urging the House passed a Federal Elections Bill to protect the rights of black voters. Democrats denounced it as a "force bill" and filibustered it to death in the Senate. Yet by the end of Harrison's term in 1892, Congress had completed its most productive term of the era, including the first billion-dollar peacetime budget. To Democratic taunts of an extravagant "Billion Dollar Congress," Republican House Speaker Thomas Reed shot back, "This is a billion-dollar country!"

Ferment in the States and Cities

It would be misleading to focus only on Washington. Most people expected little from the federal government. It was closer to home that public pressure mounted. Ambivalence about the growth of big business, discontent over discriminatory shipping rates, and widespread anxiety about political corruption and urban decay produced a ferment in the states and cities. Experimental and often effective, state programs set important precedents for later action and represented some of the era's boldest initiatives in public policy.

Starting in 1869 with Massachusetts, states established commissions to investigate and regulate industry. By the turn of the century, almost two-thirds of the states had them. The first commissions gathered and publicized information on shipping rates and business practices and furnished advice on public policy. In the Midwest, on the Great Plains, and in the Far West, merchants and farmers upset over unfair railroad rates and rebates to large shippers pressed state governments for action. In Sacramento, California, one newspaper published a schedule of freight rates to various places in Nevada, showing that lower rates had been charged by wagon teams before the railroads were built. On the West Coast and in

the Midwest, state legislatures empowered commissions to end rebates and monitor rates. In 1870 Illinois became the first of several states to define railroads as
public highways subject to regulation, including setting maximum rates.

Concern over the condition of cities and their politics led to state municipal
conventions, the first in Iowa in 1877. Philadelphia sponsored a national conference on good city government in 1894, and a year later reformers founded the
National Municipal League. Within two years it had over 200 branches. Its model
city charter advanced such far-sighted reforms as separate city and state elections,
limited franchises for utilities, and more authority for mayors. Meanwhile cities
and states in the Midwest enacted pietistic laws closing stores on Sundays, prohibiting the sale of alcohol, and making English the language of public schools—all in
an effort to control the habits of newcomers from abroad.

THE REVOLT OF THE FARMERS

In 1890 the politics of complacency cracked. Lavish expenditures of the "Billion-
Dollar Congress" on pensions and public works, together with the overall expansion of federal authority, angered many voters. Beginning in the late 1880s, a
severe agricultural depression hit. In 1887 and again in 1889 droughts withered
crops. Yet overproduction caused prices to fall, and a wave of foreclosures drove
thousands of desperate farmers from the western plains.

Farmers had no trouble explaining why. "We went to work and plowed and
planted," said one woman. "The rains fell, the sun shone, nature smiled, and we
raised the big crop they told us to; and what came of it? Eight cent corn, ten cent
oats, two cent beef and no price at all for butter and eggs—that's what came of it.
Then the politicians said we suffered from over-production." Overproduction
there had been, but as the previous chapter made clear, farmers suffered from a
great deal more—declining prices, discriminatory railroad rates, heavy mortgages, and widespread poverty. It was only in 1890 that the political resentment
building up for a decade or more boiled over on a national scale. "The farmer fed
all other men," an angry speaker concluded, "and lived himself upon scraps."

The Harvest of Discontent

The revolt of the farmers, which came eventually to be known as Populism, first
stirred on the southern frontier, swept eastward from Texas to the other states of
the Old Confederacy, and then spread through the western plains. The exaspera-
tion from which it sprang was global. Farmers found the labor-saving machines
that plowed their fields, harvested their crops, and hauled the crops to market
were also producing price-deflating surpluses. Between 1860 and 1890, wheat
output in the United States leaped from 173 million to 449 million bushels, cotton
from 5.3 million to 8.5 million bales. By the late 1880s the price of wheat had
dropped by 50 percent; that of cotton, 80 percent. In Kansas prices fell so low that
families burned corn for heat.

Farmers blamed their troubles on obvious inequalities: manufacturers were
protected by the tariff; railroads charged high rates; bankers held their mounting
debts; and expensive middlemen stored and processed their goods. All seemed to

profit at the expense of farmers. The true picture was fuzzier. The tariff protected industrial goods but supported many agricultural commodities. Railroads rates, however high, actually fell from 1865 to 1890. And it was true that mortgages were heavy, yet most were short, no more than four years. Farmers often refinanced them, using the money to buy additional land and machinery that increased their output and their incomes as well as their debts. Middlemen did make handsome profits, but increasingly millers and grain elevator operators were coming under state regulation.

In hard times, of course, none of this mattered. And in the South many poor farmers seemed condemned to hard times forever. Credit lay at the root of their problem. To plant and harvest their crops, southern farmers had to borrow money. When prices fell, they borrowed still more, stretching the financial resources of the South beyond their meager limits. Within a few years after the Civil War, Massachusetts' banks had five times as much money as all the banks of the Old Confederacy. The South became a giant debtors' pen.

The burden of debt fell most heavily on poor farmers. Increasingly they labored under the vicious crop–lien system, which operated throughout the South (page 726). From start to finish this debasing system shackled poor southern farmers to a single crop and a single merchant, in the process depriving them of land and liberty. Beginning in the 1870s, nearly 100,000 farmers a year picked up stakes throughout the Deep South, scrawled the initials "GTT" (Gone to Texas) on their doors, and fled west to escape the system—only to find it waiting for them. Others stood and fought, as one pamphlet exhorted in 1889, "not with glittering musket, flaming sword and deadly cannon, but with the silent potent and all-powerful ballot, the only vestige of liberty left."

The Alliance Movement

Before farmers could vote together, they had to get together. Life on the farm was harsh, drab, and most of all isolated. As late as 1900 an average farmer worked 68 hours a week (the average industrial worker put in 56 hours). Their clothes were mostly homespun, meals mainly potatoes, bread, and salt pork. On the Great Plains, weeks might pass before someone happened by. The Sears, Roebuck catalog was the only link many farmers had to the world outside their communities.

The earliest impulses to organize grew out of such social conditions. In 1867, Oliver Hudson Kelley, a government clerk stunned by the dullness of rural southern life, founded the Patrons of Husbandry. It was designed to brighten the lives of farmers and broaden their intellectual horizons. Local "granges"—neighborhood chapters of a few dozen members—brought farmers and their families together to pray, sing, and learn new farming techniques. The Grangers sponsored fairs, picnics, dances, lectures—anything to break down the loneliness of farm life. After a slow start the Grange grew quickly as the depression of 1873 sent farmers in search of solace. By 1875 there were 800,000 members in 20,000 locals, mostly in the Midwest, South, and Southwest.

Generally the Grangers swore off politics, but in a pattern repeated again and again among farmers, socializing soon led to economic and political action. Grangers began to pool their money to create cooperatively owned enterprises for buying and selling, for milling and storing, and for banking and manufacturing. In the early 1870s they lobbied midwestern legislatures to adopt "Granger laws" regulating rates charged by railroads, grain elevator operators, and other middlemen.

Eight "Granger cases" came before the Supreme Court in the 1870s. In *Munn v. Illinois* (1877), the most important, the justices upheld the right of Illinois to regulate private property (in this case, giant elevators used for storing grain) so long as it was "devoted to a public use." Later decisions limited regulation of railroads, ruling that states could not determine rates of carriers that crossed state lines. Congress responded in 1887 by creating the Interstate Commerce Commission, a federal agency that could regulate commerce among the states. It was supposed to investigate railroad rates and practices and stop rebates and pooling arrangements. It had little real power of enforcement, but it was a key step toward establishing the public right to control private corporations.

As the depression of 1873 waned, the Patrons of Husbandry lost members. By the end of the 1880s, stimulated by another slump in prices, a host of new organizations had blended into what the press called the Alliance Movement. The Southern Alliance, formed in Texas in 1875, spread rapidly after Dr. Charles W. Macune took command in 1886. A doctor and lawyer as well as a farmer, Macune was a tireless organizer and innovative thinker. What he had in mind was expanding Texas' network of local chapters, or suballiances, into a national network of state Alliance Exchanges. Together they would avoid the high charges of middlemen by pooling their resources to buy supplies and equipment and to store and market their crops. Hostile business leaders called the idea socialism, but Macune was no socialist. Like other farmers, he merely wanted to increase his profits, protection, and freedom to maneuver.

Soon the Southern Alliance was publicizing its activities in local newspapers, publishing a journal, and sending lecturers to 43 states and territories. By 1890 it claimed more than a million members. Hoping at first to stay within the framework of the traditional party system, the Southern Alliance tried to win over the Democratic party. "Pitchfork" Ben Tillman in South Carolina and Tom Watson in Georgia—still a loyal Democrat—successfully challenged regular Democrats.

Across the South, Alliance cooperatives sprang up, and at first the results seemed marvelous. Macune claimed that his new Texas Exchange saved farmers 40 percent on plows and 30 percent on wagons. When the jute trust—the manufacturers who made the bags used in the cottonfields—raised prices in 1888, Alliance leaders organized a boycott that brought prices back down. But most Alliance cooperatives were managed by farmers without the time or experience to succeed. Usually opposed by irate local merchants, the ventures were bound to fail. For a brief period, however, between 1886 and 1892, the cooperatives multiplied throughout the South, challenging accepted ways of doing business.

Although the Southern Alliance admitted no blacks, it did encourage African-American farmers to organize. Founded by a small group of white and black Texans in 1886, the Colored Farmers' National Alliance and Cooperative Union maintained branches in every southern state. By 1891 there were about a quarter of a million members. Activities were largely secret, since public action often brought swift, sometimes deadly, retribution from white supremacists. When Ben Patterson organized a strike of black cotton pickers near Memphis in 1891, white mobs hunted down and lynched 15 strikers, including Patterson. The murders went unpunished and the Colored Farmers' Alliance began to founder.

The idea of farm cooperation swept northward to the states of the Midwest and Great Plains in the form of the National Farmers' Alliance, or Northwestern Alliance, created in 1880. In June 1890 Kansas organizers formed the first People's party, a local political alternative that would respond to grassroots needs. Meanwhile the Southern Alliance changed its name to the National Farmers' Alliance and Industrial Union, incorporated the strong Northern Alliances in the Dakotas and Kansas, and made the movement truly national in scope.

The key to Alliance success was not organization but leadership, not simply from a few at the top but from hundreds in the middle. Specially trained Alliance lecturers traveled across states, organized suballiances, and taught members about complex national issues such as money and finance and local issues like building and expanding cooperatives. Rugged, red-haired William Lamb in Texas, Georgia firebrand Tom Watson, Ignatius Donnelly, the utopian novelist and orator from Minnesota, and "Sockless" Jerry Simpson in Kansas founded new branches throughout the South and Great Plains, reminding farmers who stood for them, who against them.

In a movement remarkably free of gender prejudice, women were as important as men. "Wimmin is everywhere," noted one observer of the "wonderful picnicking, speech-making Alliance summer of 1890." The observation seemed literally true of Mary Elizabeth Lease. In the summer of 1890 alone she gave some 160 speeches, several over two hours long. An indomitable supporter of temperance, woman's suffrage, union labor, and the Alliance, she hurled sentences, said one woman, "like Jove hurled thunderbolts." Seeing wasted corn burned for heat or piled along railroad tracks, she told farmers to "raise less corn and more hell." And she attacked northeastern financiers: "It is no longer a government of the people, by the people, and for the people," she told farmers eager for easy answers, "but a government of Wall Street, by Wall Street, and for Wall Street."

In 1890 members of the Alliance meeting in Ocala, Florida, produced the "Ocala Demands," a platform that urged reduced tariff rates, an end to national banks, rigid regulation of railroads, free coinage of silver, a federal income tax, and popular election of senators—this last designed to make government more responsive to public opinion. Its most innovative feature came again from the inventive Charles Macune. His "subtreasury system" called on the federal government to build warehouses where farmers could store their crops until prices rose, instead of having to sell them on a glutted market, as they did under the crop–lien system. To tide them over, farmers would receive greenbacks covering 80 percent of the market value of the crop, a government loan to be repaid when the crops were sold.

In the elections of 1890 the old parties faced the challenge of hostile farmers across the nation. Working within the Democratic party, southern Alliancemen measured candidates by the "Alliance yardstick" (their willingness to support Alliance demands) and nearly gained control. They elected four governors, gained control of eight legislatures, and sent 44 congressmen and three senators to Washington. In the Great Plains, the Alliance drew farmers from the Republican party. Newly created farmer parties elected five congressmen and two senators in Kansas and South Dakota and took over both houses of the Nebraska legislature. Where they did not elect their own candidates, their presence helped to account for Democratic victories over Republican incumbents.

Mary Elizabeth Lease, the "Kansas Pythoness," was admitted to the bar as a young woman but soon turned to radical activism. A charismatic speaker, she campaigned for Populist candidates in the 1890s, on one occasion warning the industrial Northeast that "the people are at bay, let the bloodhounds of money beware."

The People's Party

The successes of 1890 raised the ambitions as well as the political consciousness of farmers. In the West especially, Alliance organizers began to dream of a national third party, free from the corporate influence, sectionalism, and racial tensions that split both Republicans and Democrats. It would be a party not just of farmers but of the downtrodden, including industrial workers.

As the presidential election approached, a convention of 900 labor, feminist, farm, and other reform delegates (100 of them black) met in St. Louis in February 1892. "The fruits of the toil of millions," Ignatius Donnelly told the audience,

> are boldly stolen to build up colossal fortunes, unprecedented in the history of the world, while their possessors despise the republic and endanger liberty. From the same prolific womb of governmental injustice we breed two great classes—paupers and millionaires.

Moved to wild enthusiasm, delegates rushed the podium to grasp Donnelly's hand. They founded the People's, or Populist, party and called for a convention to nominate a ticket for the presidential election. At first southerners held back from such independence, clinging to their strategy of boring from within the Democratic party. When newly elected southern congressmen failed to support Alliance programs, southern leaders like Tom Watson abandoned the Democrats and began recruiting black and white farmers for the Populists.

The national Populist convention met in Omaha, Nebraska, on July 4, 1892. "It was a religious revival," exclaimed one observer, "a crusade, a pentecost of politics in which a tongue of flame sat upon every man." The Populists adopted a platform that harkened back to Ocala two years earlier. Its preamble, the impassioned work of Ignatius Donnelly, promised to restore government "to the hands of the people." Planks advocated the subtreasury plan, unlimited coinage of silver and an increase in the money supply, direct election of senators, an income tax, and government ownership of railroads, telegraph, and telephone. To attract wage earners the party endorsed the eight-hour workday, restriction of "undesirable" immigration, and a ban on the use of Pinkerton detectives in labor disputes—for the Pinkertons had engaged in a savage gun battle with strikers that year at Andrew Carnegie's Homestead steel plant. The interests of "rural and civic labor," the platform declared, were the same, "their enemies . . . identical." The only somber note was struck before the convention opened when Leonidas Polk, president of the Farmers' Alliance and the leading candidate for the presidential nomination, died. Delegates turned to the old greenbacker and Union general, James B. Weaver, carefully balancing the ticket with a one-legged Confederate veteran as his running mate.

The Populists enlivened the otherwise dull campaign, as Democrat Grover Cleveland and Republican incumbent Benjamin Harrison refought the election of 1888. Mary Elizabeth Lease joined Weaver on trips through the South and West, where they drew crowds that "could only be counted by the acre." In the Northwest, Ignatius Donnelly, running for governor of Minnesota, made 150 speeches to nearly 10,000 voters in a campaign he described as the "liveliest ever seen" in the state. Meanwhile Tom Watson campaigned in Georgia, bringing white and black supporters together.

The results were mixed. Weaver polled over a million votes, the first third-party candidate to do so. He carried Kansas and four western states with 22 electoral votes. Populists ran strongest among western farmers and silver miners, who found the party's stand on currency particularly appealing. When local votes were tallied, Populists elected 3 governors, 5 senators, 10 congressmen, and nearly 1500 members of state legislatures.

For all the Populists' successes, the election revealed dangerous weaknesses in the party. Ignatius Donnelly ran a disappointing third in the Minnesota gubernatorial race. In the Northeast and most of the Midwest Weaver lost badly. In southern states Weaver won more than a quarter of the vote only in Alabama. Worst of all for the southern Populists, Tom Watson lost his seat in Congress through the traditional tactics of fraud and intimidation. (In Augusta alone, his Democratic opponent received twice as many votes as there were legal voters.) For all of Watson's determination to fight on, southern conservatives were appalled by his open courtship of blacks.

Across the nation thousands of voters changed political affiliations in the election of 1892, but most often they switched from the Republican to the Democratic party, and not to the Populists. No doubt the campaign of intimidation and repression hurt the People's party in the South. In the North, the Populists also failed to win over labor and most city dwellers. Both were more concerned with family budgets than low farm prices, high farm debt, and limited supplies of money. Inflation, after all, was bound to hurt consumers, especially those workers whose wages could not keep pace with rising prices. And the darker side of Populism put off many Americans. Its rhetoric was often violent; it spoke ominously of conspiracies and stridently in favor of immigration restriction. Ignatius Donnelly might expound on the ills of farmers one moment, but the next he might be publishing an anti-Semitic novel like *Caesar's Column*, prophesying a depraved world ruled by an international Jewish oligarchy. Most fatal for the Populists, they failed to attract a majority of farmers. Even the Alliance lost members.

In 1896 and 1900 Populists nominated candidates for the presidency; neither won. The party's moment had passed. It left an exhilarating momentum and a legacy of unfinished business, including proposals for a subtreasury system, popular election of senators, and an income tax. In one form or another all would be enacted into legislation in the future. For the present, the People's party demonstrated two conflicting truths: how far from the needs of many ordinary Americans traditional parties had drifted and how difficult it would be to break their hold on the political system.

THE DEPRESSION OF 1893

In 1892 Grover Cleveland won an impressive victory in his third race for the White House, carrying seven northern states as well as the Solid South. For the first time since the Civil War Democrats also controlled both houses of Congress. Helped by working-class voters who had been revolted by the pitched battles, gunfire, and deaths in the Homestead Steel Strike, the Democrats increased their strength in industrial cities and among wage earners. Business executives remained calm. "I am very sorry for President Harrison," wrote Henry Clay Frick, manager of the Homestead plant and normally a Republican, "but I cannot see that our interests are going to be affected one way or the other by the change of administration."

The economy, not the new administration, soon shattered business confidence. In the recovery from the depression of 1873, the economy had gradually but relentlessly overexpanded: railroads overbuilt, businesses borrowed to finance expansive new projects, farmers increased their production by purchasing farm machinery on credit. The capability to borrow was essential for economic expansion, of course; but under the new industrial order, the fortunes of industry, labor, and farmers became tied so closely to one another and to international developments that a major downturn in one area affected other sectors of the economy. Even before Cleveland's inauguration ominous signs appeared that credit was crumbling. The Philadelphia and Reading Railroad, deeply in debt to finance the building of new stations, bridges, and tracks, declared bankruptcy. A major British banking firm had already failed spectacularly in 1890, causing British investors to retrench by selling their American investments for gold. This in turn contributed to a drain in U.S. gold reserves as the depression in Europe steadily worsened. In mid-February a flurry of panic selling hit the New York Stock Exchange. Stockholders sensed that uncertain currency values, glutted markets, depressed agricultural prices, and declining exports had sapped economic strength. By April the gold reserves of the U.S. Treasury had dropped below the critical $100 million mark.

On May 5, 1893, after a wave of bankruptcies had destroyed major firms across the country, stock prices sank to all-time lows. By the end of the year, 600 banks and 15,000 businesses had failed, among them such symbols of stability as the Northern Pacific, Union Pacific, and Santa Fe railroads. Officials considered closing the Stock Exchange. The new industrial order had brought prosperity to some farmers by opening larger markets to them and tied Americans closer together with better communications and transportation networks, but the price of interdependence now became obvious. Without some way to control the excesses of the boom-and-bust business cycle, depression would be visited upon the nation on as large a scale as the booming prosperity had been. The economic costs were all too quickly paid in human currency.

The Depths of Depression

The depression of 1893, the deepest to that date in the nation's history, lasted until 1897. Charles Francis Adams, Jr., railroad baron and descendant of two presidents, called it a "convulsion." The depression revived doubts about the price of industrialization, sparked labor violence and near class warfare, and produced a new awareness of how intertwined American society had become.

The most obvious problem was the sheer lack of jobs, the effect of a failing industrial economy. In August 1893 unemployment stood at 1 million; by January 1894, 2 million; by the middle of 1894, 3 million. At the end of the year nearly one worker in five was out of a job. Washington, D.C., newspapers reported "a vast army of unemployed, and men pleading for food who have never before been compelled to seek aid." Every night at every police station in Chicago, from 60 to 100 people sought shelter. In Detroit the needy transformed vacant lots into "Pingree Potato Patches" (named for the mayor of the city). In Pasadena, California, they dined at soup kitchens bitterly nicknamed "Cleveland Cafes." In the South and Great Plains states, farm prices fell below the cost of production. Western cattle went to market for a few dollars; repossessed machinery sat in sheriffs' lots. As one desperate Kansas farmer bluntly put it, "The problem is how to live."

The federal government had no program at all. "While the people should

The Massachusetts-born illustrator Charles Dana Gibson, famous for his portraits of well-bred young women in the 1890s, tackles a different subject in this ink drawing, a bread line of mixed classes during the terrible depression of 1893.

patriotically and cheerfully support their Government," President Cleveland had said at his inauguration, "its functions do not include the support of the people." The states offered little more. Relief, like poverty, was considered a private matter. The burden fell on local charities, benevolent societies, churches, labor unions, and ward bosses. In city after city, citizens organized relief committees to cope with distress. They distributed bread and clothing until their meager resources gave out under the weight of want. At one point Chicago saloons were giving free lunches to an estimated 60,000 people a day. Others were less generous. As the popular preacher Henry Ward Beecher told his congregation, "No man in this land suffers from poverty unless it be more than his fault—unless it be his sin."

The scale of hardship began a slow change in thinking about poverty. "The individual crawled as best he could, through the wreck," wrote historian Henry Adams, "and found many values of life upset." People saw that anyone could be thrown out of work—an industrious neighbor, a factory foreman with 20 years on the job, a bank president. One survey of the working class revealed that as late as 1901 half the heads of households had no jobs. Working- and middle-class families took in boarders, laundry, and sewing to make ends meet. With so many fathers and husbands unemployed, more and more wives and children left home to work. In the 1890s the number of laboring women jumped from 4 million to 5.3 million, mainly in exploitative fields such as domestic and clerical work.

In the South, where half the nation's working children were employed, child labor rose by 160 percent in textile mills during the decade. Concern over the young became so acute that middle-class women created the League for the Protection of the Family in 1896. Among other things it advocated compulsory education to keep children out of factories and mines. Older attitudes were gradually giving way to new ideas about the social causes of poverty and the responsibilities of public and private agencies.

The Rumblings of Unrest

Even before the depression, rumblings of unrest rolled across the land. The Great Railway Strike of 1877 touched off nearly two decades of labor unrest. In the late

1880s and early 1890s violence erupted at the Haymarket Square in Chicago, at the Carnegie steel plant in Homestead, Pennsylvania, and in the silver mines of Coeur d'Alene, Idaho, where federal troops finally crushed the strike. After 1893 discontent mounted as wages were cut, employers laid off employees, and factories closed. During the first year of the depression, 1400 strikes sent more than half a million workers from their jobs. The worst one idled 170,000 coal miners in Pennsylvania and the Midwest, where strikers bombed mine shafts, dynamited coal trains, and fought state militias.

Uneasy business executives and political leaders saw the hand of radicals in these uprisings. Harking back to a popular revolt in Paris in 1871 that had toppled the government and instituted a "Commune," or worker-controlled regime, American businessmen became convinced that only force could keep peace and preserve the republic. When a strike at George Pullman's Palace Car factory in 1894 led thousands of western rail workers to walk out in sympathy, a young Theodore Roosevelt, then serving as a Civil Service commissioner, advised his fellow citizens, "The sentiment now animating a large portion of our people can only be suppressed as the Paris Commune was suppressed, by taking ten or a dozen of their leaders out, standing . . . them against a wall and shooting them dead. These leaders are plotting a social revolution and the subversion of the American Republic." Roosevelt, however, was hyperventilating. Although radicals had been involved in many of the strikes, they were a tiny minority. Anarchism, which sought to abolish government entirely, had never attracted more than a handful of Americans, and socialism suffered from internal dissension and lack of strong leadership in the United States.

The depression of 1893 had unleashed another force: simple discontent with government inaction. By the spring of 1894 masses of unemployed—perhaps 10,000 in all—were wandering the roads, some slowly forming into small armies. On Easter Sunday, "General" Jacob Coxey, a 39-year-old Populist and factory owner, launched the "Tramps' March on Washington" from Massillon, Ohio. His "Commonweal Army of Christ" of some 500 men, women, and children descended on Washington at the end of April to offer "a petition with boots on," in Coxey's words, for a public works program of road-building. The government jobs would be financed through the issuance of $500 million in paper money.

The press covered the march as if it were a foreign invasion. "For every two sloggers in Coxey's ranks there was at least one reporter," recalled an amused journalist. Along the way Secret Service men mingled with the army's privates to report on their progress. In Washington President Cleveland's staff tightened security around the White House. Other "armies" mobilized across the country: an 800-person contingent left from Los Angeles; a San Francisco battalion of 600 swelled to 1500 by the time it reached Iowa.

On May 1 Coxey's troops, armed with "clubs of peace," massed at the foot of the Capitol. When Coxey entered the Capitol grounds, 100 mounted police routed the demonstrators and arrested him for trespassing on the grass. Nothing came of the protest, save unmistakable evidence of growing demand for federal action. Faced with a sputtering industrial economy, ordinary citizens had sought in Washington, rather than their state capitals, the court of last resort.

Democrats Under Fire

Grover Cleveland had barely entered office when the depression struck. The country blamed him; he blamed silver. In his view the Sherman Silver Purchase

Act of 1890 had cut business confidence by forcing the government to buy silver. The new silver reserve, in turn, had pushed the gold reserves out of the Treasury and brought on panic. Repeal of the act, Cleveland believed, was the only way to recovery. When India dropped silver as a basis for its currency late in June 1893, Cleveland called Congress into special session to roll back the Sherman Act. Congress did, after considerable debate, in November. But this bit of economic tinkering only strengthened the resolve of the "silverites" in the Democratic party to overwhelm Cleveland's conservative "gold" wing.

Even worse for the president, who had staked his reputation on it, repeal of silver purchases brought no economic revival. In the short run abandoning silver hurt the economy by contracting the money supply just when some inflation might have helped stimulate it. Worst of all, the battle over repeal had siphoned off the support Cleveland needed for his principal goal, reducing the tariff. The best Democrats in Congress could do was the Wilson–Gorman Tariff Act (1894), which reduced some schedules, raised others, and enacted a modest income tax to make up for lost revenues. A year later even the tax provision fell when the Supreme Court invalidated it.

As panic and unemployment spread across the country, Democrats were buried in state after state in the congressional elections of 1894. They lost both the House and Senate. "The truth is," said one senator, "there was hardly an oasis left in the Democratic desert." The Democrats' disaster did not favor the Populists, who elected only four senators and four representatives. Everywhere disgruntled voters had turned to the Republicans. Dropping moralistic reforms and stressing national activism, Republican candidates cut deeply into traditional sources of Democratic support. With the Democrats confined to the solid South, the politics of stalemate was over and the Republicans reigned. All that remained for them was to capture the White House in 1896.

THE NEW REALIGNMENT

Despite occasional praise for handling crises like the Pullman strike and mediating a dispute over Venezuela's boundary, Cleveland's popularity wilted. He enjoyed no practical relations with Congress; he seldom spoke or traveled; his mail shrank to that of an average citizen. Cancer of the jawbone (for which he had undergone a secret operation) also took its toll on his health and energy. By the end of 1895 the president was spending his remaining days in the White House on family matters, routine paperwork, and plans for retirement. His would-be successors, however, were lining up for the campaign of 1896, which proved to be one of the five or six most critical elections in the republic's history.* Its results, coming in the midst of a deep depression, ended by reordering the political landscape and leaving behind the "Gilded Age" of bloody shirt politics, slim party margins, and low-profile presidents.

---

*Political scientists consider five elections, in addition to the contest of 1896, as critical shifts in voter allegiance and party alignments: the Federalist defeat of 1800, Andrew Jackson's rise in 1828, Lincoln's Republican triumph of 1860, Al Smith's Democratic loss in 1928; and—perhaps—Ronald Reagan's conservative tide of 1980.

The Battle of the Standards

From the start, the campaign of 1896 was a "battle of the standards," with both major parties absorbed in the question of whether gold or silver should become the nation's monetary standard. As the self-proclaimed promoters of business interests, most Republican leaders saw gold as the stable base upon which to build confidence and prosperity. At their nominating convention in St. Louis, the party enthusiastically adopted a platform calling for "sound money" supported by gold. Senator Henry M. Teller of Colorado, a lonely dissenter, rose with tears in his eyes to offer a silver substitute, then led 23 followers from the convention hall when it was voted down almost 8 to 1.

Marcus Alonzo Hanna, a shrewd Ohio industrialist and party leader, had carried the gold plank to the convention and had been maneuvering for almost a year to win the nomination for William McKinley, former congressman and now governor from Ohio. Patient, principled, and tolerant, McKinley was no pawn of Hanna's but a power in his own right. He had championed every aspect of Republican nationalism, mastered the arts of political management, and stood firmly for the high protective tariff that bore his name. Cautiously he endorsed gold. Thanks to Hanna's organizational skills, McKinley was nominated on the first ballot. As a result, the convention spent far less time in contentious wrangling among regional party chieftains. Increasingly, the issues being raised at political conventions encompassed the whole nation, rather than sectional concerns.

As for the Democrats, four years of agitation, depression, and party fragmentation had left them in disarray. Throughout Cleveland's term, disappointed silverites wanted nothing to do with his conservative policies, pressing instead for "free and independent" coinage of silver. They argued that if the Treasury freely minted all the silver presented to it, independent of other nations, the supply of money would increase, prices would rise, and the economy would revive. "The blood of commerce," wrote one silverite, "will again flow through the arteries of business; industry will again revive; millions of men will find employment; (and) the hand of greed will be stricken from the throat of prosperity."

As much as anything, free silver was a social protest of the South and West against the financial aristocracy of the gold-bound Northeast. Associated with rural, debt-ridden farm folk (whose debts would be diminished by currency inflation), silver implied the superiority of country life over city life. Most of all, in the words of young Nebraska congressman William Jennings Bryan, it stood for the "work-worn," "dust-begrimed" people against arrogant wealth. In speech after speech, article after article, silverites pressed their case, nowhere more effectively than in William Harvey's best-selling pamphlet, *Coin's Financial School* (1894). It reached tens of thousands of readers with the common sense of Coin, its young hero. Fighting for silver, he "was like a little monitor in the midst of a fleet of wooden ships."

As Democrats assembled in Chicago for their convention, William Jennings Bryan was ready to seize the hour. Just 36 years old, Bryan was steeped in the rural virtues of grassroots democracy. He looked, reformer Robert La Follette remembered, "like a young divine"—"tall, slender, handsome," with a rich melodic voice that could reach the back rows of the largest halls (no small asset in the

"Gold Bug" pin worn by supporters of McKinley's gold standard in the election campaign of 1896.

days before electric amplification). He had served two terms in Congress and worked as a journalist. He favored a low tariff, opposed Cleveland, and came out somewhat belatedly for free silver. Confessing total ignorance of the issue in 1892, he explained, "The people of Nebraska are for free silver and I am for free silver. I will look up the arguments later." Slowly, systematically, he organized a quiet boom for his nomination in 1896.

Silverites controlled the convention from start to finish. They paraded with silver banners, wore silver buttons, and won a plank in the anti-Cleveland platform calling for the free and unlimited coinage of silver. The high point came when Bryan stepped to the lectern, threw back his head, and offered himself to "a cause as holy as the cause of liberty—the cause of humanity." The audience rose as one, cheered wildly, then listened as Bryan spoke for "the plain people of this country," for "our farms" and against "your cities," for silver and against gold. The crowd was in a near-frenzy as he reached the dramatic climax and spread his arms in mock crucifixion:

> Having behind us the producing masses of this nation and the world, supported by the . . . toilers everywhere, we will answer their demand for a gold standard by saying to them: You shall not press down upon the brow of labor this crown of thorns, you shall not crucify mankind upon a cross of gold.

The next day the convention nominated him for the presidency.

Populists were in a quandary. They had expected the Democrats to stick with Cleveland and gold, sending dissident silverites headlong into their camp. Instead, as they saw it, the Democrats had plagiarized their platform and stolen their

---

William Jennings Bryan made the first of his three presidential bids in 1896, when he ran on both the Democratic and Populist tickets. Passionate in his convictions and devoted to the plain people, the "Great Commoner" is depicted in this hostile cartoon as a Populist snake devouring the Democratic party.

thunder. "If we fuse [with the Democrats] we are sunk," complained one Populist. "If we don't fuse, all the silver men we have will leave us for the more powerful Democrats." At a convention racked with bitter debate, the fusionists nominated Bryan for president. The best antifusionists could do was drop the Democrats' vice presidential candidate, Maine shipbuilder Arthur Sewall, in favor of that agrarian rebel who had set Georgia aflame, Tom Watson.

Campaign and Election

Bryan waged an extraordinary campaign on limited financial resources. He traveled 18,000 miles by train, gave as many as 30 speeches a day, and reached perhaps 3 million people in 27 states. The nomination of the People's party actually did more harm than good by labeling Bryan a Populist (which he was not) and a radical (which he definitely was not). Devoted to the "plain people," Bryan spoke for rural America and Jeffersonian values: small farmers, small towns, and small government. Anticipating a new, more active campaign style, he tried to "educate" voters, but in the end he preached largely to the converted.

McKinley knew he could not compete with Bryan's barnstorming, so he stumped sedately from his front porch in Canton, Ohio. This gave his campaign a folksy appearance, which belied the reality. Marcus Hanna, a politician of the industrial age, relied on modern techniques of organization and marketing to put his candidate across. He advertised McKinley, in Theodore Roosevelt's words, "as if he were patent medicine." Hanna constructed a well-oiled campaign machine that brought tens of thousands of delegations by train into Canton and paraded them to McKinley's doorstep. On one day alone, McKinley addressed some 80,000 people with promises of a "full dinner pail." Hanna saturated the country with millions of leaflets, along with 1400 speakers attacking free trade and free silver. Conservatives, frightened by what they viewed as Bryan's dangerous radicalism, poured at least $4 million into McKinley's campaign.

Bryan's silver-tongued oratory proved no match for Republican money and organization. On election night, Bryan sat at home in Lincoln, Nebraska, as three telegraph operators brought him bulletin after bulletin spelling defeat. Both candidates tallied more votes than any of their predecessors. Bryan had 6.5 million, McKinley 7.1 million, making him the first candidate since Grant to receive a clear majority. More important than numbers was where the votes came from. McKinley carried the Northeast and the Midwest, four border states, and California and Oregon in the Far West. In the industrial cities he routed Bryan. The Republicans combined old support from businessmen, farmers and veterans with broader backing from wage earners to create a national coalition that dominated politics for the next 30 years. As in 1892, blacks continued to vote mainly for Republicans, when they were permitted to vote at all.

Jim Crow Politics

The violence that threatened Tom Watson's biracial campaign was the crest of a wave of racism that engulfed America in the late 1800s. "New" immigrants from eastern and southern Europe and new overseas colonies of Hispanics, Filipinos, and Hawaiians helped breed a powerful race hatred to justify control. In the South longstanding racism deepened and was enlisted into a political purpose—preventing a biracial alliance that might topple white conservative Democrats from power. But the white supremacy campaign, ostensibly directed at African-

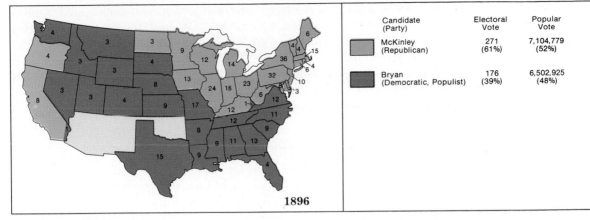

Candidate (Party)	Electoral Vote	Popular Vote
McKinley (Republican)	271 (61%)	7,104,779 (52%)
Bryan (Democratic, Populist)	176 (39%)	6,502,925 (48%)

1896

THE ELECTION OF 1896

Americans, had a broader target, political insurgents from below, as much white as black. When Mississippi designed a new constitution in 1890 to disfranchise blacks and many poor whites as well (page 732), some southern states hesitated to follow suit, because conservatives feared losing the fraudulent black votes that often gave them victory in elections. Conservatives, badly shaken by the Populist uprising of poor whites in the 1890s, demanded that if African-Americans were disfranchised (which would hurt conservatives, who controlled the votes of their black tenants and sharecroppers), the vote of potentially radical poor whites had to be reduced too.

After the defeat of Populism in the mid-1890s, the only question was which whites would be supreme, insurgents like the poor farmers who joined the People's party or conservative landholders. Eventually an all-white combination of conservatives and "reformers"—those disgusted by the frequent spectacle of election-stealing by using blocks of black votes—passed disfranchisement laws throughout the South. Between 1895 and 1908, the disfranchisement campaigns won out in every southern state. Sometimes the disfranchisement laws relied on the complicated procedure of charging poll taxes and demanding that receipts be shown at the polls, as in Mississippi. Sometimes literacy tests were used as a barrier. Where African-American voters were concentrated in large numbers, some states gerrymandered, or remapped the boundaries of election districts, to render black votes ineffective. "Grandfather clauses" allowed citizens to vote only if their grandfathers had cast ballots in elections held before 1860 (or 1866 in some cases)—a provision that excluded all blacks. By charging blacks with petty crimes, the states could often make them ineligible to vote. If these devices did not remove enough voters, politicians sometimes arranged for circuses and other entertainments to tour black districts before elections and collect poll tax receipts as the price of admission. Without these receipts, black voters would not be permitted to cast their ballots.

Populists and other reformers who agreed to the disfranchisement movement hoped that loopholes would permit poor whites to vote despite poll taxes and literacy tests. In practice, however, many whites were barred from the polls. In Louisiana, for example, under the new provisions the number of citizens voting was cut from 294,000 to 93,000, excluding virtually all the black voters and almost half the whites. The disfranchisement campaign also succeeded in splitting insurgent whites from blacks, as the tragic fate of Tom Watson demonstrated. Only a dozen years after his biracial campaign of 1892, Watson was actively promoting black disfranchisement in Georgia. "What does Civilization owe to the negro?" he asked bitterly. "Nothing! *Nothing!!* NOTHING!!!" In 1920, after more than a decade of baiting blacks (as well as Jews and Catholics), the Georgia firebrand was finally elected to the Senate. Watson, who began with such high ideals, gained power only by abandoning them.

The African-American Response

White reformers who supported disfranchisement claimed that race relations would actually improve, because blacks would learn their proper "place" in southern society. But to mount a successful campaign for disfranchisement, its supporters constantly inflamed racial passions. They staged "White Supremacy Jubilees" and complained, as the Atlanta *Journal* did, that the black man grew "more bumptious in the street. More impudent in his dealings with white men." The number of lynchings peaked during the 1890s, almost tripling in the first three years and averaging over a hundred a year for the whole decade. Most took place in the South. In Atlanta and New Orleans, white mobs terrorized blacks for several days in the new, heightened atmosphere of tension.

Under such circumstances, African-Americans were forced to work out a response to the climate of intolerance. It came in 1895 from Booker T. Washington. Born a slave, Washington struggled after the war to survive as a laborer and coal miner while attending school. In 1872 he learned of the Hampton Institute, founded by a former Union general to teach blacks skilled trades. After working his way through Hampton, Washington vowed to extend a similar opportunity to blacks in the lower South. In 1881 he accepted an offer from Alabama to establish an industrial and agricultural school at Tuskegee, Alabama. Its debut was far from auspicious, for the Tuskegee Institute opened in a log shack with 30 students and a single instructor.

Washington persevered, achieving almost overnight fame when he spoke to an audience of whites and blacks about race relations in Atlanta in 1895. "I love the South," he reassured white listeners. He conceded that white prejudice existed throughout the region but suggested that blacks should not try to fight it. "The agitation of questions of social equality is the extremist folly," he concluded. Instead, African-Americans should work for economic betterment. Every laborer who learned a trade and increased his savings through hard work would earn respect from whites. And those earnings would amount to "a little green ballot" that "no one will throw out or refuse to count." Thus Tuskegee's curriculum was designed to provide blacks with vocational skills for farming, manual trades, and industrial work.

Whites in both the North and the South hailed Washington's "Atlanta Compromise" as a solution to racial harmony. For blacks, it made the best of an increasingly difficult situation; for whites, it struck the note of patient humility they were so eager to hear. Washington, himself an astute politician, discovered that philanthropists across the nation hoped to make Tuskeegee an example of their generosity. He was the honored guest of Andrew Carnegie at his imposing Skibo Castle; Collis Huntington, one of the California "Big Four" rail magnates, became his friend; aboard the yacht of a Standard Oil executive he discussed "public and social questions." Throughout, Washington preached accommodation. He accepted segregation (so long as separate facilities were equal) and qualifications on voting (if they applied to whites as well). Above all Washington preached economic self-improvement designed to reach common black folk in fields and factories. In 1900 he organized the National Negro Business League to help establish black businessmen as the leaders of their people. The rapid growth of local chapters (320 by 1907) helped him extend his influence over the affairs of African-American communities across the country.

Not all black leaders accepted Washington's call for racial self-effacement. The most outspoken critic was W. E. B. Du Bois, a scholar with a far different vision. Born in western Massachusetts, Du Bois received training in history and economics at Fisk, Harvard, and the University of Berlin. In 1903, as a professor at Atlanta University, he leveled a broad attack on Washington's philosophy in *The Souls of Black Folk.* Du Bois saw no benefit for African-Americans in sacrificing intellectual growth for narrow vocational training. Nor was he willing to abide the permanent stigma that came from the South's discriminatory caste system. A better future would come only if blacks struggled politically to achieve suffrage and equal rights.

Instead of exhorting black folks to pull themselves slowly from the bottom up, Du Bois called on the "talented tenth," a cultured black vanguard, to blaze a trail of protest. In 1905 he founded what became known as the Niagara movement, to press for immediate political and economic equality. By 1909 a coalition of blacks and sympathetic whites had transformed the Niagara movement into the National Association for the Advancement of Colored People (NAACP). Middle class and elitist, it mounted legal challenges to the Jim Crow system of segregation. For sharecroppers in southern cotton fields and laborers in northern factories—the mass of African-Americans—the strategy offered little relief.

In keeping with Booker T. Washington's emphasis on manual training, Tuskegee Institute, opened in Alabama in 1881, was training 1400 students in 30 trades by 1900. Academic subjects received attention, too, as evidenced by this photograph of a history class (segregated by gender) learning about Captain John Smith and Pocahontas.

Neither accommodation nor legal agitation would suffice, but in the "Solid South" (as well as an openly racist North) it was Washington's patient approach that articulated an agenda for most African-Americans. The ferment of the early 1890s, among black Populists and white, was replaced by a lily-white Democratic party that dominated the region but remained largely a minority party on the national level.

McKinley in the White House

The Republican party came out of the election of 1896 not only as the grand new party but also as a dynamic instrument of government in Washington. The Republicans built an organization that could command votes, raise money, and mobilize public opinion. It combined traditional conservatives with forward-thinking leaders from the professions, education, business, and journalism. In William McKinley Republicans had a skillful chief with a national agenda. Unlike his Gilded Age predecessors, he began to reorganize the executive branch and make it more vigorous. McKinley cultivated news reporters, openly walked the streets of Washington, and charmed the public with warm handshakes and flowers from his own lapel. With a firm but delicate touch, he curbed the power of old-time state bosses like Thomas Platt of New York and Matthew Quay of Pennsylvania. When need be, he prodded Congress to action. In all these ways, he foreshadowed "modern" presidents, who would lead their party rather than act as executive caretakers.

Fortune at first smiled on McKinley. When he entered the White House the economy had already begun its recovery, as the cycle of economic retrenchment hit bottom. Factory orders were slowly increasing, causing a drop in unemployment; farm prices climbed. New discoveries of gold in Alaska and South Africa expanded the supply of money without causing the "gold bugs" to panic that it was being destabilized by silver. Freed from the burdens of the economic crisis, McKinley called a special session of Congress to make good on a campaign promise—tariff revision. In July 1897 the Dingley Tariff raised protective rates still higher but allowed the tariffs to come down if other nations lowered theirs.

McKinley also sought a solution for resolving violent railroad strikes, like the Pullman conflict, through government mediation. The Erdman Act of 1898 set up the machinery for doing so. Reformers had been complaining that the large industrial monopolies and trusts needed regulation as well, and McKinley laid plans for moving in that direction. But the same expansiveness that had pushed an industrial nation across the continent and shipped grain and cotton to international markets also drew the country into conflict and war. McKinley soon found himself facing a crisis with Spain that monopolized the attention of his fellow citizens. Regulation—and a true age of reform—would have to await the next century.

On New Year's Eve at the State House in Boston a midnight ceremony ushered in the twentieth century. The crowd celebrated with psalms and hymns. There was a flourish of trumpets, and everyone sang "America." The Reverend Edward Everett Hale, too deaf to hear anything but the brass, nonetheless recorded his sober impression: "The whole service was very satisfactory and I am writing under the influence of its solemnity."

Solemn and patriotic, the American people had weathered a decade of partisan jockeying, disorder, and violence. The conflicts arrayed a discontented South and West against the industrial Northeast and Midwest; whites against blacks, striking miners and workers against Pinkerton guards and hard-nosed industrialists. The political system, which through a policy of laissez faire had mostly ignored the social forces of urbanization and industrialization that were changing America, took the first steps of adjustment. In the race between Bryan and McKinley, it seemed that an older agrarian America was facing off against the new industrial order. The soul of the nation, divided just 30 years earlier by a civil war, had again been at stake.

The dawn of the new century brought an end to an era of political uncertainty and a decade of social upheaval. Prosperity returned at home; empire beckoned abroad. Still, deep divisions—between rich and poor, farmers and factory workers, men and women, native-born and immigrant—split America. A younger generation of leaders stood in the wings, fearful of the schisms but confident it could forge ties to bridge them. As Theodore Roosevelt looked eagerly toward war with Spain and the chance to expand American horizons, he did not mince words with one of his older opponents. "You and your generation have had your chance. . . . Now let us of this generation have ours!"

SIGNIFICANT EVENTS

1867 — Patrons of Husbandry ("Grange") founded

1869 — Prohibition party founded; Massachusetts establishes first state regulatory commission

1874 — Greenback party organized

1874 — Women's Christian Temperance Union formed

1875 — First Farmers' Alliance organized

1877 — *Munn v. Illinois*

1878 — Bland–Allison Silver Purchase Act

1881 — President James Garfield assassinated; Chester Arthur sworn in as president; Booker T. Washington founds Tuskegee Normal and Industrial Institute in Alabama

1887 — Interstate Commerce Commission created

1890 — National Woman Suffrage Association created; Sherman Antitrust Act; Wyoming enters the Union as the first state to give women the vote; Sherman Silver Purchase Act; McKinley Tariff; Southern and Northwestern Alliances adopt "Ocala Demands"

1892 — Populist party formed; Grover Cleveland elected president

1893 — Panic of 1893; Sherman Silver Purchase Act repealed

1894 — "Coxey's Army" marches on Washington to demand public works for the unemployed

1895 — National Municipal League founded

1896 — League for the Protection of the Family organized, William McKinley elected president

1903 — W. E. B. Du Bois' *The Souls of Black Folk* published

1909 — National Association for the Advancement of Colored People founded

22

The New Empire

mericans found the British wherever they looked abroad, or so it seemed. Through their navy, through missionaries from the Church of England, through manufacturers, merchants, and bankers, the British had footholds in India, Africa, the Middle East, China, the Pacific. But Americans after the Civil War were particularly galled by the influence Great Britain wielded in their own backyard. The Monroe Doctrine might assert that the United States was supreme in the Western Hemisphere, but around the Caribbean the British Navy piped the tune.

If the United States hoped to build a canal across Central America—and many Americans did—they had to share it with the British under the terms of the Clayton–Bulwer Treaty of 1850. Year after year British pounds flowed into Nicaragua, El Salvador, Guatemala, Honduras, and Costa Rica to pay for railroads and to finance their governments. When Honduras refused to pay its debts in 1872, the British navy shelled a Honduran port. Even after the government in Tegucigalpa caved in, the British decided to take over nearby Belize and turn it into British Honduras. In so doing they simply ignored the claim of Nicaragua to the same territory. In fact, the British even assumed control over the Miskito Coast of Nicaragua, which, very conveniently, offered one of the most promising sites for the eastern end of an isthmian canal. By 1900 British investors had placed all five Central American governments in the thrall of debt.

Perceptive and ambitious Americans recognized that if the British could use their navy and bankers to muscle into Central America, the United States could too. The profits from American factories and farms could open doors of trade and influence and a modern navy could help keep them open. Although English investors might buy up government securities and public utilities, Americans could gain control over the productive facilities and transportation upon which the economies of developing nations increasingly depended. For an American with the proper enterprise and bold enough plans—someone like Minor Keith, for instance—the reward might prove immense.

In 1871 this "apple-headed little man with the eyes of a fanatic," as he would later be described by the writer John Dos Passos, had arrived in Costa Rica to build railroads for which the British supplied the financing. Costa Rica had a classic one-crop colonial economy based on coffee beans. As Keith supervised construction of the railroads, he also began to tap a new market by buying bananas to ship to the United States for sale at a hefty profit. He used some of his earnings

In 1858 the United States signed its first commercial treaty with Japan. The Japanese were not especially impressed with people they viewed as barbarians; only after forceful intervention in 1867 by Western powers did Japan permit substantial commerce.

in 1884 to refinance the Costa Rican debt of $12 million to the British. The grateful government in return granted him a 99-year lease on the railroad, 800,000 acres of fertile land, and freedom from import duties on the equipment he needed for railroad and plantation construction projects.

As soon as he received the land, Keith began to create banana plantations under the control of his Tropical Fruit Company. The railroads he built, like those of southern planters in the United States, linked the plantations to the coast rather than connecting key towns and cities. Despite its huge debt for construction, Costa Rica was left without a viable internal transportation network. At the same time, Keith complemented his economic influence by cultivating political connections. Marriage to the daughter of a former president increased his sway over a government already receptive to his financial inducements. In 1899 he extended his private empire even further by merging Tropical Fruit with Boston Fruit to create the United Fruit Company.

By the early twentieth century Keith had almost single-handedly turned Costa Rica into the prototypical "banana republic" and the United States into the dominant foreign power. The country imported five times more from the Americans than from the British. United Fruit had almost equal influence in Guatemala, and Honduras would fall under the influence of Keith's company by the 1920s. Central Americans came to call the company, with its vast landholdings, railroads, and steamship lines, "the octopus."

Keith's direct involvement in the affairs of Central American states was not the only way to use economic resources to expand American influence. Numerous Americans had products they wanted to sell in foreign markets. Southern farmers exported half their cotton crop, western wheat farmers earned some 30 to 40 percent of their income from overseas markets, John D. Rockefeller's Standard Oil Company shipped about two-thirds of its refined products abroad, Cyrus McCormick supplied Russian farmers with the reaper, and Thomas Edison and Alexander Graham Bell established England's telephone service in the 1880s. But no American product sold more widely than the sewing machines of the Singer Company. All over the globe Singer found markets for a machine that was practical, profitable, and labor saving for its users.

The lure of overseas profits took Singer to Europe in the 1850s. The depressions of the 1870s, 1880s, and 1890s convinced the company that foreign sales were essential to smooth out domestic ups and downs. "We never get tired of ding-donging this matter of exports . . . for we hope we will wake [the sewing machine trade] up and make them go to work as eagerly abroad as they ever did at home," one industry journal stated. By 1900 Singer had 60,000 sales agents spread out over every inhabited part of the globe and its name had entered some foreign languages as the word for sewing machine. For many of the world's people, that little machine was their sole contact with the United States, its economy, and its culture.

Singer's most coveted market lay in China, but it was a difficult one to penetrate because the culture was so strange to most Americans. From John MacIntyre, a sympathetic Scotch Presbyterian missionary stationed there, Singer representatives learned that every business deal would involve a complex web of "compradors," or middlemen. If strangers bargained, a mutual friend or relative was needed to settle differences and guarantee the contract. Tailors, the most promising customers, had a deep aversion to innovation. Accustomed to loosely stitched seams, they disdained the tight stitching the Singer machine produced. But spurred on by the depression of 1893, the company made a concerted effort to sell Chinese officials on the virtues of the "iron tailor." Machines were introduced into the Dowager Empress Tzu Hsi's industrial training schools, free schools were established to teach machine sewing, and new machines were developed to produce a loose chain stitch. Singer had learned that in China one had to become Chinese to succeed. Although the vast market of Americans' dreams never materialized, Singer established the presence of the United States and the missionaries of its cultural, economic, and religious gospel in Asia.

VISIONS OF EMPIRE

By the grand plans of Minor Keith and the small stitches of Singer; by sales of Iowa grain and the salvation of Indochinese souls; even, finally, by navy gunboats and political strong-arming, the United States entered the new imperial race. Since the 1840s expansionists had spoken of a divine and Manifest Destiny to overspread the North American continent from the Atlantic to the Pacific. Even after the Civil

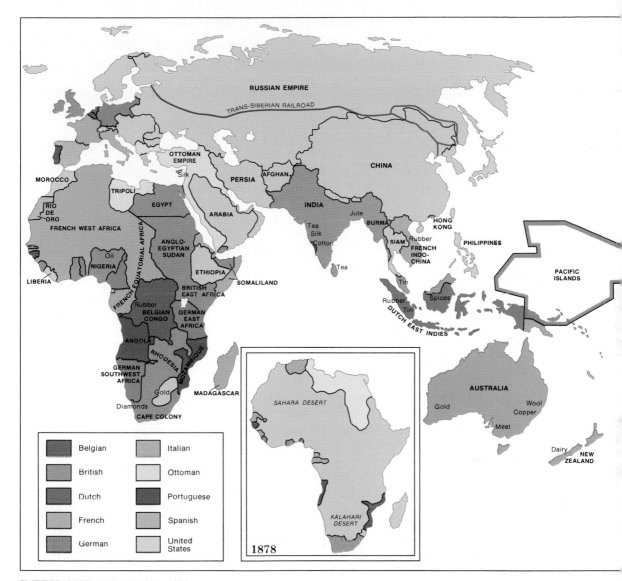

IMPERIALIST EXPANSION, 1900
A comparison of Africa in 1878 (inset) and 1900 shows how quickly Europeans extended their colonial empires. Often resource-poor countries like Japan and England saw colonies as a way to acquire raw materials, such as South African diamonds and tin from Southeast Asia. Closer scrutiny shows that four of the most rapidly industrializing countries—Germany, Japan, Russia, and the United States—had few if any overseas possessions, even in 1900. And while China appears to be undivided, all the major powers were eagerly establishing spheres of influence there.

War, some Americans still cast covetous glances at Canada to the north and Mexico and Cuba to the south. More often, however, their interest came to center on distant lands, which, unlike the Louisiana and Gadsden purchases or the territories acquired after the Mexican War of 1846, did not border on the United States.

Imperialism, European-Style and American

Spain and Portugal maintained the shrinking remnants of colonial empires dating to the age of exploration in the fifteenth and sixteenth centuries. England, France, and Russia had accelerated their efforts to control foreign peoples and lands. But toward the end of the nineteenth century, the technology of arms and the networks of communication, transportation, and commerce made the prospect of effective, truly global empires especially attractive. The race for overseas empire was well under way by the time the Americans, Japanese, and Germans entered in the late nineteenth century.

For many Americans accustomed to a heritage of continental expansion, overseas imperialism raised some difficult issues. The tradition growing out of the American Revolution painted the nation as an exceptionally free and democratic one, untainted by the corrupting influences of Old World monarchies, aristocracies, or hierarchical churches. Whereas Americans tended to see narrow and selfish interests directing the expansion of European powers, they were more likely to imagine themselves the bearers of a selfless Protestant Christianity, the economic benefits of free enterprise capitalism, and the blessings of democracy. No doubt a majority of Americans felt the world's far reaches would benefit from an expansion of such values. Even so, differences arose over how aggressive and self-interested American imperialism ought to be. The naked way in which Great Britain, France, and Germany scrambled for possessions in the Niger and Congo basins of tropical Africa in the 1880s certainly stirred popular opinion in America toward a more competitive approach. But other Americans preferred a more indirect imperialism that simply exported ideas, commerce, and influence. To them the paths of Minor Keith or Isaac Merritt Singer seemed more practical.

While Americans more than Europeans wrestled with the problem of justifying imperial control in the name of the ideals of democracy, similar social, economic, and political forces drew them into the imperial race. The growth of industrial networks linked more and more Americans to international markets, whether they were Arkansas sharecroppers depending on the price of cotton in world markets or Pittsburgh steelworkers whose jobs might continue only so long as orders for railroad steel from entrepreneurs like Minor Keith kept their factories in business. The development of efficient transoceanic steamship lines greatly facilitated international commerce. Singer was only one of many corporations, in Europe as well as America, looking to world markets. As economic systems became more tightly knit and integrated and political systems became more responsive to the interests of industrialists and finance capital, a scramble for domination of markets and distant lands was perhaps inevitable. Nations looked to project their interests, economically, militarily, and culturally.

The Shapers of Foreign Policy

Although the climate for expansion and imperialism was present at the end of the nineteenth century, the small farmer or steelworker had little if any concern about how the United States might advance its ends abroad. A small minority of informed interest groups shaped the debate over foreign policy and imperialism. They were Christian missionary groups, the navy lobby, business interests, commercial farm interests, and a small intellectual and political elite who followed American affairs in the wider world.

American overseas missionary work began in earnest in the 1840s with Protestant missions in China, which set out to convert the "heathens" to Christianity. By the late nineteenth century American missionaries had spread out to other parts of the western Pacific region and the Middle East, where they encountered people with profound cultural differences that often made them unreceptive to the Christian message. The missionaries came to believe that the natives first had to become Western in culture before becoming Christian in belief. To that end they sought to introduce Western goods, education, and systems of governmental administation—any "civilizing medium," as the Reverend McIntyre had remarked when he helped Singer gain a foothold in China. Yet most American missionaries, especially those to China, were not territorial imperialists. They assumed instead "the white man's burden" of introducing civilization to the "colored" races of the world. To that end they set up vocational training schools and Western-style universities, stores, and hospitals, but they opposed direct military or political intervention. At home their representatives lobbied in Congress and from the pulpit for expanded commercial activities to support their evangelical efforts.

In the 1870s a young American woman complained to English wit Oscar Wilde that her country, unlike Europe, had no classical ruins, no curiosities. "No ruins! No curiosities!" Wilde countered. "You have your Navy and your manners." Certainly, American naval officers could agree with Wilde's scathing sarcasm. By 1880 the once-proud Civil War fleet of over 600 warships was rotting and rusted with neglect. Only 48 could actually fire a gun. In effect, the United States had no functional navy to protect overseas interests.

Budgetary deprivation also spelled disaster for the graduates of the Naval Academy bent on a military career. Without ships, they could not find commands or avenues for promotion. Such dead-end prospects did not suit the temperament of young men drawn from the nation's elite. The average navy officer came from an upper-middle class business or professional family, belonged to an establishment Protestant denomination like the Episcopalians or Presbyterians, and married a woman from a respected eastern family. Many of these young and discontented officers joined with similarly inclined business leaders to lobby Congress to establish a modern navy with steam-powered, steel-hulled ships. Half a century later, this growing combination of business, military, and political lobbyists would become known as the military-industrial complex, and it would influence the nation significantly.

In the 1880s it was Captain Alfred Thayer Mahan who formulated the ideas of these officers and business leaders into a theory of navalism that exerted a powerful influence over the thinking of his generation. The United States, Mahan argued, required a navy prepared to do more than protect coastal waters. Great nations had always relied on foreign trade to enhance their wealth and power, especially in times of chronic industrial overproduction and sharp depressions, as had occurred repeatedly after the Civil War. The United States thus needed to make a concerted effort to expand foreign trade. And the only way to protect access to foreign markets was with large cruisers and battleships. These ships, operating far from American shores, would need coaling stations and other resupply facilities throughout the world.

Mahan's logic and the benefits that a shipbuilding program would bring American factories persuaded Congress in the 1880s to begin rebuilding the navy. Steel ships replaced those with wooden hulls. Between 1882 and 1893 the United States went from the world's twelfth to its seventh naval power and ten years later

Daily Lives

TIME AND TRAVEL

The New Navy

Early on February 3, 1874, a fleet of chunky monitors and steam frigates and sloops lumbered out of Key West at a tortoiselike 4.5 knots. It was the largest assembly of American naval power since the Civil War, but to the officers watching from shore, the overage armada was a lamentable sign of weakness. "It became painfully apparent to us that the vessels before us were in no respect worthy of a great nation like our own," declared one commodore. "Two modern vessels of war," a future admiral later observed, "would have done us up in thirty minutes."

During the Civil War the United States Navy had reached its pinnacle with over 600 ships, 65 of them ironclads. But almost immediately after the war the country began dismantling the fleet. War debts, Reconstruction, and industrial development dominated national interest. With 3000 miles of ocean as protection and no colonies to defend, a large blue-water fleet seemed unnecessary. Even steamships, though superior to vessels under sail, seemed unwarranted since the United States had no coaling stations in foreign waters to fuel them. All naval vessels were therefore required to have full sail power. The number of propeller blades on steamships was reduced from four to two to improve sailing ability. Boilers and engines were replaced by smaller ones or removed entirely. By 1878 the number of sailors had shrunk to 6000, the smallest force since the presidency of Andrew Jackson, and the United States Navy ranked twelfth in the world—behind Denmark and Chile.

Meanwhile technology was transforming the navies of Europe. Compound engines, improved armor plating, self-propelled torpedoes, and large rifled guns revolutionized naval warfare. In 1873, as the United States Navy fell into disrepair, the British launched the *Devastation*, a single-masted, steam-driven vessel with heavy armor and powerful twin turrets. A forerunner of the modern battleship, it could steam across the Atlantic and back without stopping for coal. Less than a decade later, a British fleet smashed Alexandria, Egypt, whose fortifications were sturdier than those of American ports.

Anxieties about foreign navies and dreams of empire led Congress in 1883 to appropriate $1.3 million for four modern vessels—the cruisers *Atlanta, Boston,* and *Chicago,* 3000 to 4500 tons; and the 1500-ton dispatch boat *Dolphin.* The "ABCD" ships were the first of a new steel fleet designed to raise the United States Navy to world-class status. These early "protected" cruisers (so named for the armored deck built over boilers, engines, and other machinery) were an odd mix of old and new. All three had full sail rigs yet were completely electrified and contained watertight compartments and double bottoms. The *Chicago* had twin propellers but engines and boilers so antiquated that one observer compared them to a saw mill. The steel breechloading guns were vast improvements over the iron muzzle-loaders; yet gunners still aimed them the old-fashioned way, by looking down the barrels through open sights.

Before the turn of the century, the navy had commissioned additional protected cruisers, larger armored cruisers, and its first full-sized battleships—the *Indiana, Massachusetts*, and *Oregon*, each over 10,000 tons. (Soon after 1900 giant battleships were displacing 20,000 tons; on the eve of World War I they reached

Daily Lives

Passengers on riverboats and yachts saluted the new steel-hulled, steam-powered American fleet as it steamed triumphantly up the Hudson River after naval victories in the Spanish–American War. Within a few years, these modern ships would be obsolete, as rapid innovations in naval warfare fed an international arms race.

over 30,000 tons.) With five more first-class battleships commissioned by 1896, the United States Navy rose to fifth place in the world. The prestige of naval service had risen, too, and with it the number of sailors: nearly 10,000 in uniform. A Naval War College had been created in 1884 to train officers in the science of naval war, and in 1891 states established naval militia units, which became the nucleus of the Naval Reserve.

Service aboard the new navy, as always, reflected the privileges of rank. Commanders lived in wood-paneled luxury and dined on specially prepared cuisine, capped by coffee, brandy, and cigars. The crew ate salted meats, beans, and potatoes. Officers had private quarters, while enlisted men, so the saying went, lived under the place where they slept and slept under the place where they ate. At night the tables and benches used for dining in the common quarters were stowed between overhead beams from which hammocks were hung. Battery drill was held twice a day, but under fire American marksmanship proved poor. During one battle in the Spanish–American War, Americans fired more than 8000 shells at four fleeing Spanish crusiers. An examination of their hulks later revealed only 120 hits.

By 1907 the new navy had come of age, and in that year President Theodore Roosevelt sent 16 of its newest battleships on a 46,000-mile, 14-month world tour. Ironically the Great White Fleet (named for the gleaming white hulls of its ships) was already out of date. In 1906 Great Britain had commissioned the *Dreadnought*, a warship whose gunnery rendered all of its competitors obsolete. Unlike conventional battleships with guns of varying sizes, the *Dreadnought* carried mostly big guns that gave it more than twice the firepower of anything afloat. In a single stroke the new American navy, the product of a quarter-century of effort, was outclassed—but not for long. By the end of World War II, another quarter-century away, the United States Navy would outclass the world.

BALANCE OF U.S. IMPORTS
AND EXPORTS, 1870–1910
The green areas indicate an unfa-
vorable balance of trade.

to third. Navy officers had already taken the initiative to establish a greater American presence in Korea, Haiti, Samoa, and Hawaii. With a modern navy, the
United States had both the motive and means to become an imperial power. Only
the question of method remained to be solved.

The majority of the business class had little concern with foreign trade in the
late nineteenth century. They had, after all, ample opportunity to find new markets and cheap raw materials in burgeoning urban areas with the opening of the
West and the rise of the New South. The expansion of the railroads offered seemingly endless opportunities for profitable investment of surplus capital. All the
same, at least three groups from the business community did pursue overseas
interests. Most obviously, shipbuilders, import–export businesses, and steamship
lines looked abroad, since all of them had a direct stake in foreign commerce. Any
steps that promoted foreign trade served their interests. Second, adventurers like
Minor Keith recognized that, although the risks of investment in underdeveloped
economies were greater, the potential profits were spectacular. Most investments
went into developing raw materials from mining and foodstuffs. Railroads and
shipping lines to move those goods were also popular. Finally, as in the case of
Singer, there were manufacturers who saw hundreds of millions of Chinese and
other native people as potential customers for their products. Foreign sales were
especially alluring to manufacturers in industries suffering from chronic overproduction.

Perhaps even more vocal in generating pressure to expand American overseas
markets was a fourth group: the large commercial farmers and the industries that
processed farm produce. The rapid growth of urban markets had encouraged an
even more rapid increase in farm production. When farmers began producing
more than urban markets could absorb, they began to look abroad for relief from
depressed prices.

In addition to missionaries, navy careerists, and certain members of the business class, a small, generally well-educated, influential group of individuals also
promoted the cause of imperialism. This elite group—widely traveled, politically
well connected—communicated with one another through books, journal articles,
lectures, and informal social contacts. It included such lights as Henry and Brooks
Adams, sons of diplomat Charles Francis Adams, grandsons of former President

and Secretary of State John Quincy Adams, and great-grandsons of John Adams. Brooks and Henry were almost born to assume a role in guiding the destiny of the United States, but neither had any taste for active political life. They exercised their influence through their writing and political friends like Henry Cabot Lodge, the Massachusetts senator and one of America's first holders of a doctorate (in political science from Harvard); young Theodore Roosevelt, the patrician son of one of New York City's most distinguished merchant families; and John Hay, an Illinois lawyer who had the good fortune to befriend Abraham Lincoln and inherit a large fortune through his wife's father. By the 1890s Alfred Mahan, too, was a respected member of this circle.

All these men were expansionists. They accepted and in one way or another helped define and popularize most of the era's theories on culture, race, and economics that justified the American drive toward empire. By a curious irony of history, many of these same ideas were used by anti-imperialists, who often favored expansion but felt it was a tactical mistake to acquire colonies.

The Ideology of Imperialism

It is an unusual culture indeed that does not fancy its own ways superior to those of foreign peoples. To take one example among many, the Cheyenne of the Great Plains called themselves "the people," or simply "the human beings," implying that no one else had fully achieved that rank. So, too, the civilizations arising out of western Europe at the end of the Middle Ages generally assumed the superiority of their cultures. But because of their remarkable expansion across the globe, the confidence and aggressiveness of Western beliefs became especially marked in the late nineteenth century. Not surprisingly, Americans and Europeans who sought to explain their successes over nonwhite or aboriginal populations gave themselves credit for superior government, the spread of a system of international markets, dynamically expanding industrial capacity, and technological advances in weapons and communications. All these seemed material symbols confirming the favor of divine providence.

Yet as we have also seen, the success of western European expansion into colonial North America also benefited from ecological factors (page 157). European diseases, animals, and plants often devastated and disrupted the new worlds they entered. The coming of smallpox and measles; of pigs, cattle, and horses; and of sugar and wheat played equally important roles in opening the Western Hemisphere and the Pacific basin to European domination. In areas like the Middle East, Asia, and Africa, where populations already possessed hardy domesticated animals and plants (as well as their own devastating disease pools), European penetration was far less complete. Still, journalist Finley Peter Dunne's Irish characters Mr. Hennessy and Mr. Dooley best expressed the confidence with which Americans and Europeans viewed their self-proclaimed superiority. "'We're a gr-reat people,' said Mr. Hennessy earnestly. 'We ar-re,' said Mr. Dooley. 'We ar-re that. An' the best iv it is, we know we ar-re.'"

With a confidence so sublime, scholars, academics, and scientists soon developed a number of theories justifying European and American expansion in terms of race. Charles Darwin's *On the Origin of Species* (1859) had popularized the notion that among animal species, the fittest survived through a process of natural selection, and Social Darwinists like Herbert Spencer in England and William

Graham Sumner in the United States argued that the same laws of survival governed the social order. By natural as well as divine law, the fittest people—those descended from Anglo-Saxon and Teutonic stock—would assert their dominion over the lesser peoples of the world. When applied aggressively, the theory of white supremacy could rationalize the wholesale slaughter and enslavement of native populations who resisted. When combined with the somewhat more humane notions of the "white man's burden," conquest included not only the "burden," or obligation to impose order, but also the opportunity to uplift the "lower" races by teaching them Western ideas, converting them to Christianity, and introducing law and government. Patricians like Theodore Roosevelt and Henry Cabot Lodge eagerly accepted such notions.

Perhaps more compelling than either cultural or racial motives for American expansion was the commercial imperative. The recurrent depressions of the late nineteenth century reminded Americans of the unpredictable disorder in the nation's economy. The Populists had proposed a monetary solution to depression: inflate the currency with free silver. The business community generally attempted to limit the swings of the free market through consolidation into monopolies and trusts, which would then avoid overproduction and destructive competition. High protective tariffs to keep out foreign goods was yet another solution. But as the National Association of Manufacturers explained, "Our manufacturers have outgrown or are outgrowing the home market" and "expansion of our foreign trade is [the] only promise of relief." In and out of government, leading public figures called for a campaign to "find markets in every part of the habitable globe" and to "open trade wherever we can." Imperialist policies, whether defined as an expansion of United States boundaries, the acquisition of colonies, or merely the achievement of a controlling influence, offered the opportunity to increase foreign trade, enhance American prestige, and guarantee future security.

STIRRINGS OF EMPIRE

Even when the inhabited United States encompassed little more than a baker's dozen of former colonies clustered along the Atlantic seaboard, Thomas Jefferson had dreamed of an American "empire of liberty" that one day would stretch from sea to sea. Jefferson supposed it might take a thousand generations before American pioneers had vaulted the continent, but it took a mere 40 years, and the wines of such expansionist fruits proved sometimes heady. The dream of a truly continental American republic—one that absorbed Canada and Mexico to boot—had not died out after the Civil War.

Canada

To the north lay Canada, still a British colony and still a target for American expansionists like Lincoln's secretary of state, William Henry Seward. Canadian territory took in a landmass second in size only to Russia, though its population was largely clustered in the areas of Ontario and Quebec, bordering the United States. Political unrest in 1837 had led the British by 1841 to merge French-speaking Lower Canada (Quebec) with English-speaking Upper Canada (Ontario) to form a united Canada Province. At the time of the American Civil War the Canadians were prepared for a peaceful separation from England and the creation of an independent Canada.

The continuing interest of American expansionists in the territory to the north also spurred the British to redefine Canada's status. In 1866 Congress had put financial pressure on Canada by cutting back on the amount of free trade and fishing privileges that had been negotiated between the two countries. With enough pressure, the expansionists in Congress speculated, Canadians hurt by the loss of American markets might favor annexation. In addition, neither President Andrew Johnson nor Ulysses S. Grant made any attempt to stop raids into Canada conducted periodically by the Irish Fenian Brotherhood. Canadians correctly suspected that annexation was the price the United States would extract for calling off the Irish. At the same time, the United States made extraordinary demands on Britain to pay indemnities for damages caused by Confederate raiding vessels built in England. The only way Britain could repay those damages, proponents in Congress recognized, was to cede Canada to the United States.

But in 1867 Britain eased the discontent in Canada over its colonial status by adopting the British North America Act, which organized Ontario, Quebec, New Brunswick, and Nova Scotia into a single confederation possessing greater power for self-government and an independent foreign policy. Under the Anglo-American Treaty signed in 1871 the United States settled its claims for compensation. Canada, like the United States, experienced increasing immigration from Europe and expansion into its western plains. By 1871 Manitoba and British Columbia had both achieved provincial status, comparable to American statehood. Even though disputes erupted between the United States and the new Canadian government over questions of boundaries, fishing rights, seal hunting, and tariffs, most Americans decided that it was more profitable to trade with Canada than to annex it.

Mexico

Mexico posed possibilities and problems of a different sort. During the Civil War, France's new emperor, Napoleon III, had occupied Mexico City with a French army and soon after established a puppet monarchy under Austria-Hungary's Archduke Maximilian, now Emperor Maximilian of Mexico. Only French bayonets kept the ineffectual Maximilian in power. Once the distractions of the Civil War eased, the United States made increasingly menacing noises about the new regime. Napoleon III quickly realized that social unrest in Mexico, coupled with the threat of invasion by the battle-hardened Union army, rendered his North American ambitions chancy at best. As soon as he withdrew his troops, the puppet government fell and Maximilian was executed by Mexican partisans.

Freedom from the French did not bring stability to Mexico or free it from the designs of diehard American continentalists. These included a group of veteran army officers who had suddenly found themselves without any wars to fight, Texas Rangers who coveted Mexican cattle and grazing lands, and a number of political opportunists. If a border war could be provoked, these schemers reasoned, the officers would have new commands, the Rangers could legally steal Mexican stock, and Texas would gain new lands to govern. Commercial and business interests, however, opposed such schemes. They preferred friendly economic ties with the new regime of Porfirio Díaz to the uncertainties of war and the conquest of a potentially hostile people. In 1881 Secretary of State James G. Blaine laid continentalism to rest forever. The United States had no territorial designs whatsoever in Mexico, he announced. It sought only the opportunity to invest its "large accumulation of capital."

William Henry Seward

No one did more to initiate the idea of a "New Empire" for the United States than William Henry Seward. Possessed of "a slouching, slender figure," as Henry Adams once described him, Seward had "a head like a macaw; a beaked nose; shaggy eyebrows; unorderly hair and clothes; hoarse voice; offhand manner; free talk and perpetual cigar." As secretary of state under Lincoln and Andrew Johnson, his skillful diplomacy averted direct European interference in the Civil War, and the breadth of his intellect and vision led him to dream dreams beyond those of most politicians. Though his own efforts to shape a new American empire ran into opposition in Congress, he glimpsed the course American expansion would take over the next 40 years.

Seward rested his expansionist policies on what he perceived as two central political laws. The first, based on his reading of history, was that "empire has, for the last three thousand years . . . made its way constantly westward . . . until the tides of the renewed and decaying civilizations of the world meet on the shores of the Pacific Ocean." In his view, the surge of industrialization had only accelerated that pace of westward movement. Seward thus concluded that the United States needed to be prepared to win the great battles among the commercial nations for supremacy in the Far East. His second maxim underscored how that battle should be won: the great empires of the future, he believed, would be commercial, not military. "The nation that draws the most materials and provisions from the earth, and fabricates the most, and sells the most of productions and fabrics to foreign nations, must be, and will be, the great power of the earth." Thus the American empire would not require colonies. Rather the United States asked only for unrestricted access to Asian markets on nondiscriminating terms. That idea formed the basis of the "open-door" concept, which guided both British and American Far Eastern policy.

Seward assiduously pursued American links to Japan, Korea, and China. For him, a transcontinental railroad served to tie eastern factories to western ports and, from there, to the western Pacific. His diplomatic efforts led to the Burlingame Treaty of 1868, which made it possible for the railroads to recruit Chinese labor to build the western half of the first transcontinental line. For similar reasons Seward pressed for the construction of a canal across the Central American isthmus. And though he opposed direct colonialism in Asia, he advocated that the United States acquire a string of Pacific island colonies, protectorates, or naval stations, through which the United States could defend a canal and the sea lanes to China.

Seward's dreams of opening the Far East to American commerce bore little fruit in his lifetime. Chinese society and Chinese markets remained for the most part tightly closed to American penetration, as the Singer Sewing Company's difficulties demonstrated. Moreover, the shabby treatment of the Chinese in California, compounded by the insulting restrictions placed on Asian immigrants in 1882, aggravated Sino-American relations. The efforts of American missionaries often aroused antiforeign resentment among Chinese nationalists. What access Americans had to the China market was largely the result of British determination to prevent other powers from further carving China into exclusive spheres.

Commodore Matthew Perry, seen by a Japanese artist and by the Western eye of the camera.

Japan proved an even more elusive prize. Earlier in the century, novelist Herman Melville referred to Japan as the "double-bolted land." Except for a single port at Nagasaki open to Dutch traders, Japan's ruling feudal lords kept their isolated, agricultural land closed to foreigners. That lasted until 1853, when an American naval unit under Commodore Matthew Perry arrived to "open" Japan to the West. Perry specifically sought ports for trade and refueling ships as well as protection for American sailors off wrecked whaling ships. The Japanese had never seen steam-powered ships before. To them Perry's flotilla was an invasion by "barbarians in floating volcanoes."

Despite the terror he had inspired, Perry had opened the door to Japanese trade no more than a crack. Thus in 1867 the American warship *Wyoming* joined British and French naval units determined to break Japanese resistance to foreign trade, by force if necessary. Unwilling to suffer the fate of China by becoming a dependent colonial economy, the Japanese launched an internal revolution under the Meiji restoration (1868–1912), which in little more than a decade transformed Japan into a modern power and a rival to Western hegemony in the Pacific. In its subsequent diplomatic efforts with Japan, the United States concentrated not on dominating the Japanese home market, but in securing Japanese support for an open door in China.

Korea at first seemed a more promising Asian market for American penetration. Some commercial opportunities opened in the 1860s, and in 1882 Navy Commodore Robert Shufeldt made the United States the first Western country to have formal trade and diplomatic ties with a country so isolated that Westerners called it the "hermit kingdom." Though technically a dependency of China, Korea became more vulnerable to other nations as Chinese control weakened. A remarkable American diplomat, business promoter, and missionary, Horace Allen, worked diligently to protect Korean autonomy from foreign predators while maintaining an open door to trade. Other nations had little incentive to see Allen's efforts succeed. The Russians wanted to dominate Korea to protect the eastern terminus of the Trans-Siberian Railroad in Vladivostok (see map, p. 793). The Japanese viewed an independent Korea as a knife pointed at their home islands. As the fruit of victory in successive wars with China (1894–1895) and Russia (1904–1906), Japan established exclusionary dominion over Korea.

The meager success of American initiatives in the Far East demonstrated that Seward's vision was far ahead of both opportunity and domestic political support. Even close to home he had difficulty transforming vision into policy. The transcontinental railroad, Atlantic cable, and high tariffs he supported did become realities. But when he tried in 1865 to buy the Virgin Islands with their fine harbors, Denmark insisted on more than the $5 million Seward offered. Congress balked at paying a higher price. President Grant finally killed the proposed treaty. Seward's hopes to buy Iceland, Greenland, and Samana Bay on Santo Domingo and to annex revolution-riddled Cuba, European-controlled Caribbean islands, Tiger Island off Honduras, and Hawaii all ran into domestic and foreign opposition.

Seward did make two notable territorial acquisitions. An American naval officer raised the Stars and Stripes over Midway Island in 1867. Though of no great importance by itself, Midway was a way station to Asia and close to Hawaii, where missionary planters were already establishing an American presence. More notably, Seward engineered the purchase of Alaska, a territory of some 591,000 square miles, twice the size of Texas. By the 1850s the Russian government had lost enthusiasm for its beachhead in North America. Besides, St. Petersburg sensed that if it did not sell Alaska, the Americans might seize it.

Following the Civil War, Seward opened negotiations with the Russians without informing either President Johnson or Congress; then, in March 1867 he simply presented Congress with a treaty and a bill of sale for $7.2 million. Critics derided the acquisition of the "Polar Bear Garden," or "Frigidia," when the United States had not even settled the vast western lands it owned. But key senators and congressmen, like Charles Sumner of Massachusetts, recognized that Alaska, with its vast potential natural resources, was cheap at many times that price. And other members of Congress, unpersuaded by high-minded arguments of imperial strategy, accepted the logic of bribes liberally dispensed by the Russian ambassador. Within 10 days the Senate approved the Alaskan purchase, though the House stalled for over a year.

The United States and Latin America

Many Americans did not accept Seward's conviction that history's future lay in the Far East. They thought Latin America offered the best opportunity for new markets—if obstacles to American penetration could be overcome. One impediment, as we have seen, was the British presence in Central America. James G. Blaine, "the plumed knight" from Maine, who became secretary of state under James Garfield and again under Benjamin Harrison, believed the time had come to establish American supremacy under the Monroe Doctrine in fact as well as in principle. Blaine tried to persuade Great Britain to cancel the Clayton–Bulwer Treaty and give the United States exclusive control over any canal built in the region. More important, he looked for some means to shift the region's import market from British to American goods.

At the same time Blaine sought some way to end the political disruptions and constant warfare that threatened to undermine hemispheric markets. Mexico against Guatemala, Chile against Argentina, Nicaragua against Honduras, Chile against Peru and Bolivia, and even a threat of war between Chile and the United States in 1891 demonstrated the quarrelsome nature of hemispheric relations. Internal factional rivalries, unstable governments, and British and American meddling all contributed to unrest.

The best way to ease tensions, Blaine believed, as well as promote regional trade, was a conference among the nations of the hemisphere. For nearly a decade his idea went unheeded, but in 1889 the secretary of state presided over the first Pan-American Congress, with delegates from 17 nations. Blaine suggested a "customs union," designed to reduce trade barriers in the Americas and, conveniently, allow the United States to exploit its less developed neighbors. He also urged arbitration as a way to prevent the escalation of tensions into armed conflict. Hindered by the Argentinian and Chilean delegates, who were deeply suspicious of American motives, the meeting ended only with an agreement to establish a Pan-American Union to foster peaceful understanding. Blaine thus found himself forced to pursue separate talks and use less subtle arm-twisting in order to gain the tariff reductions he sought. If a nation balked, he threatened to invoke provisions of the 1890 McKinley Tariff to ban the products of their single-crop economies. Only three nations—Colombia, Haiti, and Venezuela—had the will to resist.

Prelude in the Pacific

Preoccupation with Latin America did not quiet all interest in the Pacific, where the United States vied with Great Britain and Germany for the islands of Samoa. In 1878 a treaty gave America the rights to the harbor at Pago Pago. When the Germans sent marines to secure their interests in 1889, the British and Americans reinforced their naval presence. Only a fortuitous typhoon, which destroyed the rival ships, staved off an escalating conflict. The three powers then peacefully carved up the islands, with the United States retaining Pago Pago.

The primary target for American expansionists was not Samoa but Hawaii, earlier known as the Sandwich Islands. If the United States wanted to fashion a bracelet of trade across the Pacific to China, Hawaii was the jewel in the middle. It would afford a fine naval base and a way station along the route to Asia. As early as the 1780s an American merchant ship had stopped at the Sandwich Islands on its journey to China. By the 1840s missionaries and merchants so dominated the port at Honolulu that one historian described it as "Yankee as New Bedford." Though Polynesian culture and local rule survived for several more decades, the process of political, economic, and cultural absorption was under way. The missionaries were godly, but their descendants were a remarkably practical lot: they saw the possibilities for a harvest not only of Polynesian souls but of sugar as well. Thus they undermined local culture by converting the islanders to Christianity while they acquired large tracts of property on which they produced sugar for export to the United States.

European imperialists, eager for their own way stations in the Pacific, would have been happy to possess Hawaii. But the United States, while not yet ready to annex the islands, had by the 1880s asserted virtual control over them. Although an 1875 treaty admitted Hawaiian sugar duty-free into the states, Hawaiians paid a high price for that advantage, for their prosperity now depended on the American

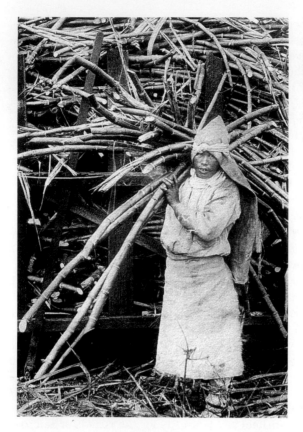

Sugar was the key to Hawaii's English- and American-dominated plantations. Polynesians were culturally ill-suited to the backbreaking labor sugar cultivation demanded. Planters filled their labor needs by recruiting Japanese workers like this one.

market. In 1886 they granted the United States naval rights to Pearl Harbor. Finding themselves hopelessly outmaneuvered, the British could only ask the Americans to keep the islands neutral and trade open to all nations.

The McKinley Tariff of 1890 changed matters dramatically, however, by removing sugar from the list of exempt items. Hawaiian planters recognized that if the islands were annexed, the tariffs would no longer apply to them. Unfortunately for their cause, in 1891 Queen Liliuokalani brought to the throne a nationalist rule much less sympathetic to American ways. As a nationalist, she firmly believed that Hawaii should remain in the hands of its native peoples. And as a monarchist, she firmly believed those hands should be hers, and not those of planter interests dominating a constitutional legislature. So the sugar planters began plotting and in January 1893 staged a revolt. Their success was conveniently assured when the American minister to Hawaii, John Stevens, ordered ashore sailors of the U.S.S. *Boston* on the pretense of protecting Americans. Faced with heavily armed opposition, the queen capitulated, leaving a commission of planters, four American and one British, in control.

While Stevens had acted without direct orders from Washington, President Harrison and Secretary of State Blaine supported his efforts. On his own initiative he also recognized the new government, placed it under the protection of the United States, and urged President Harrison to annex the islands, though the native Hawaiians had given no indication they desired to become Americans. Eager to preempt any British designs, Harrison signed an annexation treaty with the American-dominated commission from Hawaii.

Before the Senate could act to ratify, Grover Cleveland took office and immediately put the treaty on hold. Cleveland was hardly a foe of expansion, but as his
secretary of state, Walter Gresham, expressed it, the administration was "unalter-
ably opposed to stealing territory, or of annexing people against their consent, and
the people of Hawaii do not favor annexation." The idea of incorporating the
nonwhite population also troubled Cleveland. So matters stood, for a time, at a
stalemate. But given the strength of expansionist sentiments in the rising generation of Americans, the stalemate could not last indefinitely.

Crisis in Venezuela

Gold, with its universal capacity to muddy the waters out of which it was panned,
stirred trouble again in the jungles of Venezuela. In the 1880s prospectors unearthed a 32-pound nugget in the region between Venezuela and British Guiana.
Almost 10 years earlier the Venezuelans had begun to complain about British
incursions on their borderlands. Not coincidentally, those lands included the
mouth of the Orinoco River, a potential gateway to trade in the interior of South
America's northern coastal region.

Determined to preserve the sanctity of the Monroe Doctrine but lacking the
navy to oppose British actions, the United States unsuccessfully recommended
that the disputed claims be arbitrated. In 1895, with the British still threatening to
adjust the border unilaterally, the United States sent a stiffly worded protest that
Britain's expansive claims against Venezuela impinged on the "safety," "honor,"
and "welfare" of the United States. The mood in Washington had become much
more truculent now that a naval building program was under way, and, in the
midst of economic depression, Congress was hardly in the mood to see Great
Britain close off a promising market. Arbitration, the Cleveland administration
insisted, was the only way for Britain to avoid more forceful American intervention
in an area where the United States was "practically sovereign" and "practically
invulnerable as against any or all other powers." What form that intervention
might take Secretary of State Richard Olney was careful not to say.

Secretary of State Olney's cable arrived when much of the Foreign Office was
away on summer vacation. Not until November did Britain's prime minister issue
another tepid rejection of arbitration. The outraged Cleveland, unwilling to back
down but unwilling to risk war, issued what amounted to an ultimatum. The
United States would send a commission to set the boundary, and if the British did
not arbitrate, more forceful American action would follow. The British ambassador
warned London that "in Congress and among the public [exists] a condition of
mind which can only be described as hysterical." Theodore Roosevelt, the pugna-
cious police commissioner of New York City and usually a foe of Cleveland, applauded the president's menacing posture: "Let the fight come if it must; I don't
care whether our sea coast cities are bombarded or not; we would take Canada."

But cooler heads found the prospect of war with Great Britain unacceptable.
The scare had disrupted American financial markets as British investors withdrew
funds. Believers in the superiority of the Anglo-Saxon race saw no reason why
people of the same background should fight one another. Nor, in fact, did Cleveland. He wanted only to force the British to accept peace on terms acceptable to
the United States. In that he succeeded. Eager to avoid conflict with the United
States, the British agreed to arbitrate and in the end a compromise settlement left
Venezuela with what it most wanted, control of access to the Orinoco.

In reality few Americans, including Cleveland, had ever cared much about Venezuela's interests. What the administration most wanted was an opportunity to assert American power and influence in world affairs. Venezuela offered an outlet for the jingoistic spirit of the age: many nations, including the United States, adopted a belligerent posture on foreign policy issues both large and small. That aggressive tone in newspapers and political speeches reflected the expansionary nationalism of most Americans in the late nineteenth century. The Venezuelan crisis thus put new teeth into the Monroe Doctrine, as the United States moved to assume hegemony in the Western Hemisphere.

Ironically, the dispute marked the end, rather than the increase of tensions between Great Britain and the United States. Once dominant among European powers, Great Britain increasingly found itself facing a formidable rival, Germany, which had been unified under Otto von Bismarck's iron hand and was now rapidly industrializing. In Asia, both Russia and Japan threatened to close off markets Britain sought, while the 1899 Boer War with white Afrikaaners in South Africa drained British energy and resources. The Foreign Office recognized that allowing Americans a free hand in the Western Hemisphere was a small price to pay for friendly assistance in keeping trade doors open around the world. The treaty Secretary of State John Hay concluded with British Ambassador Sir Julian Pauncefote in 1901 symbolized the new era of Anglo-American friendship. Under the Hay–Pauncefote Treaty, Britain ceded its interest in building a canal across the Latin American isthmus, while the United States pledged to leave such a canal open to ships of all nations.

THE IMPERIAL MOMENT

The year 1895 signaled a major shift in relations among the imperial powers. The United States had confronted Britain over Venezuela, Japan humiliated China in the Sino-Japanese War, and revolution in Cuba threatened the last bastion of Spain's shrunken New World empire. Americans had long cast a covetous eye on that sugar-rich island some 90 miles southwest of the tip of Florida. Outside the small white Spanish minority, few Cubans benefited from the island's plantation economy. In the wake of an unsuccessful revolutionary struggle from 1868 to 1878 the majority of the island's black and mulatto population suffered from dire poverty and severe political repression from their Spanish overlords.

After almost 15 years of planning and plotting from exile in the United States, Cuban revolutionary leader José Martí returned to Cuba in 1895 to renew the struggle for independence. With cries of *Cuba libre,* the rebels on February 24 began their fight by cutting railroad lines, destroying sugar mills, and burning the cane fields. The Cuban economy was already staggering from a drop in sugar exports resulting from duties imposed by the United States in 1894, in the midst of a severe national depression. That crisis made the local populace sympathetic to Martí's cause. By 1896 the rebels controlled more than half the island. All that time Martí and his followers worried about what the United States might do. They knew their island had long been a target of American expansionists and economic interests. "I have lived in the bowels of the monster," Martí said in reference to the United States, "and I know it."

The Spanish struck back with brutal violence. Governor-General Valeriano Weyler instituted a reconcentration program, under which his soldiers herded a half million Cubans from their homes into fortified camps. Filth, disease, and starvation killed as many as 200,000 of these prisoners. Outside the camps, Weyler's forces made war on the countryside, polluting the drinking water, killing farm animals, and burning crops.

Mounting Tensions

Americans had toyed with the notion of annexing Cuba since before the Civil War, when the island's slave-driven sugar plantations offered southerners a way to add slave territory to the United States to balance the increasing number of free states. During the 1890s the Cleveland administration had little sympathy for Martí's revolution. Cleveland doubted that the predominantly black Cuban population was capable of self-government and feared that any move for independence from Spain might lead to chaos. Already the revolution had caused widespread destruction of American-owned property. Cleveland settled on a policy that would throw American support to neither Spain nor the rebels: opposing the rebellion, but pressuring Spain to grant Cuba a measure of autonomy.

That halfway approach did not satisfy Republicans in Congress, who pressed Cleveland to recognize the Cuban belligerents. As a result, when Spain refused to lighten its oppressive hand in Cuba, Cleveland found himself trapped. He wanted to end Spanish brutality, but he did not want war. He wanted to continue the commercial penetration of Cuba, but he did not want to annex the island. So Cleveland and Secretary of State Olney continued to warn Spain of American interest in Cuba, doing little more than rattling teacups.

Ardent expansionists like Theodore Roosevelt, Henry Cabot Lodge, and John Hay had already convinced Republicans in their 1896 platform to call for American annexation of Hawaii, the construction of a Nicaraguan canal, purchase of the Virgin Islands, and further naval expansion. For Cuba they called for recognition of independence, a step that, if taken, would likely lead to war with Spain. The new president, however, was only a moderate expansionist. Like Blaine, William McKinley believed that the United States had dominant interests in Latin America. Like Mahan, he favored a large navy, insular bases, and a vigorous foreign trade. At first McKinley acted privately to press Spain to cease its repression of the rebels and to avoid actions that sent American citizens to Cuban jails and destroyed American property.

In October 1897 Spain did promise to remove the much-despised Weyler, to end the reconcentration policy, and to offer Cuba far greater autonomy. That shift in Spanish policy encouraged McKinley to reject calls for a more belligerent course. But events soon proved that dominant elements of the Spanish army in Cuba were renewing their efforts to crush the rebels and uphold Spain's honor. Conservative and pro-army elements opposed to reform rioted in the streets of Havana. McKinley dispatched the battleship *Maine* to show that the United States might take stiffer measures.

Then in February 1898 the State Department received a stolen copy of a letter to Cuba sent by the Spanish minister in Washington, Enrique Dupuy de Lôme. So did William Randolph Hearst, a pioneer of sensationalist, or "yellow," journalism. "WORST INSULT TO THE UNITED STATES IN ITS HISTORY," screamed the headline of Hearst's New York *Journal*. What had de Lôme actually said? It was insulting enough that he had dismissed McKinley as "a would-be politician," but, more tellingly, he admitted that Spain had no intention of reforming its Cuban policies. It intended to fight until the rebels were beaten. Spain immediately recalled de Lôme, but the damage had been done. Most Americans believed Spain had purposely deceived the United States. McKinley recognized that he had few options short of war.

It was at this point, on February 15, 1898, that a series of explosions ripped through the hull of the *Maine* as it lay at anchor in Havana harbor. Some 260 American sailors died. The cause of the blasts to this day remains unclear, but most Americans of the day irrationally concluded that Spanish agents had sabotaged the ship. The reality that Spain had little reason to provoke a war it could ill afford to fight did not penetrate the popular emotional outcry. The cautious McKinley sought a diplomatic solution, but he also asked Congress to appropriate $50 million "to get ready for war."

Meanwhile Theodore Roosevelt, the bumptious assistant secretary of the navy, sought to overcome the caution of the president and John Long, his boss in the Navy Department. With Long away, Roosevelt ordered Commodore George Dewey to prepare his Asiatic naval squadron to attack the Spanish fleet in the Philippines should war break out. That has led to the myth that Roosevelt secretly promoted war in the Pacific. In fact, the navy in 1896 had developed plans for a Philippine attack, so though Roosevelt acted a bit precipitately, his order was consistent with administration policy. McKinley was not as bellicose as ardent imperialists like Roosevelt, but, like most of the leaders of his party, he did consider overseas expansion a way to revive the economy in the aftermath of the 1890s depression.

The pressures for war simply proved too strong for McKinley to resist for long. On April 11 he asked Congress to authorize "forceful intervention" by the United States to establish peace in Cuba. Congress responded nine days later with a resolution that recognized the independence of Cuba, insisted on the withdrawal of Spanish forces, and gave the president authority to use the army and navy to enforce American demands. In the midst of this war rhetoric Congress adopted another measure, the Teller Amendment, with almost no fanfare. The amendment renounced any aim to annex Cuba, a gesture that seemed to cast the decision for war in a humanitarian rather than an imperialist light. "We cannot look idly on while hundreds of thousands of innocent human beings . . . die of hunger close to our doors," argued Senator George Hoar of Massachusetts. In truth, many supporters of the amendment feared the burden the United States would be forced to assume for Cuba's debts and its deeply impoverished black population. Certainly idealism and moral outrage had led many Americans down the path to war. But in this instance, less lofty ambitions for empire, expanded trade, and military glory offer a better explanation for what John Hay would call a "splendid little war."

The Imperial War

Many Europeans expected war between Spain and the United States to be an even fight. Most Americans thought otherwise. They welcomed the Spanish–American War as if it were a sporting event like a heavyweight prizefight. The army was swamped with volunteers, including an unlikely cavalry troop of cowboys and eastern college dudes put together by Theodore Roosevelt. Ohio alone had almost 100,000 volunteers. Beating a decrepit Spain would be no harder than "robbing an old gypsy woman in a vacant lot after a night fair," jested the young writer Sherwood Anderson.

For the 5462 men who died in the Spanish–American War there was little splendid about the event. Only 379 of the dead actually gave their lives in battle. The rest suffered from accident, disease, and the mismanagement of an unprepared army. Its total force numbered only 30,000, none of whom had been trained for fighting in tropical conditions or dealing with tropical disease. The sudden expansion to 60,000 troops and 200,000 volunteers overtaxed the supply system, which operated largely through graft and inefficiency. Troops often fought with weapons left over from the Civil War, sweltered in winter wool uniforms, and were given tinned rations that were diseased, rotted, or poisoned. Thus American soldiers went to war facing more dangerous conditions on their own bases than under enemy fire.

Fortunately for the United States, naval battles largely determined the outcome of the Spanish–American War. The decision to modernize the fleet during the 1890s paid almost immediate dividends. Prepared by orders from Theodore Roosevelt (which had been blessed, after the fact, by the approval of President McKinley), Admiral George Dewey ordered his battle squadron from China toward the Philippines as soon as war was declared. Few Americans had heard of the islands; fewer still could easily have located them on a globe. McKinley himself actually followed the news from the southwest Pacific on an old textbook map. The navy, however, had marked the Philippines as a key target, and on April 30, under cover of darkness, Dewey's squadron slipped by the shore guns of Corregidor in Manila Bay (see map on p. 812).

The battle that followed was one of the most one-sided and decisive in American military history. It began on May 1, 1898, with Dewey's laconic command at 5.40 a.m., "You may fire when ready, Gridley." And fire they did, until 8 a.m., when the Americans stopped briefly for breakfast. Five hours later the entire Spanish squadron of 10 ships lay at the bottom of Manila Bay. Three hundred eighty-one Spaniards had died; only eight Americans were wounded, and one sailor died of a heart attack. Dewey had no plans to follow up his victory with an invasion. In fact, his fleet carried no troops with which to take Manila. Only after he learned of Dewey's success did President McKinley order American troops to the Philippines.

News did not reach the American people until May 7, but then the entire nation went wild. Victory seemed to confirm American military prowess. In Dewey people found the hero for whom they thirsted. As one bit of newspaper doggerel exulted:

> Oh, dewy was the morning
> Upon the first of May,
> And Dewey was the admiral,
> Down in Manila Bay.
> And dewy were the Spaniards' eyes,
> Them orbs of black and blue,
> And dew we feel discouraged?
> I dew not think we dew!

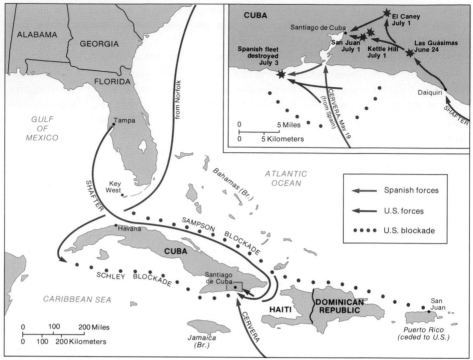

THE SPANISH-AMERICAN WAR
Had the Spanish-American War depended largely on ground forces, the ill-prepared U.S. Army might have fared poorly. But the key to success, in both Cuba and the Philippines, was naval warfare, in which the recently modernized American fleet had a critical edge. Proximity to Cuba also gave the United States an advantage in delivering troops and supplies and in maintaining a naval blockade that isolated Spanish forces.

Meanwhile, another Spanish fleet had slipped into Santiago harbor in Cuba before the U.S. Navy reached the area. American forces under Admiral William Sampson soon set up a blockade, assuming that the Spanish would try to sneak out at night. After being bottled up for five weeks, the Spanish instead made a desperate daylight dash for the open seas on July 3. So startled were the Americans that several of their ships nearly collided in an effort to sink their hopelessly exposed foes. All seven Spanish ships were sunk with 474 casualties, compared with only one dead and one wounded among the Americans. Cuba was now effectively cut off from Spain and the war virtually over.

The Cuban War

Before the outbreak of hostilities, Tampa was a sleepy coastal Florida town with a single railroad line. As the port of embarkation for the Cuban expeditionary force it became a hive of activity. Its overtaxed facilities soon broke down, with the inevitable unhealthy food and unsafe sanitation, as well as an ineffable miasma of plain human stench.

Into this scene of disease and chaos came yet another source of tension. President McKinley had authorized the army to raise five volunteer regiments of black soldiers. Despite the resistance of most state governors, the army finally accepted about 10,000 soldiers the Spanish came to call "smoked Yankees." But as Sergeant Frank Pullen of the black 24th Infantry Regiment remarked, to most white Americans, "we were 'niggers.'" Like most southern towns, Tampa and Lakeland were largely segregated, so that the 4000 blacks stationed there could sail off to die freeing the peasants of Cuba, but they could not buy a soda at the local drugstore. "Is America any better than Spain?" one dismayed black chaplain wondered. As the expeditionary force prepared to leave in early June, anger turned to violence. After drunken white troops shot at a black child, black troops in Tampa struck back. The ensuing riot left 3 whites and 27 blacks wounded.

Matters were scarcely less chaotic as the disorganized troops and hundreds of reporters finally scrambled aboard ships. There they sat for a week; on June 14 they sailed toward Santiago and battle. By June 30 the 17,000 regulars and volunteers had landed, to challenge some 24,000 Spanish troops, many equipped with more modern rifles. The following day 7000 Americans stormed up heavily fortified San Juan Hill and nearby Kettle Hill. Their objective was the high ground to

---

By the time of the Spanish-American War, blacks had been largely disfranchised and segregated; one of the few rights they preserved was the right to die for their country. Black veterans of the western Indian wars along with volunteers, segregated and commanded by white officers, made up almost a quarter of the American force that invaded Cuba. The Spanish soldiers dubbed them "smoked Yankees." Here, the all-black Tenth Cavalry supports a charge by Colonel Teddy Roosevelt's Rough Riders at the battle of San Juan Hill.

the north and east of Santiago. Among them Lieutenant Colonel Theodore Roosevelt thrilled at the experience of battle as he yelled to his Rough Riders (most of whom could not hear his rather high, squeaky voice), "Gentlemen, the Almighty God and the just cause are with you. Gentlemen, *Charge!*" After Roosevelt had repeated the call a second time, charge they did, though the battle cost the Americans over 1500 casualties. Without a fleet to cover them or any way to escape, the Spanish garrison surrendered on July 17. In the Philippines, a similar brief skirmish preceded the American taking of Manila on August 13. John Hay's "splendid little war" had ended in less than four months.

Peace and Empire

Conquering Cuba and the Philippines proved easier than deciding what the United States should do with them. The Teller Amendment renounced any American intention to exercise sovereignty over Cuba. But clearly the United States had not freed the island to see chaos reign or American business and military interests excluded. And what of the Philippines—and Puerto Rico, which American forces had taken without a struggle? Powerful public and congressional sentiment pushed McKinley to claim empire as the fruits of victory.

The president himself favored such a course. The battle in the Pacific highlighted the need for naval bases and coaling stations. "To maintain our flag in the Philippines, we must raise our flag in Hawaii," the New York *Sun* insisted. And on July 7 McKinley did just that as he signed a joint congressional resolution annexing Hawaii.

The Philippines presented a far more difficult problem. Filipinos had greeted the American forces as liberators, not colonial successors to the Spanish. The popular leader of the rebel forces fighting against Spain, Emilio Aguinaldo, had returned to the islands on an American ship. But to the rebels' dismay, McKinley insisted that the islands were under American authority until the peace treaty settled matters. Such a settlement no doubt would include permanent American control. McKinley had no intention of leaving Spain in charge and no desire to see the islands fall to such imperial rivals as Britain, Germany, and Japan. Without control of the entire island of Luzon, American military advisors warned, its capital, Manila, was indefensible as a naval base. Nor, McKinley felt certain, were the Filipinos in any way capable of self-government. Aguinaldo and his rebels understandably thought otherwise. In June Aguinaldo declared himself president of a new Philippine republic.

Many influential Americans took a strong stand against annexation. This was not, however, simply an argument for or against empire. Most members of the anti-imperialist movement, which included such prominent figures as former president Grover Cleveland, steel baron Andrew Carnegie, and novelist Mark Twain, did favor expansion in some form. Rather, business leaders among the anti-imperialists believed the United States could enjoy the economic fruits of the Philippines without the cost and consequences of incorporating the islands into the American system. Annexation would involve the United States far more deeply and undesirably in the politics of Asia. More important, a large fleet would be necessary to defend the islands. To the imperialists that was precisely the point. The United States should seek markets in Asia; and a large fleet was crucial to the interests of a powerful commercial nation.

Racist ideas shaped both sides of this argument. Imperialists believed that the

THE UNITED STATES IN THE PACIFIC

In the late nineteenth century both Germany and the United States emerged as major naval powers and as contestants for influence and commerce in China. The island groups of the Central and Southwest Pacific, though of little economic value, had potential strategic significance as bases and coaling stations along the routes to Asia. Rivalry (as in the case of Samoa) sometimes threatened to erupt into open conflict. Control of Hawaii, Midway, Samoa, Guam, and the Philippines gave the United States a string of strategic stepping-stones to the Orient.

racial inferiority of nonwhite peoples made the Philippine occupation necessary. But where the imperialists were willing to assume the "white man's burden" by annexing the Philippines, the anti-imperialists feared racial intermixing and the possibility that Asian workers would flood the American labor market.

Moreover, they believed that dark-skinned people could never develop the capacity for self-government. The Constitution made no provision for governing people without representation or equal rights. Rule in the Philippines would be successful only at the point of bayonets wielded by permanent troops of occupation. The precedent of government by force might imperil American liberties at home. Imperialists envisioned a benevolent government under which the United States would teach the virtues of democracy, Western civilization, and Christianity,[*] thus preparing the Philippines for self-rule.

*In point of fact, most Filipinos were already Catholic after many years under Spanish rule.

Still, in the Senate debate over the Treaty of Paris, the imperialists had the overwhelming support of the president, Congress, and public opinion. Even an anti-imperialist like William Jennings Bryan, defeated by McKinley in 1896, supported the treaty, in which Spain surrendered title to Cuba, ceded Puerto Rico and Guam to the United States, and for $20 million ceded the Philippines as well. Eager to see war ended, Bryan believed that once the United States possessed the Philippines it could free them.

The imperialists had other notions. Having acquired an empire and a modern navy to protect it, the United States could rightfully assert its claim as one of the great powers of the world. But managing a new empire proved far more difficult than acquiring it.

America's First Asian War

Conflict between the American occupation forces and the Philippine rebels erupted even before the capture of Manila. The Americans might hold the city, but the rebels controlled the countryside. As the Senate debated annexation, a rebel and an American patrol clashed outside the city. The guerrilla war that followed lasted more than three years, claiming 5000 American lives, 25,000 rebel soldiers, and 200,000 Filipino civilians.

The savagery of the fighting was spurred on by the deep racial antagonism on the part of most American soldiers toward people they described as "cross-eyed kakiak Ladrones." Successful resistance by such a supposedly inferior people too often turned frustration to brutality and torture. To avenge a rebel attack on unarmed troops, one American officer swore he would turn the surrounding country-

---

The American decision to occupy the Philippines rather than give it independence forced Filipino nationalists to fight U.S. troops, as they had already been fighting the Spanish since 1896. Forces like the ones pictured at the right were tenacious enough to require more than 70,000 Americans (left) to put down the rebellion. Sporadic, bloody guerrilla fighting continued until 1902 and other incidents persisted until 1906.

side into a "howling wilderness." Before long the 70,000 American troops had resorted to a garrison strategy that was embarrassingly reminiscent of the recon- centration policy of "Butcher" Weyler in Cuba. The war came to an unresolved end in 1902 only after the Americans managed to capture Aguinaldo, and his Filipino supporters finally lost hope.

In contrast to the bitter guerrilla war, the United States did practice a rela- tively benevolent colonial rule. Directed by Governor William Howard Taft, a program of modernization brought new schools, improved roads, cleaner cities, more productive agriculture, and factories, which won the support of the Filipino elite. The United States played a similar role in Puerto Rico, where, as in the Philippines, executive authority resided in a governor appointed by the president. Under the Foraker Act of 1900 Puerto Ricans were given a voice in their govern- ment, a nonvoting representative in the U.S. House of Representatives, and tariff advantages. All the same, many Puerto Ricans chafed at the idea of permanent second-class status. Some favored eventual admission to the United States as a state, while others advocated independence, a division of opinion that persists to the present day.

An Open Door in China

Interest in Asia had spurred the United States to annex the Philippines; annexa- tion of the Philippines further whetted American interest in Asia. As always, the possibility of markets in China—whether for Christian souls or consumers— proved the greatest attraction. But both the British, who had garnered most of China's export trade, and Americans were worried about China being carved up by other imperial powers. Japan had gone to war with China in 1895 and defeated it, encouraging Russia, Germany, Japan, and France to demand additional trading concessions. Each nation sought to establish a "sphere of influence" in which its commercial and military interests were supreme. Often this meant discrimination against the interests of rival powers. Since Britain and the United States hoped only for the benefits of trade rather than new colonies, they sought some means to limit further foreign demands while leaving China open to the trade of all nations.

At the urging of a British customs official from China, Secretary of State John Hay in 1899 circulated the first of several "open-door" notes to the imperial pow- ers. Hay asked only that the powers keep their spheres of influence in China open; he did not ask them to relinquish those spheres or to refrain from extending them. All of the powers accepted Hay's proposal with qualifications, but he announced that the open door was now an international policy.

Americans less familiar with imperial ambitions believed that Hay's note might actually protect China. In reality, it reflected the gap between American ambitions and power in Asia. The United States lacked the military, economic, or diplomatic means to create the fabled China market or to prevent other powers from partitioning China. Only the fear that the United States might tip the deli- cate balance by siding with a rival power led the Japanese and European powers to respond to Hay's note.

Events soon threatened the balance Hay sought to maintain. Disgruntled Chinese nationalists, known to Westerners as Boxers (their symbol was a fist), formed secret societies to drive the the *fon kwei*, or foreign devils, from their country. The Manchu empress secretly supplied them with arms and political support. Egged on by the empress, the Boxers murdered hundreds of Christian missionaries and their followers and besieged foreign diplomats and citizens in Beijing. All of the European nations sent troops to quell the uprising. Hay and McKinley sent 2500 Americans to join the march to the capital city. Along the way the angry armies did not restrain themselves against those they viewed as "slanty-eyed Celestials," confiscating valuables and committing atrocities against the civilian population.

Fearful that once in control of Beijing the conquerors might never leave, Hay dispatched a second open-door note. This time he asked the foreign powers to respect China's territorial and administrative integrity as well as access to its markets. At the same time he encouraged local Chinese authorities to suppress the Boxers and withdrew American troops once the rebellion had ended. No other foreign power endorsed this proposal, but many Americans assumed it now had the same status as the Monroe Doctrine: a principle recognized in theory and practice by other imperial powers.

Yet Hay never committed the United States to upholding the open door with anything more than words; he even briefly explored the possibility of America carving out a naval coaling station in China. It took a note from the imperial Japanese to remind him that such a step contradicted the principle he himself had enunciated. The open-door notes amounted to no more than an expression of American interests and an announcement that the United States was now committed to the preservation of stability in Asia.

THE ROOTS OF RUSSIAN–AMERICAN CONFLICT

"There are two great nations in the world which, starting from different points, seem to be advancing toward the same goal: the Russians and the Anglo-Americans. . . . Each seems called by some secret design of Providence one day to hold in its hands the destinies of half the world." To people living after World War II, such an observation seems self-evident, but when Alexis de Tocqueville made it in 1835, both Russia and the United States stood on the periphery of world affairs.

For much of the nineteenth century, in fact, Europe's most reactionary monarchy and the revolutionary New World republic maintained cordial relations. They did so by stressing their mutual interests rather than their profound ideological and cultural differences. As peripheral powers separated by great distances, they had few points of potential geographical conflict. Russian–American commerce benefited both nations and each nation viewed the other as a potential counterweight to a common enemy—Great Britain. Thus the United States maintained a sympathetic attitude toward Russia in 1854 as it battled England and France during the Crimean War. The Russians returned the favor by frustrating French and British proposals to interfere in the American Civil War. The sale of Alaska to the United States in 1867 marked the high point of Russian–American cooperation. From then on, however, their interests began to diverge and conflicting ideologies soured their once cordial ties.

Conflicting Ideology

As American power increased and British–American rivalry eased, many Americans began to see Russia as a rival power. Where Britain supported the open door in China, the Russians clearly had imperial designs on Manchuria. And the more they learned about the czar's government, the more Americans objected to its repressive policies and its secret police. They were shocked to learn about the horrors of exile in the Siberian labor camps. But no issue did more to arouse American popular opposition to the czarist government than anti-Semitism. Official Russian policy restricted Russian Jews to an area of settlement in eastern Poland and western Russia called the Pale. Other laws limited Jewish educational and economic opportunities. Young Jewish men at the age of 12 faced over 30 years of forced military service. When revolutionaries assassinated Czar Alexander II in 1881, a bad situation became worse. The government condoned pogroms that for the next 30 years led to the beating and killing of Jews, the looting of shops, and illegal confiscation of property.

In the 1880s the population of the United States included only 250,000 Jews, mostly of German extraction. Their vocal protests, however, aroused the sympathies of other Americans as well as the State Department, which interceded when the pogroms affected American Jews traveling or living in Russia. On other occasions the State Department reminded the Russian government of the American commitment to religious freedom. The Russians replied that since the United States did not see fit to treat its minorities equally, the principle should not be binding on Russia either.

By the 1890s the pogroms had turned Jewish immigration to the United States from a trickle to a torrent. American Jewish leaders and humanitarians became more insistent that the government take some action to curtail Russian anti-Semitism. At first John Hay and President Theodore Roosevelt (who succeeded McKinley in 1901) refused. "What possible advantage would it be . . . to the Jews of Russia, if we should make a protest against these fiendish cruelties and be told it's none of our business?" Hay asked Jewish financier Jacob Schiff.

Insistent public protest led the politically shrewd Roosevelt in this case to let domestic concerns reverse his support for nonintervention. He agreed to forward a petition to the Russian government, which the Russians refused to accept. All the same, the United States had taken an important step. An ideological principle rather than a material interest had influenced American relations with Russia. If anything, American protests worsened the treatment of Russian Jews and certainly aggravated Russian–American relations. Roosevelt, however, reaped political benefits from a grateful American Jewish community. Jewish leaders, in turn, had demonstrated that influential pressure groups could affect the course of American foreign policy.

Diverging Interests

By the 1890s Russian and American economic interests had begun to diverge as well. As the United States came to work more closely with Britain, both powers began to regard Russia as a threat to the open door in China. Manchuria, a Chi-

This Russian-Jewish immigrant was one of millions who fled anti-Semitic violence in the region of Russia and Poland known as the Pale. Immigration officials placed the "K" on his coat to indicate a suspected hernia condition. Some diseases and disabilities were grounds for refusing immigrants' admission to the United States.

nese province southeast of Siberia, became an area in which American and Russian geographic interests clashed. Part of the Trans-Siberian Railroad, built in the 1890s, passed through Manchuria, and the new transportation link gave the Russians a commercial advantage in Asia over its European rivals. In the wake of the Boxer Rebellion, the Russians had occupied the entire province and then refused to withdraw. In 1902 Britain responded by forming an alliance with Japan.

The United States did not formally associate itself with this anti-Russian pact, but Americans supported it as a barrier to Russian ambitions. The American consul in Manchuria had recently warned that Russia "will annihilate American trade here . . . become a serious obstacle to the extension of our trade in all the Orient, and eventually a menace to our higher civilization." Thus when the Russians extended their occupation in 1903, Secretary of State Hay called the action "injurious to our legitimate interests" and characteristic of "a government with whom mendacity is a science." Rumors quickly spread in Washington of a possible Russian–American war, encouraged by traveler, writer, and lecturer George Kennan among others. Kennan (a distant relative of the well-known Soviet expert George F. Kennan) was one of the few Americans familiar with Russia and an archfoe of the czarist regime. Kennan knew that war was unlikely, but he recognized that the new course of American empire had forever ended "the sentimental friendship that has long been supposed to exist between the governments of Russia and the United States."

That was more the choice of American than Russian leaders. The goals of Russian foreign policy remained what they had long been: secure frontiers, access to the open seas (beyond merely the Baltic and Black seas), ethnic and religious solidarity at home, and a stable balance of power in Europe. In the late nineteenth century it was the United States whose goals had changed. A nation once content with continental expansion had set its sights across the seas. Foreign markets beckoned to its merchants and manufacturers. It had transformed its feeble navy into a force capable of projecting power into distant lands. Traditionally tied by culture and history to western Europe, its people now included those who had called eastern and southern Europe home. This gave the United States more reason to involve itself in the internal affairs of foreign nations, as it did increasingly with Russia in the twentieth century. Here lay the distant roots of the Russian–American conflict that has dominated international affairs since World War II.

To men like Alfred Thayer Mahan, Brooks and Henry Adams, Theodore Roosevelt, and John Hay, American interests would be secure only when they had been established worldwide. These expansionists were confident that as a world power the United States had embarked on the course destined for it by divine providence. It could maintain its high principles of democracy and equality without descending to the cynical power politics of imperialism. But to one French diplomat, perhaps more accustomed to the corrosive effects of wheeling and dealing in the corridors of international power, it seemed that the Americans had tempted fate rather than destiny. With a whiff of Old World cynicism he remarked, "The United States is seated at the table where the great game is played, and it cannot leave it."

SIGNIFICANT EVENTS

1850	Clayton–Bulwer Treaty
1853	Commodore Perry visits Japan
1867	Alaska acquired; British North America Act creates Canadian confederation; fall of Maximilian in Mexico
1871	Minor Keith arrives in Costa Rica
1878	Samoan Treaty
1881	Revolutionaries assassinate Czar Alexander II; anti-Jewish pogroms begin in Russia
1882	Chinese Exclusion Act; Commodore Shufeldt negotiates treaty with Korea
1889	First Pan-American Congress
1890	Mahan's *The Influence of Sea Power Upon History, 1660–1783* published; Naval Appropriations Bill launches modern navy
1891	Chile–United States war threat
1893	Controversy over annexation of Hawaii
1893–1896	Depression encourages expansionist policies
1894–1895	Sino-Japanese War
1895	Venezuelan boundary dispute; Martí revives Cuban revolution
1898	Sinking of the U.S.S. *Maine*; war with Spain; Teller Amendment; Dewey captures the Philippines; Tampa riots; Treaty of Paris; Hawaii formally annexed; Anti-Imperialist League established
1898–1902	Philippine insurrection
1899	First open-door notes
1900	Boxer Rebellion; second open-door notes; Foraker Act establishes civil government in Puerto Rico
1901	Hay–Pauncefote Treaty
1902	British–Japanese anti-Russian pact

23

The Progressive Era

uitting time, March 25, 1911. The streets of lower Manhattan were just beginning to swell with people. Glancing upward, a passer-by noticed "a great swirling, billowing cloud of smoke," sweeping "like a giant streamer out of Washington Square and down upon the beautiful homes in lower Fifth Avenue." The Asch Building, home of the Triangle Shirtwaist Company, was on fire.

Five hundred people, largely Jewish and Italian immigrants, had been working at the Triangle factory for nearly 12 hours as smoke began to fill the evening sky. Since half past seven in the morning they had been making "shirtwaists," the tailored blouses worn by young women working in offices. Most of the factory workers were young women, too, many under 25. Some were children as young as 8. In fact, so many youngsters could be found laboring in the city's garment factories, recalled one seamstress, that "the corner of the shop would resemble a kindergarten."

Throughout the industry wages and working conditions were horrid. Adults earned from $3 to $15 a week, children as little as $1.50, without overtime pay no matter how heavy the schedule. Workers sat on chairs without backs and bought their needles and thread—even the electric power—from their bosses. If employees arrived late or made a mistake on the job, they were fined or sent home with no pay.

Two years earlier Triangle workers had struck the company because it routinely fired union members. Some 18,000 dressmakers and waistmakers from the city's 600 manufacturers joined them. In mid-February 1910, while New Yorkers were buying sheet music for "Heaven Will Protect the Working Girl," the companies finally settled. The largest firms made concessions on wages and hours but refused to recognize the union. At Triangle dangerous working conditions remained: fire escapes stayed broken; no sprinkler system was installed; and doors were locked each morning to keep union organizers out and workers in.

The Triangle blaze broke out in the lofts and spread quickly from floor to floor. Terrified seamstresses groped through fire and smoke toward exits, only to find them shut tight. All the fire escapes but one collapsed in the heat. Children with hair on fire jumped from top-floor windows. "Spectators saw again and again pitiable companionships formed in the instant of death—girls who placed their arms around each other as they leaped," one news story read. They fell 10 stories before their bodies hit the sidewalk or were impaled on the building's iron guard rails.

Personal magnetism, expansive vision, and shrewd use of the press enabled Theodore Roosevelt to transform the presidency into a vital center of public action. This cartoon detail depicts him as an American Caesar, triumphantly parading through Washington.

One hundred forty-six people, mainly young women, died. A few days later 80,000 New Yorkers joined the silent funeral procession as it moved slowly up Fifth Avenue in the rain. A quarter of a million watched. "This is not the first time that girls have been burned alive in the city," union leader Rose Schneiderman told a mass meeting at the Metropolitan Opera House. "Every year thousands of us are maimed." New York's governor appointed a commission to investigate the tragedy. Over the next four years its recommendations produced 56 state laws—the most far-reaching labor code in the country—regulating fire safety, hours, machinery, and home work.

The Triangle fire horrified the nation and underscored what many Americans already knew: modern industrial society had created profound strains, widespread misery, and deep class divisions. Corporations and trusts grew to sizes previously unimagined, bought and sold legislators, dictated the terms of their own profit. Men and women worked around the clock in unsafe factories for wages that barely supported them. Eight- and nine-year-olds went into coal mines and came out missing fingers or limbs. Some never came out at all. If they survived to adulthood, they faced an early death from lungs blackened by coal dust.

Americans everywhere felt the pinch of the new industrial order. In cities tenement-bred tuberculosis took the lives of the disadvantaged. Violent criminals threatened people and property; saloons tied the poor and working class to dishonest political machines. In the countryside even successful farmers could not control the high rates of shippers. Sharecroppers and tenants helplessly suffered the poverty and ignorance that stripped them of dignity and opportunity. Across prosperous America, a mild but relentless inflation, averaging about 3 percent a year, shrank the wallets of the middle class. "It was a world of greed," concluded one disillusioned garment worker; "the human being didn't mean anything."

But human beings did mean something to adherents of the great reform movement that had already begun to reshape America. Progressivism had emerged in the mid-1890s and would last through World War I. It sprang from many impulses: desires to curb the advancing power of corporations and end widespread corruption; efforts to bring order and efficiency to economic and political life; attempts by new interest groups to make business and government more

In 1911 the fiery deaths of 146 people at the Triangle Shirtwaist Company shocked the nation. Firefighters arrived within minutes, but their ladders could not reach the top stories. Trapped by locked doors, those who failed to escape perished within or leaped to their deaths on the streets below. Following the horrifying episode New York enacted the most ambitious labor code in the country.

responsive to their needs; moralistic urges to rid society of such perceived evils as drink and prostitution. The ideology of progressivism mixed elements of liberal concern for the poor and working class with conservative efforts to stabilize business and avoid social chaos. At times progressivism embraced such diversity that historians have despaired of finding any coherence in it.

If progressivism did anything, it tried to reduce the dangerous effects of industrialization, immigration, and urbanization by softening their impact on people. The aftermath of the Triangle fire offers a case study of progressivism in action. Tragedy led to publicity and investigation, which generated the outrage and evidence necessary for change. Amid the clamor for reform, legislators adopted laws to set things right. To keep things right, progressives looked to an aroused public opinion and to government, often in the form of strong executive agencies staffed by impartial experts.

Progressivism began in the cities, where the wellspring of misery was fullest, political corruption deepest, and social division clearest. Organized mostly by angry, idealistic members of the middle class, it percolated up from neighborhoods to city halls and state legislatures. Though usually pursued through the medium of politics, the goals of progressives were broadly social. Progressives wanted nothing less than to create a "good society" (shaped largely in a middle-class mold) where people could live decently, harmoniously, and prosperously.

Progressives understood that only government had the resources for such a broad-based reformation. Under their leadership the modern activist state was born. It emerged at the national level in the presidencies of Theodore Roosevelt and Woodrow Wilson. No one political party monopolized progressivism; no single group controlled it. In 1912 it gave birth to the Progressive, or "Bull Moose," party, but by then it extended well beyond politics into every realm of American life.

THE ROOTS OF PROGRESSIVE REFORM

The wrenching depression of 1893 forced reformers to focus on the need to humanize the industrial system. They came to realize that despite differences in their social backgrounds and political concerns, they shared a common goal: the improvement of society. Ordinary people found common causes that cut across lines of class, religion, and ethnicity. If streetcar companies raised fares while service deteriorated, if processors doctored food with harmful additives, all consumers suffered.

The result was not a coherent progressive "movement" but a set of loosely affiliated movements. Some progressives struggled to provide efficient government and honest politics. Others attempted to widen the regulation of business. Some fought for social justice for the urban poor, others for social welfare to protect children, women, factory workers, or consumers. Still others wanted to purify society by prohibiting alcohol and drugs, restricting immigration, stamping out slums, and ending prostitution. Although independent forces, these groups often combined when their causes overlapped.

Progressivism had its nostalgic streak, for some progressives aimed at redeeming such traditional American values as democracy, opportunity for the individual, and a spirit of public service. In this quest progressives were often paternalistic, seeking to impose their ideals no matter what the less "enlightened" poor or oppressed might view as their own best interests. Yet if the ends of progressives were traditional, their means were modern. They made use of the latest techniques of organization, management, and science—fighting the excesses of the new industrial and urban order with its own systems and methods.

The Progressive System of Beliefs

Moderate modernizers, progressives accepted the American system as sound, in need only of adjustment. In adopting this gradual approach, many drew on the increasingly popular Darwinian theories of evolution. With its notion of slowly changing species, evolution undermined the acceptance of fixed principles that had guided social thought in the Victorian era. Progressives saw an evolving landscape and ever-shifting values; thus they placed less emphasis on absolute truths and more on the relativity of ideas. With an eye to results, their prime concern was not so much "Is it true?" but "Does it work?" Philosopher Charles Peirce called this way of thinking "pragmatism," and William James, the Harvard psychologist, became its most famous popularizer. For James, the new philosophy meant "looking away from first things, principles, 'categories,' supposed necessities; and of looking towards last things, fruits, consequences, facts."

Progressives also denied the traditional Calvinist doctrine of innate sinfulness or depravity—sheer "human cussedness." They viewed human potential as more good than evil and spoke of "the essential nobility of man." But human advancement and social improvement were only possible, never automatic. One skeptical wit remarked that Theodore Dreiser, an eminent novelist of the era, possessed an abiding faith in humanity—then saw Pittsburgh and lost all hope. The barb was in jest, but it had its hook. Progressives, having seen the mean side of the industrial city, somehow had to deal with the existence of crime and vice. Some progressives agreed that evil and ugliness were "largely, if not wholly, products of environment." People went wrong, as Fremont Older of the San Francisco *Bulletin* explained it, because of "what happens to them."

Progressives thought they could change people by changing "what happens to them." Social reformer Jane Addams liked to tell the story of Marcella, a poor but decent girl who stole some silk to make a dress for a fancy ball. Neither the authorities nor the girl's mother could understand, but Addams felt she did. Marcella had been driven to crime by circumstances—poverty and temptation. Improve her environment, and she would flower. "Life in the Settlement," Addams wrote, "discovers above all what has been called 'the extraordinary pliability of human nature,' and it seems impossible to set any bounds to the moral capabilities which might unfold under ideal civic and educational conditions."

Pragmatism led educators, social scientists, and lawyers to adopt new approaches to reform. John Dewey, the preeminent educator of the progressive era, along with his wife, Alice, founded a new School of Pedagogy at the University of Chicago in 1896; it was based on the notion that human thought evolved in relation to the environment in which it was developed. Instead of forcing students to memorize abstract and unconnected facts at a teacher's command, Dewey wanted to "make each one of our schools an embryonic community life, active with the types of occupations that reflect the life of the larger society." By letting students unbolt their desks from the floor, move their chairs around, and learn by doing, schools could teach real life. Education would be a fountainhead of reform—in Dewey's words, "the deepest and best guarantee of a larger society which is worthy, lovely, and harmonious."

The blending of environmentalism and expertise led John B. Watson to "behavioral" psychology and the belief that human beings could be shaped at will. "Give me a dozen healthy infants," Watson later wrote, ". . . and my own specified world to bring them up in, and I'll guarantee to take any one at random and train him to become any specialist I might select, doctor, lawyer, artist, merchant, chief, and yes, even beggarman and thief, regardless of his talents, tendencies, abilities, vocations and race of his ancestors."

Most environmentalists were less extreme than Watson. Sociologist Edward A. Ross in *Social Control* (1901) looked at industrialized life—"its wolfish struggle for personal success, its crimes, frauds, exploitation and parasitism"—and stressed the need for restraints. In *The Theory of the Leisure Class* (1899) Thorstein Veblen, an economist, outraged genteel Americans by describing them with the detachment that an anthropologist might have reserved for some exotic tribe in Borneo. Reclusive and defiant, Veblen irreverently rejected the notion that the rich and respectable labored primarily to produce valued goods and services. Rather, he claimed, they strove to outdo each other in showing off their wealth ("pecuniary emulation") and expending labor to buy, maintain, and display their many-roomed mansions, multicourse banquets, and multilayered evening dresses ("conspicuous consumption"). Indeed, he concluded, the business class promoted an economy of waste and scarcity as they scrambled for profits. In *The Engineers and the Price System* (1921) Veblen argued that only expert planning could create an efficient and orderly industrial system.

Lawyers and legal theorists applied their own brand of pragmatism and environmentalism. Justice Oliver Wendell Holmes, Jr., appointed to the Supreme Court in 1902, rejected the idea that the traditions of American law ought to be regarded as universal and unalterable, interpreted in an august manner from the bench. "Long ago," Holmes remarked, "I decided I was not God." To him law was a living organism to be interpreted according to the needs of a changing society. The "life of the law," he wrote in *The Common Law* (1881), "has not been logic; it has been experience."

Experience was where Denver Judge Ben Lindsey looked when he handed down a verdict. Presiding over one of the first juvenile courts in the country, the "Kids' Judge" examined the home life of youthful offenders before he ruled. All too often he discovered poverty, illness, and joblessness. Environment, not heredity, produced juvenile delinquents, Lindsey believed, so he used the new authority of his court to take them from dysfunctional homes and make them wards of the state. In several states, supervised probation replaced suspended sentences to ensure that bad habits stayed broken. Yet in this urge to do good, progressives revealed an uncomfortable inclination to intrude into private lives and to limit individual choice.

"Sociological jurisprudence," as this environmental view of the law came to be known, found its most creative practitioner in Louis D. Brandeis. Brandeis believed that law must "guide by the light of reason," which meant bringing the conditions of everyday life to bear in any court case. Shaken by the Homestead steel strike, Brandeis turned away from his corporate practice to become the self-proclaimed "people's lawyer." When laundry-owner Curt Muller challenged an Oregon law limiting the working day of women to 10 hours, the National

Consumers' League retained Brandeis to defend the law before the Supreme Court in 1908. Surrounded by boxes of reports from social workers, doctors, factory inspectors, and other experts, Brandeis documented the damaging effects of long hours of work on the health and morals of women. His brief in *Muller v. Oregon* (prepared by his sister-in-law Josephine Goldmark) contained only 2 pages of legal precedents; the remaining 102 pages detailed the sociology of working women. The Supreme Court upheld the Oregon law and in so doing gave legal sanction to the "Brandeis Brief."

The Progressive Method

Seeing the nation riven by diverse ethnic and interest groups, progressives tried to restore a sense of community and common purpose through the ideal of a single public interest. Christian ethics were the guide, applied expertise and planning the instruments. "There are two gospels I always want to preach to reformers," Theodore Roosevelt told a conference on city improvement. "The first is the gospel of morality; the next is the gospel of efficiency." From the physical and social sciences progressives borrowed the latest methods for systematically gathering and analyzing data, making diagnoses, and prescribing solutions. In the modern corporation they found an appealing model for organization. Like corporate executives, progressives relied on careful management, coordinated systems, and specialized bureaucracies to carry out reforms.

Between 1902 and 1912 a new breed of investigative reporters publicized wrongdoers by name and described their deeds in vivid detail. Most exposés began as articles in mass circulation magazines. Samuel McClure, publisher since 1893 of a magazine bearing his name, sent Lincoln Steffens out to discover the unsavory ties between business and politics. Steffens' startling exposé, "Tweed Days in St. Louis," appeared in the October 1902 issue of *McClure's*. The first installment of Ida M. Tarbell's *History of the Standard Oil Company*, another stinging, well-researched indictment, followed in November. As *McClure's* annual circulation jumped to 370,000, competitors quickly adopted the new style. *The Ladies Home Journal* exposed the evils of patent medicines; *Everybody's* featured Thomas W. Lawson on crooked finance and Charles Edward Russell on the beef trust. Soon a full-blown literature of exposure was covering everything from prostitution and health care to insurance companies, urban poverty, and child labor.

Theodore Roosevelt called the new breed of journalists "muckrakers," after the man who raked up filth and ignored beauty in John Bunyan's seventeenth-century classic, *Pilgrim's Progress*. Journalist Ray Stannard Baker chose to differ: muckraking flourished, and deserved to, he argued, "because the country for years had been swept by the agitation of soap-box orators, prophets crying in the wilderness, and political campaigns based upon charges of corruption and privilege which everyone believed or suspected had some basis of truth, but which were largely unsubstantiated." By documenting dishonesty and blight, muckrakers helped to arouse public indignation. Most likely, no broad reform movement of American institutions would have taken place without them.

To move beyond exposure to solutions, progressives stressed volunteerism and collective action. They drew on the organizational impulse that seemed everywhere to be bringing people together. Between 1890 and 1920 nearly 400 new organizations appeared. Some, like the National Consumers' League, grew out of

John D. Rockefeller, oil baron and multimillionaire, was a favorite target of the investigative journalists Theodore Roosevelt dubbed "muckrakers." A sympathetic cartoon in the magazine *Judge* beseeches them to relent. "Boys," reads the caption, "don't you think you have bothered the old man just about enough?"

efforts to promote general causes, in this instance protecting consumers and workers from exploitation. Others, such as the National Tuberculosis Association, aimed at solving a specific problem. Reflecting the new emphasis on expertise, the professions also organized. Groups like the American Medical Association and the American Society of Mechanical Engineers standardized their procedures, licensed their members to keep out charlatans, and informed the public about their professional goals.

When voluntary action failed to produce results, progressives looked to government as the agent for protecting the public welfare. Disdainful of legislators controlled by special interests and political bosses, they tried to strengthen the executive branch by enhancing the power of mayors, governors, and presidents. At all levels—local, state, federal—new agencies and commissions staffed by impartial experts began to investigate and regulate society—from the activities of lobbyists and railroad companies to the state of public health.

THE SEARCH FOR THE GOOD SOCIETY

If progressivism ended in politics, it started with social reform: the shock of excesses in slums, the need to reach out, to do something to bring the "good society" a step closer. In 1890, a year after Jane Addams founded her famous settlement house in Chicago, the New England Kitchen opened in downtown Boston. Ellen Richards, a chemist-turned-home economist, designed the Kitchen to sell cheap, wholesome food to the working poor. For a few pennies, customers could choose from a menu that included beef broth, boiled hominy, cracked wheat, and spiced beef. To ensure the highest nutrition, Richards had every dish tested in her laboratory at the Massachusetts Institute of Technology.

The New England Kitchen was an exercise as much in social as in nutritional reform. Women freed from the drudgery of cooking could seek gainful employment. As a "household experiment station" and gathering place for information on "the food supply of the masses," the Kitchen tried to educate the poor about how best to prepare wholesome meals. It also sought to Americanize immigrants with standard foods and, according to philanthropist Pauline Shaw, to produce a "rival to the saloon." As she saw it, poor diets fostered drinking, especially among the lower classes.

For all these good intentions, the New England Kitchen usually served as an inexpensive eatery for middle-class working women and students rather than a resource for the poor or an instrument of Americanization. ("Oh!" one Irish mother reported her son saying when she served an Indian pudding. "You can't make a Yankee of me that way!") Still, the New England Kitchen reflected the pattern of reform that characterized so many progressive ventures: the mix of middle-class professionalism with lower-class uplift, the hope of creating the outlines of a new and better world.

The Rediscovery of Poverty

Social reformers often chose to live in slums, among the poor. There they saw poverty in a new light. During the 1890s urban reformer and pioneer photographer Jacob Riis (page 693) used lantern slide shows to introduce middle-class urbanites to the look of poverty. The slides appeared artless—merely recording the desperate poverty before the camera—but Riis' moralistic narrative used them much the way the earlier English novelist Charles Dickens had used his melodramatic tales to attack the abuses of industrialism. Riis' photographic essays were followed by an even greater naturalism in fiction and painting. Novelists such as Theodore Dreiser and Frank Norris spun tales of city dwellers struggling to survive with body and soul intact. The "Ashcan School" painted city life in all its gritty realism. Several artists of this group had been illustrators on metropolitan dailies and many—photographer Alfred Stieglitz and painters like John Sloan, George Luks, and George Bellows—chose slums, tenements, and dirty streets as subjects. Poverty began to look less ominous and more heart-rending.

Between 1908 and 1914 the Russell Sage Foundation produced six large volumes of facts and figures documenting how wretchedly urban workers lived, how dangerously they labored in factories, how poorly they were paid, how relentlessly disease struck them down. The gathering weight of evidence indicated a vicious social cycle that trapped its victims for generations. The children of paupers would likely be paupers themselves, not because of heredity but because of deprivation. No one did more to publicize this view than Robert Hunter. In researching his book *Poverty*, Hunter discovered no fewer than 10 million Americans (out of a population of about 80 million) living in poverty. As a cure he recommended a hodgepodge of progressive social legislation: prohibition of child labor; public day nurseries; pensions for the sick, the unemployed, and the elderly; sanitary legislation for tenements and factories; maximum hour and minimum wage laws; and limitations on immigration.

A new profession—social work—developed out of the settlement house movement. Like doctors (from whom they drew inspiration), social workers studied hard data to diagnose the problems of their "clients." Unlike nineteenth-century philanthropists, the new social workers refused to do things to or for people. Instead they worked with their clients, enlisting their help to solve their own problems. A social worker's "differential casework" attempted to treat individuals case by case, each according to the way the client had been shaped by environment.

No amount of middle-class goodwill and scientific endeavor could entirely eradicate poverty. Most progressives continued to see the problem as a by-product of political and corporate greed, of the evil environment of urban slums, and of "institutions of vice" like the saloon. They saw less clearly how deeply rooted poverty had become in rural areas made marginal by large-scale, mechanized agriculture, in urban areas where the unskilled congregated, and in individuals suffering from a range of pathologies—alcoholism, drug addiction, mental illness—that defied cure by even the most enlightened policies. Poverty was in reality a single symptom of a host of personal and social ills.

Expanding the "Woman's Sphere"

Progressive social reform attracted a disproportionate number of women, seeking what Jane Addams called "the larger life." Like most Americans, women were living longer and becoming better educated. Between 1870 and 1910, the proportion of women among college students had doubled to 40 percent of all American students. Meanwhile more women remained unwed and the divorce rate skyrocketed—from 1 in 21 marriages in 1880 to 1 in 9 by 1916. (Two-thirds were instigated by wives, most of them unhappy with the quality of married life.)

Single, well-educated women turned most often to professions that involved the traditional role of nurturer—nursing, library work, and teaching. Custom and prejudice barred them from other choices. The faculty at the Massachusetts Institute of Technology refused to allow Ellen Richards, the first woman in America to earn a degree in science, to pursue a doctorate, even though they hired her to run the gender-segregated "Woman's Laboratory" for training public school teachers. Only about 1500 women lawyers practiced in the whole country. In 1910 women comprised barely 6 percent of licensed physicians. That figure rapidly declined as male-dominated medical associations grew in power and discouraged the entry of women. Professions dominated by women began to define themselves in modern terms just as those largely consisting of men did. In a manner characteristic of other women's activities, teaching (still the occupation of 9 of 10 professional women) increasingly set standards of admission and monitored its members. In 1905 teachers created the National Education Association, which lobbied for government certification of teachers.

Educated women frequently discovered that their families stood in their way. "All my plans for a 'career' have been knocked to atoms," wrote one Wellesley College graduate, forced to stay home to care for her mother. "You can put me down as still alive, though." Some educated and professional women tried not simply to widen the boundaries of their sphere but to destroy them. In *Women and Economics* (1898) feminist Charlotte Perkins Gilman condemned the conventions of womanhood—femininity, marriage, maternity, and domesticity—as enslaving and obsolete. She argued for a radically restructured society with large apartment houses, communal arrangements for child rearing and housekeeping, and cooperative kitchens to free women from economic dependence on men.

Margaret Sanger, a visiting nurse on the Lower East Side of New York, sought to free women from the bonds of chronic pregnancy. "Women," she believed, "cannot be on equal footing with men until they have complete control over their reproductive functions." The insight came as a revelation one summer evening in 1912, when she was called to the home of an immigrant family on Grand Street. Sadie Sachs, a mother of three who had nearly died after an earlier self-induced abortion, had succeeded this time in killing her unborn child—and herself. Sanger vowed that night to "seek out the root of the evil, to do something to change the destiny of mothers whose miseries were as vast as the sky." She became a crusader for what she called "birth control." By distributing information on contraception, she hoped to prevent unwanted pregnancies among poor women. Some middle-class women joined the movement, largely to control the size of their own families and those of new immigrants.

For many middle- and upper-class women, it was often women's clubs that extended their sphere into the world at large. Founded in the 1880s and 1890s, over 500 women's clubs totaled some 160,000 members by the turn of the century. Banding together in the General Federation of Women's Clubs, they began to turn their attention from cultural self-improvement to social improvement— funding libraries and hospitals, supporting schools and settlement houses, eventually endorsing such controversial causes as woman suffrage and unionization.

Single or married, militant or moderate, professional or lay, more and more middle-class urban women thus became "social housekeepers." From their own homes they turned their attention to the homes of their neighbors and from there to all of society.

Social Welfare and Social Justice

In this "bigger family of the city," as one reformer called it, settlement workers bridged traditional charity and progressive reform. Like old-style philanthropists, they volunteered to staff the settlement houses, where the urban poor and foreign-born were exposed to middle-class virtues: thrift; cleanliness; orderliness; refinement; manners; culture; responsibility; and citizenship. They also offered language and cooking classes, day nurseries, and clubs for men and women. All were designed to teach immigrants American ways, lift the destitute from the slums, and help those who failed to make it out. In 1891 there were 6 settlement houses in the country; by 1910 there were over 400, most located in the worst slums and united by a national organization. Increasingly, however, settlement reformers turned to government to supplement individual charity by passing laws and establishing public agencies to promote improved housing, safer factories, parks, and playgrounds, and the abolition of child labor.

As settlement workers became more organized and professional, they helped to shape government policy. Lawrence Veiller worked at the University Settlement in New York before Governor Theodore Roosevelt named him as secretary of the newly created Tenement House Commission. In 1901 New York enacted a new tenement code based on a bill Veiller had drafted. Other states soon copied the law, which required fire escapes, a window in each room, and a water closet for each apartment. Julia Lathrop, a Vassar College graduate, spent 20 years at Hull-House in Chicago before becoming the first head of the new federal Children's Bureau in 1912. By then two-thirds of the states had adopted some child labor legislation, although loopholes exempted newsboys and countless other

By 1900 one-fourth of the nonfarm labor force was female. On average, women industrial workers made three dollars a week less than unskilled men. Here at a Labor Day parade in San Diego in 1910 women demand equal pay for equal work.

youngsters from coverage. Under Lathrop's leadership, Congress was persuaded to pass the Keating–Owen Act (1916), forbidding goods manufactured by children to cross state lines.*

Florence Kelley, who, like Addams and Lathrop, had worked at Hull-House, spearheaded the campaign that led the Illinois legislature to pass an eight-hour workday law for women in 1893. The state supreme court invalidated it, so Kelley began a nationwise crusade to mobilize public opinion and local consumers' groups. As general secretary of the National Consumers' League, she organized boycotts of companies that treated employees inhumanely. In the wake of the *Muller* decision in 1908, most states enacted laws restricting the number of hours women could work.

Woman Suffrage

Ever since the conference for women's rights held at Seneca Falls in 1848, women reformers had been pressing for the right to vote on the grounds of simple justice and equal opportunity. The suffrage campaign continued sporadically for another half century, but it was firmly opposed by a host of antisuffrage organizations that included many men and women, the Catholic church, and assorted liquor interests (which feared that giving women the vote would strengthen the drive for prohibition).

Progressives embraced women's suffrage as one means to clean up government. Many reformers believed the "purer sensibilities" of women would help cleanse the political process of selfishness and corruption. Such an argument accommodated traditional views of gender differences, not gender-equality. The suffrage movement benefited, too, from new leadership. In 1900 Carrie Chapman Catt, a woman of great personal charm, political finesse, and organizational skill,

---

*The Supreme Court struck down the law in 1918 as an improper regulation of local labor; nonetheless, it focused greater attention on the abuses of child labor.

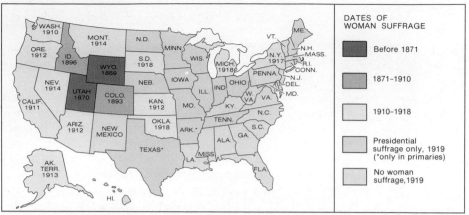

DATES OF
WOMAN SUFFRAGE

- Before 1871
- 1871–1910
- 1910–1918
- Presidential suffrage only, 1919 (*only in primaries)
- No woman suffrage, 1919

WOMAN SUFFRAGE

Western states were the first to grant women the right to vote. Sparsely populated and more egalitarian than the rest of the nation, the West was used to women participating fully in settlement and work. Other sections of the country, notably the Midwest, granted them partial suffrage that included voting for school boards and taxes. Suffragists encountered the most intractable resistance in the South, where rigid codes of social conduct elevated women symbolically but shackled them practically.

became president of the National American Woman Suffrage Association. Along with Anna Howard Shaw (a Boston social worker who succeeded her in 1904), Catt mapped a strategy of education and persuasion at the state level. Less traditional and more accustomed to having women work side by side with men, western states came around first, with victory in Washington in 1910. By 1914 California, Oregon, Arizona, Kansas, Nevada, and Montana had granted women the vote in state elections, as Illinois had in presidential elections.

The slow pace of progress drove some suffragists to more militant tactics. In 1903 women in England chained themselves to lampposts, engaged in hunger strikes while in prison, and physically attacked politicians. In 1913 Alice Paul, a young Quaker activist who had worked with English suffragists, organized 5000 women to parade in protest at President Woodrow Wilson's inauguration. Half a million people watched as a near-riot ensued. The suffragists were hauled to jail, stripped naked, and thrown into cells with prostitutes. A year later Paul formed the Congressional Union, dedicated to passing a constitutional amendment through disruptive pressure if need be. The Suffrage Association came to support the amendment, too, but Paul would not settle for their more sedate lobbying techniques. Allying her Congressional Union with western women voters in the militant National Woman's party, her forces picketed the White House in 1917. When jailed, the protesters refused to eat. The resulting attention and sympathy, plus the need for support from women once the United States entered World War I, led the House of Representatives to pass a woman suffrage amendment in 1918, and in 1920 the Nineteenth Amendment granting women the right to vote became law.

CONTROLLING THE MASSES

The drive for social justice reflected the optimistic, tolerant impulses of progressivism; the pursuit of social "welfare" for the masses, its paternalistic instincts. But more than a few progressives feared they were losing their country to aliens, ethnics, and city low-lifes. To maintain control they sometimes went beyond their basic strategy of education and sought restrictive laws to uplift and refashion the behavior of the masses. In doing so, the progressive custodians of culture sometimes allied themselves with more traditional evangelical Protestants.

To such uneasy reformers, cities seemed the place where sin flourished: races jostling uneasily, strange Old World cultures clashing with "all-American" customs, long Chinese pigtails or Hasidic Jewish sidelocks lending a discordant air to city crowds; saloons and dance halls luring youngsters and impoverishing laborers; prostitutes walking the streets; vulgar vaudeville shows and motion pictures pandering to uneducated audiences. The city challenged reformers possessed of Protestant, middle-class values to convert this riot of diverse customs and ways into a homogeneous society conceived in their own image.

Stemming the Immigrant Tide

During the late nineteenth century, racism in the form of Jim Crow laws restricted the social and economic opportunities of blacks in the South, but that region was hardly the only area where discrimination flourished. Asians, Hispanics, and Indians faced similar restrictions in the West, as did "new" immigrants from southern and eastern Europe in the North. By 1900 more than 10 million Americans out of a total population of nearly 80 million had been born in Europe. Another 26 million had foreign-born parents, largely from Mediterranean and Slavic countries. Under these conditions a new science called "eugenics" quickly lent respectability to ideas popular among "older stock" middle-class Americans that the newcomers were biologically inferior. By 1914 more magazine articles discussed eugenics than slums, tenements, and living standards combined. Eugenicists, who advocated selective breeding for human improvement, believed that heredity determined everything. "Observe immigrants," wrote sociologist Edward A. Ross in 1912; "you are struck by the fact that from ten to twenty percent are hirsute, low-browed, big-faced persons of obviously low mentality. . . . They clearly belong in skins, in wattled huts at the close of the Ice Age."

For some old-line Americans, assimilation was not only undesirable—it was impossible. "What can you expect of the Americanism of a man whose breath always reeks of garlic?" sneered a member of the Daughters of the American Revolution. Middle-class urban reformers, despairing over the link between immigrants and political machines, reduced immigrant voting power by increasing residency requirements. In many states only native-born and fully naturalized citizens could vote. Madison Grant, a Park Avenue patrician and amateur zoologist, helped to popularize the notion that the "lesser breeds" threatened to "mongrelize" America. In *The Passing of the Great Race* (1916) Grant warned that "race suicide" threatened the United States. Mixing with inferior immigrants, he argued, "gives us a race reverting to the more ancient, generalized and lower type."

More enlightened reformers such as Jane Addams stressed the "gifts" immi-

Daily Lives

PUBLIC SPACE/PRIVATE SPACE

"Amusing the Million"

In May 1903 an opening-night crowd of 45,000 patrons poured through the massive gates of Luna Park at Coney Island, just south of Brooklyn. Before them, one journalist reported, was "an enchanted, storybook land of trellises, columns, domes, minarets, lagoons, and lofty aerial flights . . . a world removed—shut away from the sordid clatter and turmoil of the streets." Those who spent their days in crowded tenements rolling cigars or sleeping nights in stuffy apartments might well blink in awe at the scene. A quarter of a million electric lights, strung like shimmering pearls, studded the buildings. At the flick of a switch, night turned into day: "Tall towers that had grown dim suddenly broke forth in electric outline and gay rosettes of color, as the living spark of light traveled hither and thither, until the place was transformed into an enchanted garden, of such a sort as Aladdin never dreamed."

Everywhere spectacle greeted the crowds. Fantastic winged griffins adorned "The Dragon's Gorge"; a huge dolphin fountain gushed water from the base of the main tower. Barkers with megaphones extolled a Venetian city with actual gondoliers, Irish and Eskimo villages, a Japanese garden, and a bustling Asian Indian celebration complete with gilded chariots, exotic dancers, soldiers, and "real Eastern people." There were sideshows and rides galore: the "Switchback" Railroad, a forerunner of the roller coaster; and the immensely popular "Shoot-the-Chutes," which sent flat-bottom boats careening down a steep incline into a lagoon. As if that were not enough, visitors could witness a genuine disaster. In "Fire and Flames," a four-story building burst into flames on cue, as mock firefighters doused the blaze and mock residents jumped from top floors to safety nets below.

Luna Park was the second of three new amusement parks that together formed Coney Island. And Coney Island was but one (albeit the largest and most famous) of a host of similar parks that popped up across the country at the turn of the century. Soaring urban populations, increases in leisure time and spending money, and new trolley systems that made for cheap excursions from the city led to the opening of Boston's Paragon Park and Revere Beach, Philadelphia's Willow Grove, Cleveland's Euclid Beach, Atlanta's Ponce de Leon Park, Denver's Manhattan Beach, and Los Angeles' Venice Beach.

All traded in entertainment, but of a sort different from earlier forms of urban recreation. In the second half of the nineteenth century Victorian reformers had promoted two influential models of public entertainment, the spacious city park and the grand public exposition. Both were intended to instruct as well as amuse, reducing the potential for urban disorder by raising public taste and reforming public conduct. When it opened in 1858, New York City's Central Park became a model pastoral retreat in the midst of the city. Its rustic paths, tranquil lakes, and woodsy views were designed as respites from the chaos of urban life. Becalmed by such natural beauty, even the rudest fellows would feel, said designer Frederick Law Olmsted, "a distinctly harmonizing and refining influence."

The World's Columbian Exposition of 1893 in Chicago also reflected an elevated

Daily Lives

The Venice Amusement Park in California was dubbed by its founders "the Coney Island of the Pacific."

vision of society. The most impressive of a host of "world's fairs," it was a fully planned neoclassical "White City" (named for the fake marble used to construct it) built on the shores of Lake Michigan, a symbol of order, unity, and civic virtue. Exhibits were housed in buildings that looked as if they had been transplanted from Renaissance Italy. They encircled an enormous basin whose shimmering waters highlighted "The Republic," a 100-foot statue draped in a toga and holding an eagle perched on a globe. Here was the Victorian ideal of a city—modern yet classic, planned and unified, inspiring to all who gazed on it.

Some amusement parks, like Venice Beach in California, self-consciously mimicked the Chicago Exposition, though on a much smaller scale. Others, like Coney Island, built dream worlds all their own. But wherever they operated, amusement park owners knew what the planners of Chicago's fair only reluctantly learned: people wanted to have fun. Adjacent to the White City had stood the Midway Plaisance, a mile-long recreational area bustling with theaters, restaurants, exotic Indian tepees, German castles, and the Persian palace of Eros where "Little Egypt" danced the "hootchy-kootchy." A gigantic steel wheel, designed especially for the Exposition by George Ferris, carried visitors 250 feet into the air for only 50 cents. The Midway's privately sponsored attractions easily lured more people than the free public exhibits of the White City.

Amusement parks expressed not the civic values of the White City but the commercial values of the Midway. Parks were in the business, said one owner, of "amusing the million." Coney Island's Luna Park claimed 5 million paying customers in a single season, drawing patrons from all social classes and ethnic groups. Jostling with crowds, eating ice cream and hot dogs, riding "Shoot-the-Chutes," even the new immigrant could feel gloriously American. A sense of solidarity drew visitors together, and the zaniness of the setting loosened social restraints. Instead of the genteel values of sober industry, thrift, and orderly conduct, amusement parks encouraged abandon, extravagance, and gaiety. They heralded the rise of mass culture, invading public space with the private dreams of multitudes.

grants brought to their adopted culture: folk dances, music, handicrafts, and of course exotic foods. With characteristic paternalism, reformers hoped to "Americanize" the foreign-born (the term was newly coined), especially through education. Peter Roberts, a progressive educator, developed a lesson plan for the Young Men's Christian Association that taught immigrants to dress, tip, buy groceries, and vote. In Milwaukee factories English was taught so immigrant workers could read safety signs. But some lessons were far from practical. In 1916 burly men who labored by day could be found nightly in Cleveland schools copying "I am a yellow bird. I can sing. I can fly."

Progressive reformers revealed their intolerant side as they sought an end to unrestricted entry for immigrants. Here, too, they employed organization, investigation, education, and legislation. Active since the 1890s, the Immigration Restriction League pressed Congress in 1907 to require a literacy test for admission into the United States. Instead the Senate appointed the Dillingham Commission to study the matter. Despite evidence that no correlation existed between the new immigrants and feeble-mindedness, crime, epilepsy, or tuberculosis, the commission's 42-volume report concluded that unlimited immigration created unmanageable social problems. The commission endorsed a literacy test to stem the tide. To the delight of many ethnic groups, Presidents Taft and Wilson vetoed it in 1913 and 1915. Congress nonetheless overrode Wilson's second veto in 1917.

The Curse of Demon Rum

Tied closely to concern over immigrants was an attack on saloons. Part of a broader effort to clean up cities, the antisaloon campaign also drew strength from the century-old crusade to ban alcohol. By 1900 the danger seemed greater than ever. Consumption had increased to over two gallons a year per person. By 1909 there was one saloon for every 300 city dwellers. Over half the population of Boston and Chicago visited a bar at least once a day. In inner cities, immigrants and the working-class poor made up most of the clientele.

Whether drinkers or teetotalers, progressives or conservatives, reformers agreed that saloons were the societal equivalent of "a nest of rats." Taverns and social clubs seemed to be at the center of a host of social problems—gambling and prostitution, political corruption, drug trafficking, unemployment, and poverty. Few temperance reformers recognized the complex cycle of social decay that produced such problems, fewer still the important social role played by saloons as "workingmen's clubs." The saloon was often the only place to cash a check, borrow money, find out about jobs, eat a cheap meal, take a bath, or sit with a group of friends.

Led by the Anti-Saloon League, reformers concentrated efforts to prohibit the sale of alcohol at local and state levels. A massive publicity campaign bombarded citizens with pamphlets and advertisements. Doctors cited scientific evidence linking alcohol to cirrhosis, heart disease, insanity, and other serious illnesses. Social workers connected drink to the deterioration of the family; employers, with accidents on the job and lost efficiency. By 1917 three out of four Americans lived in dry counties, and nearly two-thirds of the states had adopted laws that outlawed the manufacture and sale of alcohol, to stop profiteering from human pain and corruption (most reformers considered a ban on drinking unrealistic and intrusive).

Prostitution

No urban vice worried reformers more than prostitution, the "social evil" that threatened a generation of young city women with a fate reformers thought much worse than death. The Chicago Vice Commission of 1910 estimated the city had 5,000 "full-time" and 10,000 occasional prostitutes. Even Muncie, Indiana, a city of just 11,000 people, had 20 to 25 brothels, each with four to eight women. Along the urban frontier the low wage scale of women workers encouraged the increase in prostitution. "I don't propose to get up at 6:30," wrote Maimie Pinzer, a Philadelphia prostitute, "to . . . work in a stuffy room . . . until dark, for $6 or $7 a week, when I could . . . spend an afternoon with a congenial person and in the end have more than a week's work could pay me." On average, prostitutes earned five times the income of a factory worker. Most needed only to walk the streets to find willing customers. For many the risks of being exploited by pimps or "uncongenial" clients seemed worth taking.

An unlikely group of reformers united to fight the vice: feminists who wanted husbands to be as chaste as their wives; social hygienists worried about the spread of venereal disease; and immigration restrictionists who regarded the growth of prostitution as yet another sign of inferiority in the new arrivals. Progressives naturally saw the problem in economic and environmental terms. Most agreed with the conclusion of the Illinois Vice Commission of 1916 that "poverty causes prostitution."

Other Americans—and some progressives—considered prostitutes the victims of city life and male predators. Rumors of a vast and lucrative "white slave trade" spread across the country. Men armed with hypodermic needles, so the story went, traveled crowded streetcars and stalked amusement parks, dance halls, and vaudeville shows seeking likely targets to drug and abduct. While the average female rider of the streetcar was hardly in danger of villainous abduction, every city had cribs with locked doors where a substantial fraction of women (at least 10 percent of all prostitutes by conservative estimates) were held in bondage and forced into prostitution. As real abuses blended with sensationalism, Congress passed the Mann Act (1910), prohibiting the interstate transport of women for immoral purposes. By 1918 reformers succeeded in getting states to close previously tolerated "red light" districts in most cities. As with prohibition, progressives went after those who made money from misery.

Vaudeville Cleans House

Some targets of reform chose to police themselves, as in the case of vaudeville show proprietors. Vaudeville enjoyed its heyday from 1890 to the mid-1920s. The mix of rowdy performers—singers, jugglers, acrobats, magicians, animal acts, and comics—reflected urban vitality and tastes. Skits often drew on the experience of immigrants, and early comedy teams had names like "The Sport and the Jew," "Irish by Name but Coons by Birth," and "Two Funny Sauerkrauts."

Seeing housewives with children as a source of new profits, resourceful theater managers began to specialize in "straight, clean variety shows" to attract the middle-class family trade. Tony Pastor, a former choir boy and circus performer, opened the first vaudeville theater on Fourteenth Street in New York in 1881. Within a few years he was producing the kind of show, as comedian Fred Stone later said, "to which any child could bring his parents." By 1910 other owners

Balconies at vaudeville shows, like this one depicted by Charles Dana Gibson, attracted a wide variety of customers. Most seats cost $1, and theater owners scheduled performances from morning until night. "After breakfast go to Proctor's," read one advertisement, "after Proctor's go to bed."

went even further to attract families. The Keith–Albee Circuit, the most powerful and far-flung of the vaudeville chains, tacked notices backstage that warned performers not to say "slob" or 'son-of-a-gun' or 'hully-gee' . . . unless you want to be canceled peremptorily." In the interest of good taste, all of its chorus girls wore stockings.

Not all owners were so puritanical. The bare midriffs of "Ziegfeld girls" and the ethnic jokes of Webber and Fields packed houses through the 1920s. Nevertheless, vaudeville had become middle-class, mass entertainment. It was also big business. Nearly one in five city dwellers went to a show once every seven days. The self-imposed purity policies allowed theater owners to broaden appeal, avoid outside censorship, and attract citizens as solid as Woodrow Wilson, a regular customer during his tenure as governor of New Jersey.

THE POLITICS OF MUNICIPAL AND STATE REFORM

The reform of character, the cure for poverty, the movement to liberate women and care for slum children, the need to take the profit out of human misery—all these problems seemed soluble with reform in government. Jane Addams learned as much literally outside the doors of her beloved Hull-House. For months during the early 1890s, garbage piled up all along Halstead Street, until the filth and stench finally drove Addams and her fellow workers to city hall in protest—700 times in one summer—but to no avail. Like most cities, Chicago was ruled by a corrupt band of city fathers for whom garbage collection was a plum, awarded to the company that paid the most for the job. City garbage inspectors won their posts by serving the machine, and garbage collection remained erratic, especially in poor neighborhoods, where boxes overflowed with stinking refuse.

Having normally avoided politics, Addams submitted a bid for garbage removal in the ward. It was thrown out on a technicality. She then got herself appointed as a garbage inspector and dogged collection carts for almost a year, but boss politics kept things dirty. So Addams ran candidates against local ward boss Johnny Powers in 1896 and 1898. The flamboyant Powers, tossing cigars to the men and nickels to the children, won both times. Undaunted, Addams continued her campaigns for honest government and social reform, not only at city hall but in the Illinois legislature and in Washington as well. Politics turned out to be the only way to clean things up.

The Reformation of the Cities

"Sometimes, I think they'se poisonin' the life in the big city," said Mr. Dooley, the philosophical barkeep who was the creation of political satirist Finley Peter Dunne. "The flowers won't grow there." On the other hand, corruption blossomed: mayors and city councils controlled by boss-dominated machines; city contracts for sale to the highest corporate bidders; city offices filled with political hacks and cronies. Party rule seemed always at the heart of the trouble, and for middle-class reformers, the urban battleground furnished the first test of political reform.

A series of colorful mayors demonstrated that cities could be run humanely, even without changing the structure of government. In Detroit, shoe factory magnate Hazen Pingree squeaked to victory in the mayor's race of 1889 on the immigrant votes of Germans and Poles. Moral but never self-righteous, he opposed child labor, tolerated Sunday drinking, and attacked Bible reading in public schools. He cut costs and fought city bosses, a utility overcharging for street lighting, and a monopolistic street railway company. By the end of his fourth term, Pingree had built parks and public baths, modernized transit and taxes, created a city-owned light plant, and started a work-relief program to combat the depression of 1893. Similarly, Tom Johnson, mayor of Cleveland from 1901 to 1909, launched an educational campaign from a portable tent that held 4000 people. Among other things, he limited municipal franchises to a fraction of their previous 99-year terms. Like Pingree and Johnson, Mayor Samuel Jones of Toledo also put his city in the utility business. By 1915 nearly two out of three cities across the nation had copied some form of this "gas and water socialism."

Tragedy sometimes dramatized the need for effective government and led to change. On a hot summer night in 1900 a tidal wave rolled in from the Gulf of Mexico and smashed the port city of Galveston, Texas. Flood waters killed one out of every six residents. The municipal government sank into confusion and partisan wrangling. In reaction business leaders won approval of a new city charter under which a special commission replaced the mayor and city council. Each of its five commissioners controlled a municipal department, and together they enacted ordinances to run the city. By 1920 nearly 400 cities had adopted the commission plan to enhance efficiency and check party rule in municipal government.

In some cities also concerned about raising efficiency and reducing partisanship, elected officials appointed an outside expert or "city manager" to run things. At lower levels experts took charge of services: engineers oversaw utilities; accountants, finances; doctors and nurses, public health; specially trained fire fighters and policemen, the safety of citizens. Broad civic reforms attempted to break the corrupt alliance between companies doing business with the city and the bosses who controlled poor and immigrant voters. City-wide elections replaced the old ward system, while civil service laws helped to create a nonpartisan bureaucracy. Most urban reforms resulted in stronger middle-class rule. Ethnic voters lost power, but city government gained efficiency.

Progressivism in the States

"Whenever we try to do anything, we run up against the charter," complained the reform mayor of Schenectady, New York. Charters granted by the state governments defined the powers of cities. The rural interests that generally dominated state legislatures rarely gave cities adequate authority to levy taxes, set voting requirements, draw up budgets, control penal and mental institutions, or legislate moral reforms. State legislatures under the influence of business interests, party machines, and county courthouse rings were often as corrupt as city halls. Reformers therefore tried to place their candidates where they could do some good—in the governors' mansions.

State progressivism found its fullest scope in the Midwest, largely under the charismatic leadership of Robert La Follette. A graduate of the University of Wisconsin, La Follette early in his career won election to Congress by toeing the party line of high tariffs and the gold standard. But after being buried in 1890 by a Democratic landslide, the "regular" Republican was soon transformed. Practicing law in Wisconsin, La Follette was outraged when a Republican boss offered him a bribe to sway a judge in a railroad case. "The power of this corrupt influence . . . should be broken," he recalled deciding. In 1900 he won the governorship as an uncommonly independent Republican.

Over the next six years "Battle Bob" La Follette made Wisconsin, in the words of Theodore Roosevelt, "the laboratory of democracy." A magnetic stump speaker, La Follette could reach the public more easily than party insiders. So he rooted out the old Republican machine and pressed for the "Wisconsin idea," the most comprehensive program of state reform in American history. His legislation calling for a direct primary, a mechanism designed to break the hold of state machines and party bosses, transferred party nominations from back rooms at conventions and caucuses to the voters at large. Under his relentless urging, Wisconsin established a railroad rate commission, forced railways to lower charges, and raised railroad taxes. The legislature passed laws to control lobbyists, conserve the environment, and expand the civil service. Among his most notable "firsts" were a state income tax, a state commission to oversee factory safety and sanitation, and a Legislative Reference Bureau at the University of Wisconsin. La Follette transformed the university into a superb educational institution as well as an employment service and advisory board for state government.

Other states copied the Wisconsin idea or hatched reform schemes of their own. By 1916 all but three had direct primary laws. To break the power of party organizations and make officeholders directly responsible to the public, progressives worked for three additional reforms: the initiative (which allowed voters themselves to introduce legislation), the referendum (which allowed them to enact or repeal it), and the recall (which allowed them to remove elected officials). By 1912 a dozen states had adopted initiative and referendum, seven recall. That same year the Seventeenth Amendment to the Constitution permitted the direct election of senators, previously selected by state legislatures. Somewhat ironically, many city bosses supported the amendment, since it gave their voters a larger role while limiting the power of their rival state bosses and legislative cronies to hand pick the members of the United States Senate.

Almost every state established regulatory commissions, especially for railroads and utilities. Through them reformers curtailed favoritism shown to certain businesses and mediated conflicts among interest groups. Commissions had the power to hold public hearings, subpoena executives, and examine company books. Some could set maximum prices and rates. Yet it was not always easy to define, let alone serve the "public good." All too often commissioners found themselves refereeing battles within industries—between carriers and shippers, for example—rather than between "the interests" and "the people." In such cases, especially if the commission staff itself came from the business community, the "regulators" found themselves doing the bidding of the industries they were supposed to regulate.

Social welfare received special attention from the states. The lack of workers' compensation for injury, illness, or death on the job had long drawn fire from reformers and labor leaders. In Germany and England, accident insurance had guaranteed payment since the nineteenth century. American courts, however, still operated on the common-law assumption that employees assumed the risks of work. When hurt, maimed, or killed, workers and widows collected damages only if they proved employer negligence. Most victims received nothing. In 1902 Maryland finally adopted the first workers' compensation act. By 1916 most states had laws requiring insurance for factory accidents. Following the lead of New York in 1910, more than half the states passed employer liability laws by 1914. Thirteen states also provided pensions for widows with dependent children.

More and more it was machine politicians who pressed for such welfare reforms. Progressives had attacked the power of parties to control elections (and in the process reduced party loyalty and hence voter turnout). Boss politics, however, survived, in part because it adapted to the climate of reform. In New York City, where Tammany Hall dominated politics, the infamous Democratic machine promoted statewide legislation to safeguard working children and end industrial hazards. After the Triangle fire of 1911, it was Senator Robert F. Wagner and Assemblyman Alfred E. Smith, both Tammany Democrats, who led the fight for a new labor code. Working class "urban liberalism" thus became a powerful instrument of reform.

PROGRESSIVISM GOES TO WASHINGTON

On September 6, 1901, Leon Czolgosz stood nervously in line, among a crowd of well-wishers waiting to shake hands with President William McKinley at the Pan-American Exposition in Buffalo, New York. Unemployed and bent on murder, Czolgosz shuffled toward McKinley, eyes downcast, a bandage concealing the pistol in his hand. As the president reached out, Czolgosz fired two bullets into his chest. "Don't let them hurt him," cried McKinley as he slumped into a chair. Doctors searched in vain for the bullets, one of which was lodged near his spine. No one thought to use the new X-ray machine on display at the exposition. Eight days later the president was dead.

The mantle of power passed to Theodore Roosevelt, at 42 the youngest president ever to hold the office. His succession was an accident, for party leaders had seen the vice presidency as a way of removing him from political power. Accident or not, Roosevelt made the most of it. "It is a dreadful thing to come into the presidency this way," he remarked, "but it would be a far worse thing to be morbid about it." When Roosevelt entered the White House in 1901, the presidency was weak and rudderless, despite McKinley's best efforts. Both houses of Congress lay in conservative hands. National reform was a distant dream. When Roosevelt left the office in 1909, the president had become the center of attention and his powers had grown broader than at any time since Lincoln. Surely progressivism would have come to Washington without Roosevelt, and while there he was never its most daring advocate. In many respects, he was quite conservative. Yet without Roosevelt progressivism would have had neither the broad popular appeal nor the buoyancy with which he infused it.

TR in Action

"TR," as so many Americans called him, was the scion of seven generations of wealthy New Yorkers. A small and sickly boy, he suffered from fits of asthma that sent him running into the cold night air for relief. His eyes were so bad that he saw the world as a blur until he got his first pair of glasses at age 14. Through rigorous exercise and boxing lessons he built his body. He learned to ride and shoot, roped cattle in the Dakota Badlands, mastered judo, and later in life climbed the Matterhorn, hunted African game, and explored the Amazon. While vigor ruled his life, a

---

Bull-necked and barrel-chested, Theodore Roosevelt was "pure act," said Henry Adams. T.R. may have had the attention span of a golden retriever, as one critic charged, but he also embodied the great virtues of his day—honesty, hard work, constancy, courage, and, while in power, self-control.

hard moralism guided his conscience. He disciplined his emotions with obsessive denial. When his wife died in childbirth (ironically on the same day his mother died), he banished her from memory by destroying their love letters and ripping her photographs from their frames.

In choosing politics, Roosevelt defied the traditions of the American gentry. Well-bred families like the Roosevelts saw politics as a dirty business for more ordinary folk. But at the age of 23, barely out of Harvard, Roosevelt won election to the New York State Assembly. At 28 he ran unsuccessfully for mayor of New York, then in rapid succession became a civil service commissioner in Washington, New York City police commissioner, assistant secretary of the navy, and the Rough Rider hero of the Spanish–American War. At the age of 40 he won election as reform governor of New York and two years later as vice president. Arms flailing, fists pounding, his mouth locked in a toothy grin, TR remained a solid Republican, personally flamboyant but committed to mild change only.

To the Executive Mansion (which he officially renamed the "White House"), Roosevelt brought a passion for order, a commitment to the public, and a sense of presidential possibilities. Most presidents believed the Constitution set specific limits on their power. As Roosevelt saw it, the president could do anything not expressly forbidden by the Constitution. Recognizing the value of popular support, he gave reporters the first press room in the White House and fed a favored few all the stories they could write. He was the first president to play tennis, ride in an automobile, fly an airplane, and dive in a submarine—and everyone knew it.

To dramatize racial injustice, Roosevelt invited black educator Booker T. Washington to lunch at the White House in 1901. Southern journalists called it "treason," but for Roosevelt the gesture served both principle and politics. His lunch with Washington was part of a "black and tan" strategy to build a biracial coalition among southern Republicans. He denounced lynching and appointed blacks to important federal offices in Mississippi and South Carolina. Understanding the limits of political feasibility, Roosevelt went no further. In 1906, when

Atlanta exploded in a race riot that left 12 people dead, he said nothing. Later that year he discharged "without honor" three entire companies of black troops because a few unidentified soldiers had shot up Brownsville, Texas. All lost their pensions, including six winners of the Medal of Honor.

The Square Deal

"My business," said Roosevelt, surveying his presidency as he left the White House in 1908, "was to take hold of the conservative party and turn it into what it had been under Lincoln, that is, a party of progressive conservatism." Underneath it all, Roosevelt feared extremes and was bent on heading off radical change. In his hands government would use mild reform to save conservatism from its sometimes hidebound resistance to change.

That course was not easy in Washington, where an archconservative "Old Guard" dominated the Republican party and Congress in 1901. In the Senate the "Big Four"—Nelson W. Aldrich of Rhode Island, John Spooner of Wisconsin, Orville H. Platt of Connecticut, and William B. Allison of Iowa—protected business, resisted reform, and looked suspiciously at the young presidential upstart. In the House, power revolved around Speaker Joseph G. Cannon of Illinois, a politician dedicated to protecting the status quo.

Roosevelt could not long follow the cautious course McKinley had charted. He had more energetic plans for government. He accepted growth—whether of business, labor, or capital—as natural. In his pluralistic system, big labor would counterbalance big capital, big farm organizations would offset big food processors, and so on. Big government would mediate among them all. That way, he believed, everyone could count on a fair result. Later, as he campaigned for a second term in 1904, Roosevelt named this program the "Square Deal."

In a startling display of presidential initiative, Roosevelt in 1902 intervened in a strike that idled 140,000 miners in the hard coal industry. Operators, led by coal magnate George Baer, refused workers' demands for higher wages and fewer hours and would not even recognize their union, the United Mine Workers. As Americans faced a winter without heat, public anger at the operators' inflexibility mounted. When Roosevelt summoned both sides to the White House, John A. Mitchell, the young president of the United Mine Workers, agreed to arbitration, but owners balked. In desperation Roosevelt leaked word to Wall Street that the army would take over the mines if the owners did not come to terms. Never before had the government intervened on behalf of labor; seldom had a president acted so boldly. In late October 1902 the owners settled, granting miners a 10 percent wage hike and a nine-hour day in return for increases in coal prices and no recognition of the union. Roosevelt was equally prepared to intervene on behalf of management, as he did when he sent federal troops to end strikes in Arizona in 1903 and Colorado in 1904. His aim was to establish a vigorous presidency prepared to deal squarely with both sides.

Roosevelt especially needed to face the issue of economic concentration, since financial power had become increasingly consolidated in large trusts following a wave of mergers at the end of the century. As large firms swallowed smaller ones, many Americans feared that monopoly would destroy individual enterprise and free competition. A series of government investigations revealed a rash of corporate abuses—rebates, collusion, "watered" stock, and payoffs to government officials. The courts, with judges sympathetic to business interests, showed little inclination to dismember the giants or blunt their power. In *United States v. E. C. Knight* (1895), the Supreme Court crippled the Sherman Antitrust Act by ruling that the law applied only to commerce and not manufacturing. The decision left the American Sugar Refining Company in control of 98 percent of the nation's sugar factories.

In his first State of the Union message, Roosevelt told Congress that he did not oppose business concentration per se. As he saw it, large corporations were both inevitable and beneficial. He wanted to regulate, not destroy them, to make them fairer and more efficient. Only then would the economic order be humanized, its victims protected, and class violence forestalled. "Trusts are creatures of the State, and the State not only has the right to control them, but it is in duty bound to control them wherever the need of such control is shown," he said in 1902. Trusts, like individuals, had to be held to strict standards of morality. Conduct, not size, was the yardstick TR used to measure "good" and "bad" trusts.

Because he shared progressive faith in the power of publicity to marshal public opinion and keep business in line, Roosevelt moved immediately to strengthen the federal power of investigation. He called for the creation of a Department of Commerce with a Bureau of Corporations that could compel companies to hand over their records. Congressional conservatives shuddered at the prospect of putting corporate books on display. Finally, after Roosevelt charged that John D. Rockefeller was orchestrating the opposition, Congress enacted the legislation and added two assistant attorneys general to the Justice Department to prosecute more antitrust cases. In 1902, without prior warning, Attorney General Philander Knox filed suit under the Sherman Act against the Northern Securities Company, a mammoth holding company with a virtual monopoly over railroads in the Northwest. Not only was the holding company unpopular with farmers and travelers, but its founders, Morgan, Rockefeller, James J. Hill, and E. H. Harriman—all notorious business barons—also had bloated the company stock with worthless certificates. Here, clearly, was a symbol of the "bad trust."

Stunned by the suit, Morgan himself hurried to the White House. "If we have done something wrong," he told Roosevelt and Attorney General Knox, "send your man [the attorney general] to my man [Morgan's lawyer] and they can fix it up." "We don't want to fix it up," said Knox. "We want to stop it." A trust-conscious country cheered as the Supreme Court ordered the company to dissolve in 1904. "Even Morgan no longer rules the earth," declared one journal, "and other men may still do business without asking his permission." Ultimately, the Roosevelt administration brought antitrust suits against some 44 behemoths, including the Standard Oil Company, the American Tobacco Company, and the Du Pont Corporation.

Roosevelt always preferred regulation to antitrust action. The old problems of the railroads, for example, were newly underscored by a recent round of consolidation that had contributed to higher freight rates and higher prices. Roosevelt pressed Congress to revive the ineffective Interstate Commerce Commission (ICC). In 1903 Congress enacted the Elkins Act, which gave the ICC power to end rebates. On this occasion, as on others, business supported reform because it served its interests. At last railroads were saved from the costly practice of granting special reductions to large shippers.

By the election of 1904 bold initiatives had won the president broad popular support. He trounced two rival candidates, conservative Democrat Alton B. Parker, a lackluster jurist from New York, and Eugene V. Debs of the Socialist party.

It was the most lopsided victory since the election of James Monroe in 1820. No longer, Roosevelt boasted, was he a "political accident." Having strengthened his hold on the Republican party, he returned to reforming the railroads. Within weeks of the election, he launched new suits against roads and corporations that still granted rebates. Standard Oil alone, he declared, had profited "enormously" from secret rail rates. Meanwhile he put steady pressure on Congress to grant the ICC power to set maximum rates.

Conservatives in his own party opposed such federal meddling in the private sector; staunch progressives, goaded by Robert La Follette, demanded the addition of a controversial provision for disclosing the value of all rail property. In 1906, after two years of struggle, the president negotiated a compromise, typical of his cautious approach to reform. The Hepburn Railway Act enlarged the ICC, empowered it to set a ceiling on rates, and broadened its jurisdiction to include sleeping car companies, ferries, bridges, and terminals. Nestled among the fine print was a provision for ICC control of interstate pipelines—aimed, no doubt, at Rockefeller's Standard Oil Company. No provision for valuation appeared. La Follette and other progressives were furious, but with the Hepburn Act Roosevelt drew nearer to his goal of continuous federal supervision of business.

Bad Food and Pristine Wilds

Extending the umbrella of government regulation to consumers, Roosevelt belatedly threw the weight of the presidency behind two campaigns for healthy foods and drugs. In 1905 Samuel Hopkins Adams, a reporter for *Collier's Weekly*, wrote that in its patent medicines "Gullible America" would get "huge quantities of alcohol, an appalling amount of opiates and narcotics," and even worse additives—axle grease, acid, and glue. The concoctions, claimed advertisers, could cure everything from abscesses and cancer to tumors and ulcers. In 1905 industry lobbyists had succeeded in blocking several pure food and drug bills in Congress, despite a presidential endorsement.

Adams sent the samples he had collected to Harvey Wiley, chief chemist at the Agriculture Department. Wiley's "Poison Squad" produced scientific evidence supporting Hopkins' charges. Then the appearance of Upton Sinclair's *The Jungle* early in 1906 drove Congress to act. Intended to recruit people to socialism with an indictment of the exploitative labor system in the meat packing industry, the novel contained vivid descriptions of the slaughter of cattle infected with tuberculosis, of meat covered with rat dung, and of men falling into cooking vats and going out to consumers as "Durham's Pure Leaf Lard." Readers paid scant attention to the plight of the workers, but their stomachs turned at the thought of what they might be consuming at the breakfast table. The Pure Food and Drug Act of 1906 sailed through Congress in the wake of the book. The Meat Inspection Act soon followed. Even industry leaders realized that more effective government regulation was one way to restore public confidence in their products and enlarge their market abroad.

Roosevelt came late to the consumer cause, but on conservation he led the nation. An outdoors enthusiast, he galvanized growing public concern over the reckless exploitation of natural resources. His chief forester, Gifford Pinchot, persuaded him that rational, planned management under federal regulation was needed to protect the natural domain.

In the western states water was the problem. Economic growth, even survival, depended on access to it. Inequitable local and state water policy repeatedly provoked controversy and violence, and many progressives campaigned for a federal program of water distribution to replace the chaotic web of rules. Senator Frederick Newlands, a Democrat from Nevada, introduced the Reclamation Act of 1902 to set aside proceeds from the sale of public lands in the South and West for irrigation projects. Though the self-financing provisions of the bill cost western politicians some political leverage, the Reclamation Act applied progressive means to the conservationist end of putting federal resources behind western development.

The conservationist concept of efficient water use often conflicted with the more radical vision of preservationists, led by naturalist and wilderness philosopher John Muir. Muir, the founder of the Sierra Club (1892), hoped to maintain such natural wonders as Yosemite and its neighboring Hetch-Hetchy valley in a state "forever wild" to benefit future generations. Many conservationists saw such valleys only as sites for dams and reservoirs. Controversy exploded after 1900 when San Francisco announced plans to establish a reservoir in the Hetch-Hetchy valley. For 13 years Muir waged a publicity campaign against the "temple destroyers" and "devotees of ravaging commercialism." Pinchot enthusiastically backed San Francisco's claim; Roosevelt, torn by his friendship with Muir, did so more tepidly. Not until 1913 did President Woodrow Wilson finally decide the issue in favor of San Francisco. Conservation had won over preservation.

Still, Roosevelt advanced many of Muir's goals. Over the protests of cattle and timber interests, the president added nearly 200 million acres to government forest reserves, placed coal and mineral lands, oil reserves, and water-power sites in the public domain, and enlarged the national park system. When Congress tried to block Roosevelt, he relied on his own ample view of executive authority to get the job done, appropriating another 17 million acres of forest before Congress could pass a bill limiting him. He also set in motion national congresses and commissions on conservation, mobilizing governors from across the country and, like a good progressive, setting hundreds of experts to work applying science, education, and technology to the problems.

As Roosevelt grew bolder in his assertion of public interests, conservatives, many from his own party, lashed back. Roosevelt's record, so far, had been modest, but his chief accomplishment—invigorating the presidency—had the potential for promoting deeper reform. When a financial panic hit Wall Street in 1907, business leaders and conservatives blamed the president. Roosevelt, in turn, pointed to the "speculative folly and the flagrant dishonesty of a few men of great wealth." But having declared he would not run again in 1908, Roosevelt (just 50 years old) prepared to hand the reins of his party and office to William Howard Taft.

The Troubled Taft

Early on the morning of March 4, 1909, while snow swirled outside the White House, Taft readied himself for his inauguration. Over breakfast with Roosevelt, he warmed in the glow of recent Republican victories. Taft had decisively beaten William Jennings Bryan in the "Great Commoner's" third and last run for the presidency. Republicans had retained control of Congress as well as a host of legislatures in northern states. Reform was at high tide, and Taft was ready to continue in the Roosevelt tradition.

William Howard Taft (left), a full-bodied 300 pounds, enjoyed golf more than politics.

"Will," as Roosevelt liked to call him, was his hand-picked successor. A distinguished jurist, the first governor-general of the Philippines under American rule, and Roosevelt's secretary of war, Taft had demonstrated great administrative skill. He could be charming, was often funny, and was always honest. His size—nearly 300 pounds—reflected his tastes and temperament. He ate too much, slept too long, and disliked strife and political maneuvering. He preferred conciliation to confrontation. Even Roosevelt had doubts. "He's all right," TR had told a reporter on inauguration day. "But he's weak. They'll get around him. They'll"—and here Roosevelt pushed the reporter with his shoulder—"lean against him."

The standard-bearer of conservative Republicans was Joseph G. Cannon, the Speaker of the House. Every committee assignment, every patronage appointment, every bill required "Uncle Joe's" approval. Thirty progressive House members were hoping to curb these dictatorial powers—and they had Taft's blessing. But Cannon had no intention of backing down without a fight. He threatened to block any reduction of the tariff if the congressional revolt continued. Taft, who wanted tariffs lowered, caved in so that the tariff bill would pass. When progressives later broke Cannon's power without the president's help, they scorned Taft's lack of backbone. And Taft's compromise went for naught, since Senate protectionists led by Nelson W. Aldrich peppered the tariff bill with some 800 amendments, which raised rates nearly to their old levels. With both wings of the party disenchanted with his waffling, Taft lost control of Republicans in Congress.

The ties between Taft and the progressives were stressed even further in a dispute over conservation. Taft had appointed Richard Ballinger as secretary of the interior over the opposition of Chief Forester Pinchot. Ballinger and Taft, like Pinchot, were genuine conservationists. Through their efforts more land was protected than Roosevelt had saved during all his years in office. But Taft and Ballinger sought to weaken the centralized federal power that Roosevelt and Pinchot used to pursue their goals. When Ballinger opened a million acres of Pinchot-protected public lands for sale, Pinchot rebelled. He unearthed a report that claimed shady dealings had led to the transfer of Alaskan public coal lands to a syndicate that included J. P. Morgan. Taft stood by Ballinger. Out of frustration Pinchot took his case to the press and to Congress early in 1910, whereupon Taft fired him for insubordination. The Ballinger–Pinchot controversy, as it became known, led some progressives to label Taft the "friend of thieves and the enemy of honest men." They began to look longingly across the Atlantic, where TR was stalking lions in Africa.

In the off-year elections of 1910, Republicans—conservative and progressive alike—were swept from office. Democrats won the industrial Northeast and Midwest. The new state lawmakers, largely from the ranks of immigrants, advanced social welfare in the form of worker's compensation, utilities regulation, and pro-labor laws. For the first time in 16 years Democrats controlled the House of Representatives. Republicans clung to a nominal majority in the Senate. There a small band of independent-minded progressives held the balance of power.

Despite the failures of his leadership, Taft was no conservative apologist. For the next two years he pushed Congress to enact a progressive program regulating safety standards for mines and railroads, creating a federal children's bureau, and setting an eight-hour workday for federal employees. Taft's support of a constitutional amendment permitting graduated income taxes was sometimes ardent, sometimes tepid, but in the end proved decisive. Early in 1913 the Sixteenth Amendment was added to the Constitution. Many historians have viewed it as the most important reform of the century, for it eventually gave the federal government the financial resources to increase the scope of its responsibilities. Yet no matter what he achieved, Taft somehow managed to alienate conservatives and progressives without retaining the support of either. That spelled trouble for the Republicans as the presidential election approached.

The Election of 1912

In June 1910 Roosevelt had come home, exuberant as ever and laden with hunting trophies. He was confronted with an unhappy Taft and a fractious party. Angry progressives were threatening to bolt. Party loyalty kept Roosevelt quiet through most of 1911, though in private he described Taft as a "flubdub with a streak of the second-rate." Roosevelt could not contain himself any longer when, in October 1911, Taft pricked him on the particularly sensitive matter of busting trusts. Taft, like TR, accepted trusts as natural, but he failed to make Roosevelt's distinction between "good" and "bad" ones. He demanded, more impartially, that all trusts be prevented from restraining trade. In his four years as president, Taft initiated nearly twice as many antitrust suits as Roosevelt had in seven years.

In October 1911 the Justice Department filed suit against U.S. Steel, charging the company with having violated the antimonopoly clause of the Sherman Act by acquiring the Tennessee Coal and Iron Company. Roosevelt, while president, had personally accepted the acquisition to stave off a financial collapse. To see the Taft administration now prosecuting U.S. Steel irked him immensely, for the suit not only blurred his distinction between "good" and "bad" trusts but also seemed to censure his behavior as president. Taft, complained Roosevelt confidentially, "was playing small, mean, and foolish politics."

TR decided to play big, high-minded, and presidential. Already, in a speech at Osawatomie, Kansas, in 1910, he had called for a "New Nationalism," a sweeping program that stressed planning and efficiency at the hands of a powerful national executive. The New Nationalism recognized the value of collectivism—big business, big government, big labor—but insisted on protecting the interests of

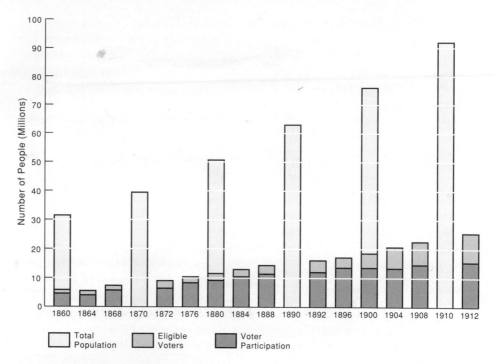

THE VOTING PUBLIC, 1860–1912

Between 1860 and 1910 the population and the number of eligible voters increased nearly threefold. As reforms of the early twentieth century reduced the power of political machines and parties, the percentage of voter participation actually declined.

individuals. The community, Roosevelt declared, had the right to regulate property "to whatever degree the public welfare may require."

Based partly on the ideas of progressive theorist Herbert Croly, the New Nationalism harked back to Alexander Hamilton's brand of federalism, with its reliance on a strong central government. But it hoped to combine that brand of federal leadership with a respect for the rights of individuals at the core of Thomas Jefferson's republicanism. As Roosevelt elaborated his New Nationalism, he defended economic concentration so long as government could control it by national incorporation and regulation. His program would support labor through compulsory investigation of labor disputes and limits on court injunctions against unions. It would control wealth by taxing income and inheritances. It embraced social justice in the eight-hour workday, workers' compensation, child labor laws, minimum wages for women, and "equal suffrage"—a nod to women and loyal black Republicans. Occasionally Roosevelt even suggested that conservative judges might be curbed by putting in place a "recall" system for judicial decisions.

All that remained was to find some stalwart, energetic president to put the New Nationalism into effect. "My hat is in the ring!" Roosevelt announced in February 1912, to the surprise of few. "The fight is on and I am stripped to the buff!" Taft responded by claiming that the New Nationalism had won support only from "destructive radicals," "political emotionalists," and "neurotics." In fact, the enormously popular Roosevelt won most of the primaries; but by the time Repub-

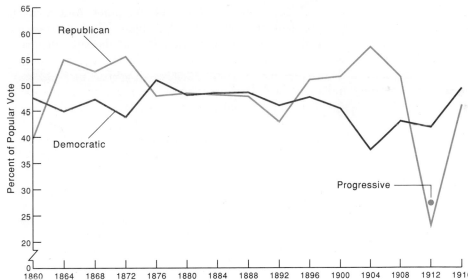

REPUBLICAN AND DEMOCRATIC PARTIES' SHARE OF POPULAR VOTE, 1860–1912
In the last quarter of the nineteenth century the Republican and Democratic parties were
deadlocked until the Republicans became the majority party in 1896. In 1912 the parties
splintered, TR ran as a Progressive, and Republican fortunes plummeted.

licans met in Chicago in June 1912, Taft's use of patronage and promises had won
him the nomination.

A frustrated Roosevelt bolted and took progressive Republicans with him.
Two months later, amid choruses of "Onward Christian Soldiers," delegates to the
newly formed Progressive party nominated Roosevelt for the presidency. "We
stand at Armageddon," he told a crowd of nearly 10,000, "and we battle for the
Lord." At one point Roosevelt bellowed at reporters, "I'm feeling like a bull
moose!"—and Progressives had a symbol for their party. The Democrats met in
Baltimore, jubilant over the prospect of facing a divided Republican party. On the
verge of regaining the White House after a 16-year absence, delegates chose as
their candidate Woodrow Wilson, the reformist governor of New Jersey.

Wilson saw Roosevelt, not Taft, as his major opponent. He immediately countered the New Nationalism with his "New Freedom," a reiteration of Louis Brandeis' program to free the American people from the control of large concentrations
of wealth and power. Wilson rejected the managed economy of the New Nationalism. He wanted to free the marketplace. Instead of Roosevelt's "regulated monopoly," Wilson proposed a "regulated competition." Only by enforcing strict limits
on size and removing artificial barriers to commerce could concentration be controlled and free enterprise preserved. Nothing less than liberty was at stake. "If
America is not to have free enterprise," he said in October 1912, "then she can
have freedom of no sort whatever." Though he accepted social justice as an admi-
rable goal, Wilson feared that government-sponsored social welfare programs
would threaten constitutional freedoms. "Liberty," he warned, "has never come
from government," only from the "limitation of governmental power"—
sentiments Jefferson no doubt would have endorsed.

Increasingly voters found Taft's conservatism beside the point. And in an age of reform, even the socialists looked good. Better led, financed, and organized than ever before, the Socialist party had increased its membership to nearly 135,000 by 1912. Socialist mayors ran 32 cities, from Schenectady, New York, to Berkeley, California. The party also had an appealing candidate in Eugene V. Debs, a home-grown Indiana radical. Crisscrossing the country on a train dubbed the "Red Special," Debs had won 400,000 votes for president in 1904. Now, in 1912, he summoned voters to make "the working class the ruling class of the nation and the world." As for trusts, he proposed simply to nationalize them.

On election day voters gave progressivism a resounding endorsement. Wilson won 6.3 million votes, Roosevelt 4.1 million. Debs received almost a million votes, whereas the conservative Taft attracted just 3.6 million. Thus the progressive candidates combined had a 3 to 1 margin, and the Democrats won control of both houses of Congress. Though shaken by his defeat, Roosevelt remained optimistic about reform: "The Progressive movement must and will go forward even though its progress is fitful."

Woodrow Wilson and the Politics of Morality

Soon after the election Woodrow Wilson told William McCombs, chairman of the Democratic National Committee, "I wish it clearly understood that I owe you nothing." Taken aback, McCombs reminded Wilson of his sturdy service during the presidential campaign. Wilson replied: "God ordained that I should be the next President of the United States. Neither you nor any mortal could have prevented that!"

Born in Virginia in 1856, Woodrow Wilson grew up believing, as he put it, "in predestination and election." A minister's son and a devout Presbyterian, he dismissed those who disagreed with him as plain "wrong." Gyrating between Christian love and Calvinist severity, he could be warm and generous one moment, cold and petty the next.

To compensate for a learning disability (probably dyslexia), Wilson developed a near-photographic memory. He studied the words and cadences of great speakers, then wandered the woods reciting their speeches. Like most southerners, he loved the Democratic party, hated the tariff, and accepted the necessity of racial separation. Under his presidency, segregation would return to Washington for the first time since Reconstruction.

Bored and disheartened by a career in law, Wilson turned to political science, earned a doctorate from Johns Hopkins, and taught at Bryn Mawr, Wesleyan, and Princeton. Political science persuaded him that a president must act as a "prime minister," directing and uniting the party, shaping legislation and opinion, exerting continuous leadership. In 1902 he became president of Princeton and helped to transform it into one of the nation's finest schools. His tenure was often controversial, however, and as in later crises in Washington, if pushed, Wilson retreated into a sanctimonious moralism that made compromise difficult. He escaped academic politics in 1910, when Democratic party bosses helped elect him governor of New Jersey, and after a successful term of reform, president in 1912.

The New Freedom in Action

In power Wilson was a model of executive leadership. He went to Congress, the first president since John Adams to appear in person. He kept party discipline

Candidate (Party)	Electoral Vote	Popular Vote
Wilson (Democratic)	435 (82%)	6,293,454 (42%)
T. Roosevelt (Progressive)	88 (17%)	4,119,538 (28%)
Taft (Republican)	8 (1%)	3,484,980 (24%)
Debs (Socialist)	—	900,672 (6%)

1912

THE ELECTION OF 1912

tight, threatened to veto bills he did not like, and mobilized public opinion when confronted with congressional obstruction. During his presidency progressivism peaked.

Lowering the high tariff was Wilson's first order of business. Progressives regarded the tariff as yet another example of the unrestrained power of trusts, and in Wilson's view it weakened competition by protecting American manufacturers. Roosevelt had avoided the tariff; Taft had bungled its revision; Wilson moved quickly and forcefully to reduce it. Addressing Congress directly he declared, "We must abolish everything that bears even the semblance of privilege or of any kind of artificial advantage." When protectionists in the Senate threatened to raise rates, Wilson appealed directly to the public. "Industrious" and "insidious" lobbyists had descended on Washington to block reform, he told the press. A "brick couldn't be thrown without hitting one of them."

The Underwood–Simmons Tariff of 1913 marked the first downward revision in 19 years and the biggest since before the Civil War. It lowered most rates from 40 percent to 25 percent and placed many new items on the free list. To compensate for lost revenue, Congress enacted a graduated income tax, permitted under the newly adopted Sixteenth Amendment. It applied solely to corporations and the tiny fraction of Americans who earned more than $4000 a year. It nonetheless began a momentous shift in government revenue from its nineteenth-century base—public lands, alcohol taxes, and customs duties—to its twentieth-century base—personal and corporate incomes.

Wilson turned next to the knotty problem of money and banking. Early in 1913 the Pujo Committee, created by Congress to investigate the "money trust," revealed "a spider web of interlocking Wall Street directorates" that concentrated control of the nation's credit system in a few powerful investment firms. Without a stable but flexible currency, Wilson's free market would be enslaved to the great investment banks, which could choke industry and commerce with high interest rates or tight money. As a banking reform bill moved through Congress in 1913, opinion split sharply over its design. Wall Street wanted a privately controlled, centralized banking system that could issue currency and set interest rates. Rural Democrats, led by Senator Carter Glass of Virginia, favored a decentralized sys-

Woodrow Wilson, 28th president of the United States, was the first Ph.D. in the White House and the first president to hold open press conferences.

tem of regional banks run by local bankers. Populists and progressives, including Bryan, La Follette, and Brandeis, wanted public control.

Wilson reconciled their differences in the Federal Reserve Act of 1913. The new Federal Reserve System contained not one central bank, but 12 regional banks (scattered deliberately around the country) that held reserves for commercial banks. A central Federal Reserve Board in Washington, appointed by the president, supervised the whole system. It could regulate credit and the money supply by setting the interest rate it charged member banks, by buying or selling government bonds, and by issuing paper currency (called Federal Reserve notes) backed by a combination of gold and government credit. Each Federal Reserve Bank was owned and directed by local member banks. Thus the Federal Reserve Act sought to stabilize the existing order by making currency more elastic and credit easier to obtain. As it turned out, the conservatives Wilson appointed to the Federal Reserve Board failed to understand how their power to expand and contract the nation's money supply influenced the health of the economy. Later financial upheavals would show that mistakes made by the Federal Reserve System could be as devastating as those made by private bankers on Wall Street.

When Wilson took on the trusts, he moved a bit closer toward the New Nationalism of Theodore Roosevelt. The Federal Trade Commission Act of 1914 created a bipartisan executive agency to oversee business activity. The end—to enforce orderly competition—was distinctly Wilsonian, but the means—an executive commission to regulate commerce—were pure Roosevelt. The Federal Trade Commission (FTC) had wide investigatory powers, could order corporate compliance, and had the power to prosecute against "unfair trade practices." The FTC proved to be more of a guide than a sheriff. It gave advance warning of government disapproval and, through consent decrees, persuaded companies to make changes without having to convict them of anything. Wilson, like Roosevelt, was no extremist. He chose commissioners sympathetic to the business community and accepted a revision in the law that gave the conservative courts power to review all FTC decisions.

Roosevelt would have stopped there, but Wilson complemented regulation with the Clayton Antitrust Act of 1914. The Clayton Act outlawed some of the worst corporate malpractices—price discrimination, holding companies, and interlocking directorates—but only when they "tend to create a monopoly." Action on these practices was at the government's discretion. More and more, the Wilson administration chose to regulate rather than break up bigness. The Justice Department filed fewer antitrust suits than the Taft administration had and negotiated more "gentlemen's agreements" (voluntary agreements by companies to change practices) than had Roosevelt.

By November 1914, tariff and banking reform, regulatory legislation, a graduated income tax, and a new antitrust law—all impressive and important accomplishments—adorned Wilson's two-year-old presidency. Yet voters seemed lukewarm toward the New Freedom. In the elections of 1914 Republicans cut Democratic majorities in the House and won important industrial and farm states. To strengthen his hand in the presidential election of 1916, Wilson began edging slowly toward the social programs of the New Nationalism he had earlier criticized as paternalistic and unconstitutional. He signaled the change in 1915 when he nominated his close adviser Louis D. Brandeis to the Supreme Court. The "people's lawyer," Brandeis had fought for the very social reforms lacking from Wilson's agenda. With Wilson's staunch support, Brandeis broke the tradition of conservatism and anti-Semitism that had previously kept Jews off the Court.

Wilson had been cool to labor and social reform and was unwilling to exempt strikes and boycotts from antitrust prosecution. But in 1916 he effectively dropped his opposition to such "class legislation" by signing the Seamen's Act, to provide federal protection for the rights and working conditions of merchant seamen. Wilson maneuvered for passage of the Keating–Owen Child Labor Act (declared unconstitutional in 1918) and workers' compensation for federal employees. Just before the election he intervened to avert a nationwide strike of rail workers. Despite his reservations about federal intrusion in the economy, he later signed the Adamson Act, mandating an eight-hour day for workers on all interstate railroads.

Farmers and women also gained his support. The Federal Farm Loan Act and the Warehouse Act furnished farmers with long-term, federally supported, low-interest loans based on the value of their crops and land. The Federal Highway Act of 1916 helped farmers on their way to market by granting aid to states that improved their roads. In 1915 Wilson even endorsed state action to grant women the right to vote.

"The future," Woodrow Wilson had written in 1914, "is clear and bright with promise of the best things." As the presidential campaign of 1916 approached, the future looked brighter still. Under Wilson's administration, progressivism had reached high tide. He himself had come reluctantly to accept big government and big business. He had also learned the value of protective social legislation. Like Theodore Roosevelt, Wilson harnessed the chief executive to change. Together they made the presidency newsworthy and the president noteworthy. For good or ill, Americans thereafter looked to the White House for leadership and direction.

The Mixed Legacy of Progressivism

Reform, then, had taken the country far during the first heady decade and a half of the twentieth century. Seeing chaos in the modern industrial city, progressives worked to reduce the damage of poverty, eliminate the dangers of industrial work, control the rising immigrant tide, and spread a middle-class ideal of morality. In city halls and state legislatures, they looked to break the power of special corpo-rate interests and entrenched political machines. In Washington, they enlarged government and broadened its mission from simple caretaker to promoter of pub-lic welfare. Progressivism did not always succeed, in part because powerful forces opposed it, in part because the progressive vision was limited and fuzzy. Progres-sives sometimes betrayed their own reformist ideals by denying blacks, Asians, and other minorities racial equality and by attempting to Americanize foreigners rather than accept the rich contributions of their cultures. And efforts to regulate business fell short of the protection intended. Too often regulatory agencies were captured by the very interests they were supposed to oversee.

For all its sweeping claim to reform, progressivism left the system of market capitalism largely intact. But the Gilded Age's philosophy of laissez faire—of giv-ing private enterprise a free hand—had been clearly rejected. Both state and federal governments had established their right to regulate the actions of private corporations for the public good. That public good, progressives believed, could be exposed through vigorous publicity brought about by commissions, investiga-tive hearings, activist presidents. The reforms achieved through these means—the eight-hour day, woman suffrage, direct election of senators, graduated income taxes, public ownership of utilities—began to address the problems of an urban industrial society. Under progressive leadership, the modern state—active and interventionist—was born. A sense of mastery, so characteristic of twentieth-century reform, replaced the awful feeling of drift that had dominated the 1890s.

Such accomplishments invigorated American faith in progress as the new century unfolded. A higher civilization of enlightened culture, peace, and pros-perity seemed within reach. But in 1914, as progressivism crested in America, the guns of a hot August shattered an uneasy calm in Europe and plunged the world into war. Few people anywhere were prepared for the carnage that followed.

SIGNIFICANT EVENTS

1890 — New England Kitchen opens; General Federation of Women's Clubs organized

1892 — Sierra Club founded

1893 — Illinois legislature enacts eight-hour workday law for women; Anti-Saloon League created

1895 — *United States v. E. C. Knight*

1899 — National Consumers League founded

1900 — Galveston, Texas, creates first commission form of government

1901 — Leon Czolgosz assassinates President William McKinley; Theodore Roosevelt becomes president; Robert La Follette elected reform governor of Wisconsin; Socialist Party of America founded

1902 — Bureau of the Census created; Northern Securities Company dissolved under Sherman Antitrust Act; anthracite coal miners strike in Pennsylvania; Maryland adopts first workers' compensation law

1903 — Department of Labor and Commerce created; Elkins Act passed; Wisconsin is first state to enact direct primary; Wright brothers' flight

1904 — Lincoln Steffens' *The Shame of the Cities* published; Robert Hunter's *Poverty* published; Theodore Roosevelt elected president

1906 — Hepburn Act strengthens Interstate Commerce Commission; Upton Sinclair's *The Jungle* published; Meat Inspection and Pure Food and Drug acts passed

1907 — William James' *Pragmatism* published

1908 — Henry Ford introduces the Model T; *Muller v. Oregon*; William Howard Taft elected president

1909 — Payne–Aldrich Tariff; Ballinger–Pinchot controversy

1910 — Mann Act passed

1911 — Triangle Shirtwaist fire

1912 — Progressive ("Bull Moose") party nominates Theodore Roosevelt for presidency; Woodrow Wilson elected president

1913 — Sixteenth Amendment and Seventeenth Amendment passed; Underwood–Simmons Tariff enacted; Federal Reserve Act passed; Keith–Albee Circuit opens Palace Theater in New York

1914 — Clayton Antitrust Act passed; Federal Trade Commission created

1916 — Margaret Sanger organizes New York Birth Control League; Keating–Owen Child Labor Act passed; Woodrow Wilson reelected president

1917 — Congress enacts literacy test for new immigrants

1920 — Nineteenth Amendment passed

24

The United States and the Old World Order

n 1898, when the battleship *Oregon* steamed from San Francisco Bay to its battle station in the Caribbean during the Spanish–American War, it had to travel around the tip of South America, a journey of over two months. The delay was more than embarrassing; it was dangerous. As an emerging naval power, the United States needed a canal farther north to link the Atlantic and Pacific. A path between the seas, most likely across Central America, would also speed American trade; between 1890 and 1900 the value of American exports had jumped from $845 million to nearly $1.4 billion.

From the days of the sixteenth-century conquistador Francisco Pizarro, travelers had crossed through the jungles of the Panamanian isthmus (later acquired by Colombia) on foot, horseback, or mule train, taking their chances with muddy trails and tropical diseases. Only in the 1850s, when the first true transcontinental railroad cut through Panama, did the trip cease to be a nightmare.

The commercial and strategic possibilities of a canal had long inspired dreamers. A French diplomat who had been involved in building the Suez Canal, Ferdinand de Lesseps, planned to cut across the isthmus in the 1880s. The venture was brought low by yellow fever and problems insuperable without more advanced engineering. Teddy Roosevelt was equally visionary about the possibility of a canal and even more energetic at mustering the resources and confidence to complete the task. "With Roosevelt," said one engineer, "anything is possible."

"I took the isthmus," Roosevelt later told a crowd of cheering students at Berkeley. In a way he did. In 1901 Roosevelt persuaded Britain to give up its rights to a joint canal enterprise, then authorized Secretary of State John Hay to negotiate with Colombian chargé d'affaires Tomas Herran. The Hay–Herran Convention (1903) leased to the United States a strip across the Panamanian region of Colombia, the site of the earlier French attempt to link the Atlantic with the Pacific. Meanwhile Roosevelt agreed to pay the old de Lesseps Company $40 million for its equipment and other assets.

Suddenly the Colombians drew back. Hoping for more money and a firmer guarantee of sovereignty, their senate refused to accept the treaty. The Colombi-

On November 11, 1918, six hours after the armistice was signed in a railroad car in the forest of Compiègne, France, the guns of World War I fell silent. At 3 a.m. news reached the United States, which burst into wild celebrations.

ans, fumed TR, were "highwaymen," "blackmailers," and "inefficient bandits," barring "one of the future highways of civilization." He convinced himself that the order and stability of the region required action. Privately, Roosevelt talked of seizing Panama; instead he settled on fomenting a revolution.

Phillipe Bunau-Varilla, a French engineer with the de Lesseps Company, told Roosevelt of a budding independence movement in Panama. Roosevelt let it be known that he would welcome a revolt. On November 3, 1903, on schedule and without bloodshed, the Panamanians took over. The next day the cruiser *Nashville* dropped anchor offshore to prevent Colombia from landing troops on the isthmus. Two days later, far quicker than diplomatic convention dictated, the United States recognized the new Republic of Panama; and within two weeks, Bunau-Varilla, acting for the Panamanian government, signed a treaty with the United States for a renewable lease on a canal zone 10-miles in width. Panama received $10 million plus an annual rent of $250,000 (the same terms earlier offered to Colombia). The Chicago *American*, one of the few critics of this affair, called it "a rough-riding assault upon another republic over the shattered wreckage of international law and diplomatic usage." Roosevelt never apologized, but in 1921, when oil had been discovered there, Congress voted $25 million to Colombia. One historian later dubbed it "canalimony."

To underscore the importance of the canal, Roosevelt himself traveled to Panama, the first president ever to leave the country while in office. Arriving early in November 1906 on the new 16,000-ton *Louisiana*, the largest battleship in the

PANAMA CANAL—OLD AND NEW TRANSOCEANIC ROUTES
Tropical forests cover three-fourths of Panama, including the Canal Zone. Vegetation is denser at high elevations, but tightly packed even below 1000 feet. The terrain is rugged, but the distance saved by the canal (nearly 8000 miles) made the ordeal of construction worthwhile.

fleet, he timed his visit with the rainy season in order to see the canal site at its foulest. "If we shrink from the hard contests," he once said, "then the bolder and stronger people will pass us by."

Soaked from head to toe, his huge panama hat and white suit sagging about his body, Roosevelt made the canal tour a public event. He had Dr. William Gorgas, exterminator of the deadly yellow fever–bearing mosquito, take him in person through the hospital at Ancon. At the cuts, he asked black workers about their complaints, walked railroad ties, splashed through labor camps, and made speeches in the pouring rain. "This is one of the great works of the world," he boasted to an assembly of diggers.

As Roosevelt clambered aboard a giant 95-ton Bucyrus steam shovel, he saw proof of his boast—the largest trench yet cut in the earth's surface. When completed in 1914 it stretched some 40 miles across the Isthmus of Panama. Three years of planning and seven years of construction went into it, and its final cost, $352 million, was four times what had been spent on the Suez Canal when it opened in 1869. Crews working on the Panama Canal dug the equivalent of a Suez Canal every three years. "Everything," reported one journalist who visited the site in 1911, "is on a colossal scale." The locks of the canal, used to raise and lower water levels, were 1000 feet long and rose higher than a six-story building. Three Statues of Liberty could be laid end to end in any one of them with room to spare. The volume of concrete poured to make just one of the three main locks was enough to build a wall 8 feet high, 12 feet thick, and 133 miles long.

Nearly 6000 men lost their lives from disease and accidents. About 4500 were blacks, among 30,000 black laborers imported from the West Indies for the back-breaking job of digging the canal. They worked 10 hours a day, 6 days a week, for 10 cents an hour (considered good wages at the time). To emphasize the difference between black and white workers, blacks were paid in silver, whites in gold.

The Panama Canal embodied Roosevelt's muscular policy of respect through strength. "I do not believe," he told Taft after leaving office, "in our taking any position anywhere unless you mean to shoot." He tripled the size of the army and doubled the navy's strength. He modernized the armed forces, created a general staff for military planning and mobilization, and established the Army War College. As a pivot point between the two hemispheres, his canal would allow the United States to flex its strength across the globe. These widening horizons came about largely as an outgrowth of its commercial and industrial expansion in the world, just as the imperialist drives of England, France, Germany, Russia, and Japan reflected the spread of their own industrial and commercial might.

In the ensuing rivalry, the industrialized powers often contested with one another for spheres of influence. The United States, steeped in democratic ideals, frequently seemed uncomfortable with the dirty business of "spheres of influence" or baldly stated dreams of empire. Roosevelt's embrace of the canal showed how far some progressives had come, however, in being willing to intervene, influence, and actively shape the world order. In domestic affairs TR did not oppose big trusts, only "bad" ones. Abroad, he saw no problem with the United States exercising power globally, so long as power was wielded in a "good" way. As in the matter of judging trusts, the distinction between good and bad was not always easy to make, and control was not easy to maintain. The expansionist diplomats, whether idealistic or cynical, had convinced themselves they could maintain global order by a series of political alliances. In the end, that system of alliances and spheres of influence did not suffice, and the old order collapsed in a terrible world war.

PROGRESSIVE DIPLOMACY

The progressive era was the busiest period in American diplomacy since the eve of the Civil War. In the aftermath of the war with Spain, the United States intervened in China and Latin America, dominated the Caribbean and Central America, and fought a world war. American diplomacy became assertive and nationalistic. Diplomatic and defense budgets climbed steadily, from less than $200 million in 1900 to $1 billion in the war year of 1917.

Progressive diplomacy, like progressive politics, stressed moralism and order. Progressives pursued these aims abroad as they had at home—by stretching executive power and shaping the environment. In their hands manifest destiny, once confined to the continent, assumed global proportions. "Of all our race," Albert Beveridge told his fellow senators in 1900, "[God] has marked the American people as His chosen nation to finally lead in the redemption of the world." A widely held belief in the superiority of Anglo-American institutions lay at the core of Beveridge's faith. Implicit in his remark was the growing notion—shared by all leaders—that northern Europeans were superior in other ways as well. The darker peoples of the tropical zones, observed educator and anti-imperialist David Starr Jordan, dwelled in "nature's asylum for degenerates."

Aggressive economic expansion underlay the commitment to a "civilizing" mission. Shocked by the depression of 1893, American manufacturing and agricultural interests looked to markets abroad to ease the burdens of overproduction at home. By 1900 the United States stood first in the world among industrial nations. Five years later tractors, sewing machines, and other manufactured goods replaced agricultural commodities as America's chief exports. When World War I ended in 1918, the United States found it had become the largest creditor in the world. American-based corporations like Singer Sewing Machine and Standard Oil of New Jersey operated all over the globe. Every administration in the twentieth century committed itself to opening the doors of trade to American interests and keeping them unobstructed.

The Big Stick in the Caribbean

"Walk softly and carry a big stick," Roosevelt once remarked, but in the Caribbean he and his successors moved both loudly and mightily. The Panama Canal gave the United States a commanding strategic and commercial position in the Western Hemisphere. Its existence required the country to "police the surrounding premises," explained Secretary of State Elihu Root. Roosevelt moved promptly to make the Caribbean an American lake. Before granting Cuba independence in 1902, the United States reorganized its finances and included in the Cuban constitution the so-called Platt Amendment. According to its terms, the United States could intervene if Cuban independence were threatened or internal disorder broke out. Under its provisions, American troops occupied the island from 1906 to 1909 and again from 1917 to 1923.

Apart from his higher aim of encouraging stable governments that would be fiscally responsible and open to investment, Roosevelt worried quite practically that instability would open the Caribbean to deeper European penetration. Ever since the Monroe Doctrine of 1823 asserted American opposition to further European colonization of the Western Hemisphere, the United States had sought to keep foreign powers out of the region. In the early twentieth century the rising

Theodore Roosevelt visited the site of the Panama Canal in 1906. Relentlessly curious, he had to know everything, from the salary of engineers to the proper techniques for operating this giant Bucyrus steam shovel. "It is greater work than you, yourselves, at the moment realize," he told workers.

scale of Latin American debts to European powers invited their intervention. "If we intend to say hands off to the power of Europe," Roosevelt told Elihu Root, "then sooner or later we must keep order ourselves." Roosevelt did not shrink from the challenge. The great powers could minimize dangers by counterbalancing each other, much as big government offset big business at home, and each of them, including the United States, had an obligation to keep order in its own sphere of influence while avoiding encroachment on another's. Going well beyond Monroe's concept of resisting foreign intrusions, Roosevelt asserted an American hegemony over the Caribbean.

An early test of resolve came when British and German gunboats blockaded Venezuela for refusing to pay debts in 1902. Roosevelt successfully urged arbitration on both sides. When the Dominican Republic defaulted on its debts in 1904, Roosevelt stretched the Monroe Doctrine from a warning to keep Europe out into an American pledge to move in. Decrying "chronic wrongdoing or impotence," the president appointed the United States "policeman of the West." If Latin American nations failed to keep their affairs in order, the United States would do it for them. Under this "Roosevelt Corollary," the United States assumed responsibility for the internal affairs of several Caribbean states. In 1905, with the navy just off the coast, American agents took control of Dominican customs and tax services to ensure payment of debts. Within two years the United States established protectorates over Cuba and Panama.

A "Diplomatist of the Highest Rank"

Roosevelt exercised ingenuity rather than force in Asia. He did not consider it within the American sphere, and in any event few of his countrymen would have supported armed intervention half a world away. Roosevelt, therefore, committed himself only to maintaining an "open door" of equal commercial access to China and to protecting the Philippines, "our heel of Achilles." The key lay in offsetting Russian and Japanese ambitions to dominate the region. When Japan launched an attack on Russian holdings in the Chinese province of Manchuria in 1904, Roosevelt privately cheered the audacious Japanese, "a great civilized nation." To his way of thinking, the Russians were little more than "a menace to the higher life of the world." Still, he worried that an unchecked Japan might threaten American interests in China and the Philippines. He looked for an end to the war that would balance power in the region.

In 1905 both sides accepted Roosevelt's offer to mediate. At the U.S. Naval Base in Kittery, Maine, just across the river from Portsmouth, New Hampshire, he tried to keep angry diplomats from each other's throats. "I am having my hair turned gray by dealing with the Russian and Japanese peace negotiators," the president complained to his son. Roosevelt's skillful intercession finally produced the Treaty of Portsmouth in August 1905, leaving Japan as the dominant naval power in the Far East. Further negotiations secured a Japanese promise not to invade the Philippines in return for recognition of Japan's control over Korea. Roosevelt thus agreed to shut the open door in a portion of Asia in order to secure American interests throughout the Far East. For his efforts in ending the Russo–Japanese War he received the Nobel Peace Prize in 1906.

The Japanese government signed the peace treaty, but not without resentment among Japanese nationalists. Anger surfaced in a protest lodged not against Roosevelt, but against the San Francisco school board. In 1906 San Francisco school authorities, succumbing to racial prejudice, segregated the city's 200 Asian students. In Japan citizens talked of war over the insult to national honor. Roosevelt, fuming at those "infernal fools in California," summoned the mayor of San Francisco and seven school board members to the White House. In exchange for an end to the segregation order Roosevelt offered to arrange a mutual restriction of immigration between Japan and the United States. In 1907 all sides accepted his "gentlemen's agreement."

Relations between the two nations reached a new peak of harmony in 1908 when the Root–Takahira Agreement affirmed the status quo in the Pacific, the independence of China, and the open door in the Far East. In case Japan or other nations thought of upsetting the Pacific balance, Roosevelt conceived of a grand gesture of American might. He sent 16 sleek white battleships, many of them launched during his administration, on a global tour in the summer of 1907. The "Great White Fleet," as Roosevelt cheerfully called it, made its most conspicuous stop in Japan in 1908. Some Europeans predicted armed disaster. Instead, cheering crowds turned out in Tokyo and Yokohama. The show of force heralded a new age of American naval might but had an unintended consequence: it spurred Japanese navalists to expand their fleet, thus threatening the balance of Pacific power Roosevelt had sought to secure.

Roosevelt's policies toward Japan reflected two of his central beliefs: American interests were global and armed conflict between great powers should be avoided. When Germany and France seemed on the verge of war over control of the North African colony of Morocco in 1905, Roosevelt arranged for an international conference in Algeciras, on the coast of Spain. Breaking a century of isolation from European affairs, he sent American delegates. The peaceful outcome, favorable to France and the stability of Europe, pleased him. In the summer of 1908 the United States and 43 other nations again met at the Hague in the Netherlands to set limited rules for war. Horrified at the destructiveness of new weaponry, they outlawed poison gas but held back from banning aerial balloons, battleships, airplanes, and submarines.

Watching Roosevelt in his second term, an amazed London *Morning Post* dubbed him a "diplomatist of the highest rank." Abroad and at home his brand of progressivism was grounded in an enthusiastic nationalism, mixed force with finesse, and sought always to achieve balance and order. For all his strenuous efforts, however, disorder still threatened. Imperial rivalries, empires both rising and falling, an unchecked naval arms race, and domestic unrest in Europe threatened to plunge the world into war.

Taft and Dollar Diplomacy

Roosevelt's hand-picked successor, William Howard Taft, was TR's opposite—prudent, legalistic, and cooperative. Rather than wielding force or finesse, Taft preferred to promote American interests by encouraging private corporations to invest abroad, particularly in the Caribbean and China. American capital, managed wherever possible by American financiers, would help to achieve prosperity, keep peace, and tie debt-ridden nations to the United States instead of Europe. "Dollar diplomacy," Taft explained, simply amounted to "substituting dollars for bullets." As it turned out, he and his prickly secretary of state, Philander Knox, relied on both.

South of the Rio Grande Taft and Knox (himself a corporation lawyer) treated the restless nations of Latin America like ailing corporations, injecting capital and

AMERICAN INTERVENTIONS IN THE CARIBBEAN, 1898–1930
In the first three decades of the twentieth century, U.S. diplomacy transformed the Caribbean into an American lake as armed and unarmed intervention became part of the country's diplomatic arsenal.

reorganizing management. Aided by the State Department, American money flowed across the border. One-half of all American investments abroad were in Latin America by the time Taft left office in 1912. Taft and Knox convinced American investors to supply credit to Honduras to pay off European bondholders in 1909. A year later Taft got American bankers to take over the national bank of chronically unstable Haiti.

In Nicaragua dollar diplomacy was not enough. An American-supported revolt against the unfriendly dictator José Zelaya had brought Adolfo Díaz to power in 1909. When the Nicaraguan legislature balked at American demands to take over its customs house and national bank, a U.S. warship dropped anchor off the coast. The lawmakers changed their minds, but in 1912 a revolution reinstated Zelaya. Taft sent 2000 marines to protect American lives and property, an assignment that lasted on and off for more than a dozen years.

Taft found he could assure American influence in the Caribbean far more easily than in Asia. Where Roosevelt had tried to conciliate Japan, Taft tried to strengthen China with American capital and increased American trade. Dollar diplomacy, in the words of New York banker and diplomat Willard Straight, would become the financial expression of the open door. Knox and Taft saw an end to foreign control of Manchuria as their first goal. So dominant were the Japanese that they collected taxes, appointed police, and supervised Chinese all along the railroads they operated. Knox tried to organize an international syndicate through which China could buy back the railroads from Japan and Russia. When Russia, England, and Japan refused to cooperate in 1910, the scheme fell apart. Encouraged by the Chinese, Knox then elbowed his way into a British, French, and German venture to finance a new rail line across the province of Hukuang. The Japanese and Russians also demanded entry, then paralyzed the resulting consortium to protect their spheres of influence. The best Taft and Knox could do was dragoon American bankers into lending a paltry $2 million to China.

Failure dogged Taft overseas as it did at home. In the Caribbean his dollar diplomacy was linked so closely with unpopular regimes, corporations, and banks that Woodrow Wilson dissociated himself from it as soon as he took office. In the Far East Taft's initiatives only intensified rivalry with Japan and made China more suspicious of all foreigners, including Americans. In 1911 the southern Chinese provinces rebelled against foreign intrusion and overthrew the monarchy. Only persistent pressure from the White House kept "dollar diplomacy" in Asia alive at all.

WOODROW WILSON AND MORAL DIPLOMACY

Before running for public office Woodrow Wilson had devoted his academic life to studying politics, Congress, and the presidency. His political touch was therefore surest at home. Abroad he felt his way through unknown territory. Just before his inauguration in 1913 he confessed to a friend, "It would be the irony of fate if my administration had to deal chiefly with foreign affairs." Wilson, it turned out, lacked the sense of irony to deal with what fate had in store.

To the diplomacy of order, force, and finances he brought a commitment to justice, democracy, and Christian values. He revived Jefferson's notion of the United States as a beacon of freedom for the world and then went a step beyond: he wanted the country, with its newfound power, to become an active promoter of peace, human rights, and social progress. "We are chosen, and prominently chosen," Wilson asserted in 1910, "to show the way to the nations of the world how they shall walk in the paths of liberty." Such paternalism only thinly masked the assumption of Anglo-American superiority that Wilson shared with his predecessors and other Western leaders.

Wilson's evangelical democracy had a practical side. In the twentieth century foreign markets would serve as America's new frontier. "Our industries have expanded to such a point," he warned in the campaign of 1912, "that they will burst their jackets if they cannot find free outlets in the markets of the world." Wilson's genius lay in reconciling this commercial self-interest with global interests. As he saw it, exporting American democracy and capitalism would promote stability and progress throughout the world.

Missionary Diplomacy

Solitary and self-assured, Wilson served as his own vicar of foreign policy. Circumventing the State Department, he sent personal emissaries to foreign leaders and often typed his own dispatches. Sometimes he even left his secretary of state uninformed about important initiatives. When in doubt, Wilson usually turned to his trusted personal friend, Edward M. House. A private citizen and presidential kingmaker, the honorary "Colonel" House had seen in Wilson's ascent his own road to power and influence behind the scenes. Those who sought to reach the president learned first to go to New York to see the man who had become his alter ego.

In his secretary of state, William Jennings Bryan, Wilson found an ardent public preacher for spreading the blessings of democracy and Christianity. As an evangelical and a pacifist, this thrice-frustrated presidential candidate served mineral water and grape juice at State Department receptions. Like Wilson, Bryan had no experience in foreign affairs. He distrusted the elite corps of foreign affairs experts and appointed politically "deserving Democrats" to key posts around the world. All too often they were as ill equipped and unsophisticated as Bryan himself.

In 1913, many progressives harbored a utopian hope that nations could settle their differences peaceably, if given the chance. Bryan offered that chance through treaties of conciliation with some 30 nations, including Great Britain, France, and Italy. (Ominously, Germany refused to sign one.) Completed in 1914, on the eve of World War I, these "cooling-off" agreements placed disputes before international commissions of investigation, usually for a year. Commissions of "experts," after all, had been at the heart of so many progressive domestic reforms. According to these agreements, neither disputant could further arm itself or declare war until the commission rendered an opinion.

In Asia and the Pacific Wilson gave early signals of his desire to put "moral and public considerations" ahead of the "material interests of individuals." Soon after entering the White House he pulled American bankers out of the Chinese railroad consortium. Observing that the terms of its loan required foreign control of tax collection and expenditures, he pledged to aid China without undermining its sovereignty. The United States became the first major power to recognize the new Republic of China after a revolution in 1911 toppled the last Manchu emperor, and in 1915 strongly opposed Japan's "Twenty-one Demands" for control of the country. At the end of Wilson's first administration the Philippines gained limited self-government, the first step toward the eventual independence granted in 1946.

In the Caribbean and Latin America, despite promises of change, Wilson found himself resorting to armed intervention. Like Taft and Roosevelt, he failed to appreciate the near impossibility of trying to graft American-style democracy and capitalism onto countries with indigenous traditions and aspirations. In August 1914 he convinced Nicaragua, already occupied by American troops, to yield control of a naval base and grant to the United States an alternative canal route. By the end of his administration U.S. troops were still stationed there and also in the Dominican Republic, Haiti, and Cuba. All of them were economically dependent on the United States and all were virtual American protectorates. Missionary diplomacy, like its predecessors, spread its gospel with steel and cash.

Intervention in Mexico

A lingering crisis in Mexico made a final mockery of Wilson's moral diplomacy in Latin America. In 1911 President Francisco Madero, an aristocratic reformer, overthrew the aging dictator, Porfirio Díaz. Despite efforts to modernize his country, Díaz had succeeded mainly in enriching himself and a few powerful families. Most Mexicans remained poor and uneducated in a population deeply divided among whites, Indians, and mestizos. Díaz kept Mexico financially afloat by encouraging foreign investment in oil, railroads, land, and mines. United States corporations owned nearly half the investment property.

Backed by the middle class, Madero set about raising taxes on foreign holdings, canceling concessions, and nationalizing properties. His reforms plunged the country into political turmoil for two years. The climax came on February 22, 1913, when General Victoriano Huerta surrounded the presidential palace, arrested Madero, and had him killed. Foreign investors endorsed Huerta, a conservative militarist likely to protect their holdings. Most European nations recognized the new regime immediately, but Wilson refused to accept the "government of butchers." He wanted to extend into Mexico the same principles progressivism fostered at home: orderly government and a democratic rule of law. So he threw his support to rebel leader Venustiano Carranza, on the condition that Carranza participate in American-sponsored elections. No Mexican, least of all Carranza and his "constitutionalists," was ready to lose face by tolerating such heavy-handed interference. They rejected the offer. Having few options, Wilson supplied the rebels with arms anyway.

Wilson's distaste for the Huerta regime was so great that he used a minor incident as a pretext for armed intervention. In April 1914 the paymaster and crew of the U.S.S. *Dolphin* landed without permission in the Mexican port city of Tampico. Local police promptly arrested them, only to release the sailors with equal speed. Unappeased, their squadron commander demanded a 21-gun salute to the American flag to salve the honor of the United States. Huerta refused to salute a nation that did not recognize his regime unless the Americans returned the salute to Mexico. Learning of a German shipload of weapons about to land at Veracruz; Wilson broke the impasse by ordering American troops to take the port city, expecting a bloodless occupation. Instead, marines encountered stiff resistance as they stormed ashore; 126 Mexicans and 19 Americans were killed before the city fell. The intervention accomplished the unlikely feat of uniting the rival Mexican factions in a moment of shared rage.

With Mexico and the United States edging toward war, Wilson accepted an offer from Argentina, Brazil, and Chile (the "ABC powers") to mediate. As talks convened, a bankrupted Huerta resigned and Carranza formed a new constitutionalist government. Under the guidance of the ABC powers the United States evacuated Veracruz in November 1914. Wilson, still irked by Carranza's hostility over American intervention, threw his support to Francisco "Pancho" Villa. The wily, peasant-born general had broken from the government, and with Emiliano Zapata, another peasant leader, he kept a rebellion flickering.

A year later, when Wilson finally accepted reality and recognized the Carranza regime, Villa turned against the United States. In January 1916 he abducted 17 Americans from a train in Mexico and executed them. In March, after months of shooting up border towns, he galloped into Columbus, New Mexico, killed 19 people, and left the town in flames. While Senator Henry Cabot Lodge denounced Villa as a murderous peon, Wilson sent 11,000 troops into Mexico to capture him.

Led by General John "Black Jack" Pershing (who would later command the American Expeditionary Force in Europe), the army chased Villa across northern Mexico on horseback, in automobiles, and with airplanes. There were bloody skirmishes with Mexican troops, but not Villa; he and his rebels eluded the Americans for several months. As the goose chase turned wilder and wilder, Carranza withdrew his consent for U.S. troops to invade Mexican soil. Early in 1917 Wilson ordered Pershing home. The "punitive expedition," as the president called it, poisoned Mexican–American relations for the next 30 years.

Like a good progressive, Wilson had wanted "to teach the South American republics to elect good men." Condescending and impatient, he failed to realize the irrelevance of his bright vision and the presumptuousness of his methods. Imposing progressive ideals of law, democracy, and gradual reform on an impoverished country like Mexico, riven with class, racial, and ethnic strife and torn by revolution, virtually guaranteed a hostile reception.

THE ROAD TO WAR

In the century before the world order shattered in 1914, Europe's population had more than tripled. As the ranks of its middle and working classes swelled, discontent with industrial society deepened. Antagonisms among rival empires grew; nationalism rose and militarism flourished alongside it. These profound social strains led Europe down the road to war.

In theory—the theory of hard-nosed, "realistic" diplomats—war should not have come. A system of interlocking alliances, fashioned by Europe's great powers

General John J. "Black Jack" Pershing led U.S. forces into Mexico on a "punitive action" to catch rebel leader Pancho Villa "dead or alive." Villa (pictured below) eluded the Americans for several months before they abandoned the expedition. Audacious and ruthless, he was worshiped by Mexican peasants, who extolled his exploits in folktales and ballads after his assassination in 1923.

at the turn of the century, was designed to maintain a reasonable balance of power. But what was reasonable? Led by the stiff-necked Kaiser Wilhelm II, Germany dreamed of a glorious empire and allied itself with Turkey and Austria–Hungary. The established imperialist powers—England and France—had committed themselves to Germany's foe, Russia, promising one another guns and troops in case of war. By the summer of 1914 Europe was a powder keg ready to explode.

The Guns of August

The unlikely spark was Archduke Franz Ferdinand, benign heir to the Austro–Hungarian throne. On June 28, 1914, the archduke and his wife were gunned down by a Slavic nationalist. Austria–Hungary mobilized to punish Serbia, which was rumored to be responsible for the assassination. Mobilization prompted a protective response from Russia (with 6 million men, the largest army in Europe) on behalf of the Serbs and led Germany and France to call out their troops. On July 28, after a month of insincere demands for apologies, Austria attacked Serbia. Early in August German siege cannons with barrels the size of freight cars and shells a yard long hammered the forts of neutral Belgium. The Germans were marching on France, and these guns of August heralded the first global war.

Germany's plan for a quick knockout blow against France not only failed but also set in motion a chain of events that ultimately brought most of the world's major powers into the war. By early August, five German columns were slicing west through Belgium toward Paris. "The smell of half a million unbathed men," wrote a news reporter, hung about Belgian towns for days, nauseating evidence of an invading army again on the move. Meanwhile 11,000 trains carrying nearly 2 million soldiers sped across eastern Europe to Russia. Great Britain, responding to the violation of Belgium's neutrality and rallying to aid the French, declared war on Germany on August 4, 1914.

One by one the other industrial nations were drawn in: Japan and Italy to the side of "Allies" Britain, France, and Russia; Bulgaria, Rumania, and Greece to "Central Powers" Germany, Austria–Hungary, and Turkey. Armies fought from the deserts of North Africa and the Near East to the plains of Flanders; fleets battled off the coasts of Chile and Sumatra. Soldiers came from as far away as Australia and India. Nearly 8 million never went home.

American Neutrality

The outbreak of war in Europe shocked most Americans. Few were prepared to do anything about it. Among them was President Wilson, who called an emergency cabinet meeting to issue a declaration of neutrality and to approve a plan for evacuating Americans stranded in Belgium. Then he hurried to the bedside of his wife, whose failing health absorbed him throughout the crisis. Early in August, as Germany marched on France and Russia, Ellen Wilson died. For an instant the president seemed near collapse. Personal grief mixed with contempt as he watched Europe disembowel itself. "The more I read about the conflict across the seas," Wilson wrote a friend, "the more open it seems to me to utter condemnation."

Wilson slowly came to see in the calamity an opportunity for a new world order. Neutral America would lead warring nations to "a peace without victory."

THE COURSE OF WAR IN EUROPE, 1914–1917
When World War I erupted between the Central and Allied Powers in 1914, few countries in Europe remained neutral. The armies of the Central Powers penetrated as far west as France and as far east as Russia, but by 1917 the European war had settled into a hideous standoff along a deadly line of trenches on the western front.

Selfish nationalism would give way to cooperative internationalism, Christian charity and fellowship would replace power politics, progressive faith in reason and gradual change would triumph over irrational conflict. Everything hinged on American neutrality. Only if the country stood above the fray could America achieve a higher peace. Americans, Wilson declared in 1914, must remain "neutral in fact as well as in name, impartial in thought as well as action."

Neutrality would be difficult, but impartiality was impossible. Nearly 9 million Americans of German and Austrian descent naturally had sympathy for the Central Powers, while Irish-Americans, almost 5 million in number, shared those sympathies on the grounds of England's centuries-old domination of Ireland. On the other hand, the bonds of language, culture, and history tied the majority of Americans to Great Britain. Wilson himself, who had long venerated British institutions of government and law, could not escape feeling tugged toward the Allies. Meanwhile gratitude for French aid during the American Revolution still lived. When the first American division marched through Paris years later, its commander stopped to salute Lafayette's tomb with the cry, "Nous voilà, Lafayette!"— Lafayette, we are here!

Germany aroused different sentiments. Although some progressives admired German social reforms, most Americans saw Germany as an iron military power bent on world conquest. For years newspapers had featured photographs of the uniformed Kaiser, strutting arrogantly, a monocle clutched in his eye, looking like an imperial robber baron. Americans read British propaganda—some based on real events, some manufactured, some merely embellished—of the pillage of innocent Belgium, the rape of its women, the murder of its children, and the destruction of its national treasures, all by spike-helmeted, bayonet-wielding "Huns."

Even though hundreds of young Americans slipped across the border to enlist in the Canadian army, most of their fellow citizens felt that neutrality was the wisest course. Before the war a peace movement had taken seed in the United States, nourished in 1910 by a gift of $10 million from Andrew Carnegie. In 1914 a host of social justice reformers, led by Jane Addams, Charlotte Perkins Gilman, and Lillian Wald, condemned the war as the offspring of militarists, munitions makers, and imperialists. They founded the Women's International League for Peace and Freedom and the American Union Against Militarism. Calling on Wilson to convene a peace conference, they lobbied for open diplomacy, disarmament, an end to colonial empires, and an international organization to settle disputes.

Even as pacifists pressed for peace, American economic ties to Britain and France created a tangible investment in Allied victory. Commanding the seas, Great Britain drew on American resources—munitions, arms, food, and fibers. Between 1914 and 1916 trade with the Allies more than tripled, from $800 million to $3 billion. After faltering briefly in 1914, the American economy boomed with the flood of war orders. The Allies eventually borrowed over $2 billion from American banks to finance their purchases. By contrast, a British blockade reduced American "contraband" commerce with the Central Powers to a trickle.

The Diplomacy of Neutrality

The blockade sorely tested Wilson's patience with Great Britain. British warships forced American vessels into port and seized cargoes. The British navy mined the North Sea. British censors opened American mail to Europe. British authorities refused to allow the United States to trade with Germany's neutral neighbors. They even barred British companies from dealing with "blacklisted" American firms that did business with Germany. Wilson insisted that the Allies respect the trading rights of neutral nations, but he never forced the issues of freedom of the seas and commercial rights to the point of rupture. He feared that strong retaliation, such as embargoing arms to the Allies, would deprive Britain of its most powerful weapon—the navy—and tip the balance toward Germany, a land power.

Dependent on American supplies, the British pursued a policy of reducing German–American trade without souring British–American relations. When Britain forbade cotton from being sold to the Central Powers in 1915, it arranged to buy American surpluses. It also agreed to compensate American firms for their losses when the war was over. By the end of 1915 the United States had all but accepted the British blockade of Germany, while American supplies continued to flow to England. True neutrality was dead as America became the quartermaster of the Allied war effort.

While Wilson looked for diplomatic leverage to bring the belligerents to the peace table, Secretary of State Bryan called for "real neutrality," evenhanded treatment of all combatants. On those grounds he opposed loans to the Allies. "Money," Bryan said in 1914, "is the worst of all contrabands because it commands everything else." Later that year he gave in, only to become embroiled in a hot debate over a dreadful new weapon—the submarine.

Early in 1915 Germany mounted a counterblockade of Great Britain with two dozen submarines, or *Unterseeboote*, called U-boats. Before submarines, sea raiders generally were required to stop their targets, examine their cargoes, and allow crews and passengers to escape. If the U-boats surfaced to obey these conventions, they risked being rammed or blown from the water. So submarines attacked without warning and spared no lives. In February 1915 Berlin announced that U-boats would torpedo enemy vessels within a war zone around the British Isles. Even neutral ships were at risk, since British vessels often flew neutral flags as cover. Invoking international law and national honor, President Wilson threatened to hold Germany to "strict accountability" for any American losses. Germany promised not to sink any American ships, but within a month a new issue—the safety of American passengers on belligerent vessels—claimed the headlines.

On the morning of May 7, 1915, the British passenger liner *Lusitania* appeared out of a fog bank off the coast of Ireland on its way from New York to Southampton. The commander of the German U-20 could hardly believe his eyes as the giant ship, displacing some 30,000 tons, filled the viewfinder of his periscope. He fired a single torpedo. A tremendous roar followed as one of the *Lusitania*'s main boilers exploded. The ship stopped dead in the water and soon listed so badly that lifeboats could barely be launched. Within 18 minutes it slid beneath the waves with a sound, recalled one survivor, "like a terrible moan." Nearly 1200 men, women, and children perished, including 128 Americans.

Former President Theodore Roosevelt charged that such an "act of piracy" demanded war against Germany. Wilson, horrified at this "murder on the high seas," still urged restraint. "There is such a thing as a man being too proud to fight," he said a few days later. "There is such a thing as a nation being so right that it does not need to convince others by force." Instead he sent three notes of protest demanding that Germany disavow submarine warfare, compensate the victims, and agree to stop sinking passenger liners. Secretary Bryan wanted equal protests lodged against both German submarines and the British blockaders. He suspected that the *Lusitania* carried munitions and was thus a legitimate target. To "rely on passengers to protect her from attack," Bryan argued, was "like putting women and children in front of an army." In Wilson's mind the two were scarcely equivalent. The blockade killed only trade; submarines killed people. Rather than endorse the policy, Bryan resigned and was replaced as secretary of state by Robert Lansing, a pro-Allied lawyer in the State Department.

Germany, battling on two fronts in Europe, wanted to keep the United States out of the war. When two Americans died in August 1915 after the torpedoing of the British steamer *Arabic*, Germany apologized, offered an indemnity, and pledged not to sink passenger liners without warning. But in February 1916 a desperate Germany declared submarine warfare on all *armed* vessels, belligerent or neutral. A month later a U-boat commander mistook the French steamer *Sussex* for a mine layer and torpedoed the unarmed vessel as it ferried passengers and freight across the English Channel. Several Americans were injured. The *Arabic* pledge seemed suddenly empty.

Pressed to the breaking point, Wilson issued an ultimatum on April 18. If Germany failed to stop sinking nonmilitary vessels, the United States would cut diplomatic relations. War would surely follow. Without enough U-boats to control the seas, the Kaiser accepted. According to the *Sussex* pledge of May 4, 1916,

The ideal of neat, sharply defined spaces for living and fighting is exemplified by these model trenches in northern France (left). Trench warfare, wrote one general, was "marked by uniform formations, the regulation of space and time by higher commands down to the smallest details . . . fixed distances between units and individuals." The reality (below) was something else again.

Germany agreed to Wilson's terms, all but abandoning the submarine campaign. For a time tensions between the two countries eased. The *Sussex* pledge gave Wilson a major victory, but with a grave risk. His ultimatum was so tough that if Germany resumed unrestricted submarine attacks, the honor and prestige of the United States would require war. "Any little German [U-boat] commander," Wilson told his cabinet, "can put us into the war at any time by some calculated outrage."

Preparedness

While pacifist groups condemned the war and any hint of involvement in it, corporate leaders and Republican party spokesmen claimed the nation was woefully unprepared to fight or even to keep peace. The army numbered only 80,000 men in 1914, the navy just 37 battleships and a handful of new "dreadnoughts," or supercruisers. Advocates of "preparedness" called for a navy larger than Great Britain's, an army of millions of reservists, and universal military training.

Wilson at first resisted efforts to "turn America into a military camp," even when Theodore Roosevelt criticized him for "milk and water" diplomacy. As his frustration with German submarines rose, Wilson ordered the War Department to plan for military expansion. In November 1915 he proposed a volunteer army of 400,000, and in January 1916 he toured the country promoting preparedness and promising "a navy second to none."

By the middle of 1916 Wilson's steady pressure persuaded Congress to double the army, increase the National Guard, and begin construction of the largest navy in the world. To foot the bill progressives pushed through new graduated taxes on incomes and estates as well as additional levies on corporate profits. Higher rates on the wealthy would largely underwrite the preparedness program. Whoever paid for it, most Americans in 1916 were thinking of preparedness for peace, not war.

The Election of 1916

As the Democratic National Convention opened in St. Louis in June 1916, former New York Governor Martin Glynn was determined to talk of Americanism and preparedness, just as President Wilson had instructed. Glynn began what he expected to be a dull recitation of the precedents for American neutrality. Warming to his audience, he cited case after case of Wilson's diplomatic maneuvers, each one punctuated with screams of "What did we do? What did we do?" from the crowd. "We didn't go to war! We didn't go to war!" Glynn shouted back. The next day Wilson was renominated by acclamation. Within weeks his campaign had taken up "He Kept Us Out of War" as its slogan. The Democrats had discovered the political power of peace.

The Republicans had already nominated Charles Evans Hughes, a moderate progressive, the former governor of New York, and later a Supreme Court justice. With his endorsement of "straight and honest" neutrality, Hughes too endorsed

THE ELECTION OF 1916

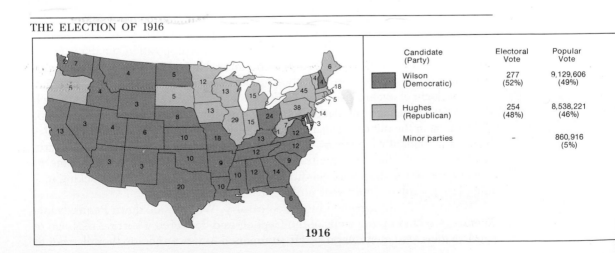

Candidate (Party)	Electoral Vote	Popular Vote
Wilson (Democratic)	277 (52%)	9,129,606 (49%)
Hughes (Republican)	254 (48%)	8,538,221 (46%)
Minor parties	–	860,916 (5%)

1916

peace. It won the loyalty of German-American voters, whether he liked it or not. Hughes also turned away from the saber rattling of Theodore Roosevelt, whose presidential overtures were spurned by party leaders. "The country wasn't in a heroic mood," Roosevelt wrote soon after the Republican convention. As the election approached, Democrats took full-page advertisements in newspapers across the country: "If You Want WAR, Vote for HUGHES! If You Want Peace with Honor VOTE FOR WILSON!" Voters liked the pledge enough to give Wilson a slender majority. He carried the South and key states in the Midwest and West on the tide of prosperity, progressive reform, and promises of peace. As the British ambassador reported, "Americans desire nothing so much as to keep out of war."

The Final Peace Offensive

Twice since 1915 Wilson had sent Colonel House to European capitals in behind-the-scenes attempts to negotiate a peace settlement. With the election over, Wilson opened his final peace offensive. But when he asked the belligerents to state their terms for a cease-fire, neither the Allies nor the Central Powers accepted. Total war had committed both sides totally to victory. Frustrated, fearful, and genuinely agonized, Wilson in a dramatic speech to the Senate on January 22, 1917, called for "a peace without victory." There could be no victor or vanquished, only "a peace among equals."

As Wilson spoke a fleet of U-boats cruised north toward the British Isles. Weeks earlier German military leaders had persuaded the Kaiser to take one last gamble to starve the Allies into submission in six months. On January 31, 1917, the German ambassador in Washington informed Secretary of State Lansing that unrestricted submarine warfare would be resumed the next day.

The collapse of his dream to keep the country from war shook Wilson, but still he clung to it. As he told Secretary of State Lansing, the future of "'white civilization' and its domination over the world rested largely on our ability to keep this country intact." On February 4 Wilson severed relations with Germany, though later that month Congress refused his bill to arm merchant ships. Then British authorities handed him an intercepted telegram from the German foreign secretary, Arthur Zimmermann, to the Kaiser's ambassador in Mexico. In the event of war, the ambassador was instructed to offer Mexico guns and money to attack the United States. After victory, Mexico would receive its "lost territory in Texas, New Mexico, and Arizona." Wilson released the Zimmermann telegram to the press on March 1. Stunned and outraged, the House of Representatives passed Wilson's bill immediately, but La Follette and other opposition senators stalled until the session ran out. On March 9, acting on his own, Wilson ordered gun crews aboard merchant ships and thereafter told them to shoot U-boats on sight.

The logic of events now propelled a reluctant nation toward war. On March 12 U-boats torpedoed the American merchant vessel *Algonquin*. On March 15, with Russia in the midst of a shattering revolution, the abdication of Czar Nicholas II threw a major ally into chaos. By the end of the month U-boats had sunk nearly 600,000 tons of Allied and neutral shipping. For the first time reports came to Washington of the desperate condition of Allied armies and of their cracking morale. The president could wait no longer.

On April 2, accompanied by armed cavalry, Wilson rode down Pennsylvania Avenue, trudged up the steps of the Capitol, and delivered a stirring message of war to a joint session of Congress. He summoned Americans not to their flag but to a higher purpose: "the ultimate peace of the world and for the liberation of its people, the German people included: for the rights of nations great and small . . . to choose their way of life." "The world," he said, "must be made safe for democracy." The United States had to enter "the most terrible and disastrous of wars." "God helping her, she can do no other."

Despite opposition (6 votes in the Senate; 50 in the House), the war resolution passed quickly. American entry into the war boosted Allied confidence at a critical moment. Wilson had not wanted war, but now it seemed the only way to realize his vision of a higher peace.

WAR AND SOCIETY

The first "world war" enlisted whole societies in the pursuit of victory. Governments not only fielded armies, but they mobilized industry, controlled labor, and rationed food as well. For the first time civilians died in air attacks. In 1915 the German Zeppelin L-13, hovering at 8000 feet, dropped a load of bombs that killed 17 Londoners. In the United States, despite substantial opposition to the war, traditions of cooperation and volunteerism led people to pull together. Even though its citizens never came under direct attack, war still shaped American society in peculiarly progressive ways.

The Slaughter of Stalemate

While the United States prepared to win the Great War, the Allies were coming perilously close to losing it. They had halted the initial German assault at the River Marne, north of Paris, in September 1914. The war then settled into a grisly stalemate. A continuous, immovable front stretched from Flanders to the border of Switzerland. Troops dug ditches, six to eight feet deep and four to five feet wide, to escape bullets, grenades, and artillery. Twenty-five thousand miles of these "trenches"—enough to circle the globe—cut a muddy scar across Europe. Men lived in them for years, prey to disease, lice, and a plague of rats. One British sergeant left a tomcat in the mess hall overnight to dispose of the rodents. He returned the next morning to find the cat disposed of, fur and all.

The military fruits of industrial technology turned all assaults into bloodbaths. Soldiers bravely charged "over the top," only to be shredded by machine guns that fired 600 rounds a minute. Poison gas choked them in their tracks. Barbed wire strung them out and made them easy targets. Giant howitzers lobbed shells on them from positions too distant to see. "The advantage is all with the shell," wrote one veteran, "and you have no comeback." The German siege of Verdun in 1916 cost 680,000 lives; later that year a million men died in the valley of the Somme River during four months of fighting. Even in quiet times 7000 British soldiers were killed or wounded every day. Only late in the war did new armored "landships"—code-named "tanks"—return the advantage to the offense by surmounting the trench barriers with their caterpillar treads.

By then Vladimir Lenin, a revolutionary Marxist exiled to Switzerland during the early stages of the Russian Revolution, was speeding home to Petrograd aboard a special train provided by the Germans. In November 1917 he led the

Bolshevik party to power in Russia, and in December his lieutenant, Leon Trotsky, opened peace negotiations with Germany in the Polish city of Brest-Litovsk. While Russia lapsed into civil war, Germany transferred a million soldiers to the western front in preparation for the spring offensive. A dispirited Allied army settled in for another cold winter. "We will wait," said a French commander, "for the tanks and the Americans."

"You're in the Army Now"

Many Americans went to war assuming their role would be limited to economic and military aid. "Congress," a prominent senator had declared in mid-April 1917, "will not permit American soldiers to be sent to Europe." The Allies' desperate plight forced the General Staff of the Army into a crash program for sending a million men to Europe by the spring of 1918. To raise such a fighting force, Congress passed the Selective Service Act in May 1917. Feelings about the draft ran from strong opposition to enthusiastic support. "There is precious little difference," protested Democratic House Speaker "Champ" Clark in 1917, "between a conscript and a convict." Progressives were more inclined to see military service as an opportunity to overcome class antagonisms in America: "Universal [military] training will jumble the boys of America all together, . . . smashing all the petty class distinctions that now divide, and prompting a brand of real democracy."

After local draft boards opened their doors, 24 million men registered. Almost 3 million Americans were drafted; another 2 million volunteered. Most were white, and all were young, between the ages of 21 and 31. Several thousand women served as clerks, telephone operators, and nurses. But there were people who opposed the war and military service. A handful of tenant farmers, blacks, and Indians in two Oklahoma counties protested in the "Green Corn Rebellion." Official reports put the number of draft evaders at 300,000, though many more went unreported. Others, including some 4000 conscientious objectors, simply requested exemptions.

Most of the 2 million American troops who landed in Europe looked forward to service. "Here was our one great chance for excitement and risk," wrote a volunteer later. "We could not afford to pass it up." In a nation of immigrants, nearly one draftee in five had been born in another country. Training often aimed at educating and Americanizing ethnic recruits. In special "development battalions" drill sergents barked out orders while volunteers from the YMCA taught American history and English. Not all camps sought assimilation. "We are not in this war to make American citizens," read a staff report, "we are in to win the war." At Camp Gordon in Georgia, Italians and Slavs drilled full-time in two distinct units. Commanders spoke their languages; chefs cooked them Italian and Slavic dishes; and no one bothered with Americanization.

African-Americans volunteered in disproportionately high numbers and quickly filled the four rigidly segregated Regular Army and eight National Guard units that already existed for them. White officers commanded almost every one. A training program at Fort Des Moines graduated a single class of 639 black officers, all below field rank and all assigned to one experimental division—controlled by whites. Historically barred from skilled trades and often too poor to support their families, blacks failed to get exemptions at the same rate as whites. They made up about 10 percent of the population but 13 percent of the draftees. Only one in five sent to France actually saw combat (compared to two of every three whites). Southern Democrats had opposed training African-Americans to arms, fearful of the prospect of putting "arrogant, strutting representatives of black soldiery in every community." Most were trained for menial tasks, serving as stevedores aboard navy ships in the Atlantic and common laborers in support units in Europe.

Racial violence sometimes exploded among the troops. The worst episode occurred in Houston in the summer of 1917. Seasoned black regulars, harassed by white soldiers and the city's Jim Crow laws, rioted and killed 17 white civilians. Their whole battalion was disarmed and sent under arrest to New Mexico. Thirteen troopers were condemned to death and hanged within days, too quickly for appeals even to be filed.

The progressive impulse did not ignore an army often in need of reforming. Testing intelligence became a standard procedure for all recruits, most of whom had fewer than seven years of education (for immigrants, fewer than five; for southern blacks, fewer than three). One in four could not read at all. "Mental meddlers," as one general called the psychologists, administered new intelligence tests to inductees. The impersonal tests were an improvement over impression, prejudice, and personal influence. Yet what at the time seemed such a scientific advance in organizational management often measured little more than class origins. Questions such as "Who wrote 'The Raven'?" and "Where was the Overland car manufactured?" exposed background rather than intelligence. More than half the Russian, Italian, and Polish draftees and almost 80 percent of blacks showed up as "inferior." The army stopped the testing program in January 1919, but schools across the country adopted it after the war, reinforcing prevailing ethnic and racial prejudices.

New recruits, including these black ones at Camp Meade in Maryland, were each issued a clothing slip, which was then stamped with a number.

While war raged in Europe, moral crusaders waged a war against sin at home. Temperance leaders pressured the War Department to prohibit the sale of liquor to anyone in uniform in the vicinity of training camps. The army also declared war on venereal disease. "A Soldier who gets a dose is a Traitor!" warned one poster. The Commission on Training Camp Activities produced thousands of pamphlets, films, and lectures on dangers of sexual misconduct. The drive constituted the first serious sex education many young Americans had ever received. When Premier Clemenceau generously offered to establish licensed houses of prostitution, customary for French troops, Secretary of War Newton Baker exclaimed, "My God . . . don't show this to the President or he'll stop the war."

Mobilizing the Economy

To arm, clothe, feed, and transport an army of nearly 5 million required a coordinated national effort. The production of a single ammunition shell brought more than a dozen components from every section of the country (plus vital nitrates shipped from Chile through the Panama Canal) to assembly plants in New Jersey, Virginia, and Pennsylvania and from there to military installations or Atlantic ports. At the Treasury Department Secretary William Gibbs McAdoo fretted over how to finance the war, which cost, finally, $32 billion, at a time when the entire national debt ran to only $2 billion. New taxes paid about a third of the war costs. The rest came from loans financed through "Liberty" and "Victory" bonds and war savings certificates.

Bond drives served a dual purpose. They raised national fervor as well as money. "We capitalized the profound impulse called patriotism," McAdoo explained. At huge rallies, celebrities exhorted Americans to buy bonds. Boy Scouts sold them under the slogan "Every Scout to Save a Soldier." All five bond issues were oversubscribed—and no wonder. "Every person who refuses to subscribe," McAdoo told a crowd in California, ". . . is a friend of Germany." The Federal Reserve System expanded the money supply to make borrowing easier. By 1920 the national debt climbed to $20 billion, and, through inflation, the consumer price index nearly doubled from 1916.

With sweeping grants of authority under the Overman Act (1918) and other new statutes, President Wilson constructed a massive bureaucracy to run the home front. What actually emerged was a managed economy, similar to the New Nationalism envisioned by Theodore Roosevelt. Nearly 5000 new executive agencies employed thousands of business leaders, the readiest source of expert managers. For a nominal "dollar-a-year," they served their country and built a partnership between business and government. Industrial and trade associations such as the Chamber of Commerce tied industry to a network of federal agencies. It was never clear who gained most. Antitrust suits, as the attorney general later recalled, were simply put "to sleep until the war was over." Business influence grew, and corporate profits tripled.

With rapid conversion on such a grand scale, bottlenecks inevitably occurred. In March 1918 mounting criticism led Wilson to name Wall Street wizard Bernard Baruch to the War Industries Board (WIB) with orders to sort out the mess. Under Baruch's leadership, the WIB had the authority to set production schedules, allocate resources, standardize procedures, and coordinate government purchases. Aware that such broad powers might be deemed unconstitutional, Baruch worked indirectly. Lucrative contracts helped him persuade manufacturers to shift to war goods. The WIB covered all costs and guaranteed a profit. When a businessman refused WIB requests, Baruch threatened to marshal public opinion to make him "such an object of contempt and scorn in your home town that you will not dare to show your face there."

As war made battlefields out of wheat fields in Europe, the government encouraged American farmers to make up the loss. The Lever Act (1917) authorized Wilson to create the Food Administration. Herbert Hoover, who had saved starving refugees as chairman of the Commission for Relief in Belgium in 1914, was appointed administrator. Like Baruch, Hoover mobilized what he called "the spirit of self-sacrifice." Huge publicity campaigns promoted "wheatless" and "meatless" days each week and encouraged families to plant "victory" gardens. Half a million people went door to door to enlist housewives in the cause of food conservation. "Do not permit your child to take a bite or two from an apple and throw the rest away; nowadays even children must be taught to be patriotic to the core," joked *Life*. Spurred by high prices, farmers brought ever more marginal lands into cultivation, as their real income increased 25 percent. When in later years prices fell and rain did not, both farmers and their land would suffer from the rush to maximize profits and production.

A Fuel Administration met the army's energy needs by increasing production and limiting domestic consumption. Transportation snarls required more drastic action. In December 1917 the U.S. Railroad Administration simply took over rail lines for the duration of the war. Government coordination, together with a new system of permits, got freight moving. Federally imposed "daylight savings time" stretched the workday and saved fuel as well. Railroad workers turned out to be among the chief beneficiaries of nationalization. Their wages grew by $300 million. Treasury Secretary McAdoo, a master organizer who also served as railroad administrator, ordered equal pay for women and fought discrimination against blacks. Railroad unions won government recognition, an eight-hour day, and a grievance procedure. For the first time in decades labor unrest subsided and trains finally ran on schedule.

The size and scope of government increased enormously during the 18 months of American participation in the war. The number of federal employees soared from just under 400,000 in 1916 to over 850,000 by 1918. The modern bureaucratic state received a powerful boost. Speeding trends already under way, a host of federal agencies and committees centralized authority and cooperated with business and labor to meet the demands of war. The wartime bureaucracy was quickly dismantled at the end of the war, but it set a powerful precedent for the future.

War Work

The war benefited working men and women, though not as much as their employers. Government contracts guaranteed high wages, an eight-hour day, and equal pay for comparable work. To keep people on the job, federal contracting agencies encouraged employers to "manage" personnel. Arsenal officers and munitions contractors attended special classes at Dartmouth College to learn the young science of personnel management. American industry moved one step closer to the

War posters exhorted Americans to pull together for victory.

"welfare capitalism" of the 1920s, in which employers used profit-sharing, company unions, and personnel departments to forestall worker discontent.

During the war, personnel management was not enough to guarantee industrial peace. In 1917 American workers called 4450 strikes, the most in American history. To keep factories running smoothly, President Wilson created the National War Labor Board (NWLB) early in 1918. The NWLB arbitrated over 1000 labor disputes, helped to increase wages and decrease hours, and established overtime pay. In return for pledges not to strike, it guaranteed the rights of unions to organize and bargain collectively. NWLB examiners oversaw elections for shop committees in the steel industry, long impervious to unionization. When the Smith and Wesson arms plant in Springfield, Massachusetts, and the Western Union telegraph company discriminated against union employees, the government commandeered both firms.

Given such sympathetic federal support, organized labor grew. President Samuel Gompers of the American Federation of Labor (AFL), the nation's largest union, represented labor on Wilson's National Defense Council and later on the War Labor Board. Membership in the AFL increased from 2.7 million members in 1916 to nearly 4 million in 1919. On Armistice Day Gompers complained that labor had yet to achieve all the gains it needed. What rights had been won, Gompers justifiably feared, would end with peace.

War work sparked massive internal migrations of labor to meet shortages as the war choked off immigration from abroad and the draft depleted manpower at home. Factory owners scoured the country for a fresh labor supply. Industrial cities, no matter how small, soon swelled with newcomers. Between 1917 and 1920, some 100,000 Mexicans crossed the border into Texas, California, New Mexico, and Arizona. Some Mexican-Americans left segregated barrios in the West for northern war plants. Most worked on farms and ranches, freed from military service by the deferment of all agricultural labor.

Northern labor agents fanned out across the South to recruit young blacks. African-American newspapers like the Chicago *Defender* summoned them north to the "Land of Hope." "I beg you, my brother, to leave the benighted land," urged one editor. "Get out of the South." Over the war years more than 400,000 migrated to the booming industrial centers of the North. The number of African-Americans in Chicago more than doubled. In Cleveland it quadrupled; in Detroit it jumped sixfold. Towns like Hattiesburg, Mississippi, were decimated by the drain. Finally, under pressure from southern politicians, the U.S. Employment Service suspended its program to assist blacks moving north.

Largely unskilled and semiskilled, blacks took factory jobs in the steel mills of Pennsylvania, the war plants of Massachusetts, and the brickyards of New Jersey. Mostly rural backgrounds left them unprepared for life in the city. The new arrivals, noted one magazine, were often "crowded into dark rooms, . . . shivering with the cold from which they do not know how to protect themselves." The Urban League and other voluntary organizations tried to meet the housing shortage, but the basic problems—high rents and low wages—remained unresolved.

W. E. B. Du Bois and other African-American leaders urged their followers to "forget our special grievances and close our ranks shoulder to shoulder with our own white fellow citizens." So they did, deferring dreams of equality and material gain until the war was over. In France, where 200,000 blacks served, only 42,000 saw combat. Four regiments of the all-black 93rd Division, brigaded with the French army, were among the first Americans in the trenches and among the most decorated units in the U.S. Army. Three of the regiments later received the Croix de Guerre for heroism.

At home the war aggravated racial tensions. Southern lynching parties murdered 38 blacks in 1917 and 58 in 1918. In 1919, after the war ended, more than 70 were hung, some still in uniform. Housing shortages and job competition helped to spark race riots across the North. In almost every city blacks, stirred by war rhetoric of freedom and democracy, showed new militancy by fighting back. In mid-1917 some 40 blacks and 9 whites died when East St. Louis erupted in racial violence. During the bloody "red summer" of 1919 race wars broke out in Washington, D.C., Omaha, Nebraska, and New York City. In July a two-week reign of racial terror began in Chicago after whites stoned a black who had drifted into their section of a segregated beach. Thousands were burned out of their homes, hundreds injured, and 38 killed—15 whites and 23 blacks.

Just as the war lured African-Americans to northern factories, it brought as many as a million more women into the labor force. Most were young and single. Sometimes they took over jobs once held by men as railroad engineers, drill press operators, and electric lift truck drivers. The prewar trend toward higher paying jobs temporarily intensified. More and more women worked in offices, schools, hospitals, and telephone exchanges. Some of the most spectacular gains in defense and government work evaporated after the war. When the country demobilized, tens of thousands of women lost jobs as army nurses, defense workers, and war time administrators. Agencies such as the Women's Service Section of the Railroad Administration, which fought sexual harassment and discrimination, simply went out of business, while organized labor remained hostile.

The constraints of war brought more women than ever into the job market. These women work on a production line manufacturing bullets. The novelty of the situation seems evident from the fashionable high-heeled high-button shoes that they wear—ill-suited to the conditions in an armaments plant.

Propaganda and Civil Liberties

"Once lead this people into war," President Wilson said before American entry into the conflict, "and they'll forget there ever was such a thing as tolerance." Americans did succumb to a ruthless hysteria during World War I, but they had help. Intense prewar opposition to American participation coupled with pressing fears over public apathy led the president to create the Committee on Public Information (CPI), headed by George Creel, a California newspaperman. Surrounding himself with old muckrakers such as Ida Tarbell and Ray Stannard Baker, Creel launched what he called "a fight for the *minds* of men, for the 'conquest of their convictions.'" The CPI mobilized artists to design colorful war posters, including James Flagg's famous "I Want *You* for the U.S. Army." It distributed 75 million pamphlets, issued 6000 press releases, and sponsored war expositions attended by 10 million people in two dozen cities.

Initially committed to a simple "faith in the fact," the CPI soon developed into the most powerful propaganda mill the nation had ever known. An army of "Four-Minute Men," 75,000 fast-talking orators, invaded movie theaters, lodge halls, schools, and churches to keep patriotism at "white heat" with four minutes of war tirades. The CPI organized "Loyalty Leagues" in ethnic communities and sponsored parades and rallies, including a much-publicized immigrant "pilgrimage" to the birthplace of George Washington. Such propaganda often worked. People whose anthem had been the pacifist song "I Didn't Raise My Boy to Be a Soldier" were singing George M. Cohan's patriotic "Over There" six months later.

The line between patriotic appeal and intolerance proved impossible to maintain. Overly enthusiastic parents enlisted their five-year-olds in paramilitary clubs like the "Khaki Babes." As war hysteria mounted, volunteerism blossomed into an orgy of "100-percent Americanism." Immigrants, aliens, radicals, and pacifists came under suspicion as a coercive urge to conformity took hold. German-Americans naturally became special targets. Local influenza epidemics were blamed on German spies contaminating water supplies. In Iowa the governor made it a crime to speak German in public. Hamburgers were renamed "Salisbury steak"; German measles, "liberty measles." In April 1918 a mob outside of St. Louis seized Robert Praeger, a naturalized German-American who had tried to enlist in the navy, bound him in an American flag, and lynched him. After deliberating for 25 minutes a jury found the leaders not guilty.

In 1917 Congress gave hysteria more legal bite. The Espionage Act provided $10,000 fines and 20-year sentences for anyone convicted of obstructing military operations (including recruitment), aiding the enemy, or mailing treasonous material. In 1918 the Sedition Act outlawed in one broad stroke "any disloyal, profane, scurrilous, or abusive language about the form of government of the United States, or the Constitution of the United States, or the flag of the United States, or the uniform of the Army or Navy." Under these acts, 1500 citizens were arrested for offenses including denouncing the draft, criticizing the Red Cross, and complaining about taxes. Opponents of the war, especially radical groups, suffered most. The Industrial Workers of the World (IWW), a militant labor union centered in western states, saw the war as a battle among capitalists and threatened to strike mining and lumber companies in an anti-war protest. In September 1917 federal agents raided the Chicago headquarters of the IWW—familiarly known as the "Wobblies"—seized membership lists and office equipment, and arrested 113 of its leaders in the name of patriotism. The crusade succeeded in destroying the union.

Similarly, when the Socialist party stridently opposed the "capitalist" war, the postmaster general banned a dozen Socialist publications from the mail, though the party was a legal organization that had elected mayors, municipal officials, and congressmen. In June 1918 government agents arrested Eugene V. Debs, the Socialist candidate in the presidential election of 1912, for an antiwar speech to the Socialist convention in Canton, Ohio. Promptly found guilty of sedition, Debs received a 10-year sentence. Running for the presidency from his jail cell in 1920, he received nearly 1 million votes.

The Supreme Court endorsed the aggressive wartime assaults on civil liberties and dissent. In *Schenck v. United States* (1919), the Court unanimously affirmed the conviction of a Socialist party officer who had mailed pamphlets urging potential army inductees to resist the draft. "When a nation is at war," wrote Justice Oliver Wendell Holmes, Jr., "many things that might be said in time of peace are such a hindrance to its effort that their utterance will not be endured." Schenck's pamphlets, Holmes concluded, created "a clear and present danger" for the safety of the nation. Holmes and his associate Louis Brandeis later sought to narrow the scope of the *Schenck* decision, but in *Abrams v. United States* (1919) the majority upheld, by 7–2, the verdict against Russian immigrant Jacob Abrams, whose pamphlets had denounced an American intervention in Russia to fight the Bolsheviks. Although Holmes saw no "clear and present danger," the Court ruled that the pamphlets tended to discourage the American war effort.

Over There

American forces began to reach France in the fall of 1917, but it was not until March 1918 and the German spring offensive that they helped to turn the tide. General John Pershing, commander of the American Expeditionary Force (AEF), wisely held his raw troops out of battle for several months of additional training. Pershing had kept his force separate, in part because American politicians wanted the AEF to preserve its identity, in part because Allied generals disagreed over strategy. Pershing understood, too, that "when the war ends, our position will be stronger if our army acting as such shall have played a distinct and definite part." But as the German army advanced within 50 miles of Paris, Pershing rushed 70,000 American troops to the front.

Early in May American units helped to block the Germans at the town of Château-Thierry. Four weeks later they met the German spearhead at Belleau Wood. When the French sounded retreat, one marine captain snorted, "Retreat, hell!" and the Americans attacked instead, even though it cost half their force to drive the Germans out of the woods. Two more German attacks, one at Amiens, the other just east of the Marne River, ended in costly German retreats. On September 12, 1918, half a million American soldiers and a smaller number of French troops overran the German stronghold at Saint-Mihiel in four days. Even as the strategic initiative shifted to the Allies, the slaughter continued. As nearly 900,000 Americans moved north along a 24-mile front between the Meuse River and the Argonne Forest, five undermanned and dispirited German divisions, just over 100,000 men, held them off for almost two months. According to one estimate 10 Americans died for every dead German in the Meuse-Argonne campaign.

As the German army retreated and war weariness drained morale at home, Germany's civilian leaders sought an armistice. They hoped in particular to negotiate terms along the lines laid out by Woodrow Wilson in a speech to Congress in

THE FINAL GERMAN OFFENSIVE AND ALLIED COUNTERATTACK, 1918
On the morning of March 21, 1918, the Germans launched a spring offensive designed to cripple the Allies. Sixty-three German divisions sliced through Allied lines for the first time since 1914 and plunged to within 50 miles of Paris. The tide turned in July, when the Germans were stopped at the Marne. The Allied counterattack, with notable American successes at Château-Thierry, Belleau Wood, Saint-Mihiel, and Meuse-Argonne, broke the German war effort.

January 1918. In it, Wilson presented his vision for a postwar peace that encompassed "Fourteen Points." The key provisions called for open diplomacy, free seas and free trade, disarmament, national self-rule, and an "association of nations" acting together to keep peace—nothing less than a new world order with an end to selfish nationalism, unilateral action, and war. Wilson the progressive was applying the tactics and goals of domestic reform to the taming of world-class rivalries.

Allied leaders were not all impressed. "President Wilson and his Fourteen Points bore me," French Premier Georges Clemenceau said. "Even God Almighty has only ten!" But Wilson's idealistic platform had also been designed to save the Allies deeper embarrassment. Almost as soon as it came to power in 1917, the new Bolshevik government in Moscow had begun publishing secret treaties from the czar's archives. Those treaties revealed that the Allies had gone to war for selfish ends such as the acquisition of territories and colonies, not the high principles they claimed. Wilson had given their cause a nobler purpose. His ideals stirred deep yearnings among German liberals. On October 6 Wilson received a telegram from Berlin requesting an immediate armistice. Within a month Turkey and Austria surrendered. Early in November the Kaiser was overthrown and fled to neutral Holland. On November 11, 1918, just before dawn, German officers filed into Allied headquarters in a converted railroad car near Compiègne, France, and signed the surrender.

The guns of August fell silent for the first time in four years. Of the 2 million Americans who had served in France, 50,000 had died in combat and 230,000 had been wounded. By comparison, the war claimed 1.8 million Germans, 1.7 million Russians, 1.4 million French, 1.2 million Austro-Hungarians, and nearly a million Britons. The American contribution had nonetheless been crucial to victory, providing vital convoys at sea and fresh, confident troops on land. The United States emerged from the war stronger than ever. Europe, on the other hand, looked forward—as one newspaper put it—to "Disaster . . . Exhaustion . . . Revolution."

THE LOST PEACE

As the S.S. *George Washington* approached the coast of France in mid-December 1918 the mist suddenly lifted, an omen of good hope. On board were the president of the United States, a group of advisers called the "Inquiry," and an entourage that included Committee on Public Information chief George Creel, there to make a movie of the historic mission. Woodrow Wilson was going to represent the United States at the peace conference at Versailles, outside Paris, where a world of problems awaited settlement. Large portions of European cities and farmlands had been shelled into ruin, scarred with trenches, barbed wire, and the debris of war. Fifty million people lay dead or maimed from the fighting. Starvation and typhus spread across the continent, eventually killing another 6 million people in the first year of peace. In eastern Europe especially, the social order had broken down and revolution unsettled the land. Poles fought with Czechs, Slavs with Italians, Turks with Greeks, Bolshevik "Reds" with czarist "Whites," Jews with Arabs. With the old world order so evidently in shambles, it seemed clear to Wilson that vigorous, immediate action was imperative.

Thus the president hand-picked the Peace Commission that accompanied him, including only loyal supporters like Secretary of State Lansing and Colonel House. Not a single member of the Republican-controlled Senate was included. What promised to make negotiations easier at Versailles, however, created a crippling liability in Washington, where Republicans cast a hostile eye on the impending Democratic peace treaty.

The Treaty of Versailles

Woodrow Wilson was the first president in office to meet with a foreign head of state; in fact, he met leaders of 27 nations from five continents. The most important were David Lloyd George, the prime minister of England, who had promised to squeeze Germany "until the pips squeak"; French premier Georges Clemenceau, nicknamed "Le Tigre" and obsessively dedicated to French security; and Vittorio Orlando, prime minister of Italy, who kept a covetous eye on neighboring

Daily Lives

The Doughboys Abroad

At ten in the morning on July 20, 1917, Secretary of War Newton Baker tied a blindfold over his eyes, reached into a huge glass bowl at the Senate Office Building, and drew the first number in a new draft lottery. The United States, with barely 180,000 men in the service, had begun to raise an army. During the first weeks after American entry into World War I, only 32,000 more volunteered. Yet by the time the conflict ended 16 months later, nearly 2 million men had donned uniforms, learned the manual of arms and close order drill, and gone off to fight in Europe. For the first time the New World was invading the Old, and for most of those who went, it was their first trip from home.

Armed against the enemy, scrubbed and clothed, drilled until they dropped, the "doughboys" marched out of their training camps and up the gangplanks of the "Atlantic Ferry"—the ships that conveyed them to Europe. The infantrymen were called "doughboys" for the "dough" of clay that soldiers had used to clean their white belts in the 1850s. Each man was outfitted with a pack, a weapon, a set of uniforms, and a "safety" razor, a new device that quickly altered American shaving habits.

Almost half the soldiers sailed on British vessels. Some were fortunate enough to ship out on refitted luxury liners, but most made the voyage in converted freighters. "Assigned quarters below decks," one private reported, "the blackest, foulest, most congested hole that I ever set foot into." A few who never made it across died from anthrax in the horsehair of their new shaving brushes. It

was a poignant taste of things to come. Disease killed more Americans than enemy fire. Nearly 50,000 troops died in the influenza pandemic of 1918.

The first American troops, a division of army regulars and a battalion of marines, arrived in France at the end of June 1917. Two months later the first volunteers landed, wearing spring parade uniforms and carrying just 10 rounds of ammunition apiece. They were squeezed into "40-and-8's"—French freight cars designed to hold 40 men and 8 horses—and carried inland to training areas. In the end the American Expeditionary Force purchased more of its supplies in Europe than it shipped from the "arsenal of democracy" in the United States. The American doughboy typically wore a steel helmet modeled on the British "Tommy" and fought with French artillery. More often than not American fliers went aloft in European-made planes.

With the United States at war for only 18 months (from April 1917 to November 1918), most American soldiers spent more time in training and on leave than in the trenches. To keep the men from becoming restless, company commanders marched their troops against imaginary enemies in never-ending exercises. "Every hill in this vicinity has been captured or lost at least ten times," wrote one weary infantryman who had to keep training even after the armistice. Soldiers complained about "cooties" (lice) and food (so bad that many reported a 10 percent weight loss within weeks of arriving). Most of all they hated military discipline. Used to freewheeling individualism and equality, Americans of all ranks abhorred hierarchy and subordination.

Enlisted men groused about army life, but touring France, whether on leave

Daily Lives

After months of training stateside, the American Expeditionary Force sailed to Europe on the troop ships of the "Atlantic Ferry." Most soldiers departed from Hoboken, New Jersey, and almost half made the journey aboard British vessels.

or in troop transports, awed them. Paris was both exhilarating and titillating, with women who danced the "Can-Can" and cried "oo-la-la." In fact, warned an army journal, too many soldiers expected France to be an "international Coney Island, a universal pleasure resort." As it turned out, the sheer beauty of the place impressed them more than the entertainment. Most of the doughboys arrived in the spring and summer of 1918, when France was awash in color. "The country is green and covered with flowers," observed a young infantryman. "It is a continuous garden."

The antiquity of Europe struck the doughboys even more. "The church here," one wrote, "is very, very old, probably built sometime in the 12th or 13th century. Saint Louis the Crusader, King of France, attended a service there on three occasions and Jeanne d'Arc was there several times." The Europeans seemed old too. Elderly women in black shawls of mourning often were the only ones left in shattered villages, deprived by war of their men. "My but the people are old fashioned," remarked a soldier. "They still harvest with cradles and sickles." Everything endorsed the American myth of the Old World as hidebound and worn and the New as modern and vital.

It was as if they had become crusaders, off on what one doughboy called "a glorious adventure" to save beleaguered Europe. They witnessed "thrilling air fights" from the ground and spectacular artillery fire—often from a distance. Up close, the shellfire could maim and kill, sometimes leave men frozen with "shell shock." Disillusion and discontent overcame British and French troops after years in the trenches, but most doughboys never fought long enough to lose their sense of wonder and delight. A year after the war ended a veteran wrote: "I know how we all cried to get back to the States. But now that we are here, I must admit for myself at least that I am lost and somehow strangely lonesome. These our own United States are truly artificial and bare. There is no romance or color here, nothing to suffer for and laugh at." Their tours of duty were short, but the doughboys traveled far.

territory. Together with Wilson they comprised the "Big Four." War had united them; now peacemaking threatened to divide them.

In December Wilson traveled to Europe to prevent, in his words, "a peace of loot or spoliation." Everywhere he went, cheering throngs greeted him. In Paris 2 million people threw flowers in his path as he made his way down the Champs-Elysées; in Italy the most enthusiastic crowds of all hailed him as the "peacemaker from America." And Wilson believed them, unaware of how determined the victors were to punish the vanquished Germans.

The sweeping reforms he proposed had taken Allied diplomats by surprise. Hungry for colonies that had been German and eager to see Germany crushed and disarmed, their secret treaties already divided the territories of the Central Powers. Germany offered to surrender on the basis of Wilson's Fourteen Points, but the Allies refused to accept them. When Wilson threatened to negotiate peace on his own, Allied leaders finally agreed—but only for the moment.

Noticeably absent when the peace conference convened on January 18, 1919, were the Russians. Fearful of the spread of revolutionary communism, none of the Western democracies had recognized the Bolshevik regime in Moscow. Instead, France and Britain were helping to finance Bolshevik adversaries in a civil war. They had blockaded Russian ports, landed troops on Russian soil, and persuaded President Wilson to send a small expeditionary force to Siberia in 1918, then another to Vladivostok on the Sea of Japan in 1919. The Soviets would neither forgive nor forget this instrusion.

During the grueling negotiations, Wilson was forced to yield several of his Fourteen Points. The European Allies resisted even putting free trade and freedom of the seas on the agenda. His "open diplomacy" was conducted behind closed doors by the Big Four themselves. Peace without victory gave way to a

On June 28, 1919, representatives of the new German republic were herded into the Hall of Mirrors in the old world palace of Louis XIV at Versailles, just outside Paris. Glumly they signed the peace treaty, which they had never seen before. The Germans, observed one reporter, suffered a "horrible humiliation." Here, Woodrow Wilson (in the red chair) sits with the other Allied leaders.

"guilt clause" that placed responsibility for the war on Germany. Worse still, the Allies saddled their enemies with reparations that eventually reached the impoverishing sum of $33 billion. The only mention of disarmament involved Germany, which was permanently barred from rearming.

Wilson did achieve a number of successes. He convinced Clemenceau to scale down demands for $200 billion in German payments in exchange for promises of aid if Germany attacked France. His pleas for national self-determination led to the creation of a dozen new states in Europe, including Yugoslavia, Hungary, and Austria. (Poland and Czechoslovakia, also carved from the empires of the Central Powers, contained millions of Germans whose national affiliation was thus violated.) Although former colonies were not granted the sovereignty Wilson desired, they gained new status as "mandates" of the victors, who were obligated to prepare them for eventual independence. The old German and Turkish empires in the Middle East and Africa became the responsibility of France and England, while Japan took over German possessions in the Far East.

Wilson never lost sight of his main concern—a League of Nations. He had given so much ground precisely because he believed such a body could correct any mistakes in the peace settlement. As constituted, the League was composed of a general Body of Delegates, a select Executive Council, and a Court of International Justice. Members promised to submit all war-provoking disagreements to arbitration and to isolate aggressors by cutting off commercial and military trade. Article X (which Wilson called "the heart of the convenant") bound members to respect one another's independence and territory and to join together against attack. "A living thing is born," the president told a general session of the conference in mid-February 1919. "It is definitely a guarantee of peace."

Wilson left immediately for home to calm congressional opposition. The previous October he had called on Americans to endorse his liberal peace plan by returning Democratic majorities to Congress. Instead, disaffected by wartime controls, attacks on civil liberties, and new taxes, voters gave both houses to the Republicans. A slim majority of two in the Senate put Wilson's archrival, Henry Cabot Lodge of Massachusetts, in the chairman's seat of the all-important Foreign Relations Committee. A Harvard-educated disciple of T.R., Lodge bristled at the notion of Wilson as the foremost intellectual in Washington. "I never expected to hate anyone in politics with the hatred I feel toward Wilson," he confessed.

While most of the country favored the League, Lodge was set against it. Lodge loved the Republican party more than world peace and certainly did not want the Democrats to win votes by taking credit for the treaty. Yet less partisan motives also moved him. For decades he had fought to preserve American freedom of action in foreign affairs. Now he believed Americans were being asked to "subject our own will to the will of other nations." Securing the signatures of 37 senators, enough to block passage of any treaty, Lodge rose in the Senate just before midnight on March 3 to read a "round robin" resolution against the League. "Woodrow Wilson's League of Nations died in the Senate tonight," concluded the New York *Sun*. Wilson began to suffer again from the mind-numbing headaches that always afflicted him under pressure.

Early in March the president returned to Paris for a final round of horse-trading with the Europeans. He withdrew often to nurse a stubborn case of influenza and bang out new amendments on his battered old typewriter. A twitch that had developed at his left eye now convulsed the whole left side of his face. Mindful of Senate critics, he engineered three changes he thought would satisfy them: keeping domestic affairs free from League interference; preserving the Monroe Doctrine; and permitting members to quit with two years' warning. The Allies exacted a price, including Japanese control of Shantung and additional reparations for the British. Forced to sign a treaty they had no role in writing, the Germans suffered a terrible national humiliation of crushing debt, impounded colonies, and war guilt.

The Battle for the Treaty

Wilson was about to suffer his own humiliation. On July 10, 1919, just one day after returning home, he drove to Capitol Hill to present the treaty to the Senate. "Dare we reject it and break the heart of the world?" he asked the senators. Fourteen Republicans and four Democrats were happy to do just that. "Irreconcilable" opponents of internationalism, they vowed to kill what one of them called "the unholy thing with the holy name." Twenty-three "strong reservationists," led by Lodge, sought to amend the treaty with major changes requiring Allied approval. Twelve "mild reservationists" wanted minimal alterations, mainly interpretive in nature.

Wilson's only hope of winning the necessary two-thirds majority lay in combining loyal Democrats with Republican "mild reservationists." But temperamentally the president could not abide compromise. Worn out by the concessions already wrung from him in Paris, he resisted more change at home and, despite his doctor's warnings, took his case to the people in a month-long railroad stump across the nation.

In Pueblo, Colorado, before a crowd of 10,000, he gave perhaps the greatest oration of his career, speaking movingly of American soldiers killed in France and American boys whom the League one day would spare from death. Listeners wept openly. That evening, utterly exhausted, the president collapsed in a spasm of pain. On October 2, four days after returning to the White House, he fell to the bathroom floor, knocked unconscious by a stroke. For six weeks Wilson could do no work at all, and for months after he worked only an hour or so a day. His second wife, Edith Bolling Wilson, his secretary, and his doctor handled the routine business of government, concealing the seriousness of his condition from the country. Wilson recovered slowly but never fully. He walked only with the aid of a cane, became more irritable, and at times broke into tears. More and more the battle for the treaty consumed his fading energies.

On November 19 Lodge finally reported the treaty out of committee, appending exactly 14 amendments (to match Wilson's Fourteen Points). The most important asserted that the United States assumed no obligation under Article X of the treaty to come to the aid of League members if their territory or political independence were violated, unless Congress consented. Whatever ill will Lodge bore Wilson, his objections did not destroy the treaty but only weakened it by protecting the congressional prerogative to declare war. Wilson believed Lodge had delivered a "knife thrust at the heart of the treaty" and refused to accept any changes. "The Senate must take its medicine," he told the French ambassador.

Under orders from the president, Democrats joined Republicans and "irreconcilables" to defeat the treaty with Lodge's reservations. An attempt to pass the unamended treaty failed. Although four-fifths of the senators favored it in some form, Wilson and Lodge stubbornly refused to compromise. When the modified treaty came before the Senate for final consideration in March 1920, 21 Democrats disobeyed the president by voting for it, enough to produce a 49–35 majority but seven votes short of the necessary two-thirds. The Treaty of Versailles was dead, and loyal Democrats had been forced to deliver the killing blow. Not until July 1921 did Congress enact a joint resolution ending the war. The United States, which had fought separately from the Allies, made a separate peace as well.

Red Scare

Peace abroad did not bring peace at home. On May Day 1919, six months after the war ended, mobs in a dozen cities broke up Socialist parades, injured hundreds, and killed three people. Later that month, when a spectator at a Victory Loan rally in Washington refused to stand for the national anthem, a sailor shot him in the back. The stadium crowd applauded. On the floor of the Senate Kenneth McKellar of Tennessee advocated sending citizens with radical beliefs to a penal colony on Guam.

The spontaneous violence and extremism occurred because Americans believed they were under attack. Rapid and unplanned demobilization had brought inflation, unemployment, and a chilling wave of strikes—3600 in 1919 alone. Over 350,000 steel workers and 450,000 coal miners struck for higher wages as the nation plunged into postwar turmoil. In Boston even the police walked off their jobs. When a strike by conservative trade unionists paralyzed Seattle for five days in January, Mayor Ole Hanson draped his car in an American flag and led troops through the streets in a show of force. Hanson blamed radicals, while Congress ascribed the national ills to Bolshevist agents, inspired by the revolution in Russia.

In truth, the menace of communist subversion was entirely overblown. With Socialist Eugene V. Debs in prison, his dwindling party numbered only about 30,000. Radicals at first hoped that the success of the Russian Revolution would help reverse their fortunes. But they discovered that most Americans found the prospect of "Bolshevik" revolution threatening, especially after March 1919, when the new Russian government formed the Comintern to foment revolution in other countries. Furthermore, in 1919 John Reed and Benjamin Gitlow deserted the Socialists to form the more radical Communist Labor party. About the same time, a separate Communist party was created, mostly by Slavic radicals (fewer than 7 percent of whom could speak English). In all, both parties could count no more than 40,000 members.

On April 28, Mayor Hanson received a small brown parcel at his office, evidently another present from an admirer of his tough patriotism. It was a home-made bomb. Within days, 20 such packages were discovered, including ones sent to John D. Rockefeller, Supreme Court Justice Oliver Wendell Holmes, and Postmaster General Albert Burleson. On June 2 bombs exploded simultaneously in eight different cities. One of them demolished the front porch of A. Mitchell Palmer, attorney general of the United States. The bomb thrower was blown to bits in the explosion, but enough remained to identify him as an Italian anarchist from Philadelphia. Americans, already edgy over Bolshevism and labor militancy, assumed they were under attack by an organized conspiracy to overthrow the government.

Palmer, a Quaker and a staunch progressive, hardened in the wake of the bombings. With an emergency appropriation of $500,000 he launched an anti-radical campaign on November 7, 1919. The Palmer raids in a dozen cities rounded up hundreds of suspects, who were held in violation of their legal rights. On December 21, 1919, a total of 249 aliens, most of whom had no criminal records, were marched aboard the army transport *Buford* (nicknamed the "Soviet Ark") and deported to the Soviet Union. Among them were radicals Emma Goldman and Alexander Berkman, several philosophical anarchists pledged against violence, and a few communists.

A new round of raids began in January 1920. In a single night, government agents invaded private homes, meeting halls, and pool parlors in 33 cities. They took nearly 2000 alleged communists into custody without warrants. Beatings often accompanied the arrests. Prisoners were marched through streets in chains, crammed into dilapidated jails, and held incommunicado without hearings. Arrests continued at the rate of 200 a week through March. State after state passed new statutes outlawing radical unions, and local vigilance committees even screened the loyalty of schoolteachers. In Centralia, Washington, vigilantes spirited radical labor organizer Wesley Everest from jail, castrated him, and hanged him from the Chehalis River bridge as they riddled his body with bullets. The county coroner ruled it a suicide.

Such wholesale abuses of civil liberties provoked a backlash. After the New York legislature expelled five duly elected Socialists in 1919, responsible politicians—from former presidential candidate Charles Evans Hughes to Ohio Senator Warren Harding—denounced the action. A revolt against Palmer by the Labor Department, where assistant secretary Louis Post refused to issue more deportation orders, ended the "deportation delirium" early in 1920. Then Palmer overreached himself by predicting a revolutionary uprising for May 1, 1920. Buildings were put under guard and state militia called to readiness. Nothing happened. Four months later, when a wagonload of bombs exploded on Wall Street, Palmer conjured up a Bolshevik conspiracy. Despite 33 deaths and over 200 injuries,

---

On September 16, 1920, as lunch-hour crowds filled the heart of New York's financial district, a wagonload of bombs exploded at the corner of Broad and Wall streets. Thirty-three people were killed and over 200 injured in the blast, probably the work of deranged anarchists. All of the dead were workers—runners, stenographers, and clerks. The nation, though horrified, saw no communist plot, as Attorney General A. Mitchell Palmer charged. The Red Scare at last was over.

Americans assumed it was the work of a few demented anarchists (which it probably was) and went about business as usual.

Not for another 20 years would the United States assume a leading position in
international affairs. And the spirit of reform at home waned as well. When war
came, progressivism had furnished the bureaucratic weapons to organize the fight,
but the push for social justice and toleration had been overshadowed by a patriotic
frenzy.

War changed Americans in important ways. They experienced a centralized
and planned economy for the first time. Propaganda shaped diverse ethnic, racial,
social class, and gender differences into a uniform set of national issues. Such
singlemindedness would not quickly disappear. War work drew millions from
country to city, from farm to factory. The army mixed millions of recruits from
thousands of hometowns. They did not simply learn to fight. Some learned to
read, to sleep in a bed, to eat regular meals, and to take regular baths. After seeing
Europe, they returned like tourists in uniform to tell of its wonders. Provincial
America became more cosmopolitan, urban, and homogenized. With the war
over, the nation turned from idealistic crusades to the practical business of getting
and spending.

SIGNIFICANT EVENTS

1901	Hay–Pauncefote Treaty authorizes U.S. to build canal across the Central American isthmus
1902	Platt Amendment ratified
1904	Roosevelt Corollary to Monroe Doctrine
1905	Treaty of Portsmouth ends Russo–Japanese War
1907	"Gentlemen's agreement" with Japan; "Great White Fleet" embarks on world tour
1911	Mexican Revolution erupts
1913	Secretary of State William Jennings Bryan begins negotiating "cooling-off" treaties
1914	U.S. Navy invades Veracruz; Archduke Franz Ferdinand assassinated; World War I begins; Panama Canal opens
1915	Japan issues Twenty-one Demands; Germany proclaims war zone around British Isles; *Lusitania* torpedoed; Secretary of State Bryan resigns; *Arabic* pledge; Wilson endorses preparedness
1916	*Sussex* pledge; General John Pershing invades Mexico in pursuit of Pancho Villa; Wilson reelected president
1917	Wilson calls for "peace without victory"; Germany resumes unrestricted submarine warfare; Zimmermann telegram released; Russian Revolution breaks out; U.S. enters World War I; Selective Service Act passed; War Industries Board created
1918	Wilson's Fourteen Points for peace; Eugene Debs jailed under Sedition Act; influenza epidemic; Germany sues for peace; armistice declared
1919	Paris Peace Conference; *Schenck v. United States* affirms Espionage Act; Red Summer; Chicago race riot; Senate rejects Treaty of Versailles
1920	Palmer raids; Red Scare

PART FIVE

THE PERILS
OF DEMOCRACY

In the wake of World War I, the editors of the American progressive journal *The New Republic* despaired that "the war did no good to anybody. Those of its generation whom it did not kill, it crippled, wasted, or used up." With the specter of Russian Bolshevism looming, parliamentary governments across Europe struggled to establish what President Warren Harding in the United States called "normalcy": a mixture of material prosperity and political stability.

By the mid-1920s despair had given way to hope. The postwar recession lifted. Woodrow Wilson's vision of a world made safe for democracy no longer seemed a naive hope. In both political and material terms democracy seemed to be advancing almost everywhere. Great Britain eliminated restrictions on suffrage for men; and between 1920 and 1928 women gained the vote in both Britain and the United States. Hapsburg Germany transformed itself into the Weimar Republic, whose constitution provided universal suffrage and a bill of rights. Across central and eastern Europe, the new nations carved out of the old Russian and Austro-Hungarian empires, along with the previously independent Romania, Bulgaria, Greece, and Albania, attempted to create governments along similarly democratic lines.

The winds of political reform blew from Europe across the Middle East through Asia. No longer were the nationalists of these areas willing to see their people and resources exploited for the benefit of foreigners. Nor were they willing to see their cultures erased by Westerners. Some Asians, like Mao Tse-tung in China and Ho Chi Minh in Indochina, saw in communism the means of liberation for their oppressed peoples. But even Asian Marxists aligned themselves with the

powerful force of nationalism. In India, the Congress party formed by Mohandas K. Gandhi (1869–1948) brought together socialists and powerful industrial capitalists. Through tactics of nonviolence and boycotts of British goods, Indian nationalists wrested concessions from the British on political representation, economic autonomy, and eventual self-government. In Turkey, Kemal Atatürk in 1923 abolished the sultanate and established the Turkish Republic with all the trappings of a Western democratic state.

The spread of democracy had a material side as well. The credibility of parliamentary governments depended heavily on their ability to restore and maintain prosperity. In the second half of the 1920s the world economy expanded. Scientific and technological discoveries created new products, while improving and lowering the costs of old ones. Some optimists suggested that innovations in manufacturing, like Henry Ford's moving assembly line, augured an era where plenty would replace want. Increased earnings encouraged a democratic culture of consumption, whether it was buying radios in France or Western-style fashions in Tokyo (below, left). Products like the automobile, once available only to the rich, were increasingly accessible to people of all classes. Ford himself became an international hero and German and Russian engineers used the term *Fordismus* to characterize modern industrial techniques.

Along with the automobile the mass media introduced a revolution in world culture. The impact of movies, radio, and mass circulation magazines, while greatest in the United States, was felt around the globe. Some social critics saw in the pervasive reach of the media a way to overcome the divisions among people and the disintegrative force of modern society. The movie camera, observed social critic Lewis Mumford, brought ordinary people into the public world. Once-remote people and places became accessible and famil-iar. Stories, names, phrases, images, and ideas could become the common property of all. "In short, it seems to be the nature of radio to encourage people to think and feel alike," two prominent psychologists concluded. Consumption of culture as well as manufactured goods seemed to walk hand in hand with the democracy of the masses.

But often the foundations upon which democracy rested were fragile. The Bolsheviks, led by Lenin and the young Joseph Stalin, demonstrated how readily talk of "the masses" and "democratic socialism" could mask an iron totalitarianism. In Japan, democracy was hampered by that nation's persistent feudal traditions. Although its parliamentary government was controlled for a time by liberal, Westernized factions, nationalists from the old samurai class joined with the nation's economically powerful families in quest of a Japanese East Asian empire. By the late 1920s those elements had embarked on a militarist course that would lead eventually to war.

While conservative nationalists tolerated democratic forms, they worried that communism would spread its infection beyond the Soviet Union's boundaries. Nowhere were those fears deeper than in Italy. With the parliamentary government seemingly paralyzed by postwar unrest, Benito Mussolini and his *Fasci di Combattimento*, or fascists, under the cover of parliamentary means, used terrorism, murder, and intimidation to defeat their enemies. Through the mass media they spread antidemocratic propaganda and promoted an "all-embracing" single-party state, outside which "no human or spiritual values can exist, let alone be desireable." They rejected both the liberals' belief in political parties and the Marxist concept of class solidarity in favor of the glorified nation-state dominated by the middle class, small business people, modest property owners, and small farmers.

Fascism thus gave a sinister twist to the liberal ideal of national solidarity, but one that others embraced as a no-nonsense means of blunting Marxism. Adolf Hitler, like many Germans, resented the stinging defeat that war brought in 1919. Like Mussolini, Hitler too used the politics of discontent to rise to power. And having achieved it in 1933, his Nazi party destroyed democracy. Under one-party rule, the Gestapo secret political police ensured that Germans expressed only those ideas that conformed to the views of their national leader, the *Führer*.

Hitler succeeded partly because the prosperity of the 1920s was shattered worldwide by the corrosive hardships of the Great Depression. Farmers were particularly hard-hit: during the 1920s the opening of new lands to cultivation had already led to overproduction. In Java, for example, the use of scientific agricultural techniques created a glut in the sugar market. By 1930 the price of wheat, measured in gold, reached its lowest point in four hundred years. And those urban unemployed who walked the street in search of a job ("I seek work of any sort," reads the German's sign on the preceding page.) were often ready to believe that only the forceful leadership of one could unite the many. Even in the United States, the business newspaper *Barron's* voiced the thoughts of more than a few when it mused that "a mild species of dictatorship" might "help us over the roughest spots in the road ahead."

Still, the rise of Hitler and Mussolini shook those who had faith in the possibilities of mass politics. While Franklin Roosevelt had used his radio "fireside chats" to bring government closer to the people, Hitler's fiery speeches and mass rallies seemed bent on encouraging racist fears and controlling public opinion. While Hollywood produced films that overwhelmingly affirmed popular faith in democratic government, a capitalist economy, and the success ethic, the German director Leni Riefensthal used her cinematic gifts to combine myth, symbolism, and documentary into an evocation of the *Führer* as a pagan god of strength and a Christian savior. The "mass" aspects of the media were a two-edged sword. Perceptive critics recognized that even in democracies, mass culture was devoted primarily to the entertainment and escapism of light comedy and melodrama rather than serious social criticism.

Thus the Depression shook both the political and material pillars of democratic culture. On the eve of World War II the number of European democracies had been reduced from twenty-seven to ten. Latin America was ruled by a variety of dictators and military juntas that differed little from the dictatorships of Europe. China suffered not only from invasion by Japan's militarists and civil war but also from the corrupt and ineffectual one-party dictatorship of Chiang Kai-shek. Almost alone, the New Deal attempted to combat the Depression through the methods of parliamentary democracy. The totalitarian states that had promised stability, national glory, and an end to the communist menace instead led the world to chaos and war from which both communism and democracy emerged triumphant.

CHRONOLOGY

AMERICAN EVENT	YEAR		GLOBAL EVENT
	1920s		Inflation plagues defeated Germany
First commercial radio station on the air (KDKA, Pittsburgh)	1920		
Prohibition takes effect			
	1921	HARDING	Washington Conference on naval armaments
Sinclair Lewis' *Babbitt* published	1922		Mussolini marches on Rome
			James Joyce's *Ulysses* published
Teapot Dome scandal exposed	1923	COOLIDGE	Atatürk establishes Turkish Republic
F. Scott Fitzgerald's *The Great Gatsby* published	1925		
Scopes trial debates evolution			
Stock market boom underway	1928		Kellogg–Briand Pact outlaws war
Stock market crash	1929	HOOVER	Stalin's power consolidated
	1931		Depression spreads to Europe
			Japan invades Manchuria
Bonus Army arrives in Washington	1932		
"Hundred days" of the New Deal	1933	ROOSEVELT	Hitler becomes chancellor of Germany
Prohibition ends			
Good Neighbor Policy announced			
"Second New Deal" program	1935		Italy invades Ethiopia
Isolationists pass Neutrality Act			
	1936		Civil war breaks out in Spain
FDR fails to enlarge the Supreme Court	1937		Japan attacks China
	1938		Germany annexes Austria
			Munich Conference placates Hitler
John Steinbeck's *The Grapes of Wrath* published	1939		Nazi–Soviet nonaggression pact
			Germany invades Poland; World War II
America First Committee formed	1940		U.S.S.R. invades Baltic nations, Finland
Roosevelt supports preparedness			German blitzkrieg sweeps Europe
Black unions press for integration of government-contract jobs	1941		Germany attacks U.S.S.R.
			Nazis begin systematic extermination of Jews and other subject peoples
Pearl Harbor attacked; U.S. enters war			
U.S. wins Battle of Midway	1942		Japan occupies the Philippines
Japanese-Americans interned			North Africa campaign
Race riots in Detroit and Los Angeles	1943		Allies invade Italy
			Jean-Paul Sartre's *Being and Nothingness* published
American war production peaks	1944		D-Day invasion of Normandy
			U.S. recaptures the Philippines
Roosevelt dies	1945	TRUMAN	Allies capture Berlin
			Atomic bomb dropped on Japan
			World War II ends

25

The New Era

On Armistice Day 1918 the "Gospel Car" pulled into Tulsa, Oklahoma. Bold letters on one side announced "Jesus Is Coming—Get Ready"; those on the other side asked "Where Will You Spend Eternity?" Aimee Semple McPherson, the vivacious red-headed driver, was on her way to conquer the West. Just before Christmas she arrived in Los Angeles "with ten dollars and a tambourine." For the next three years she wandered in and out of the state before landing in San Diego. With the highest rates of illness and suicide in California, it was the perfect place for Sister Aimee to preach the healing message of her "Foursquare Gospel." Her first revival attracted 30,000 people, who witnessed her first "miracle": a paralytic walked.

Billed as the "world's most pulchritudinous evangelist," Sister Aimee had a Pentecostal message for her flock. "I am not a healer," she readily confessed. "Jesus is the healer. I am only the little office girl who opens the door and says, 'Come in.'" After the miracle in San Diego, her fame quickly spread. She returned triumphantly to Los Angeles, at the time more of an enormous village than a real metropolis. In the decade of the 1920s almost three-quarters of a million people, many of them from the nation's rural heartland, had migrated there in search of opportunity, sun, and perhaps salvation. In heading west, most had lost touch with the traditional Protestant denominations at home. Sister Aimee put her traveling gospel tent away and attended that lost flock at her doorstep.

And what a doorstep she created. The Angelus Temple was pure Hollywood. To the blare of trumpets on New Year's Day in 1923 she unveiled a $1.5 million dollar structure graced by a 75-foot, rotating electronic cross, visible at night from 50 miles away. Inside was a 5000-seat auditorium, radio station KFSG (Kall Four Square Gospel), a wardrobe room that rivaled those of the movie studios, a "Cradle Roll Chapel" for babies, and a "Miracle Room" filled with the crutches, trusses, wheelchairs, and other aids Sister Aimee's cured faithful had discarded. Services were not simply a matter of hymn, sermon, and prayer. Aimee staged pageants, Holy Land slide shows, dramatized sermons, circuses, and healing sessions to ease the pain and boredom of the folks who flocked to see her.

Sister Aimee succeeded because she was able to blend the old with the new. Her lively sermons had a simple message, easy to remember. They carried the spirit of what people were calling the "New Era." Casting aside hellfire evangelism, wrote one observer, Sister Aimee "substituted the cheerfulness of the playroom for the gloom of the morgue." Where country preachers menaced their

The pulsating rhythms of the Jazz Age are captured in this vibrant painting by Archibald Motley. The New Orleans–born artist was one of a group of black genre painters in the 1920s who became part of the Harlem Renaissance.

congregations with visions of eternal damnation, she gave her faithful, "flowers, music, golden trumpets, red robes, angels, incense, nonsense, and sex appeal." To that she also added the sophistication of the booming media industries of the 1920s. She had a nose for publicity, a great capacity for self-dramatization, and a gift for improvising new activities to entertain her followers. Here was one brand of evangelism eminently suited to a new consumer age.

Aimee Semple McPherson was hardly the only evangelist to use technology. In Fort Worth, Texas, the Reverend J. Frank Norris of the First Baptist Church built a 6000-seat amphitheater, set aglow by spotlights. If the lights failed to bring the faithful to Christ, advertising would. Bruce Barton, founder of a major advertising agency, became concerned that Christ no longer had the proper "image." In *The Man Nobody Knows* (1925), he portrayed Jesus as the thoroughly modern businessman, a bibulous socializer who had, after all, changed water into wine at the wedding feast at Cana and whose parables of wisdom were the "most powerful advertisements of all times." Barton explained how Christ had "picked up twelve men from the bottom ranks of business and forged them into an organization that conquered the world." With the Savior himself said to be blessing mass marketing, it was small wonder that so many Americans embraced a consumer culture. Half a million of them bought Barton's book.

Modernizing the way the gospel was spread was just one symptom of the

"New Era." Writing in 1931, journalist Frederick Lewis Allen found the changes of the preceding decade so overwhelming that he could not believe that 1919 was *Only Yesterday,* as he titled his book. To give some sense of the transformation, Allen introduced his readers to "Mr. and Mrs. Smith," a moderately well-to-do couple living in a city apartment. Among the images that struck Allen (as well as disapproving conservatives) was the revolution in Mrs. Smith's fashions. No longer was she wrapped in a heavy, formless dress hanging to the floor. Her hemline exposed her ankles as it raced toward her knees. Her petticoats and corsets had vanished. Her dress was straight and long-waisted. She wore flesh-colored stockings of silk or rayon (which "flappers," the more adventurous women of her day, rolled at the top). She had "bobbed," or cut, her hair to the popular, near-boyish length, and flattened her breasts, all in an effort to gain greater freedom of movement. In 1919 Mrs. Smith had used face powder but never other cosmetics, the surest sign of "a scarlet career." By the end of the decade she was applying rouge every day, visiting a "beauty parlor" regularly, and using one of the 2500 brands of perfume and 1500 face creams on the market.

With Prohibition in full force, Mrs. Smith and other women of her day were walking into illegal "speakeasy" saloons and ordering drinks as readily as did men. In the trendy hotels she and her husband danced to "jazz" (so popular by the mid-twenties that the "Jazz Age" became another name for the decade). Modern couples like the Smiths sprinkled their conversations with references to "repressed sexual drives" and the best methods of contraception. But the most striking fact about Allen's description of these "average" Americans was that they lived in the city. The census of 1920 showed that for the first time just over half of the population were urbanites. Here, in urban America, the New Era worked its changes and sent them rippling outward.

Yet the Smiths of Frederick Allen's imagination were in many ways hardly average. According to the census tables, nearly as many Americans still lived on isolated farms, in villages, and in small towns. In fact, many "city" dwellers lived out there too. By defining a city as any place with 2500 people, the Census Bureau had created hundreds of statistical illusions. Boston with its millions of inhabitants ranked in the census tables alongside Muncie, Indiana, just under 37,000 people, and Sac Prairie, Wisconsin, whose population hovered barely above the mystical mark of 2500, and tiny Hyden, Kentucky, along the Cumberland plateau of eastern Kentucky. As late as 1927 nearly all American farms lacked electricity; two-thirds of American homes had no washing machines or vacuum cleaners and half had no telephones; 95 percent were without refrigerators; and despite the amazing growth of the medium, 70 percent had no radio. Most citizens, the Smiths aside, still clung to the values of an earlier America and still lived there too.

The poet August Derleth grew up in Sac Prairie, and as a 10-year-old in 1919 he could hear the "howl of wolves" at night. The town observed changing seasons not with new fashions but by the appearance and disappearance of plants and animals. Sac Prairie was a world of farming and gossip and fishing, of men swapping stories over potbellied stoves, of barn-raisings, and of harvest moon dances—all within a few hours' drive of the state capital at Madison. In Hyden, Kentucky, Main Street was still unpaved, livestock roamed at will, and the lots on either side

Sister Aimee Semple McPherson in her evangelical robe.

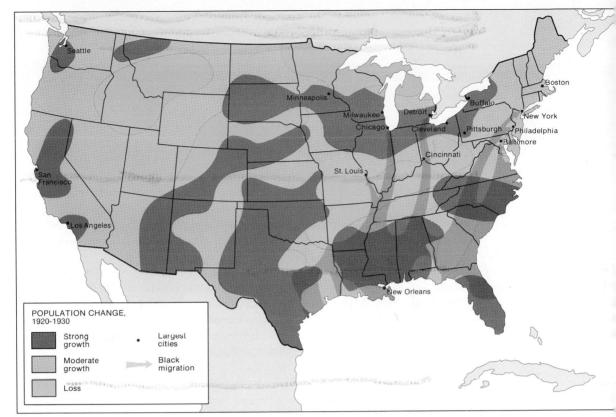

AREAS OF POPULATION GROWTH

In the 1920s the population of urban America grew by some 15 million, at the time the greatest ten-year jump in American history. Spurred first by the industrial demands of World War I and then by declining farm income, cities grew largely by depopulating rural areas. The biggest gains were in the South and West, where farmers followed opportunity to cities in climates similar to their own. In the most dramatic manifestation of the overall trend, more than a million African-Americans migrated from the rural South to the urban North in hopes of escaping poverty and discrimination.

had fences to keep front yards and gardens free of animals. By 1930 there were still only 10 automobiles in the county, and god-fearing Baptists not only worshiped together as their parents had before them but also repaired to the Middle Fork of the Kentucky for an open-air baptism when they declared their new birth in Christ. They would have nothing to do with flapper girls and "paint" or the showy miracles of Aimee McPherson.

As much as some Americans resisted the transforming forces of modern life—technology, corporatism, bureaucratization, and consumerism—the New Era could not be ignored or walled out. Modernism mixed uneasily with traditionalism in the 1920s. Automobiles had come to Hyden, no matter how few in number, and in Tennessee, a few hundred miles down the road, the mass media had flocked to a spectacular trial involving Darwinian evolution. Whether Americans embraced the New Era or condemned it, they could not ignore the changes in society that worked to develop a mass-produced consumer economy, a culture shaped more than ever by the mass media, and a more materialistic society.

THE ROARING ECONOMY

If anything roared in the "Roaring Twenties," it was industry and commerce. America was in the midst of a productivity revolution, turning out more goods with less labor. Manufacturing output rose 64 percent, output per workhour 40 percent. Between 1922 and 1927 the economy grew by 7 percent a year—the largest peacetime growth rate ever. The sale of electricity doubled; the consumption of fuel oil more than doubled.

Technology was partly responsible. All over the country old machines were being junked for new. Between 1919 and 1927 nearly half the steam engines in the United States went to the scrap heap. Steam turbines and steam shovels, electric motors, belt and bucket conveyors, dump trucks, and countless other mechanized innovations became commonplace in factories and at work sites—all improving productivity. As automatic and semiautomatic machinery replaced 200,000 workers each year, a new phrase entered the vocabulary: "technological unemployment." Even so, the labor force grew at a faster rate than the population. And for the larger percentage of the population that worked, wages improved too, climbing nearly $150 for industrial workers between 1919 and 1927.

As the industrial economy matured, more and more consumer items appeared on store shelves—cigarette lighters, wristwatches, radios, antifreeze fluids, Pyrex glass cooking utensils, panchromatic film. Given the improvement in productivity, prices were stable, and some even fell. The cost of a tire and an inner tube tumbled from $30 in 1914 to nearly half that amount by 1929. Americans enjoyed the highest standard of living any people had ever known. Yet for all the prosperity, the average American depositor increased savings by only $11 in 1928. Most people saved nothing. Personal debt was rising two and a half times faster than personal income. Sooner or later buying power would be exhausted and the roaring economy would grind to a chilling stop.

The Boom Industries

Along with technology, new "boom industries" promoted economic growth. A short recession in 1921 gave way to a massive construction boom to make up for the wartime backlog in demand for offices, homes, factories, and warehouses. During the twenties New York got a new skyline, topped in 1931 when the Empire State Building rose to the world record height of 86 stories. Soon cities the size of Beaumont, Texas, Memphis, Tennessee, and Syracuse, New York, boasted buildings of at least 21 stories. Residential construction doubled as people fanned out from cities to suburbs. Near Detroit, suburban Grosse Point grew by 700 percent; Shaker Heights, outside of Cleveland, by 1000 percent; Beverly Hills by 2500 percent. The construction of roads made settling in the suburbs possible and poured millions of dollars into the economy. In 1919 Oregon, New Mexico, and

Colorado hit on a new idea for financing road building—a tax on gasoline. Within a decade every state had one. At the end of the war only 7000 miles of hard-surfaced roads existed; by 1927 there were 50,000; and by 1928 a tourist could drive from New York as far west as St. Mary's, Kansas, and never leave a paved highway.

Construction stimulated other businesses and industries: steel, concrete, glass, lumber, wiring, home mortgages, and insurance. The demands of war already had spurred the chemical and synthetics industries. In the 1920s rayon transformed the textile business; cellophane, used to wrap everything from leftovers to cigarettes, doubled in sales each year from 1924 until the end of the decade. Meanwhile the urban diet became more varied as interest in nutrition climbed. Shipments of fresh fruits and vegetables soared, and vitamins, publicized with new zeal, appeared on breakfast tables. "Kitchenettes" in small city apartments boosted the canning industry. Between 1914 and 1929 purchases of canned milk nearly tripled. City families could dine at home on canned soup, canned meat and vegetables, and canned fruit for dessert.

The Automobile

The most important boom industry involved the automobile. The first cars had appeared on streets at the turn of the century but for many years remained expensive toys for the rich. By 1920 there were 10 million in America, a sizable number; by 1929 that had jumped to 26 million, one for every five people (compared to one for every 43 in Britain and one for every 7000 in Russia). During the decade automakers bought one-seventh of the nation's steel. They were the leading purchasers of rubber, plate glass, nickel, and lead. By 1929 it was estimated that one American in four derived employment directly or indirectly from automobiles.

Henry Ford made this revolution possible by pushing the principles of standardization and mass production to such ruthless extremes that the automobile became available to the masses at a price most could afford. At the age of 16, Ford walked away from the family farm in Dearborn, Michigan. In 1902, after a decade of tinkering and building autos, he saw his flame-shooting "999" race car roar to a world speed record of 70 miles per hour. Trading on his fame he founded the Ford Motor Company in 1903 and in 1907 announced his dream: to build a "motor car for the multitude." "Everybody wants to be somewhere he ain't," Ford said. The way to succeed was to make all the cars alike, "just like one pin is like another pin when it comes from a pin factory." In 1908 Ford perfected the Model T. It had a 20-horsepower engine and a body of steel. It was high enough to ride the worst roads, and it came in one color: black.

Priced at $845, the Model T was cheap by industry standards, but still too costly, and it took too long to build—12 hours for the chassis alone—to fulfill its designer's dream. Two Ford engineers suggested copying a practice of Chicago meat-packing houses, where beef carcasses were carried on moving chains past a line of meat dressers. In 1914 Ford introduced the moving assembly line. A conveyor belt, positioned waist high (to eliminate bending or walking), propelled the chassis at six feet per minute as stationary workers put the cars together. The process cut assembly time in half. By 1925 the process had been so well streamlined that new Model T's were rolling off the assembly line every 10 seconds. At $290, almost anybody could buy one. By 1927 Ford had sold a total of 15 million "tin lizzies," making him the giant of the automobile industry, not only in America but throughout the world.

Ford, the greatest industrialist of the twentieth century, was also a social prophet. Unlike most of his contemporaries, he praised the benefits of a "doctrine of high wages," pointing out that workers with extra money in their pockets would stimulate enough consumption—of autos, clothing, all the new products—to sustain a booming prosperity. In 1915 his plants in Dearborn established the "Five-Dollar Day," twice the going wage rate in Detroit. He reduced working hours from 48 to 40 a week and cut the work week to five days. By 1926 he employed 10,000 blacks, many of whom had advanced far enough to hire and fire whites. His methods simplified each operation so much that he could employ even the disabled.

Yet Ford workers were not happy. Ford himself admitted that the routinized operations on his assembly line were "so monotonous that it scarcely seems possible that any man would care to continue long at the same job." By 1915 labor turnover at Ford plants had reached over 300 percent a year. The Five-Dollar Day was designed partly to keep workers at Ford, and it did: within two years turnover dropped to 40 percent. Ford recouped his profits by speeding up the assembly line. Anything that reduced efficiency was barred. Ford workers could not talk, sing, whistle, smoke, or sit on the job. They wore frozen expressions called "Fordization of the Face" and communicated in the "Ford Whisper" without moving their lips. A "Sociological Department" sent company inspectors to workers' homes to encourage "thrift, honesty, sobriety, better housing, and better living generally." In Ford factories an "Education Department" ran "Americanization" classes where immigrant workers learned English, proper dress, and even etiquette, as well as plant procedures.

Sometimes Ford's paternalism led to tyranny. The company fired nearly a thousand Greek and Russian workers, who as Orthodox Christians celebrated Christmas 13 days later than other Christian sects. "If these men are to make their home in America," said a Ford official, "they should observe American holidays." Unions were barred, and when advertisements for 3000 jobs brought 25,000 men to the Rouge Assembly Plant on January 2, 1929, company guards drove them off with fire hoses. In 14-degree temperature the water froze almost as soon as it hit the men. Only 600 found employment that day. Ford didn't mind a bit of social revolution, so long as it was on his own terms.

General Motors copied Ford's production techniques but not his business strategies. Where Ford, the inventive mechanic with an eighth-grade education, operated on instinct, college-educated Alfred Sloan, manager of GM, combed statistics for market trends. Where Ford centralized operations, GM decentralized them. "Policy," Sloan liked to say, "may originate from anywhere." While Ford tried to sell everyone the same car, GM created "a car for every purse and purpose." There were Cadillacs and Buicks for the well-to-do, Chevrolets for the modest. GM cars had flashy designs, plush upholstery, self-starters, and hydraulic brakes. They came in a rainbow of colors, and every year the look changed. In an increasingly standardized society, these details allowed people to view their automobiles as symbols of distinction and social prestige. Only in 1927 did Ford realize that efficiency and economy were not enough. He dropped the Model T, retooled his factories, and introduced the upscale Model A in 1928 in an array of colors.

By making automobiles available to the masses, the growing industry

Henry Ford at the turn of the century.

changed the face of America. The spreading web of paved roads fueled urban sprawl, real estate booms in California and Florida, and a new roadside culture. Thousands of "auto camps" opened to provide tourists with tents and crude toilets. "Auto clubs" like the Tin Can Tourists Association (named for the tin can tied to the radiator cap of a member's car) sprang up to aid travelers. Automobile travel broke down provincialism and advanced standardized dialects and manners. By 1930 almost two farm families in three had cars. When asked why her family had bought a Model T when they had no indoor plumbing, a farm woman replied, "You can't go to town in a bathtub." Across the country the automobile gave the young unprecedented freedom from parental authority. After hearing 30 cases of "sex crimes" (19 of which had occurred in cars), an exasperated juvenile court judge in Indiana declared that the automobile was "a house of prostitution on wheels." It was, of course, much more. The automobile was to the 1920s what the railroad had been to the nineteenth century: the catalyst for economic growth, a transportation revolution, and a cultural symbol.

The Business of America

A generation earlier, progressives had criticized business for its social irresponsibility (even as reformers adopted business techniques and helped businesses to stabilize whole industries). Patriotic and productive service in the war enhanced the reputation of businessmen, and after a brief postwar recession, the return of prosperity in 1922 deepened respect for them. When Harvard established a graduate school of business administration in 1924, it was a sign that business had become a "profession," whose mastery required special training.

In the 1920s business also became a form of public service. A new middle class of civil servants, sales representatives, and salaried managers thrived on pep, boosterism, and good cheer. Immortalized in Sinclair Lewis' *Babbitt* (1922), they joined the Kiwanis or the Rotary Club, worshiped Henry Ford, and shared his belief that in business the "fundamentals are all summed up in the single word, 'service.'" President Calvin Coolidge echoed the theme in 1925: "The business of America is business. The man who builds a factory builds a temple. The man who works there worships there."

Encouraged by federal permissiveness, a wave of mergers swept the country. Between 1919 and 1930, some 8000 firms disappeared as large ones swallowed small. Oligopoly, where a few firms dominated whole industries, grew increasingly common. At the end of the decade, four companies packed nearly three-quarters of all American meat; another four rolled nine-tenths of all cigarettes. National chains began to replace local "mom and pop" stores. One bag of groceries in ten came from the Great Atlantic and Pacific Tea Company. A & P's chain of 15,000 red-and-gold stores did more business than the Ford Motor Company. One mammoth holding company, Drug, Incorporated, owned 10,000 Rexall drugstores, 706 Liggett stores, the Owl chain on the West Coast, and huge drug companies like Vick Chemical, Bayer Aspirin, and Bristol-Myers. Almost every pill that Americans bought over the counter came from Drug, Incorporated or a business owned by the company.

This expansion and consolidation meant that the capital of the nation was controlled not by a host of individuals, or even by a concentration of rich "captains of industry," but by large, bureaucratic organizations in which management was divorced from ownership. The economy became "corporatized." By 1929 half the total industrial income was concentrated in 100 corporations. Nearly one-fifth of all national wealth had shifted from private to corporate hands. Stocks and bonds were becoming so widely dispersed that few individuals held more than 1 or 2 percent of the shares in any company. The 20 largest shareholders in U.S. Steel owned only 5.7 percent of the stock among them.

Modern bureaucratic management made it possible for huge corporations to run their empires ever more efficiently. Control of business policy was passing from entrepreneurs to a salaried bureaucracy of executives and plant managers. They formed a new elite, which no longer aimed to own a business; instead they wanted to work their way up a corporate ladder. They were less interested in risk than productivity and stability. Mergers left them with more resources, and increasingly managers shoveled earnings back into their companies to expand physical plants and to carry on research for future development. By the end of the decade more than a thousand firms had research laboratories.

At Harvard and other new schools of business, through new journals, professional societies, and consultants, corporate leaders learned the techniques of "scientific management," an innovative system for standardizing business procedures. In the nineteenth century a Carnegie or a Rockefeller applied his quick mind and indomitable will to business. In the 1920s management was the key—to selling, budgeting, financing, even personnel. Like Alfred Sloan at General Motors, managers divided and subdivided their enterprises. Central headquarters planned for the future, while semi-independent divisions took care of daily operations. It was still experimental. Most businesses, for example, began to use budgets to plan their expenditures and capital outlays only after 1922.

Scientific management stressed good relations between managers and workers. Businesses preferred to retain laborers and avoid the expense of training new ones. A new form of labor relations emerged, designed to keep workers in factories and trouble-making unions out. In 1921, after a rash of postwar strikes, the National Association of Manufacturers, the Chamber of Commerce, and other employer groups launched the "American Plan." Backed by a million dollars in business pledges, it aimed at opening "closed shops," where only union members were allowed to work. Employers made workers sign agreements (dubbed "yellow dog contracts" by unions) disavowing union membership, infiltrated their organizations with company spies, locked them out of factories if they protested, and boycotted firms that hired union labor.

The benevolent side of the American Plan involved a social innovation called "welfare capitalism." Leading exponents such as General Electric and Bethlehem Steel built clean, safe factories, installed cafeterias and hired trained dietitians, formed baseball teams and glee clubs. Millions of workers enrolled in company unions (called by critics "Kiss-Me Clubs," for their lack of power). They nonetheless offered what few traditional unions could match: health and safety insurance, a grievance procedure, and representation for African-Americans, women, and immigrants. Several hundred firms encouraged perhaps a million workers to buy company stock. The Western Electric Company introduced rest breaks, provided free refreshments, and shortened the workday. Productivity increased immediately.

Still, such welfare capitalism embraced only about 5 percent of the work force and often gave benefits only to skilled laborers, the hardest to replace. Most companies cared more for productivity than contented workers. At a steel mill where tired workers lost their hands in steel sheet cutters, foremen handcuffed

A shop steward.

them to a lever that pulled their arms away from descending blades in the interest of safety. "There they work, chained to their machines, as galley slaves were chained to their oars," wrote one visitor. In the interest of increasing productivity, other machines displaced laborers. Throughout the decade unemployment never dropped below 5 percent, and in ailing industries like coal mining it averaged 30 percent. According to one estimate, almost one American family in six was "chronically destitute." In the 1920s a family of four could live in "minimum health and decency" on $2000 a year. The average industrial wage was $1304 a year, so many families needed more than one wage earner to just get by.

Over a million children, ages 10 to 15, still worked full-time in 1920, some for as little as 20 cents an hour. In Passaic, New Jersey, a textile town, the sons and daughters of Hungarian and Polish immigrants went into the mills at 13 so their families could survive. Some of the worst conditions existed in the textile town of Gastonia, North Carolina. Parents and children worked 10- to 12-hour shifts around the clock in 90-degree heat. To wring more production from the mill, managers imposed "stretch-outs," the textile equivalent of assembly-line speed-ups. In 1927, in the most famous strike of the decade, 2500 mill hands left their jobs, and even strikebreakers walked out. Eventually unsympathetic local authorities ended the strike, presaging a national trend. A year later there were only 629 strikes in the whole country, a record low. Union membership plummeted from almost 5 million in 1921 to less than 3.5 million in 1929. "The AF of L machinery," observed a despondent union official, "has practically collapsed."

The Consumer Culture

By the time of World War I, the network of industrial and manufacturing systems— in communications, sales, and distribution—had penetrated enough of the country to create mass markets. As the industrial base matured with the production of more consumer goods, prosperity in the 1920s hinged increasingly on consumption. Business leaders began to look at workers (in fact at all their fellow citizens) as "consumers." Henry Ford's doctrine of high wages was based on the assumption that more take-home pay would raise mass purchasing power, increase demand and production, and bring down costs. The flip side of his doctrine was low prices, which would lift mass sales still higher. If this continued, prosperity would reign without end.

Everything rested on consumers: they now had to be courted. Wives ceased to be homemakers and became purchasers of processed food and manufactured goods. Husbands were no longer just workers but bill-payers—consumers of mortgages and other forms of credit. As more employees got two-week (unpaid) vacations, even leisure became consumable. So, as one government report observed, "it is preeminently the problem of marketing, and especially the creation of demand, which has held the attention of business executives." Consumption (as reflected in sales) was the final key to prosperity, and consumption hinged on two modern innovations: advertising to increase demand and credit to help consumers buy.

Before World War I advertising had been a grubby business. Most top advertising executives were former copywriters for patent medicines. Around the turn of the century, however, advertising began a critical shift from emphasizing the virtues of products to stressing the wants of consumers. During the war the Committee on Public Information demonstrated the power of advertising as an instrument of mass persuasion, and soon businesses were shaping the tastes of consumers, convincing them that almost any want could be bought. Behavioral psychologists like John B. Watson, who left Johns Hopkins University for an advertising agency in the 1920s, showed advertisers how to develop more sophisticated techniques. Like the war propaganda, advertising copy aimed increasingly at emotions and cynically regarded the "average normal American," in the words of one executive, as having the "literate capacity of a 12- or 14-year-old."

More than anyone else, Albert Lasker developed modern advertising in America. Lasker, the owner of Chicago's largest advertising firm, Lord and Thomas, created copy that was hard-hitting, forthright, positive—and often fantastical. To boost the sales of Lucky Strike cigarettes Lord and Thomas advertisements suggested that smoking made people slimmer and more courageous. "Lucky's" became one of the most popular brands in America. Other advertisers were even less scrupulous. Bogus doctors and dentists endorsed all kinds of products, some downright dangerous. Millions were told to brush their teeth with toothpaste containing potassium chloride—eight grams of which could kill a human being. (At least one person committed suicide by eating a tube.) "Halitosis," plucked from the pages of an obscure medical dictionary, was used to sell Listerine mouthwash, and Lifebuoy soap thrived on fears of "B.O." ("body odor"). The bottom line was to sell not products, but desires: health, popularity, social prestige.

Advertisers declared war on the traditional virtues of thrift and prudence. A generation earlier debt had been considered unrespectable, the result of wantonness or disaster. When sociologists Helen and Robert Lynd completed an exhaustive study of Muncie, Indiana (*Middletown*, 1929), they found almost no family without debts. Installment buying, once confined largely to sewing machines and pianos, grew into the tenth biggest business in the United States. The automobile industry led the way. In 1919 Alfred Sloan created millions of new customers by establishing the General Motors Acceptance Corporation, the first consumer credit organization in the country. Ten years later it was the largest sales financing company in the world, and more than two-thirds of all automobile sales were on time payments. By 1929 consumer debt had jumped 250 percent, to $7 billion, almost twice the amount of the federal budget. The consumer culture encouraged Americans to borrow today so they could buy what advertising convinced them they wanted for tomorrow. At the end of the decade Americans were buying over 60 percent of their cars, radios, and furniture on the installment plan. By persuading them that what was new was also desirable, advertising also helped to propagate modernism.

A MASS SOCIETY

The increasingly consumer-oriented structure of the American economy played a central role in shaping a modern culture of consumption. During the late nineteenth century the economy had boomed, too, but a larger part of its energies went into the development of heavy industry and non–consumer goods: greater steel capacity and the growth of national rail, communications, and energy networks. As the economy shifted to consumer goods and the modern ethic of high spending and high consumption worked its way into American society, life changed. The new systems of distribution and mass marketing led not simply to a higher standard of living but also to a mass culture, with tastes less regional and diverse. More and more Americans read the same weekly magazines, saw the same films, heard the same radio programs, and had the same idols.

Other aspects of the new mass culture weakened many of the traditional ties that bound Americans together. Local communities and churches, which had often been the arbiters of what was moral and proper, sometimes found their authority undercut by the tastes of moviemakers in Hollywood or magazine writers in New York. The automobile gave families, and individuals within families, the independence to travel at their convenience. Families saw their role in educating their children decrease as the bureaucratic institution of the school steadily expanded its influence. The New Era was witness to "a vast dissolution of ancient habits," remarked columnist Walter Lippmann. In the place of those habits came many of the forces of modern life: independent women, free and easy love, standardized culture, the energy and impersonality of cities, the alienation of intellectuals.

The New Woman

The "New Woman," charged critics, was at the bottom of what Frederick Lewis Allen called the "revolution in manners and morals" that characterized the twenties. Before the war women were arrested for smoking cigarettes in public, using profanity, appearing on public beaches without stockings, driving automobiles without men beside them, and wearing slacks or shorts. Judges heard such cases not just in small towns but in cities like New York and Chicago as well. Wartime America ended many of these restrictions. With so many women bagging explo-

Daily Lives

CLOTHING AND FASHION
The Beauty Contest

On a sunlit day early in September 1921 eight young women stood nervously on the boardwalk at Atlantic City, New Jersey. For a week the seaside resort had presented a succession of swimming exhibitions, dance contests, and automobile races. A giant parade featured clowns, bands, a float carrying King Neptune escorted by mermaids, and the boardwalk's famous rolling chairs draped with flowers. With the exception of the clowns all the marchers wore bathing suits, even the mayor and the members of the city council and chamber of commerce. They had been instrumental in organizing the week's central event—a national beauty contest to select the first "Miss America."

The American beauty contest drew on a heritage that dated back to medieval festivals, which often included a competition for the most attractive woman. In colonial times the traditional May Day celebration crowned a Queen of the May as a symbol of fertility. By the middle of the nineteenth century many cities began holding festivals to publicize their virtues and attract settlers. Queens played a vital role, embodying fruitfulness and community. Though physical beauty mattered in the selection, qualities such as civic leadership and popularity also counted.

The flamboyant huckster P. T. Barnum created the modern beauty contest. In 1854 Barnum conceived of a competition among women to judge their appearance at his high-class American Museum in New York. As first prize he offered a diamond tiara (or a dowry if the winner were unmarried), but Victorian codes of conduct prohibited such public displays, and Barnum attracted only contestants of "questionable reputation." To lure middle-class women, he announced that "daguerrotypes," or photographs, could be submitted. Participants did not even have to send their names. Barnum sold his museum before he received the photographs, but the idea quickly spread to newspapers and later to the new mass-circulation dailies. When the promoters of the St. Louis Exposition advertised a beauty contest in 1905, some 40,000 women applied.

Carnivals, fairs, and "dime museums" (where for 10 cents one could see midway curiosities and stage entertainment) had begun holding beauty contests with entrants actually present. Catering to

Margaret Gorman of Washington, D.C., crowned in 1921 as the first Miss America.

Daily Lives

working-class customers whose social conventions were not rigid, the shows produced few complaints. Around the turn of the century, as mass advertising and mass entertainment spread across the country, chorus girls and models gained acceptance. "Bathing beauties" began cropping up at summer resorts and on the silver screen. The legitimate beauty contest, with middle-class audiences and participants, was simply the next step.

Despite public pronouncements, the contestants at the Miss America pageant came not from the nation at large but from eight nearby cities, each of which had conducted local competitions. Promoters had conceived of the pageant as a way of extending the summer season past September 1, but Victorian prudishness threatened the venture. The contest measured physical beauty alone, with the high point being a bathing suit competition. (Only later did the pageant add a talent show.) After the turn of the century, bathing suits had grown alarmingly scant, exposing arms and discarding billowy bloomers in favor of revealing tights. Straight-laced visitors might balk at the sight of middle-class women strutting seminude before a panel of judges.

Aware of such perils, organizers depicted entrants as wholesome, conventional, and unsophisticated. None of the contestants were permitted to wear short "bobbed" hair or makeup—both symbols of the racy modern woman. Models, theatrical performers, and other "professional beauties" competed separately. Famous women's illustrators lent legitimacy by serving as judges. Howard Chandler Christie alone judged the first contest, but the following year Norman Rockwell and two other artists joined the panel. To underscore the lightheartedness of the pageant, local police dressed like Keystone Kops, the bumbling heroes of Mack Sennett's comedy films.

As the contestants waited anxiously, officials announced the winner—Margaret Gorman of Washington, D.C. She looked like Mary Pickford, the screen star dubbed "America's Sweetheart" by the press. Like Pickford, Gorman radiated innocence and athletic vigor. "She represents the type of womanhood America needs," observed Samuel Gompers of the American Federation of Labor, "—strong, red-blooded, able to shoulder the responsibilities of home-making and motherhood."

The Miss America pageant was an immediate success. Newspapers across the country reported the results. In 1922 representatives of 58 cities competed, and a crowd of 200,000 watched the opening parade. Five years later the number of contestants had jumped to 75, including some from distant California and Alaska. The much-feared protests nonetheless materialized. In 1928 organizers were forced to cancel the pageant when hotel owners objected that their middle-class clientele found the display offensive. The pageant was revived again in 1935, and a Miss America has reigned ever since.

Miss America and other beauty contests evolved as Victorianism declined in the early twentieth century, but the lengths to which pageant organizers went to gain respect demonstrated the strength of the older social codes. The Miss America pageant in particular came to symbolize the middle-class ideal of womanhood. Physical beauty remained the chief component, marriage and motherhood the chief ends. The message was graphic: men competed in sports gear, business attire, and professional garb; women in bathing suits. That fashion would be slow to change.

sives, running locomotives, and drilling with rifles, the old taboos often seemed antiquated or plain silly.

Before the war disseminating birth control information by mail had also been a crime. By the armistice there was a birth control clinic in Brooklyn, a National Birth Control League, and later an American Birth Control League led by Margaret Sanger. Sanger's crusade had begun as an attempt to save poor women from the burdens of unwanted pregnancies. Hostile authorities confiscated the literature she mailed discussing sex education, venereal disease, and contraception, and in 1914 she fled the country to evade arrest. By the 1920s she had become less a radical crusader for the poor than a feminist advocate of "new ideals of sex," which she hoped would transform the sex act from "biological necessity" to "a psychic and spiritual avenue of expression." Her message found a receptive middle-class audience. Surveys showed that by the 1930s nearly 90 percent of college-educated couples practiced contraception.

Being able to a degree to control the matter of pregnancy, women felt less guilt about enjoying sex. In 1909 Sigmund Freud had come to America to lecture on his theories of coping with the unconscious and overcoming harmful repressions. Freud's complex ideas sailed blissfully over the heads of most Americans, but as popularized in the 1920s by crusaders like Sanger, they gave the clear impression that sexuality was a key to health. In a consumer culture preoccupied with self-gratification, sexual fulfillment became an important ingredient. Anybody could learn to free suppressed desires and consequently enjoy a richer life. To help them, Sears, Roebuck began listing books such as *Ten Thousand Dreams Interpreted* and *Sex Problems Solved*.

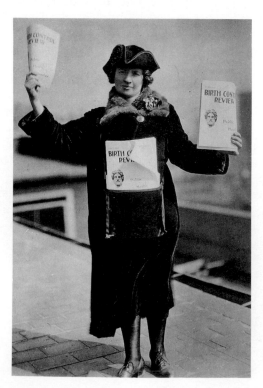

"Street selling was torture for me," Margaret Sanger recalled of her efforts to promote the *Birth Control Review*. Hecklers often taunted Sanger and her colleagues. "Have you never heard God's word to 'be fruitful and multiply and replenish the earth'?" one asked. The reply came back, "They've done that already."

Cocktail in hand, cigarette in mouth, the New Woman became a symbol of liberated womanhood. If she was up to the latest wrinkle, she wore a close-fitting felt hat and lots of makeup, had a long-waisted dress and two strings of beads, unbuckled her galoshes, and called herself a "flapper." She was, wrote F. Scott Fitzgerald, the chronicler of the decade, "lovely and expensive and about nineteen." The flapper, though, was hardly an accurate symbol of the age. Certainly women in the 1920s gained a measure of power and independence. With passage of the Nineteenth Amendment in 1920 the United States became the twenty-second nation to grant women the vote, and in 1924 two women—Nellie Ross in Wyoming and Miriam ("Ma") Ferguson in Texas—were elected governors, the first female chief executives. But the deserved fame of a few women was one thing, the daily working patterns of American life another. Over the decade, the female labor force had grown by more than 2 million, making one worker in every five female. That represented an increase of barely 1 percent. As late as 1930 nearly 60 percent of all working women were African-American or foreign-born, generally holding low-paying jobs in domestic service or the garment industry.

The new age did offer some new career choices for women. The consumer culture spawned a preoccupation with appearance that led to the opening of some 40,000 beauty parlors staffed by hairdressers, manicurists, and cosmeticians. "Women's fields" carved out by progressive reformers expanded opportunities in education, libraries, and social welfare. In many ways extensions of women's domestic sphere, these fields nevertheless became more professionalized in the 1920s. Specialized training and licensing required more education. Women earned a higher percentage of doctoral degrees (from 10 percent in 1910 to 15.4 percent in 1930) and held more college teaching posts than ever (32 percent). In most areas, professional men resisted the "feminization" of the work force. The number of women doctors dropped by almost 3000, a 50 percent decline, as medical schools imposed restrictive quotas and some 90 percent of all hospitals rejected female interns.

Having won the vote, most women did not use it, and when they did, they voted with their husbands or families along lines of class, region, and ethnicity, not gender. A few activists succeeded in winning passage of the Sheppard–Towner Federal Maternity and Infancy Act in 1921 to fight high rates of infant mortality. But by the end of the decade it had lapsed. Even the most obstreperous flapper, if she wed, ended up in a conventional marriage that tied her to home and family.

In the wake of its greatest success, the hard-won vote for women, the feminist movement splintered. The National Woman Suffrage Association disbanded in 1920, at the prompting of its most distinguished member, 65-year-old Carrie Chapman Catt. In its place the League of Women Voters was begun to encourage informed voting. For the more militant Alice Paul and her allies, that was not enough. Their National Woman's Party, founded in 1916, began to press for a constitutional Equal Rights Amendment (ERA).

Strongest support for the ERA came from middle-class women. Social workers and others familiar with the conditions under which women labored opposed it. Death and injury rates for women were nearly double those for men in the same industries. Barred from most unions, working-class women had won some protection only because they were women. To them the ERA meant losing the protection as well as the benefits they derived from mothers' pensions and maternity insurance. Joined by most men and a majority of Congress they fought the amendment to a standstill.

Mass Media

In balmy California, where movies could be made year-round, Hollywood helped to give the New Woman notoriety as a temptress and trend-setter. When Theda Bara (the "vamp") appeared in *The Blue Flame* in 1920, crowds mobbed theaters all along the East Coast. Clara Bow, the "It" girl, became a featured player. "It" was sex appeal, and the only others who had "It," explained novelist Elinor Glyn, were "Rex, the wild stallion, actor Tony Moreno, [and] the Ambassador Hotel doorman." And just as Hollywood came to dictate the standards of physical attraction, it became the arbiter of taste and fashion in countless other ways because motion pictures were a virtually universal medium: there was no need for literacy or fluency, no need even for hearing, given the simple stories parading across the silent screen.

Motion pictures, invented in 1889, had first been shown in tiny neighborhood theaters called "nickelodeons." For a nickel, almost anyone, children included, could afford to walk into the dark, overheated theater. The screen flickered with moving images as an accompanist played music on a tinny piano. The audience was anything but silent. The theater reverberated with the cracking of Indian nuts, the day's equivalent of popcorn, while young cowboys shot off their Kilgore repeating cap pistols during dramatic scenes. Often children read the subtitles aloud to their immigrant parents, translating into Italian, Yiddish, or German. After the first feature-length film, *The Great Train Robbery* (1903), productions became rich in spectacle, attracted middle-class audiences, and turned into America's favorite form of entertainment.

By 1926 more than 20,000 theaters offered customers overstuffed seats, live music, and a celluloid dream world—all for 50 cents or less. At the end of the decade, they were drawing over 100 million people a week, roughly the equivalent of the national population. In Muncie, Indiana—the "Middletown" of America—nine theaters opened their doors at 1 p.m. and closed at 11 at night, 7 days a week, 12 months a year. Every theater had two films, and each changed programs two or three times a week. Westerns were the staple of five theaters, and a comedy star named Harold Lloyd was the town favorite. Next to Lloyd comedies, movies with "sex appeal" drew the biggest audiences. *Flaming Youth* packed houses in 1924 with promotions that promised "neckers, petters, white kisses, red kisses, pleasure-mad daughters, sensation-craving mothers, by an author who didn't dare sign his name." Rudolph Valentino, whose dark good looks seduced a generation of moviegoers, traded on raw sexuality to become the era's premier matinee idol. When he died of peritonitis at the age of 31, the line of mourners stretched over a mile through the streets of New York.

Radio came into its own as a mass medium. In the spring of 1920 Frank Conrad of the Westinghouse Company in East Pittsburgh rigged up a research station in his barn and began sending out phonograph music and baseball scores to local wireless operators. An ingenious Pittsburgh newspaper began advertising radio equipment to "be used by those who listen to Dr. Conrad's programs." In October 1920 Westinghouse officials opened the first licensed broadcasting station in history, KDKA, to stimulate sales of their supplies. By 1921 the number of licensed stations had jumped to 28; half a year later there were 430. Radios—"furniture that talks," comedian Fred Allen called it—were soon being purchased by millions of Americans.

At first radio was seen as a civilizing force, an agent of cultural uplift that

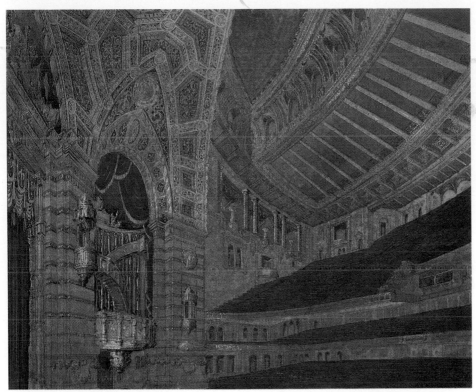

The Roxy, the largest theater in the world when it opened in 1926, in all its palatial glory. Such lavish movie houses sought to attract more prosperous middle-class audiences with splendor reminiscent of European cathedrals. On the night the Roxy opened, pealing chimes marked the beginning of the show, whereupon a man dressed as a monk strode onto center stage, pointed to the balcony, and declared, "Let there be light!" Blazing spotlights then set the orchestra aglow. "Does God live here?" asked a little girl in a *New Yorker* cartoon.

could beam high-toned programs to an audience of individuals and small groups. "The air is your theater, your college, your newspaper, your library," trumpeted one ad in 1924. After a rocky start, commercial broadcasting slowly took hold as the ownership of sets spread to less affluent listeners. By 1931 advertisers were paying $10,000 an hour for a national hook-up, and the gross income of the the National Broadcasting Company, launched only five years earlier, was $150 million. Nearly one home in three had a radio. Almost the entire nation listened to "Amos 'n' Andy," a comedy about blacks created by two white vaudevillians in 1929. People refused to answer their telephones during the program, and in smaller cities movie theaters stopped their shows to tune it in so patrons would not leave.

Radio changed national habits. At night families gathered around the radio instead of the hearth. Rather than going out to hear music people listened to it on the radio. Together with movies, radio cut deeply into the traditional audiences of vaudeville. After all, noted *Broadcasting* magazine, "You can get Eddie Cantor on the air for nothing." The aged, the sick, and the isolated could be, as one advertisement declared, "at home but never alone." Across the country, linked by nothing but airwaves, Americans were finding themselves part of a vast new community.

Print journalism also developed broader systems of distribution during the 1920s. In 1921 DeWitt Wallace, a veteran with a knack for condensing magazine stories, borrowed $5000 from friends and relatives, set up business in the basement of a Greenwich Village speakeasy, and mailed out the first issue of *Reader's Digest* to 1500 subscribers. Within a decade circulation stood at half a million. In 1923 Henry R. Luce and Briton Hadden, classmates at Yale, rewrote news stories in a snappy style, mixed them with photographs, and created the country's first national newspaper, *Time* magazine. By 1927, 55 giant chains distributed 230 newspapers with a combined circulation of 13 million. Though they controlled under 10 percent of all papers, the chains pioneered modern mass news techniques. Editors relied on central offices or newspaper syndicates to prepare editorials, sports, gossip, and Sunday features for a national audience.

"Ain't We Got Fun?"

"Ev'ry morning, ev'ry evening, ain't we got fun?" ran the 1921 hit song. As the average hours on the job decreased from 47.2 in 1920 to 42 by 1930, spending on amusement and recreation shot up 300 percent. Some of the spare time went into fads of the new mass culture. To mark their individuality and win notoriety people sat on flagpoles, swallowed goldfish, and entered dance marathons. In 1922 no home was considered complete without a mah-jongg set, a Chinese board game that had its own national association. As leisure time expanded, upper-class sports like tennis and golf spread to the middle class and created heroes—Bill Tilden in tennis, Bobby Jones in golf.

Spectator sports came of age. In 1921, some 60,000 fans paid $1.8 million to see Jack Dempsey, the "Manassas Mauler," knock out French champion Georges Carpentier. Millions more listened as radio took them ringside for the first time in sports history. Universities constructed huge stadiums for football—a 60,000-seater at Berkeley; a 64,000-seater at Ohio State. By the end of the decade college football games outdrew major league baseball, and Harold "Red" Grange, the "Galloping Ghost" of Notre Dame, became the first athlete to make the cover of *Time*.

Baseball still remained the national pastime. An ugly World Series scandal in 1919 led owners to appoint Judge Kenesaw Mountain Landis "czar" of the sport early in the decade. His iron rule reformed the game. In 1920 the son of immigrants revolutionized it. George Herman "Babe" Ruth hit 54 homers (more than any other whole team hit that year), batted .376, and made the New York Yankees the first baseball club to attract a million fans in one season. A heroic producer in an era of consumption, Ruth was also baseball's bad boy, "our national exaggeration," said one writer. He smoked, drank, cursed, and chased every skirt in sight. Under the guidance of his personal manager, Christy Walsh (the first modern sports agent), Ruth became the highest paid player in the game and made a fortune endorsing everything from automobiles to clothing.

At parties old diversions—charades, card tricks, recitations—vanished as dancing took over. The ungainly camel-walk, the sultry tango, and in 1924 the frantic Charleston were the urban standards. Country barns featured a revival of square dancing with music provided by Detroit's WBZ, courtesy of Henry Ford. And from the turn-of-the century brothels and gaming houses of New Orleans,

Memphis, and St. Louis came a rhythmic, compelling music that swept into night-clubs and over the airwaves: jazz.

The term "jazz" had illicit sexual overtones when bestowed by whites, who found its bolder style of playing and its origins in the community to be little more than immoral "race music." But jazz was a remarkably complex blend of several older African-American musical traditions. It grew most directly out of "the blues," whose haunting melodies were often sung or played with a quavering, passionate pitch:

> The moon looks lonesome when it's shining through the trees.
> Yes, the moon looks lonesome, shining through the trees.
> And a man looks lonesome when his woman packs up to leave . . .

The new jazz bands combined the soulfulness of the blues with the brighter synco-pated rhythms of ragtime music. Jazz bands usually used five to eight instruments—a few trumpets, trombones, a rhythm section of drums and a plucked string bass, a piano or perhaps a banjo. Their distinct style came from a marvellous improvising. Most music compositions, whether the symphonies of Brahms or the marches of John Phillip Sousa, were written out in advance and played note by note. A jazz piece provided only a backdrop, a kind of rough musical framework. Within these limits, musicians would embellish the melody, playing off one another, encourag-ing their partners to go them one better.

The jazz style spread when the "Original Dixieland Jazz Band" (hardly origi-nal but possessed of the advantage of being white) recorded a few numbers for the phonograph. The music became a sensation in New York in 1917 and soon spread to other parts of the country. Black New Orleans stalwarts like Joe "King" Oliver's Creole Jazz Band began touring; in Chicago Oliver introduced audiences to a young cornet player named Louis Armstrong, who became a leading jazz musician and arranger in his own right. In 1924 Paul Whiteman inaugurated respectable "white" jazz in a concert at Carnegie Hall, and George Gershwin was soon adapt-ing its rhythms to musicals and symphonic compositions like "Rhapsody in Blue." Guardians of good taste and propriety denounced such music as "intellectual and spiritual debauchery." Whiteman disagreed: "Jazz is the folk music of the machine age."

The Art of Alienation

Painters of the Ashcan School continued to find subjects, in the words of teacher Robert Henri, "anywhere, everywhere," but mostly where they always had—in the strident life of the industrial city. George Bellows painted violent prizefights, the most famous of which depicted Argentina's Luis Firpo knocking Jack Dempsey from the ring. Charles Sheeler broke with the gauzy, artistic photography of the past. He snapped the machine age, shot by raw shot, most notably in a study of Henry Ford's Rouge Assembly Plant. Georgia O'Keeffe moved in the opposite direction. As warm as Sheeler's work was cool, her paintings represented passion and sexuality in near-abstract shapes and bold colors.

Before the war a generation of young writers had begun rebelling against Victorian purity. During the war years many lost faith in reason and progress, seeking relief from a comforting "nihilism" that denied all meaning in life. When the conflict ended they launched a brilliant assault on small towns, big business, conformity, technology, and material culture. Some fled to the urban bohemia of Greenwich Village in New York City. Others, called expatriates, simply left the country for the artistic freedom of London and Paris (where the rising value of the dollar also made living cheaper). Their alienation helped to produce a literary outpouring unmatched in American history.

On the eve of World War I the poet Ezra Pound had predicted an "American Risorgimento" that would "make the Italian Renaissance look like a tempest in a teapot." From Europe the expatriate Pound began to make it happen. Abandoning rhyme and meter, he decried the "botched civilization" that had produced the war. Another voluntary exile, T. S. Eliot, bemoaned the emptiness of modern life in his epic poem *The Waste Land* (1922). Ernest Hemingway captured the disillusionment of the age in his novels *The Sun Also Rises* (1926) and *A Farewell to Arms* (1929), where resolution came as it had in war—by death.

At home Sherwood Anderson led a revolt against small-town life. In 1912, at the age of 36, Anderson walked out of his paint factory in Elyria, Ohio. After a nervous breakdown, in 1919 he published his masterpiece, *Winesburg, Ohio*, a series of short stories connected by place and mood. Compassionate but pessimistic, Anderson examined the underside of the small town. He wrote about frustrated spinsters, repressed businessmen, pimply teenagers. Some were near suicide; all had sex on their minds. No American novel of the period had greater influence on those that followed.

A year later Minnesota-born Sinclair Lewis, the first American to win a Nobel Prize in literature, wrote *Main Street*. A scathing vision of small-town life in the Midwest, the book described "savorless people, gulping tasteless food, . . . saying mechanical things about the excellence of Ford automobiles, and viewing themselves as the greatest race in the world." It sold 3 million copies. His next novel, *Babbitt* (1922), dissected small-town businessman George Follansbee Babbitt, a peppy realtor from fictional Zenith. Faintly absurd and supremely dull, Babbitt was the epitome of the average.

The novels of another Minnesotan, F. Scott Fitzgerald, glorified youth and romantic individualism but found redemption nowhere. His heroes, like Amory Blaine in *This Side of Paradise* (1920), spoke for a generation "grown up to find all Gods dead, all wars fought, all faiths in man shaken." Like most writers of the decade, Fitzgerald saw life largely as a personal affair—opulent, always self-absorbing, and ultimately tragic. It was "characteristic of the Jazz Age," he wrote, "that it had no interests in politics at all."

John Dos Passos, whose novels pulsed with the energy and edginess of the machine age, was a notable exception. The child of Portuguese immigrants, Dos Passos embraced individualism and communism equally, fought entrenched power, and saw the country as divided along class, ethnic, and racial lines. "All right," he said in *The Big Money* (1931), the last volume of his searing *U.S.A.* trilogy, "we are two nations."

A "New Negro"

As World War I seared white intellectuals, so too did it galvanize blacks. Postwar unemployment and racial violence dashed blacks' hopes for equality with white

Born in Jamaica in 1887, Marcus Garvey founded his "Back to Africa" movement in 1914. He went to prison for mail fraud in 1925, but it was like "jailing a rainbow," said one observer. President Coolidge pardoned Garvey in 1927, then deported him to Jamaica.

America. Common folk in urban slums found an outlet for their alienation in a charismatic nationalist from Jamaica named Marcus Garvey.

Garvey had come to America in 1916, bringing with him an organization and a dream. The Universal Negro Improvement Association (UNIA) was Garvey's vehicle for returning Africans to Africa and Africa to Africans. He decried racial prejudice and stressed black superiority, pride, education, and industry. "Up you mighty race," he told his followers, "you can accomplish what you will." By 1920 Garvey claimed 4 million followers. Even his harshest critics admitted there were at least half a million members in more than 30 branches of his organization. It was the first mass movement of African-Americans in history. When Garvey spoke at the first national convention of the UNIA in 1920, more than 25,000 supporters jammed Madison Square Garden in New York to hear him preach black nationalism and separatism.

In 1925 Garvey's dream shattered. He was convicted of mail fraud for having oversold stock in his Black Star Line, the steamship company founded to take Africans back to Africa. The movement fell apart, but its audacious spirit infected other African-Americans. As Garvey rose to prominence a renaissance of black literature, painting, and sculpture was brewing in Harlem. The first inklings came in 1922 when Claude McKay, another Jamaican immigrant, published a book of poems entitled *White Shadows*. McKay mixed defiance with racial pride in his most famous poem, "If We Must Die."

> If we must die, let it not be like hogs
> Hunted and penned in an inglorious spot, . . .
> Like men we'll face the murderous, cowardly pack,
> Pressed to the wall, dying but fighting back!

Often supported by white patrons, or "angels," young black writers and artists found their subjects in the street life of cities, the folkways of the rural South, or further back in the primitivism of preindustrial cultures. Though generally not promoters of racial protest, the young artists of the Harlem Renaissance drew on the new assertiveness of African-Americans as well as on the alienation of white intellectuals. In 1925 Alain Locke, a black professor from Howard University, collected a sampling of their works in *The New Negro*. The title reflected not only a new artistic movement but a new racial consciousness as well.

DEFENDERS OF THE FAITH

Like the races, America itself was divided. One part of the nation looked ahead, the other back. Modernists rushed toward a glorious future of machines, organization, middle-class urban living, and cosmopolitan tolerance. Traditionalists followed a cherished older faith, associated with rural life and valuing neighborliness, small communities, and comfortable sameness.

The two had stood side by uneasy side for decades. In the 1920s the emergence of a mass society sharpened awareness of the differences—and the dangers—each saw in the other. As modernism transformed the country, traditional culture hardened, looking on change with suspicion and diversity with dismay. If urban cosmopolitans could be patronizing about the "rubes" and "hayseeds" from the country, country folk could be mean-spirited and intolerant in return. They could draw support from their allies—rural migrants to cities and an embattled Protestant elite. All were determined to defend the older order against the modern age.

Nativism and Restriction of Immigration

In May 1920 Nicola Sacco and Bartolomeo Vanzetti, two Italian aliens and admitted anarchists, were indicted for a shoe company robbery and murder in South Braintree, Massachusetts. Most of the evidence linking them to the crime was circumstantial. In July 1921, after a jury found them guilty, Judge Webster Thayer sentenced them to death. For the next six years they appealed the decision. Each time Thayer denied their motions, even when a Rhode Island gang member confessed to the crime.

The case, seemingly a straightforward robbery and murder, became one of the most celebrated of the decade. Critics charged that Sacco and Vanzetti were innocent, convicted only for being foreign-born radicals. Whatever the merits of their case, the two never received a fair hearing. Testimony at their trial often focused on their anarchist beliefs, draft evasion, and foreign birth. Thayer himself had called them "anarchist bastards" in private. When a special commission including the presidents of Harvard and the Massachusetts Institute of Technology denied clemency, the forces of upper-class respectability seemed aligned against them. For protesters around the world, Sacco and Vanzetti were symbols of bigotry and prejudice. In August 1927, when they were executed, 50,000 marchers wearing red armbands followed the funeral procession for eight miles to bid a final farewell.

By then, nativism—a rabid hostility to foreigners—had produced the most restrictive immigration laws in American history. In the aftermath of World War I immigration was running close to 1 million a year, almost as high as prewar levels. Most immigrants came from eastern and southern Europe; the majority were Catholics and Jews. With just over half the American population white and of native-born parents, alarmists like novelist Kenneth Roberts worried that unrestricted immigration would produce "a hybrid race of people as worthless and futile as the good-for-nothing mongrels of Central America and Southeastern Europe." Appreciating the benefits of a shrunken labor pool, the American Federation of Labor supported restriction too.

Led by Henry Cabot Lodge of Massachusetts and Hiram Johnson of California, in 1921 Congress enacted emergency legislation that established an annual limit on immigration. A quota set the number of entrants at 350,000 a year and parceled them out on the basis of 3 percent of each nationality living in the United States as of 1910. Asian immigration was banned entirely. Three years later the National Origins Act cut the quota to 150,000, pushed the base year back to 1890 (before the bulk of southern and eastern Europeans arrived), and made the restrictions permanent.

The National Origins Act fixed the pattern of immigration for the next four decades. Immigration from southern and eastern Europe was reduced to a trickle, while the steady flow of northern and western Europeans continued. In Congress support for restriction was especially strong among rural members who saw limiting immigration as a matter not only of race and religion but also of beliefs and loyalties. "On the one side," declared a representative from Kansas during the debate, "is beer, bolshevism, unassimilating settlements and perhaps many flags—

on the other is constitutional government; one flag, stars and stripes." The great movement of Europeans to America, a migration of classes and nationalities that had been unimpeded for 300 years, came largely to an end.

The "Noble Experiment"

In the same years that Sacco and Vanzetti were appealing their case, the "noble experiment" of Prohibition was under way. The Eighteenth Amendment, banning the sale, manufacture, importation, and transportation of liquor, took effect in January 1920. For nearly a hundred years reformers had tried to reduce the consumption of alcohol. Progressive temperance arguments stressed efficiency, public health, and the corrupting influence of the saloon. In World War I the need to feed starving war victims prompted the conservation of grains for food. Meanwhile hysterical patriots questioned the loyalties of breweries with German names and fellow citizens who drank beer and ale.

Where in force, Prohibition was not total: as private citizens, Americans could still keep liquor in their homes and serve drinks to their friends. They simply could not make, sell, or import any "intoxicating beverage." The Volstead Act, an enforcement statute passed in September 1919, defined an "intoxicating beverage" as one containing 0.5 percent alcohol. The act permitted the use of existing stocks of liquor for religious and medicinal purposes and allowed the manufacture of industrial alcohol—but only if rendered poisonous.

Prohibition never stamped out liquor, but it did reduce consumption (as much as half by some accounts). Despite the availability of "moonshine" and hard cider, drinking declined in rural areas. Cities recorded fewer deaths from alcohol and fewer arrests for drunkenness. From the start, however, enforcement was underfunded and understaffed. The Justice Department's Prohibition Bureau consisted of 1500 agents. The entire Pacific Northwest never had more than 20 agents to cover it. Not one was given an airplane, a boat, or an automobile. Their salary of $2000 a year amounted to a license to steal. One New York agent banked over $1.6 million in four months on the job. Other agents, like Izzy Einstein and his partner Moe Smith, were honest and dedicated. Disguised as everything from rabbis to college deans, they made nearly 3000 arrests. Still others, frustrated and poorly trained, relied on quick triggers, pistol whippings, or their fists.

Prohibition had always been unpopular with a sizable minority of Americans. In southern Florida people drilled holes in coconuts, added brown sugar, waited three weeks, and enjoyed a pungent "cocowhiskey." Some citizens, like Alice Roosevelt Longworth, wife of the Speaker of the House of Representatives, made their own home brew in copper stills purchased at hardware stores. A few states never ratified the Eighteenth Amendment; others refused to enact local enforcement statutes.

The consequences of so vast a social experiment as Prohibition were often unexpected. Prohibition reversed the prewar trend toward beer and wine, since hard liquor brought greater profits to bootleggers. Ironically, it advanced the cause of women's rights: saloons had discriminated against "ladies," having them enter by a separate door; speakeasies welcomed them. A democratic air prevailed inside, where everybody broke the law together. Prohibition also helped to line the pockets—and boost the fame—of gangsters. "Scarface" Al Capone moved from New York to Chicago in 1920. Seven years later he was the best known mobster in America, with a $60 million empire of alcohol, gambling, extortion, prostitution, and drugs. Thousands of poor immigrants looked to bootlegging to move them out of the slums, and cities erupted in a mayhem of violence among rival gangs.

Prohibition worked best as cultural and class legislation. Support for Prohibition had always been strongest among Protestant evangelical churches, including Baptists and Methodists. And there had always been a strong antiurban and anti-immigrant bias among reformers. As it turned out, cities recorded the steepest decline in drinking, especially among working-class ethnics, just as reformers had hoped. Only the rich had enough money to drink regularly without risking death or blindness, the common effects of cheap, tainted liquor. Working-class Americans, concentrated like the wealthy in cities, had a strong incentive to avoid the only liquor they could afford. Not only did they find themselves deprived of alcohol, but they lost the saloon as well. The saloon had functioned as their labor exchange, union hall, and social club as well as a source of corruption, but Prohibition turned it into a speakeasy for the middle and upper classes. Workers went to the movies or enjoyed radio instead. Traditionalists might celebrate the triumph of the "noble experiment," but most urbanites either ignored or resented it.

KKK

On Thanksgiving Day 1915, just outside Atlanta, 16 men trudged up a rocky trail to the crest of Stone Mountain. Leading them was William Simmons, 35 years old, tall and thin, formerly a circuit-riding Methodist minister and fraternal organizer. As night fell the assembly gathered around a burning wooden cross and by its light swore allegiance to the Invisible Empire, Knights of the Ku Klux Klan. A week later they received a preliminary charter from the state of Georgia. The KKK was reborn.

The modern Klan, a modified throwback to the hooded order of Reconstruction days (p. 635), reflected the particular insecurities of the New Era. Any white man could join the old Klan, but the new one admitted only "native born, white, gentile Americans." No Catholics could enter the order. Members believed in 100 percent Americanism and feared "foreigners" as much as African-Americans. In Texas Klansmen fed off hatred for Mexicans; in California, for Japanese; in New York, for Jews and other immigrants. Unlike the hooded night riders of old, the reborn Klan was not confined to the rural South. By the 1920s the capital of the Klan was Indianapolis, Indiana, and it had chapters in towns and cities as well. More than half of its leadership and over a third of its members came from metropolises of more than 100,000 people. Even the urban Northeast succumbed. In May 1923, Klansmen gathered, 10,000 strong, in New Brunswick, New Jersey, barely out of sight of New York City, and set a 62-foot cross ablaze.

The new Klan drew on the culture of small-town America. It was philanthropic, patriotic, and avowedly fraternal. Its elaborate regalia and rituals included white-hooded sheets and satin robes; titles of "Imperial Wizard," "Exalted Cyclops," and "Klaliff"; songs called "klodes"; and a secret handshake. A typical Klan gathering involved whole families, drawn together by fireworks, a barbecue, hymn-singing, oaths of loyalty to flag and country—all capped by the burning of a giant cross. Often working-class Americans of old Protestant stock, Klan members usually found themselves at the bottom of an industrialized, urbanized society. With few skill , they lived on the edge of unemployment and poverty, threatened by blacks and immigrants, anxious about changing codes of conduct, "moral

A raw and brutal form of racial violence, lynching continued to be a national scourge well into the 1920s and 1930s, when Paul Cadmus drew this searing study entitled *To the Lynching!* In 1919 alone more than seventy African-Americans were lynched, some of them returning soldiers still in uniform. In 1921, at the prompting of the National Association for the Advancement of Colored People, Representative L. C. Dyer of Missouri introduced the first antilynching bill in Congress. Despite passage in the House, the bill was filibustered to death by southerners in the Senate. Later antilynching bills met similar fates.

decay," and the rise of cities. Klan membership gave them reassurance and un-dreamed-of status. They could "klasp" each other's hands, converse in secret language, and feel as secure as any small-town lodge member.

Klansmen lived with the hope of restoring an older America. They fought for laissez-faire capitalism and fundamental Protestantism; white supremacy; chastity, fidelity, and parental authority; Prohibition; law and order; and an America free of foreigners. When benign methods failed they resorted to brutality—floggings, kidnapings, acid mutilations, and murder. In Houston a woman accused of bigamy, a doctor suspected of performing abortions, and a lawyer who accepted blacks as clients were whipped, tarred, and feathered. A naturalized citizen in Alabama was lashed for marrying a native-born woman. The Klan played so heavily on a fear of Catholics that when a train rumored to be carrying the pope pulled into Kokomo, Indiana, a mob stoned it.

Klan members may have distrusted the New Era's new values, but like so many other schemes of the decade, the Klan itself was dedicated to making money. Using modern promotional techniques, two professional fund-raisers, and an army of 1000 salesmen (called "kleagles"), the Klan enrolled a million new members by the end of 1921. By 1922 some 5000 applications were pouring in every day, and soon there were perhaps 5 million members. Moving into politics, the Klan won control of legislatures in Indiana, Texas, Oklahoma, and Oregon. It was instrumental in electing six governors, three senators, and thousands of local officials. In 1924 the KKK became so powerful that it blocked the Democratic National Convention from adopting a plank condemning it.

At the height of its strength, the Ku Klux Klan began to unravel. In an attempt to prove their power, 50,000 Klansmen marched down Pennsylvania Avenue in August 1925, but a violent thunderstorm burst over the rally like an omen of doom and sent Klansmen scurrying for shelter. Across the country in elections for mayor, governor, or senator, Klan-backed candidates lost as conventional politicians fought back. Sex scandals and financial corruption rocked its leadership and embarrassed members who saw themselves as guardians of morality. In November 1925, David Stephenson, grand dragon of the Indiana Klan and the most powerful leader in the Midwest, was sentenced to life imprisonment for rape and second-degree murder. The Klan never recovered.

Fundamentalism versus Darwinism

Although Aimee Semple McPherson and Bruce Barton adapted their religions to the cultural changes of the New Era, many Protestants, especially in rural areas, felt as though they had been under steady assault over the past half century. They felt threatened by the tide of Catholic and Jewish immigrants who poured into the country demanding a place in America. Equally troubling was the secular culture of modern life and its fluid morality, as well as scientific theories about geology, the age of the earth, and a skepticism about the possibility of miracles. The number of churches steadily declined during the decade. Despite an increase of nearly 13 million in church membership, many pastors reported fewer and fewer of their flock actually in attendance. Some pastors abandoned Sunday evening services altogether. Others attempted to reconcile the Bible with the modern world by stressing Jesus' ethical teachings rather than dealing with the miracle-oriented questions of bodily resurrection and the Day of Judgment, heaven, and hell.

Troubled conservatives had combined, as early as the late 1870s, to combat modernist influences. Between 1909 and 1912 two wealthy Los Angeles laymen, Lyman and Milton Stewart, subsidized a series of booklets known as *The Fundamentals*, which were sent to "every pastor, evangelist, minister, theological professor, theological student, Sunday school superintendent, YMCA and YWCA secretary in the English speaking world." The 3 million copies distributed stressed the "verbal inerrancy" of scripture: every word of the Bible was literally true. Proponents of this view, who after 1920 were increasingly known as "fundamentalists," saw themselves as defenders of traditional religion. Yet their literal reading of scripture was hardly traditional, for many Christian theologians in the past had interpreted various passages of scripture allegorically.

Fundamentalists maintained effective ministries nationwide, and they could be found among Presbyterians, Methodists, and other denominations. They were strongest in the South, however, especially among Baptists. Nothing disturbed them more than Darwinian theories of evolution, which by definition denied the divine origin of humankind and made the creation story of Adam and Eve either fanciful mythmaking or at best a parable. In 1925 George Washington Butler, a part-time schoolteacher and clerk of the Round Lick Association of Primitive Baptists, succeeded in convincing his fellow Tennessee legislators to make it illegal to teach that "man has descended from a lower order of animals."

Tennessee was neither the first nor the last state to seek legal means to restrain the onslaught of modern scientific ideas. Oklahoma, Florida, Mississippi, and Arkansas all passed similar statutes. What made Tennessee exceptional was the decision of some skeptics in the town of Dayton to test the legality of Butler's law. In the spring of 1925 a slender, bespectacled biology teacher named John T. Scopes was charged with violating the statute by teaching evolution. Behind the scenes, Scopes' sponsors were as much preoccupied with boosting their town's commercial fortunes as with the defense of free speech. When the Scopes trial opened in July it took on the flavor of a championship boxing match. Hot dog, lemonade, and sandwich stands lined the streets; vendors sold everything from Bibles to stuffed monkeys; loudspeakers relayed court proceedings to the thousands of people who stood outside, cooling themselves with toothpaste company fans that read "Do Your Gums Bleed?" Millions more listened over the radio to the first trial ever broadcast. Inside the courtroom, trial judge John Raulston sat beneath a banner advising "Read Your Bible Daily."

On one side of the bench stood Clarence Darrow, the most famous defense lawyer in the country and a professed agnostic, who had journeyed from Chicago to act as co-counsel for Scopes. Opposing him was William Jennings Bryan, the three-time presidential candidate who had recently joined the antievolution crusade. It was urban Darrow against rural Bryan in what Bryan described as a "duel to the death" between Christianity and evolution.

When Judge Raulston ruled that scientists imported by the defense could not be called on behalf of evolution (their testimony was considered "hearsay" because they had not been present at the Creation), the defense virtually collapsed. To keep the trial going (and to save his skin from angry vendors and town boosters) Judge Raulston agreed to let Darrow put Bryan on the stand. Darrow made him admit, to the horror of many of his followers, that the Earth was not made "in six days of 24-hours." In the end, the Dayton jury took eight minutes to find Scopes guilty and fine him $100. But by then the trial had become more of a national joke than a confrontation between darkness and light. The New Era would continue to be condemned in many quarters, but it could not be repealed. The larger issue of how much religious beliefs could influence public education in a nation where church and state were constitutionally separated would remain relevant as scientific, religious, and cultural standards clashed.

REPUBLICANS ASCENDANT

On March 4, 1921, Woodrow Wilson limped from the White House to a waiting automobile, took a seat beside President-elect Warren G. Harding, and rode down Pennsylvania Avenue to the Capitol. After the inauguration Wilson returned to his S Street house and lived the remaining two years of his life in bitter seclusion. Harding, the former Republican senator from Ohio, had won a smashing victory over Ohio governor James Cox and his young running mate, Franklin D. Roosevelt. "It wasn't a landslide," said Wilson's personal secretary after the election, "it was an earthquake." The Republicans were again ascendant.

"The change is amazing," wrote a Washington reporter shortly after the inauguration. "The populace is on a broad grin." The contrast in presidents could not have been more striking. Wilson had been ill, reclusive, and austere. Harding was handsome, warm, and lovable. Wilson had kept his own counsel; Harding promised to bring the "best minds" into the cabinet and let them run things. For the first time in four years, sentries disappeared from the gates of the White House, tourists walked the halls, and reporters freely questioned the president. The reign of "normalcy," as Harding called it, began. "By 'normalcy' I don't mean the older order," he had said during the campaign, "but a regular steady order of things. I mean normal procedure, the natural way, without excess." That Christmas, in a typical gesture of goodwill, Harding released socialist Eugene Debs from jail and invited him to dinner at the White House.

The Politics of Normalcy

"Normalcy" turned out to be anything but normal. After eight years of Democratic rule, Republicans controlled the White House from 1921 to 1933 and both houses of Congress from 1918 to 1930. For the first time since Reconstruction one party ruled Washington for a decade. Fifteen years of reform gave way to eight years of consolidation and cautious uses of government. A strong executive fell into weak hands. The cabinet and the Congress set the course of the nation.

Harding and his successor, Calvin Coolidge, were content with delegating power. To the cabinet Harding appointed some men of true quality: Charles Evans Hughes as secretary of state; Henry C. Wallace as secretary of agriculture; and Herbert Hoover as secretary of commerce. He also made, as *The New Republic* put it, some "unspeakably bad appointments": his old crony Harry Daugherty as attorney general and New Mexico Senator Albert Fall as interior secretary. In the end they undermined his administration. Daugherty sold influence for cash and resigned in 1923. Three years later only a divided jury saved him from jail. In 1929 Fall became the first cabinet member to be convicted of a felony. In 1922 he had accepted bribes of over $400,000 for secretly leasing naval oil reserves at Elk Hill, California, and Teapot Dome, Wyoming, to private oil companies.

Harding died suddenly in August 1923, before the scandals came to light, leaving Vice President Coolidge to clean up the mess. Though Harding would be remembered for a lackluster reign of normalcy, his tolerance and moderation had a calming influence on the strife-ridden nation. Slowly he had even begun to lead. In 1921 he created a new Bureau of the Budget that brought modern accounting techniques to the management of federal revenues. Toward the end of his administration he averted a scandal from the Veterans' Bureau and set an agenda for Congress that included expanding the merchant marine.

To his credit Calvin Coolidge handled Harding's sordid legacy with skill and dispatch. He created a special investigatory commission, prosecuted the wrongdoers, and restored the confidence of the nation. Decisiveness, when he chose to exercise it, was one of Coolidge's hallmarks. As governor of Massachusetts, he had ended the Boston police strike in 1919 with a firm declaration: "There can be no right to strike against the public safety by anybody, anywhere, anytime." He was honest and ascetic, privately talkative but notoriously tight-lipped in public. He believed in small-town democracy and minimalist government. Practicing what he preached, he slept 11 hours a day while president, more than any of his predecessors. "One of the most important accomplishments of my administration," he observed later, "has been minding my own business." Above all Coolidge worshiped wealth. "Civilization and profits," he once said, "go hand in hand."

As president his popularity rivaled Harding's. In an age of consumption and ballyhoo, his Yankee frugality and taciturn manner reassured Americans, off on an orgy of spending. Barely half the qualified voters cast ballots in the election in 1924, but they returned Coolidge to the White House by a margin of nearly two to one. Coolidge gave the credit to "Divine Providence." In fact the victory was yet another sign that Americans had wearied of reform, delighted in surging prosperity, and approved of the business-dominated Republican government. Whether the policies served the economy or the nation well in the long term, however, was open to question.

The Policies of Mellon and Hoover

Coolidge retained most of Harding's cabinet, including two of its most powerful members, treasury secretary Andrew Mellon and commerce secretary Herbert

Hoover. Mellon, a favorite of Old Guard Republicans, revived traditional Republican conservatism; Hoover developed innovative policies that reflected the new mass-production economy. Both placed themselves in service of business; as a result, the role of government in the economy grew. After a brief postwar decline, moreover, the number of federal employees increased by over 40,000 between 1921 and 1930.

Mellon, president of aluminum giant Alcoa, was the third richest man in the country (behind Ford and Rockefeller). He believed that prosperity "trickled down" from rich to poor through investment, which in turn raised production, employment, and wages. For more than a decade he devoted himself to cutting government spending and reducing taxes on high incomes. The rich would benefit from the lower taxes, invest more, and invigorate the economy. In 1921 Mellon got Congress to repeal the excess-profits tax on corporations, but progressives blunted his efforts to slash income taxes, 75 percent of which were paid by the wealthiest 2 percent of Americans. Bolstered by the Coolidge landslide, in 1926 he persuaded Congress to end all gift taxes and halve the estate tax and to cut the maximum income tax from 40 to 20 percent. In 1928 he reduced corporation and consumption taxes still further.

Business leaders applauded the Mellon tax program, which almost completely reversed the progressive tax policies of the Wilson era. They had contributed $8 million to Harding's campaign in 1920, and they profited most from the tax cuts. They also benefited from the narrow economic nationalism pushed by conservatives—tariff revision. In 1921 Congress, worried about rising imports from Europe, passed an emergency tariff act to increase the moderate rates of the 1913 Underwood–Simmons Tariff. In 1922 the Fordney–McCumber Tariff lifted schedules even higher. Farmers, who supported the increase, won protection too—but at a price. For each dollar they gained by keeping out agricultural products, costs on manufactured goods they needed rose by $3.50.

Herbert Hoover, a mining engineer who had made himself a millionaire, transformed the lowly Commerce Department into one of the most active agencies in Washington. Among insiders he was known as "Secretary of Commerce and Under Secretary of Everything Else." Unlike Mellon, Hoover was no narrow conservative. Dedicated to efficiency, distribution, cooperation, and service, he espoused a progressive capitalism that tried to navigate between centralization

Andrew Mellon, secretary of the treasury and the millionaire head of an aluminum monopoly, is flanked by Grace and Calvin Coolidge on the lawn of the White House. A disciple of business, President Coolidge believed that what was of "real importance to wage-earners was not how they might conduct a quarrel with their employers but how the business of the country might be so organized as to insure steady employment at a fair rate of pay. If that were done there would be no occasion for a quarrel, and if it were not done a quarrel would do no good."

and laissez faire to serve public needs. Called "associationalism," it sought to bring stability and order to industry by relying on trade associations, industry-wide organizations of business firms. By 1929 there were nearly 2000 of them. Government provided advice, statistical information, and forums for business leaders to exchange ideas, set standards for industries, and cooperate in developing markets. At the same time Hoover promoted welfare capitalism, encouraging firms to sponsor company unions, pay employees decent wages, and develop responsible social programs that protected workers from factory hazards and unemployment.

In government and industry Hoover declared war on waste. To "Hooverize" meant to economize, save, and share. The newly created Division of Simplified Practices of the Commerce Department held more than 1200 conferences and helped industries standardize everything from accounting procedures to toilet paper. The real efficiencies thereby gained saved businesses millions. Meanwhile the Overseas Market Division worked to expand foreign markets and fought international cartels in raw materials such as rubber, silk, and nitrates. Government and business, building on the ties developed during World War I, dropped all pretense of a laissez-faire economy and forged a corporate commonwealth. "Never before, here or elsewhere," boasted the *Wall Street Journal*, "has a government been so completely fused with business."

Postwar trends pushed farmers outside the magic circle of Republican prosperity. By far the biggest business in America, farming had an investment value greater than manufacturing, all utilities, and all railroads combined. A third of the population relied on farming for their livelihood. Yet the farmers' portion of the national income had shrunk from 16 percent in 1919 to 9 percent by 1929. The government withdrew price supports for wheat and ended its practice of feeding refugees with American surpluses. The postwar impoverishment of Europe reduced the export market. Wartime speculation in farmland and heavy equipment purchases doubled farmers' prewar mortgage debt. New dietary habits meant that average Americans of 1920 ate 75 fewer pounds of food than they had 10 years earlier. The development of synthetic fibers like rayon drove down demand for natural wool and cotton fibers. And the 1920 harvest brought what farmers wanted least—bumper crops to drive prices down further. In one year American farmers suffered a net loss estimated at $6 billion.

In 1921 a group of southern and western senators organized the "farm bloc" to unite farm-district congressmen behind agricultural legislation. Over the next two years they brought stockyards, packers, and grain exchanges under federal supervision. The Capper–Volstead Act (1922) exempted farm cooperatives from antitrust actions, and the Intermediate Credit Act (1923) created 12 banks for low-interest farm loans. Regulation and cheap credit were not enough, so in 1924 Senator Charles McNary and Representative Gilbert Haugen proposed a radical plan to raise American farm prices by selling staple crop surpluses abroad. Since it did not address the central problem of overproduction and would have sent agricultural prices plummeting overseas, McNary–Haugenism was doomed to fail. When Congress passed the bill in 1927 and again in 1928, President Coolidge vetoed it.

For four years President Coolidge continued to run a "businessman's government." His administration balanced the budget, scaled down the federal debt, reduced corporate, estate, and income taxes, and decreased antitrust suits. Serious economic imbalances were ignored. Insulated from government regulation, corporations grew and corporate profits soared. But workers reaped far fewer gains in wages, purchasing power, and bargaining power. Although welfare capitalism promised compensating benefits, only a handful of companies put the philosophy into practice. Those that did often used it simply to weaken independent unions. Most farmers languished throughout the decade. When President Coolidge vetoed the price supports of McNary–Haugenism, he offered nothing in their place. High tariffs protected American manufacturers but left desperate Europeans with no place to send their exports. And on Wall Street shaky methods of finance and investment were leaving a dangerous legacy. "Nero fiddled while Rome burned," observed H. L. Mencken. "Coolidge only snores."

The Election of 1928

On August 2, 1927, the fourth anniversary of Calvin Coolidge's elevation to the presidency, 30 reporters assigned to cover his vacation entered a mathematics classroom at the Rapid City High School in South Dakota for a presidential press conference. As they filed past Coolidge, he handed each a slip of paper on which was typed a terse message: "I do not choose to run for President in nineteen twenty-eight."

Republicans, bowing to the will of "Silent Cal," nominated Herbert Hoover as his successor. Hoover was not a politician but an administrator who had never run for public office. His entire campaign consisted of seven speeches, delivered in typical Hoover fashion—head bent, eyes riveted to the page, left hand nervously jiggling the keys in his pocket. However flat the midwestern tones of his delivery, his message was bland: "We in America today are nearer to the final triumph over poverty than ever before in the history of any land." Republican prosperity would be difficult for any Democrat to beat. Hoover—Iowa-born Quaker, self-made millionaire, dry (he drank no alcohol), perhaps the most admired official in America—would make the task impossible.

The Democratic party, on the other hand, continued to be dangerously polarized between its rural supporters in the South and West and urban laborers in the

---

THE ELECTION OF 1928
Historians still debate whether the election of 1928 was a pivotal one that produced a significant political realignment. Hoover cracked the solidly Democratic South, which returned to the Democratic fold in 1932. On the other hand, Democrat Al Smith won the twelve largest cities in the country, all of which had voted Republican in 1924 but stayed in the Democratic fold in 1932.

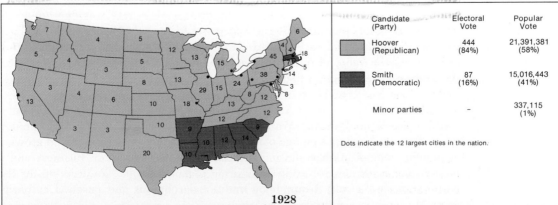

Candidate (Party)	Electoral Vote	Popular Vote
Hoover (Republican)	444 (84%)	21,391,381 (58%)
Smith (Democratic)	87 (16%)	15,016,443 (41%)
Minor parties	–	337,115 (1%)

Dots indicate the 12 largest cities in the nation.

1928

Northeast. The two factions had clashed during the 1924 convention, where rural delegates had rallied behind William Gibbs McAdoo. McAdoo, a former secretary of the Treasury and wartime head of the Railroad Administration, was as dry as a desert on the subject of Prohibition, openly criticized city life, and enjoyed the endorsement of William Jennings Bryan and the Ku Klux Klan. To boot, he was Woodrow Wilson's son-in-law, the heir apparent to the presidency. But the urban wing of the party was set on New York governor Alfred E. Smith, a Tammany Hall politician, the grandchild of Irish immigrants. As governor he combined support for social legislation with fiscal orthodoxy, administrative economy, and honest politics. The 1924 convention had deadlocked at 102 ballots before finally settling on an entirely different compromise ticket: conservative Wall Street lawyer John W. Davis and Charles W. Bryan, the radical governor of Nebraska and brother of William Jennings Bryan. The ticket was less balanced than "schizoid." It won fewer votes than any Democratic presidential team in the twentieth century. Robert La Follette, running for president in 1924 as an independent Progressive, fell only 3.5 million votes short of the Davis–Bryan total.

By 1928 the shift in population toward cities had given the urban wing control of the party. Al Smith won the nomination on the first ballot, even though his liabilities were evident. He had a jarring New York accent. When he spoke "poisonally" on the "rha-dio" to voters across America, they winced collectively. He claimed jokingly not even to know what states were west of the Mississippi River. Though he pledged to enforce Prohibition, he campaigned against it. He even took an occasional drink, which produced the spurious rumor that Smith was not only wet but a hopeless alcoholic. Most damaging of all, he was Catholic, at a time when anti-Catholicism remained virulent in many areas of the country. Baptist ministers in the South and Methodists in the North advised their flocks to "Vote as You Pray," and they did. Nearly 60 percent of the eligible voters turned out to give all but eight states to Hoover. The solidly Democratic South cracked for the first time, as the Republicans carried Texas, Florida, Kentucky, Virginia, and North Carolina. No Democrat could have beaten the Republicans, but Smith's urban roots, wetness, and Catholicism deepened defeat.

Buried in the returns were the stirrings of a major political realignment. Rhode Island and Massachusetts, industrial states that had voted Republican in 1924, voted Democratic, moved by a formidable Catholic vote. The 12 largest cities in the country had gone to the Republicans in 1924, but in 1928 the Democrats won them by slight margins. Western farmers, ignored by Republicans for a decade, also voted for Smith. The Democrats were becoming the party of the cities and of immigrants, a tangible nucleus around which to build a powerful vote-getting machine. Meanwhile a new kind of electorate was emerging. No longer were voters part of a vast partisan army. Instead they were embedded in a culture of consumption. Parties courted them with newspaper advertisements and, recognizing the value of publicity, persuaded them with radio "spots." In 1929 the Democrats created the first public relations department in American politics.

Modern times came to America in the 1920s. Changes building for half a century accelerated during World War I and converged with unprecedented force. Despite Harding's pledge of a return to normalcy, Americans faced growing economic concentration as fewer corporations controlled more business and a strong state became involved in monitoring personal habits like drinking. As the culture of mass society triumphed, traditional religious and parental authority declined, to the dismay of many Americans who clung to older ways of thought and action even as they experimented with new ones. This ambivalence between the old and the new produced paradoxes. Conventional small-town matrons coexisted with nonconformist flappers, Henry Ford's nostalgia for square dancing with his innovations in mass production. Traditional values continued to assert themselves in a modern culture. A business economy produced greater government intervention. A mass society looked to heroic individuals like Babe Ruth and Rudolph Valentino.

No greater hero existed than Charles Lindbergh. After his solo flight across the Atlantic in 1927 he and his plane, the *Spirit of St. Louis,* returned home aboard the warship *Memphis.* Eight other flyers had died trying to cross the ocean; Lindbergh alone succeeded. As he sailed up the Potomac, he received an honor previously reserved only for heads of state, a 21-gun salute. President Coolidge brought him to the White House. Four million screaming fans buried him with ticker tape as he rode through the streets of New York. Lindbergh, wrote one reporter, "fired the imagination of mankind." Never had one person mastered a machine so completely or conquered nature so gallantly. To Americans ambivalent about mass productivity and mass consumption here was a sign. Perhaps they could control the New Era without losing their cherished individualism. For a brief moment it seemed possible.

SIGNIFICANT EVENTS

1903 — First feature-length film, *The Great Train Robbery*, released

1909 — Sigmund Freud comes to America

1914 — Henry Ford introduces moving assembly line

1915 — Modern Ku Klux Klan founded

1916 — Marcus Garvey brings Universal Negro Improvement Association to America

1919 — Eighteenth Amendment outlaws alcohol use

1920 — First commercial radio broadcast; Nineteenth Amendment grants women right to vote; Warren Harding elected president

1921 — Congress enacts quotas on immigration; Budget and Accounting Act; Sheppard–Towner Federal Maternity and Infancy Act; American Birth Control League organized; first Miss America crowned

1922 — Capper–Volstead Act; Fordney–McCumber Tariff raises rates; Sinclair Lewis' *Babbitt* published; T. S. Eliot's *The Waste Land* published

1923 — *Time* magazine founded; Harding dies; Calvin Coolidge becomes president; Harding scandals break

1924 — Coolidge elected president

1925 — Bruce Barton's *The Man Nobody Knows* published; John T. Scopes convicted of teaching evolution in Tennessee; Alain Locke's *The New Negro* published

1927 — Charles Lindbergh's solo flight across the Atlantic; McNary–Haugen farm bill vetoed; Sacco and Vanzetti executed; first "talking" film, *The Jazz Singer,* released

1928 — Herbert Hoover elected president

1929 — Robert and Helen Lynd's *Middletown* published

Generations of the Republic

The Modern Family (1900–1960)

In the first half of the twentieth century the forces of modern life overwhelmed traditionalism. Urbanism, ethnicity, the progressive drive to use expertise to mold society—all these forces shaped Americans born at the turn of the century. This generation saw the demographic balance tip from farm to city, lived through unprecedented prosperity and depression, and fought two world wars. It was indeed the first modern generation.

As industrial cities grew, American families continued their century-long contraction. By 1900 the average mother was giving birth to three or four children, compared with seven or eight a century earlier. Fertility still remained higher on the farm than in the city, while birth rates among immigrants inched above those of the urban middle class.

Historians still do not know why fertility declined, but it seems likely that the growth of cities, a desire among women for greater personal freedom, and new medical advances were responsible. City living inhibited family size. On farms children could soon be put to work at home or in the fields, but in crowded urban apartments they meant more mouths to feed

and less room for other family members or rent-paying boarders. Limiting the number of newborns thus became a way to improve standards of living for the whole family.

At the same time, cosmopolitan, middle-class women believed they could gain greater personal freedom by controlling their sexual lives. After the turn of the century, they relied increasingly on contraception. In 1906, almost a decade before Margaret Sanger began her crusade for birth control, a physician reported that "hardly a single middle class family" did not expect him to help "prevent conception." By 1922 nearly three-quarters of the women questioned in one study used contraceptives. Among working-class and ethnic wives, however, knowledge of modern contraceptive techniques or access to them remained rare.

Declines in infant mortality also seem to have contributed to falling birth rates. Though still high, deaths of those under a year old dropped to one in ten, half the number a century earlier. With more children likely to survive into adulthood, there was less incentive to continue having them. Medical advances reduced infectious diseases, particularly among infants and toddlers. And after the turn of the century cities began requiring that milk be pasteurized to kill bacteria and apartments ventilated to combat tuberculosis.

Childhood diseases were by no means wiped out. A mother probably spent most of her time nursing sick children. A knife cut could easily become infected and leave a child fever-ridden for days. Measles required a month of bed rest, pneumonia six months. The global influenza pandemic of 1918 killed 550,000 people in the United States alone, 10 times the number of Americans who died in World War I.

Under the impact of progressive reforms, childbirth—like other aspects of American life—became the province of trained experts. In 1900 a woman was likely to give birth at home, without an anesthetic or even a physician; after the turn of the century, male doctors trained in obstetrics began to replace midwives. Anesthetics came into use, and the use of forceps, which in the hands of untrained attendants had mangled many newborns, was curbed. By the mid-1930s almost 4 women in 10 delivered in a hospital. (By 1945 the number was nearly 8 in 10.)

Child rearing, once left entirely to the family, became community business, as middle-class mothers found themselves bombarded with expert advice. Seeing children as active creatures with special needs, progressive professionals advanced a new ideal of "scientific mothering." They recommended imposing regularity, detachment, and control, not only to produce healthy toddlers but eventually to produce an orderly, efficient society as well. Children were to be subject to rigid eating and sleeping schedules. Thumb-sucking was discouraged and so was caressing, lest early sexual drives be overstimulated.

At school, "Little Mothers' Leagues" sent young girls home with special injunctions for their working-class and immigrant parents: "Don't give the baby herring; Don't give the baby beer to drink; Don't let the baby eat dirty things from the floor that she threw down at first; also pickle." The government's newly created Children's Bureau collected the prevailing wisdom in a pamphlet, *Infant Care* (1914), designed for the "average mother." "The care of the baby," it read, "is readily reduced to a system." Among immigrant families children sometimes became interpreters of the new regimen for parents who could neither speak nor understand English. "Please," one child wrote to the Children's Bureau, "can you send me your book 'Infant Care' in Greek. We can read American, but mother cannot."

Not all parents were inclined to follow the "experts'" often unrealistic advice. Complained one Wisconsin woman, "Most of the advice I have read says—

Fruite in plenty a bath every morning—
gentle exercise . . . music—pleasant surrounding now I have a perfectuly fine husband and a loveing home but here is my
day—get up at 5 a.m. hustle breakfast for
5, wash dishes help milk feed pigs clean
up bakeing-scrubbing washing . . . where
could I have the time for a bath every
morn?"

As blacks increasingly moved to the
city, limited opportunities placed sharp
pressures on their families. Blocked from
holding even factory jobs by discrimination in hiring, many black males remained
chronically unemployed or were forced to
work at the most menial labor. Poor housing and diet (especially a deficiency in protein) left both children and parents prey to
disease. A study in 1917 in one New York
City district showed that 90 percent of
black infants had rickets. For pregnant
mothers, rickets meant a much higher
likelihood of dying during or after birth,
due to puerperal fever or toxemia. Life
expectancy rates among blacks, especially
the women, appear to have *worsened* significantly in the half-century after the
Civil War, at a time when white rates were
improving. With families forced to endure
such conditions, black churches attempted
to provide support. By the 1920s they had
established day-care services for working
parents, scout troops for their children,
and couples clubs for young marrieds. But
urban conditions continued to be corro-

sive for those at the bottom of the social
ladder.

In an industrial society that stressed
technical skill, more children attended
school and stayed longer. By the 1920s, for
the first time in American history, a majority of teenagers went to high school instead of work. College enrollment, though
still low, reached 10 percent of the eligible
population by 1928; in 1890 it had been
less than 3 percent. The intrusion of outside institutions like schools also meant
that children spent more of their time outside the family among people their own
age. By the 1920s a full-blown "peer culture" emerged. Revolving around school
and friends, its components were remarkably modern—athletics, clubs, sororities
and fraternities, dating, proms, "bull sessions," and moviegoing.

Tolerance for premarital sex seems to
have grown in the 1920s ("necking" and
"petting" parties replaced sedate tea parties), but the new subculture of youth still
tied sexual relations to love. Casual sex
remained rare; what changed was the
point in the courtship at which sexual inti-
macy occurred. A growing minority of
young women reported having premarital
intercourse, for example, but only with
their future husbands. A rigidly supervised courtship was replaced by unsuper-
vised dating and "going together." A boy
picked up his "date" usually just by honk-
ing the horn of his car. Once on the road

they were truly on their own, free from parental control.

For all the frivolity and rebelliousness it promoted, the new peer culture of the 1920s, as historian Paula Fass observed, "also subscribed to specific work values: aggressive and directed competition, merit through association, and a carefully calibrated system of prestige." These tended to fuse young adults to the larger social culture. Conformity remained the norm. Even the notorious "flappers," who wore short skirts and short hair and rouged their cheeks, usually ended up in conventional marriages that emphasized the roles of wife and mother. Modern marriage did, however, place a new premium on "companionate" values. Compatibility, emotional fulfillment, and sexual satisfaction were lauded above financial security, status, and procreation. In the words of one survey, couples envisioned "a perfect consummation of both personalities that would involve all phases of mutual living."

As this generation approached middle age in the 1930s prosperity gave way to the greatest depression in modern history. Reflecting a sense of caution about the future, marriage and birth rates fell sharply. The rate of population increase dropped from 16.1 percent in the 1920s to 7.2 in the 1930s. More women sought employment outside their homes to supplement family incomes. For those who remained at home, household chores consumed even more of their time. "Labor-saving" devices, introduced over the previous half-century, ended up making more work for women by upgrading standards of cleanliness. Automobiles added to their burdens by transforming mothers into part-time chauffeurs for their children. And the deepening depression often led to more hours canning vegetables, making clothes, and stretching family budgets with homebound businesses like laundering and baking.

Continuing the trend of the previous hundred years, old age and dying shifted from a family to a community experience, presided over by professionals. The New Deal set in place Social Security, which would be expanded gradually to cover more older citizens. And Americans of this generation were far more likely than their parents to die in a hospital or to have their bodies prepared at a funeral home. They were also likely to pay much more for the services. In 1900 a typical undertaker recommended minimum charges of $5 for washing and dressing the body, $10 for embalming, and $8 to $10 for a hearse; in the early 1960s Americans paid an average of nearly $1500 for an elaborate funeral that included body preparation, casket, burial vault or plot, flowers, clergy, and cemetery charges. Shaped by experts and oriented toward consumers, modern life governed this generation even in death.

26

Crash and Depression

igh above Columbus Circle in New York City a gigantic electric sign blinked out the happy injunction: "You should have $10,000 at the age of 30; $25,000 at the age of 40; $50,000 at the age of 50." And in the pages of the *Ladies Home Journal* John J. Raskob, who had run the Finance Committee at General Motors and who listed his profession as "capitalist," told people how. "Everyone ought to be rich," he declared: $15 a month, "wisely invested," would be worth $80,000 in 20 years. In the 1920s, when 4 families in 10 earned less than $1500 a year, that was rich.

As the decade wore on, some people did grow rich. In 1914 there were 7000 millionaires; in 1928 there were 35,000. Between 1919 and 1928 the number of six-figure incomes doubled. Easy money obsessed the nation. The volume of sales on the New York Stock Exchange jumped 400 percent from 1923 to 1928. Other exchanges in Chicago, St. Louis, San Francisco, and Los Angeles registered similar gains. Buyers were less concerned about the assets of a company than about the prospects for a rise in the price of its stock. A simple dictum governed the market: buy low, sell high; buy high, sell higher.

Possibilities for profit were everywhere, including far-off Florida. In 1929 the Marx Brothers broke into films with *The Cocoanuts*, a zany farce about real estate scams in the Sunshine State. "You can get stucco," says Groucho as he pitches a land deal. "Oh, can you get stucco!" Thousands of investors had gotten "stucco" when "land fever" hit southern Florida in the mid-1920s. Before World War I Miami was largely mangrove jungle and bug-infested swamp. Attracted by 80-degree temperatures in winter, developer Carl G. Fisher cleared the jungle, drained the swamp, put up a sea wall, and built a three-mile causeway from the beach to the mainland. Miami became the fastest growing city in America. The Miami *Herald* carried more advertising than any other newspaper in the world. Miami, residents boasted, was "the Magic City." By 1925 city lots were going for $20,000 apiece, sight unseen.

In Palm Beach, 75 miles up the coast from Miami, oceanfront property sold for $3300 a foot, up from $4.65 just three decades earlier. "Buy anywhere," said locals. "You can't lose." Gertrude Shelby, a journalist who went to Florida to write about the boom, put down a binder of $2500 on 34.5 acres, sold it before paying the first installment, and made $13,000 in one month. The Florida boom was on. So many people arrived in the summer of 1925 that famine threatened the state, and ice could be obtained only by doctor's prescription.

In the 1930s, Dorothea Lange pioneered a new realism in photography—grim, unvarnished, and poignant. Nowhere did she better capture the shattering effects of the Great Depression than in these pictures of a heavily mortgaged Georgia cotton farmer.

One mid-September night in 1926, Miami barometers dropped to 27.75—the lowest reading to date in North America. Wind howled through the city at 130 miles per hour as 20-foot waves pounded sea walls and washed away beaches. The swamp reclaimed landfills. Speculators discovered an awful truth: southern Florida lay in the middle of the hurricane belt. In one night 100 Miamians drowned; 40,000 lost their homes. Property damage in the state ran to $300 million. Reality punctured the vast speculative bubble. The value of oceanfront lots dropped from $2000 to $700 a foot. Hundreds went bankrupt; thousands lost their land to foreclosures.

Though Florida land values plummeted, the boom laid the foundation for later development, but stock market scams and speculation did nothing except turn the financial center of the nation into a gambling den. Outright swindles in phony stocks (oil wells and mines were the most popular) netted con artists more than $600 million a year. Some stock maneuvering was legal but deceptive. Favored "insiders"—from wealthy speculators like Bernard Baruch to the president of the United States—were placed on "preferred lists" at brokerage houses and tipped off about impending issues. They bought discounted stocks in advance, then sold them on the market for a tidy profit. Insiders formed "stock pools" to drive up prices so they could make a quick killing. In 1928 a group that included John Raskob pushed Radio Corporation of America stock from $90 to $109 a share. They made $5 million by selling the stock one week later.

More middle-class people were trading too, boosting the level of ignorance almost as much as the volume of sales. Once the province of the wealthy, Wall Street buzzed with tales of the dumb luck of simple folk. An actor was said to be $40,000 richer for having bought stock in just four companies. A waiter at the Exchange's Luncheon Club was supposed to have made $90,000 by investing on the basis of customers' shop talk. A group of pages from the floor of the New York Stock Exchange captured the national mood in a song they wrote for their bosses:

> O hush thee, my babe, granny's bought some more shares.
> Daddy's gone to play with the bulls and the bears,
> Mother's buying on tips and she simply can't lose,
> And baby shall have some expensive new shoes.

The stock market dominated the news. Millions watched it as closely as they watched their favorite baseball team. Even those with no money followed sales and prices just like they counted home runs and figured batting averages. In Saginaw, Michigan, and Amarillo, Texas, people shook open their morning papers to the financial pages. In Steubenville, Ohio, and Storm Lake, Iowa, they gathered at brokerage houses to watch the daily fluctuations in stocks. Some bought and sold; a few got rich quick; most shoveled their profits into the market again. Even if they lost money it did not matter. "Everybody ought to be rich"—and anyone could be. Another Florida bubble might develop at any moment; each business day brought fresh quotations on the ticker tape; untold riches were just around the corner.

So it seemed in the late 1920s, as the New Era careened toward disaster. Behind electric signs directing the pursuit of wealth and slogans exhorting it, beneath stock deals and land booms, the economy was honeycombed with weaknesses, and in 1929 it began to collapse.

THE GREAT BULL MARKET

As the last business day of the year drew to a close in 1928, the floor of the New York Stock Exchange radiated optimism. In Wall Street parlance the "bulls"— those who buy stock—had routed the "bears"—those who sell. In fact it was the greatest bull market in history as eager buyers drove prices higher and higher. Nineteen twenty-eight had been a record year with over 90,500,000 shares traded. General Electric jumped from $124 a share to $221; American Can from $70 to $117; and the Radio Corporation of America from $85 to a breathtaking $420. More remarkable still, RCA never paid a dividend. Its skyrocketing price alone was enough to keep buyers clamoring for more.

Strolling across the quarter-acre, felt-padded floor of the New York Stock Exchange, Superintendent William Crawford welcomed the New Year with a confident assertion: "The millennium's arrived"; but Alexander Noyes, a veteran financial analyst, was worried. Despite the opulence of the New York Exchange and the swelling volume of trade, there was trouble in this financial paradise. It was built on economic quicksand. Noyes knew it could not last. "Something has to give," he told reporters in the fall of 1929. Less than a month later, the Great Bull Market fell in a heap.

The Rampaging Bull

The Great Bull Market had been building for most of the decade. In the early twenties a day when 2 million shares were traded was noteworthy; by mid-decade 3 million–share days still created a stir; by 1928 4 million–share days left smug brokers convinced the stock market bubble might never burst.

No one knows exactly what caused the orgy of speculation on the market. Speculation had infected the culture, and the market was not immune. In fact a new breed of aggressive outsiders had helped to spread the speculative fever. In search of quick profits, these traders had invaded the exchanges at the start of the decade. The "Establishment," which consisted of the leading investment bankers and their clients, had ruled Wall Street since the late nineteenth century. Its members, including such leaders as J. P. Morgan, Paul Warburg, and Otto Kahn, shared both background and outlook. They came from wealthy eastern families, went to Ivy League schools, and supported the Republican party. They stood for moral rectitude, financial stability, and sound investment practices. But in the 1920s their control of the market weakened. Rich outsiders from the Midwest— William Durant of General Motors, the seven Fisher brothers from Detroit, the flamboyant Jesse Livermore—plunged in, bought millions of shares, and helped to send prices soaring.

Rambunctious individuals may have ignited the boom, but new personnel and innovative financial devices allowed it to grow. Hundreds of young "customer men"—largely untrained "go-getters"—flooded investment houses to handle the booming business. Like automobile salesmen, they had quotas to meet and were awarded bonuses for high volume. Before long, as one student of the market put it, "uninitiated brokers were selling stocks to an uninformed public." New investment trusts allowed buyers with only a few hundred dollars to participate in a portfolio of "glamour stocks." The first such trust, International Securities Trust of

America, had been formed in 1921. By 1929 a new investment trust was opening every other day. Several were created by people who simply wanted to sell their own securities. Some owned shares in other investment trusts. In this financial house of cards if one trust failed, it could bring down others, since their only assets might be stock in other investment trusts. Profits were so great, however, that by 1927 even the Establishment had become involved in such risky ventures.

Money to fuel the market became plentiful. From 1922 to 1929, some $900 million dollars worth of gold flowed into the country, a sign of international faith in the American economy. Bankers could lend up to $13 for every $1 of gold they held, so the money supply expanded by $6 billion. Over the decade corporate profits grew by 80 percent. At interest rates as high as 25 percent, more could be made from lending money to brokers (who then made "brokers' loans" to clients buying stock) than from constructing new factories or taking on sound investments. Borrowed over the phone, lent with the purchased stock as collateral, this "call money" could be collected, or called in, at any time and was usually renewable. It provided the sort of loan speculators crave—one that did not tie up their cash. By 1929 Bethlehem Steel had over $157 million in the "call money market," and brokers' loans had almost tripled from two years earlier.

"Margin requirements," the cash actually put down to purchase stock, had dropped as low as 10 percent but hovered around 50 percent for most of the decade. Thus buyers had to come up with only half the price of a share; the rest was financed by borrowing from brokers. As trading reached record heights in August 1929, the Federal Reserve Board finally tried to dampen speculation by raising the interest, or "rediscount," rate charged by the Federal Reserve System for loans to member banks. Higher interest rates would make borrowing more expensive and, authorities hoped, gently reduce inflated stock prices. They were wrong, for it was already too late.

Chinks in the System

If the economy had been sound, nothing could have shattered it. But the economy was not sound. With national attention riveted on the stock market, hardly anyone noticed the warning signs. The construction and automobile industries, key spurs to the prosperity of the New Era, began to lose vitality by 1928 as consumer demand sagged. Residential construction slackened throughout the year, and in the last 10 months of 1929 building permits dropped by 65 percent. Construction fell to the levels of 1921, when the country had been in a deep recession. Meanwhile mortgaged indebtedness had more than doubled, from $13 billion in 1922 to $27.1 billion in 1929. Americans increasingly were gambling their futures on the soundness of the economy.

Automobile sales continued to rise, but at a much slower rate after 1925. By 1929 the automobile industry and ancillary industries like tires and oil were badly overbuilt. Automakers cut back on orders for steel, glass, and other components; industrial production declined; commodity prices dropped. An alarming growth in business inventories, from $500 million in 1928 to $1.8 billion in 1929, further dampened productivity. A deflationary cycle of sinking prices and wages took hold. Increases in consumer spending slowed to a lethargic 1.5 percent for 1928–1929.

The danger signs reflected genuine trouble. For 10 years business had increased profits at twice the rate of productivity. Without strong labor unions or government support, real wages increased only about 11 percent, far below rises in production. Mass purchasing power never kept pace with productivity and consumer demand, so people made up the difference between what they earned and what they bought by borrowing. Increasingly consumers bought "on time," paying off purchases a little each month. During the decade consumer debt rose by 250 percent. Few could afford to keep spending at that level. Nor could the distribution of wealth sustain prosperity. By 1929, 1 percent of the population owned 36 percent of all personal wealth. The savings of the top 60,000 families equaled those of the bottom 25 million families. The wealthy had more money than they could possibly spend; the working and middle classes did not have enough to keep the economy growing.

Unemployment began to increase as early as 1927, revealing growing softness in the economy. By early 1928 the director of the Charity Organization Society in New York reported that unemployment was worse than at any time since the end of World War I. In the fall of 1929 there were 3 million people out of work, many of them in textiles, coal mining, lumbering, and railroads—all "sick" industries suffering from overexpansion, reduced demand, and weak management. Most farmers had been in a recession since the end of World War I. They had 16 percent of the national income in 1919 but only 9 percent in 1929. As more of them went bust, so did many rural banks.

During the twenties nearly 6000 banks failed, mostly in rural areas. Mismanagement, greed, and the emergence of a new type of executive—half banker, half broker—led banks to divert more funds from investment to speculation. "The banks," observed one writer, "provided everything for their customers but a roulette wheel." The uniquely decentralized American banking system left no way to set things right. At the end of the decade half of the 25,000 banks in America lay outside of the Federal Reserve System. Its controls even over member banks were weak. And no government agency monitored the stock exchanges at all. Soon even elite banks were caught up in shady deals. In 1928 Charles Mitchell, president of National City Bank, sold $90 million worth of Peruvian bonds. His own auditors had reported the Peruvian government was likely to default, but Mitchell floated the bonds anyway. That year he earned over $1 million in bonuses from his bank's security-selling subsidiary. When the Peruvian government refused to pay bondholders, their holdings were as worthless as used ticker tape.

Corporations operated unchecked by any countervailing power. The federal government encouraged consolidation. Big business gained so much control over the marketplace that changes in demand had little effect on prices. Managers had so much influence over the workplace that workers received much less pay than their productivity warranted. High profits and the Mellon tax program helped to make many corporations wealthy enough to avoid borrowing, so even changes in interest rates could not control them. Free from government regulation, fluctuating prices, and the need for loans, businessmen ruled the economy. And they ruled badly.

The Great Crash

On Thursday morning, October 24, 1929, the gallery of the New York Stock Exchange was packed with visitors, including the former British Chancellor of the Exchequer Winston Churchill. Trouble was in the air. The day before, a sharp break downward had capped a week of falling prices. Speculators had begun to

On "Black Tuesday"—October 29, 1929—the stock market collapsed in the greatest single day of losses Wall Street had ever experienced. The long slide actually began in September and did not end until mid-November. In those ten weeks, the value of stocks on the New York *Times* industrial index dropped by half.

take their profits. Other traders exhausted their margins and had no more money to spend. After only an hour, millions of shares went up for sale. There were no buyers.

As a torrent of orders to sell flooded the New York Stock Exchange, prices plunged. Panic set in. By the end of "Black Thursday" the ticker tape was running more than four hours late. Nearly 13 million shares had been traded—a record. Losses stood at $3 billion, another record. Representatives of 35 of the largest brokerage houses on Wall Street issued a joint statement of reassurance to their customers across the country: "The worst has passed."

The worst had just begun. Prices rallied for the rest of the week, buoyed by a bankers' buying pool organized at the House of Morgan. The following Tuesday, October 29, 1929, the bubble burst. Over 16 million shares changed hands. Stockholders lost $10 billion. In a single day almost as much money in capital value vanished as the United States had spent on World War I. The biggest gainer of the decade, RCA, which had peaked earlier at $450 a share, eventually dropped to $32. Within a month industrial stocks lost half of what they had been worth in September. It was the greatest crash so far in history—and it continued for almost four years. At their peak in 1929 stocks had been worth $87 billion. In 1933 they bottomed out at $18 billion. The exchanges were littered with casualties, including boxer Jack Dempsey, the first millionaire athlete. He lost $3 million and went broke.

The Great Crash did not cause the Great Depression, but it did damage the economy in several ways. Although only about 500,000 people were actually trading stocks by the end of the decade, many of them were the people whose investments helped to sustain prosperity. Thousands of middle-class investors lost their savings and their futures. They had bought cars, houses, clothing, and other consumer items on the promise to pay when stock profits came in, and profits never came. The credit structure of the nation was suddenly in jeopardy. Commercial banks, some heavily loaded with corporate stocks, others sunk deeply into the call money market, reeled in the wake of the crash. Business confidence sank, and American optimism withered.

The Great Crash signaled the start of the greatest depression in the history of the nation. The gains of the twenties were wiped out in a few years. By 1933 the gross national product had fallen by almost half. Manufacturing was less than it had been in 1913. The automobile industry was operating at under 20 percent of its 1929 capacity, the steel industry at 12 percent. By some estimates 85,000 businesses failed, and major railroad systems like the Missouri Pacific went into receivership. American foreign trade fell by more than two-thirds.

The shock waves helped to topple already fragile economies in Europe. American loans, investments, and purchases had propped up a shaky Europe since the end of World War I. When they stopped, European governments defaulted on war debts. More European banks failed; more businesses collapsed. Unemployment surged. Europeans scrambled to protect themselves. Led by Great Britain in 1931, 41 nations abandoned the gold standard. With currency no longer redeemable in gold, foreign governments hoped to expand their supplies of money. Such devaluation, they hoped, would make exports cheaper and increase foreign trade. Each simultaneously raised tariffs to protect its industries from inexpensive foreign goods. So devaluation failed, and the resulting trade barriers only deepened the crisis.

Declining sales at home and abroad sent crop prices in the United States to new lows. Wheat fell from $1.05 a bushel in 1929 to 39 cents in 1932, corn from 81 cents to 39 cents a bushel, cotton from 17 cents to 6 cents a pound. In 1932 a wagonload of oats could not buy a $4 pair of Thom McCann shoes. Farm income dropped by more than half—to a paltry $5 billion. The contagion of rural bank failures spread to the cities. Nervous depositors rushed by the thousands to withdraw their cash. Even healthy banks could not bear the strain. In August 1930 every bank in Toledo but one failed. Between 1929 and 1933 collapsing banks took over $20 billion in assets with them.

Fearing that the United States would soon abandon the gold standard, foreign investors traded their dollars for gold. As gold vanished from the country, the money supply contracted. Gold reserves began to grow again only after the Federal Reserve Board raised short-term interest rates in October 1931. By then money was so scarce that the banks could not meet domestic needs. Stores in the state of Washington accepted wooden money; Iowa towns issued scrip; the city of Knoxville printed its own currency. In the first three years after the crash total productivity dropped from $103 billion to $56 billion. National income fell by half, factory wages by almost half. The economy spiraled downward, and no one could stop it. Overexpansion of major industries, uneven distribution of wealth and income, the relative decline in mass purchasing power, a weak banking and corporate structure, and plain economic ignorance were the underlying causes.

THE AMERICAN PEOPLE IN THE GREAT DEPRESSION

"When a great many people are unable to find work," said Calvin Coolidge in 1930, "unemployment results." Between 1929 and 1932 U.S. Steel laid off all of its

225,000 full-time employees. An average of 100,000 people lost their jobs every week in the first three years after the crash. By 1932 more than 13 million were jobless. At least one worker in four could find no work at all. In the industrial cities the toll was staggering. A million unemployed walked the streets of New York; over half a million roamed the streets of Chicago. In Cleveland half the working force had no jobs; in Toledo, more than three-quarters were without work. By 1931 even white-collar workers, usually safe in past depressions, were unemployed. "Time was when a white collar case was an event," wrote one social worker. "Not so today."

The Great Depression was a great leveler, reducing differences in the face of common deprivation. The New York seamstress without enough piecework to pay her rent felt the same frustration and anger as the Berkeley student whose college education was cut short when the bank let her father go. Most husbands had some job; most wives continued as homemakers; and most Americans got by as best they could, often cooperating with one another, practicing a ruthless underconsumption to make ends meet. "We lived lean," recalled one Depression victim. So did most of the American people—black and white, northern and southern, urban and rural.

Hard Times

When asked in 1932 whether there had ever been anything like the Great Depression, the economist John Maynard Keynes replied, "Yes, it was called the Dark Ages, and it lasted four hundred years." In the 1930s hard times lasted 10 years, the longest depression in American history. In 1940, some 7.5 million Americans (roughly 14 percent of the labor force) were still without jobs. Five future presidents—John Kennedy, Richard Nixon, Gerald Ford, Ronald Reagan, and George Bush—grew up during the Great Depression, and no one who lived through the ordeal forgot it. In one way or another, it changed everybody, even those who did not suffer directly. "I had been a conformist, a Southern snob," recalled Virginia Durr, who became a pioneer in the battle for civil rights. "What I learned during the Depression changed all that. I saw a blinding light like Saul on the road to Damascus."

Three years after the Great Crash nearly one American in three had no income. Half the labor force was either unemployed or underemployed. People set forest fires in Washington State so they could be hired to put them out. An Arkansas man walked 900 miles in search of work. New York City department stores required college degrees for elevator operators; professors drove taxicabs. Armtorg, the Russian trading company, received an average of 350 applications a day from Americans who wanted to settle in the Soviet Union. Throughout the decade emigration from the United States exceeded immigration into the country. Most left because they could find no work in America.

Even before the Great Crash a great many Americans were having trouble making a living. The Depression publicized their plight. In the golden year of 1929, economists at the Brookings Institution calculated that for the barest necessities a family of four required $2000 a year—more money than 60 percent of American families earned. By 1932 the average family had an annual income of $1348, barely enough to survive. Only one family in five had as much as $3000 a year to spend.

Even members of the middle class suffered a sickening descent. One defendant in Brooklyn, charged with vagrancy for sleeping in a vacant lot for 46 days,

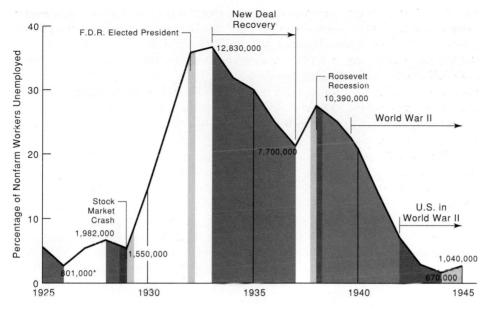

*Unemployed totals for entire labor force.
UNEMPLOYMENT, 1925–1945
The dark bands mark significant events during the era.

had served as a civil engineer for the governments of Panama, China, and Venezuela. The man who knocked at the door for a handout at night, noted a New York *Times* reporter, "might be the same fellow who a few months or a year ago had cheerfully O.K.'d your loan at the bank or had written editorials in your newspaper or had been the vice president of a leading real estate company."

National morale sank. "The energy of the country has suffered a strange paralysis," said one observer. "We are in the doldrums, waiting not even hopefully for the wind which never comes." The nation's capital looked grim. "I come home from the Hill every night filled with gloom," wrote a Washington correspondent in 1932. "I see on the streets filthy, ragged, desperate-looking men, such as I have never seen before." In New York and Boston, soup kitchens opened and bread lines formed. Midwestern schoolteachers donated their salaries to feed their students at lunch. A teacher told one haggard girl to go home and get some food. "I can't," she replied. "This is my sister's day to eat."

Millions stayed alive by foraging like animals. In Chicago people stood at local dumps, waiting for the next garbage truck. When one pulled away from the pile, read a 1932 report, a crowd of 35 "started digging with sticks, some with their hands, grabbing bits of food and vegetables." One widow always removed her glasses before eating so she would not see the maggots. In Kentucky people ate violet tops, wild onions, and weeds previously thought fit only for cattle.

Big-city hospitals began receiving new patients ill primarily from starvation. The New York City health department reported that more than one schoolchild in five suffered from malnutrition. In the coal-mining regions of West Virginia and Illinois almost every child fed by the American Friends Service Committee was underweight. Diseases associated with malnutrition, like pellagra, increased, especially in the South. Despite reassurances from public officials and chambers of commerce that "no one has starved," the New York City Welfare Council reported

Shantytowns (called "Hoovervilles" after President Herbert Hoover) sprang up around most cities as the Depression deepened. Sometimes the down-and-out turned to desperate action. In 1931 a hunger riot broke out when the unemployed stormed a grocery store in Oklahoma City. Meanwhile thousands occupied the Seattle County–City Building to protest conditions there. Two years later in Chicago, 55 citizens were arrested when they were found tearing down a four-story building and taking it away brick by brick.

29 victims of starvation and 110 dead of malnutrition in 1932. Most were children.

Unable to pay mortgages or rent, many families lived off the generosity of forgiving landlords. Some traded down to smaller quarters; others lost their homes. In 1932 some 273,000 families were evicted. In a single day in April, an estimated one-fourth of Mississippi went to auction. People sought shelter anywhere. In Oakland, California, they lived in unsold sewer pipes. Near the Salt River in Arizona miners camped under bridges. In every large city women could be found sleeping on subways. Men huddled in abandoned factories. In winter the homeless begged to be sent to a warm jail cell. A New York couple set up house in a Central Park cave and lived there for an entire year. By 1932 between 1 million and 2 million Americans were homeless wanderers, among them an estimated 25,000 nomadic families. The Missouri Pacific caught 13,745 migrants hitching illegal rides in 1929 and 186,028 in 1931. They were part of what one federal report later called a "migration of despair."

Victims of the Depression overthrew the governments of seven Latin American countries, but in the United States most citizens turned their anger inward. "People blamed themselves, not the system," said one woman. "They felt they had been at fault: . . . 'if we hadn't bought that old radio' . . . 'if we hadn't bought that second-hand car.'" Shame, self-doubt, and pessimism became epidemic. "I'm just no good, I guess," a Houston woman told a caseworker in 1934. "I've given up ever amounting to anything." Most tried to keep up appearances. Men resharpened old razor blades, rolled their own cigarettes, and used 25-watt bulbs to save electricity. Women retailored their dresses for their daughters and sewed together lengths of sheets to equalize wear. Families went through old Christmas cards so they could be sent to different friends next year.

It was often a losing battle. "The unemployed have been so long without food—clothes—shoes—medical care—dental care etc—we look pretty bad," wrote an Oklahoma woman. "And we look and feel a little worse each day." There was no escaping anxiety. "What will become of us?" wondered an Arizona man. "I've lost twelve and a half pounds this last month, just thinking." Rates of mental illness and suicide rose. "No home, no work, no money," despaired a Pennsylvania man as he pled for a "human" method to dispose of his family in 1934. "We cannot go along this way."

A few people profited from the Depression. Albert Fuller sent a corps of salesmen from home to home to sell his brushes. Business grew by $1 million a year. With crude oil selling for 10 cents a barrel in west Texas, J. Paul Getty began acquiring oil wells cheaply. In 1932 he gained control of the Pacific Oil Corporation. Each year of the Depression cigarette sales increased as smokers switched from cigars to less expensive cigarettes. The Mason family was able to keep its factory in Muncie operating at full capacity until 1935 as Americans again were canning their food in Mason jars, reversing the trend toward commercially canned goods. Fear of pregnancy and extra mouths to feed boosted sales of contraceptives to $250,000 a year. In some families sex became a form of therapy. "Life is terrible," said a California woman worried about her unemployed husband. "You must try all the time to keep him from going crazy. And many times—that's the only way."

The Depression Family

"I have watched fear grip the people in our neighborhood around Hull House," wrote Jane Addams in 1931, "men and women who have seen their margin of savings disappear; heads of families who see and anticipate hunger for their children before it occurs. That clutch of cold fear is one of the most hideous aspects." The "clutch of cold fear" led many young couples to put off having children: births per 1000 women of childbearing age dropped from 97.4 in 1929 to 75.7 in 1933, part of a long-term decrease aggravated in the early years of the Depression. For the first time in three centuries the curve of population growth was leveling off. Unable to foresee World War II and the "baby boom" to follow, experts predicted a "baby crop shortage."

After 1929 the marriage rate plunged; it did not begin to recover until 1934. An estimated 800,000 marriages were postponed—some forever. "Do you realize how many people of my generation are not married?" a Chicago educator later told an interviewer. By 1930 the number of women between the ages of 25 and 30 who never married had increased 30 percent over the previous five years. Throughout the decade divorce declined (largely because of expense) but desertion, the "poor man's divorce," increased.

Studies found that the Depression did not break up families so much as it magnified tendencies already present. Weak families languished or fell apart; strong ones hung together and grew closer. The Burtons of Saginaw, Michigan, had a steady marriage before Mr. Burton lost his business in the early 1930s. He moved his family to Ann Arbor, where he took a job as a salesman. His income dropped from $10,000 to $3000 a year. His wife took in boarders, remained cheerful and ambitious, and pulled together with her husband. Everyone regarded her as the "family heroine." The Rileys, another Michigan family—but one already on shaky ground—sank into a morass of anxiety, resentment, and debt. After his unsuccessful law practice failed, Mr. Riley turned to gambling, his wife became callous, and their 24-year old daughter took on the roles of chief breadwinner and family leader. She resented both of her parents.

When unemployment struck, such role reversals were not uncommon. Men without work grew listless and discouraged after a few weeks at home. Work had defined them as productive members of society. Suddenly they had nothing to do. "One of the worst things was occupying your time, sensibly," recalled Ward James, fired from his publishing job in 1935. "You'd go to the library. You took a magazine to the room and sat and read. I didn't have a radio. I tried to do some writing and found I couldn't concentrate. The day was long. There was nothing to do evenings. I was going around in circles, it was terrifying." Mr. Riley spent his days at the local pool hall. Other husbands put on ties and jackets each morning, but instead of going to the office they went to distant neighborhoods to sell Two-in-One shoe polish or cheap neckties door-to-door. In a culture that stressed self-reliance and self-help, such men felt like failures and blamed themselves.

Most of the country's 28 million homemakers stayed at home. During the Depression their routines were less disrupted than their husbands', but demands on them grew. Poor rural women, the wives of tenants and sharecroppers, experienced the fewest changes. They had long since adjusted to poverty. As always they did field and farm work, cared for their families, and still deferred to their husbands. In middle-class families strong women like Mrs. Burton often rose to fill roles vacated by defeated husbands. "I did what I had to do," said one woman. "I seemed to always find a way to make things work."

The role of homemaker took on added importance. The typical middle-class family in the Depression had one or two children and lived in a rented house or apartment (few Americans owned their homes in the 1930s). Between 1929 and 1933 living costs dropped almost 25 percent, but family incomes tumbled by 40 percent. Homemakers watched family budgets with a close eye. They substituted less expensive fish for red meat or dropped meat from their menus altogether. Jell-O, the cheapest all-purpose dessert, enjoyed new popularity. Corn, tomatoes, and pole beans sprang up in backyards and vacant city lots. Families took in relatives and boarders. Some wives started home businesses selling baked goods, making dresses, or operating kitchen beauty parlors. Returning to "Middletown" for a follow-up study in 1935, sociologists Helen and Robert Lynd discovered an increase in prostitution. Working-class wives were selling themselves to keep their families going.

More and more women worked outside their homes, largely to supplement meager family incomes. Some critics claimed they took jobs from men. "There are approximately 10,000,000 people out of work in the United States today," wrote Norman Cousins in 1939, "there are also 10,000,000 or more women, married and single, who are jobholders. Simply fire the women, who shouldn't be working anyway, and hire the men. Presto! No unemployment. No relief rolls. No depression." Such thinking was sheer nonsense. Past discrimination in employment had relegated most women to "women's work," traditionally secretaries, schoolteachers, and social workers. Over half the female labor force worked in domestic service or the garment trades. Most unemployed men would have been reluctant to take such jobs, even if they were available.

An evicted sharecropper stands with his child. In 1930 such children faced a grimmer future than their parents. Throughout the South, where most African-Americans lived, the difference in the quality of education accorded whites and what was available to blacks widened between 1900 and 1940. By the first year of the Great Depression more money was being spent on school buses for whites than on new schools for blacks.

In the 1930s discrimination still dogged working women. Their jobs paid little. Live-in maids, the elite of domestic servants, got $8 a week; pieceworkers in the textile mills of Lawrence, Massachusetts, got $4. It was worse for married women. Opinion polls showed more than three in four Americans believed that wives belonged at home. Frances Perkins, later secretary of labor, denounced "the pin money worker" as a "menace to society." Few school districts would hire married women, and half had a policy of firing them. Between 1932 and 1937 federal authorities prohibited more than one member of a family from working for the civil service. Three-quarters of those forced to resign were women. The proportion of women in the work force rose anyway, approaching 25 percent by 1940, and most new women workers were married. Wages for women rose, too, until they were 63 percent of men's.

The nation's 21 million children could not escape feeling some anxieties. "The children all seem to be so excitable and high-strung these days," reported a New York City kindergarten teacher. "I can't help thinking it's due to the distress at home." Enrollment in public schools and colleges grew as prospects for employment sank. By 1940 three of four high school–aged children were attending school, compared to less than half in 1930. Extended schooling now kept children out of the labor force. Universities, still reserved for a privileged few, drew 1.2 million students, or 7.5 percent of the college-age population. The long-term trend toward a highly educated public continued.

A *Literary Digest* survey in 1931 showed that eight-year-olds still wanted to be cowboys, aviators, and army officers if they were boys, movie stars if they were girls. But by age 18 they had developed a new practicality. Boys looked forward to being lawyers, engineers, and architects, girls to making careers as stenographers and secretaries. Gone were the swashbuckling, goldfish-swallowing college students of the 1920s. "The present day college generation is fatalistic," observed the editors of *Fortune* magazine. "It keeps its shirt on, its pants buttoned, its chin up, and its mouth shut."

As many as 250,000 children took to the road, some to relieve families of their support, others just to wander. Most youngsters stayed at home; indeed, for a child of unemployed parents life barely extended beyond the front door. "The unemployed man and his wife have no social life," wrote one observer in 1934. "The only visitors they have are their married children with their families." The picture was not so bleak for everyone, but after a decade of being drawn apart by automobiles and mass entertainment, the middle-class family turned inward. Church attendance declined; the spending of recreational groups dropped by half; a third of the Grange and rural women's clubs vanished; millions of telephones were taken out; even the mails lightened.

The home and family emerged as the center of recreation and companionship. People dreamed of exuberant activity—playing tennis, swimming, or boating—but surveys showed that they actually spent their free time reading newspapers and magazines, listening to the radio, and going to the movies, in that order. "There was a lot of visiting back and forth in the evenings," recalled one man, "games of penny ante poker, monopoly, and bridge, sampling the newly legal beer and whiskey, going to picnics, discovering golf at a nearby country club which had opened its course to all-comers at one dollar greens fee."

The Great Depression forever marked the generation that lived through it. Countless women came to associate working outside the home with crisis and financial distress. The middle-class dream of a wife freed from working for wages, weakened in the 1920s, reasserted itself. "Some day, Dear Sister," a union officer told one spouse unhappy about married women with jobs, "I hope we will reach that economic ideal where the married woman will find her place in the home caring for children, which is God's greatest gift to women and her natural birthright." Whether in the renewed importance of homemaking and family life or the reemergence of home industries, Americans retreated into traditionalism.

Some never forgot the humiliation of life in the Depression. "Shame? You tellin' me?" recalled a businessman. "I would go stand on that relief line. I would look this way and that and see if there's nobody around that knows me: I would bend my head low so nobody would recognize me. The only scar that is left on me is my pride, my pride." The lasting legacy of humiliation and fear—that the bottom would fall out again; that life would be leveled once more; that the next depression might not end—this was what one writer called an "invisible scar." "Security to me is not what we have," said a woman who grew up in the 1930s, "but what we can do without."

A Depression Culture

In a decade when uncertainty and fear dominated their feelings, middle-class Americans threw themselves into games that depended on rationality as well as chance. Contract bridge, with its system of bidding and play, Parker Brothers' board game Monopoly, which rewarded orderly investing in real estate, and pinball, the ultimate machine-age game that carried the injunction "Do Not Tilt," were Depression favorites. All relied on rules and skill as well as luck. In more physical games, sheer endurance became a virtue. Six-day bicycle races staged a comeback, and dance marathons, another contest for survival, kept partners on the floor 45 minutes out of every hour, 24 hours a day, sometimes for weeks on end.

The Depression produced more sober fashions: longer skirts and hair, fewer long waists, more curves. A desire to escape the here-and-now helped to make best sellers of *The Good Earth* (1931), Pearl Buck's saga of China, and Margaret Mitchell's Civil War epic, *Gone with the Wind* (1936). New skepticism about business led Fred Schlink to write *100,000,000 Guinea Pigs*, a sequel to *Your Money's Worth* (1927), his earlier exposé of false advertising. By 1935 the two books had sold half a million copies. Reflecting the new tight-fistedness, consumer cooperatives multiplied more than tenfold during the decade.

Hungry for diversions, people still flocked to spectacles, just as they had in the 1920s. A World's Fair in Chicago in 1933 and a second in New York in 1939 both attracted large crowds. Families living a limited life found cheaper pursuits than they had a decade earlier. Stamp collecting quadrupled during the 1930s. There were fads for knitting and jigsaw puzzles. Boxtop contests and other games of chance held out hope of turning bad luck good. Inaugurated in 1930, the Irish Sweepstakes became the most successful lottery in the world within five years. Nearly every adult in Colorado was involved in the chain-letter craze of 1935.

With a wider audience than ever, record sales increased a hundredfold between 1934 and 1937. Classical music enjoyed new popularity as tastes turned to a more controlled, full-bodied sound. By 1939 there were over 270 symphony orchestras in the country; only 17 had existed in 1915. More than 10 million families listened to symphonic music and opera each weekend on radio. Popular music became more melodic and cheerful. Pop hits were usually romantic ("Stardust"), often sentimental ("Red Sails in the Sunset"), and occasionally poignant ("Brother, Can You Spare a Dime?"). "Swing," a commercialized jazz, dominated the charts, and "big bands," orchestras that played popular favorites at nightclubs and theaters, capitalized on the continuing dance craze. In 1937 Benny Goodman, the "King of Swing," drew an audience of nearly 4000 when he opened at the Paramount Theater in New York City. Couples added the acrobatic "jitterbug" and exotic Latin imports like the rumba to such durable favorites as the fox trot.

By the end of the decade almost 9 families in 10 owned radios. People depended on the radio for almost everything—news, sports, and weather; music and entertainment; advice on how to bake a cake or find God. Radio entered a golden age of commercialism. At an average price of $50 (down from $100 in 1929), a radio brought variety programs like "Major Bowes' Amateur Hour," comedy shows with George Burns and Gracie Allen, and soap operas such as "One Man's Family" and "Against the Storm" to some 27 million listeners. A hair-raising adventure like "The Lone Ranger" (first broadcast in 1933) became so popular that by 1939 it was being heard three times a week on 140 stations.

Radio continued to bind the country culturally. A teenager in Splendora, Texas, could listen to the same wisecracks from Jack Benny, the same music from Guy Lombardo as kids in New York and Los Angeles. In 1938, when Orson Welles broadcast H. G. Wells' classic science fiction tale, *The War of the Worlds*, Americans everywhere listened to "Invasion from Mars," and many believed it. In Newark, New Jersey, cars jammed roads as families rushed to evacuate the city; church services in Indianapolis came to a hurried end so parishioners could scurry to safety; in a small town in Washington State the power suddenly failed and women fainted in the streets, convinced the end was at hand. The nation, used to responding to radio advertising and bombarded with continual reports of impending war in Europe, was prepared to believe almost anything, even invaders from Mars.

In Hollywood an efficient but autocratic "studio system" churned out a record number of feature films. Eight motion picture companies produced more than two-thirds of them. Color, first introduced in features in *Becky Sharp* (1935), soon

Daily Lives

FOOD/DRINK/DRUGS
The Control of Narcotics

The problem was old, and the new president intended to attack it firmly. Early in his first administration he sent his personal adviser to the federal commissioner of narcotics with an unmistakable message: no clemency for drug pushers. If the commissioner ever forwarded such a recommendation to the White House, he was to attach his own resignation. The public would stand for nothing less than strict enforcement of the law, and neither would Franklin Roosevelt.

As Roosevelt entered the White House in 1933, narcotics had been under federal control for two decades. But it had taken a half century before that to recognize the social costs of addiction. In the nineteenth century, a host of drugs offered Americans increasing control over tension and pain. Laudanum, or tincture of opium, had been used since the Renaissance to calm nerves, induce sleep, and relieve gastrointestinal illnesses such as cholera, food poisoning, and parasites. Chloroform and ether had served as anesthetics since the 1850s, and chloral hydrate (the famed "knockout drops" of sensational novels) was developed in 1868. Morphine, derived from opium in 1803, was a potent painkiller, while heroin, isolated in 1898, promised "heroic" therapy as an analgesic and sedative. Cocaine was made not from opium but from the South American coca leaf in the late 1850s. By the 1880s testimonials from authorities as diverse as Sigmund Freud and former surgeon general of the army William Hammond praised it as an anesthetic and stimulant, even as a cure for opiate addiction.

These addictive drugs became commonly available in a host of products. The exhilarating qualities of cocaine made it a favorite ingredient in medicines, wines, tonics, and, until 1903, in the soft drink Coca-Cola. Morphine and other opiates had worked their way into popular over-the-counter medicines like "Mrs. Winslow's Soothing Syrup" and "Hooper's Anodyne, the Infant's Friend." In the 1880s many doctors continued to believe that narcotics administered hypodermically were nonaddictive, and by the 1890s anyone could order a hypodermic kit from Sears, Roebuck for $1.50. Still, with drug use on the rise, the detrimental effects soon became obvious. By the turn of the century, conservative estimates placed the total number of abusers in the country at about 1 million.

As early as 1860 some states had begun regulating the use of pure narcotics, but strong traditions of individualism and privacy made control difficult and uneven. The emergence of the United States as a world power at the end of the nineteenth century gave domestic reformers a powerful boost. They had long argued that addiction was a foreign contagion, and in the early years of the twentieth century they pressed for the United States to mount an international war on drugs. Naturally such moral leadership abroad required moral rectitude at home.

As concern for public health and individual morality peaked during the progressive era, new laws brought narcotics slowly under federal control. The federal government had regulated opium through import taxes since the late nineteenth century. The Pure Food and Drug Act of 1906 required labeling of ingredients, including narcotics. In 1909 Congress excluded the

Daily Lives

The fruits of a drug raid in the 1920s. Until 1930, when the Federal Bureau of Narcotics was created, drug agents operated under the Treasury Department's Narcotics Division.

importation of opium for other than medical uses. Finally, in 1914 it enacted the more comprehensive Harrison Anti-Narcotic Act, which permitted only federally registered dealers to dispense morphine, cocaine, opium, and heroin. Physicians were allowed to issue the substances for medicinal purposes but had to file records of their prescriptions with federal authorities.

Once the prohibition of alcohol went into effect in 1920, the Treasury Department (given authority over enforcement) created a special Narcotics Division. As alcohol prohibition declined in popularity, supporters of the Harrison Act succeeded in establishing a separate Federal Bureau of Narcotics in 1930. It was this bureau's

commissioner to whom Roosevelt wrote his stern memorandum.

A disturbing pattern ran through the history of narcotics control. The most ardent campaigners often believed that certain drugs would make feared minorities unmanageable. In the late nineteenth century opium had been linked to the Chinese, raising alarm that its use would promote sexual contact with white women. At the turn of the century, cocaine was believed to endow blacks with cunning, hostility, and superhuman strength. (The fear that "cocainized" blacks could not be stopped by .32-caliber bullets is said to have led many southern police departments to arm themselves with .38-caliber pistols.) Heroin was used to explain the violence and promiscuity of adolescents in urban gangs in the 1920s. And in the 1930s, as pressure mounted for federal control of cannabis, or marijuana, local officials in southwestern states said smoking it increased crime among Mexican immigrants.

In each instance anxieties peaked amid social crisis: a glut of low-paid Chinese workers in the depression-filled 1890s; a battle for political control of blacks at the turn of the century; the rise of an unruly youth culture in the 1920s; and high unemployment among Mexican immigrants in the Great Depression of the 1930s. In 1937, despite resistance from an understaffed and underfunded Narcotics Bureau, Congress enacted the Marijuana Tax Act, which resulted in total prohibition. "America is a nation of drug-takers," wrote one authority in 1881. By the 1930s the nation had taken steps to change its habits.

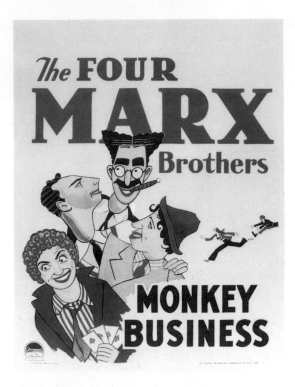

Lunatic social jesters, the Marx brothers turned convention topsy-turvy in the 1930s. Their antics made the Depression-spawned prospect of social disorder fun. *Monkey Business* (1931), their first Hollywood film, unleashed Groucho, Chico, Harpo, and Zeppo on a gang of crooks.

complemented sound, which had debuted in the 1927 version of *The Jazz Singer*. Neither alone could keep movie theaters full. As attendance waned early in the Depression, big studios like Metro-Goldwyn-Mayer, Columbia, Warner Brothers, and Universal sought to lure audiences back with films designed to shock, titillate, and just plain entertain in the midst of crisis.

Popular movies often played on deep national emotions. Horror movies such as *Frankenstein* (1931) and *Dracula* (1931) drew on anxieties about the dangers of tampering with the natural order of things. Early Depression gangster movies like *Little Caesar* (1931), *The Public Enemy* (1931), and *Scarface* (1932) allowed Americans ambivalent about the ethic of success to root for misfits who challenged it and still applaud their just demise. The Marx Brothers made fun of social disorder in *Monkey Business* (1931) and *Duck Soup* (1933), while Walt Disney's *Three Little Pigs* (1933) scoffed at it in the cartoon's hit song, "Who's Afraid of the Big Bad Wolf?" *She Done Him Wrong* (1933) catapulted Mae West to the top of box-office favorites by mixing sex with West's bawdy humor. ("Haven't you ever met a man who could make you happy?" Cary Grant asks her. "Sure, lots of times," she replies.) Busby Berkeley's choreography for *42nd Street* (1933) and *Gold Diggers of 1933* (1933) and Fred Astaire and Ginger Rogers, first paired in *Flying Down to Rio* (1933), leavened spirits in musicals that stressed teamwork and cooperation. Only toward the end of the decade did Hollywood develop a social conscience in such films as *Dead End* (1937), *Angels with Dirty Faces* (1938), and *The Grapes of Wrath* (1941).

By the mid-1930s more than 6 Americans in 10 were going to the movies at least once a week. They saw tamer films as the industry regulated movie content in the face of growing criticism. To avoid censorship and boycotts from such groups as the Legion of Decency (a watchdog group created in 1933 by the Catholic church), studios agreed to stiffen already existing regulations. "Evil and good are never to be confused," stated the Motion Picture Production Code of 1934. Producers could not depict homosexuality, abortion, drug use, or sex. Actors could utter no profanities. Even the word "sex" was banned. If they were featured in bed, couples had to be clothed and one foot of each partner had to touch the floor. Traditional middle-class morality reigned on the "silver screen." As a result most Depression movies, like most of popular culture, tended to preserve the basic social and economic tenets of American culture.

"Dirty Thirties": An Ecological Disaster

On the morning of Armistice Day 1933, the wind began to blow through Beadle County, South Dakota. Soon it was blowing at 60 miles an hour. It carried away almost everything that was not nailed down. "By noon," reported R. D. Lusk from the Karnstrum farm, "it was darker than night." When Lusk stepped outside, he ran smack into "a wall of dirt one's eyes could not penetrate, but it could penetrate the eyes and ears and nose. It could penetrate the lungs until one coughed up black." When the wind finally died down, the Karnstrum farm, like the rest of Beadle County, was changed. Lusk no longer saw any fields, "only sand drifting into mounds. . . . There was no longer a section-line road fifty feet from the front door. It was obliterated. In the farmyard, fences, machinery, and trees were gone, buried. The roofs of sheds stuck out through drifts deeper than a man is tall."

On and off the winds blew for 10 years. Between 1932 and 1939 an average of nearly 50 storms a year howled across the Great Plains. The "black blizzards" lasted anywhere from an hour to three and a half days. In 1935 one storm carried twice as much earth from the plains as had been dug out to make the Panama Canal. Visibility was so limited, said an observer, "Lady Godiva could ride thru streets without even the horse seeing her." Some cities burned their street lights 24 hours a day. In one small town a seven-year-old lost his way in the gloom. Days later he was found suffocated under a drift. "This is the ultimate darkness," despaired one Kansan in the midst of a dust storm. "So must come the end of the world."

One of the worst ecological disasters in modern history, the dust storms transformed 1500 square miles from the Oklahoma panhandle to western Kansas into a gigantic "Dust Bowl." From 1932 to 1936 drought parched fields and pastures and made sand dunes of plowed land. Record temperatures scorched the earth. The thermometer topped 100 degrees in Vinita, Oklahoma, every day for over a month in 1934. By 1936, reported *Newsweek*, the nation was "a vast simmering cauldron." That year the heat killed 4500 people. Nature alone was not to blame. "The dirty thirties," wrote one historian, "were primarily the work of man." The semiarid lands west of the 98th meridian were not suitable for intensive agriculture or livestock grazing. Sixty years of use and abuse had stripped the Great Plains of its natural vegetation. Without sod, the land lay defenseless against the elements. When the dry winds came, one-third of the Great Plains just blew away.

For protection people wore gauze masks, swabbed their nostrils with Vaseline, and covered their windows with paraffin-soaked rags, all to no avail. Tiny

"Black blizzards" dwarfed all man-made structures. The drought that gave rise to the huge dust storms lasted from 1932 until 1936, and few who lived through one ever forgot. "Noon was like night," reported a conductor on the Santa Fe railroad. "There was no sun, and, at times, it was impossible to see a yard. The engineer could not see the signal lights." In a single day in 1934, 12 million tons of western dirt fell on Chicago.

particles of dust covered everything—bedspreads, dinner plates, bread dough. Food crunched to the bite. An epidemic of respiratory infections and a new disease, "dust pneumonia," broke out among farm families in the plains states. Autopsies of dead cattle showed their lungs caked with mud; fish died from lack of oxygen in dust-coated rivers. As far east as Memphis people covered their faces with handkerchiefs to filter the air they breathed. Yellow grit from Nebraska collected on the window sills of the White House, and ships 300 miles off the East Coast found bits of Montana and Wyoming on their decks.

All told, some 3.5 million plains people abandoned their farms. As many as nature forced off their land were pushed out by landowners or corporations. Large-scale commercial farming was slowly spreading into the heartland of America. Huge "factories in the field," commercial farms were advancing east across the Great Plains from California, where 10 percent of the farms grew more than 50 percent of the crops. As in industrial America, the strategy was to consolidate and mechanize, increase production, cut labor costs, and raise profits. As farms grew in size, so did the number of tenants. In most Dust Bowl counties less than half the land was owned by the people who lived on it. American agriculture was turning from a way of life into an industry, American farmers from independent yeomen into common laborers. "We are not husbandmen," sighed an agricultural spokesman. "We are not farmers. We are producing a product to sell."

In the 1920s there had been a net migration of 6 million Americans, most of them young or black, from farms to towns and cities. During the Depression the trend reversed itself. By 1935 the largest number of people in American history—

33 million—were living on farms. The Great Plains, by contrast, were the only states that suffered a net loss of residents during the decade; 10,000 houses were left vacant on the high plains alone; 9 million acres of farmland went untended. The "exodusters" joined a growing migration of rural refugees. No one knows how many became migrants, but relief offices around the country did report a change in the typical migrant family. No longer black or brown, it was white and native-born, typically a young married couple with one child, leaving a farm or town on the Great Plains or in the South and traveling west.

Most did not travel far, perhaps to the next county. Long-distance migrants—many from Oklahoma, Arizona, and Texas—usually set their sights on California. Handbills and advertisements promised jobs picking fruit and harvesting vegetables. If they were like the Joad family in John Steinbeck's classic *The Grapes of Wrath* (1939), they drove west along Route 66 through Arizona and New Mexico, their belongings piled high atop rickety jalopies, heading for their Promised Land. Over 350,000 Oklahomans arrived in California during the decade. So many came that "Okie" came to mean any Dust Bowler, even though most of Oklahoma lay outside the Dust Bowl.

During the decade nearly two of every five migrants ended up in California, increasing its population by 1.1 million, the largest jump of any state. The poor were only a small minority of new arrivals, but enough came to make local citizens edgy. In 15 months, 86,546 destitute migrants crossed the California border, more than the total number of migrants for the first two years of the gold rush. By the middle of the decade the Los Angeles police had begun forming "bum blockades" to keep them out. "Negroes and Okies upstairs," read one sign in a San Joaquin Valley theater. Native-born whites had never encountered such discrimination before.

Only one in two or three migrants actually found work. At peak season California needed no more than 175,000 pickers. The labor surplus allowed growers to set their own terms. A migrant family could expect to earn about $450 a year, less

"Arkies" from Arkansas and "Okies" from Oklahoma fled west from the ravages of dust storms and farm tenancy.

than half the subsistence level. Those that did not work formed wretched enclaves called "little Oklahomas." The worst were located in the fertile Imperial Valley. There at the end of the decade relief officials discovered a family of 10 living in a 1921 Ford. When the mother, suffering from tuberculosis and pellagra, was told to go, she responded vacantly, "I wonder where."

The Fate of Outsiders

The Chavez family lost their farm in the North Gila River valley of Arizona in 1934. They had owned the small homestead near Yuma for two generations, but the Depression pushed them out. Cesar, barely six years old at the time, remembered only images of his family's departure: a "giant tractor" leveling the corral; the loss of his room and bed; the family piling into a Chevy for the journey west; his father promising earnestly to buy another Arizona plot someday.

The elder Chavez could never keep his promise. Instead he and his family lived on the road, "following the crops" in California. Like the Joads, the Chavez family roamed the West Coast in search of work. In eight years Cesar went to 37 schools. The whole family was forced to sell their labor to unscrupulous contractors for less than $10 a week. The father joined the strikes that hit the Imperial Valley in the mid-1930s, but they were crushed. "We were trapped," recalled Cesar. "Some people put this out of their minds and forget it. I don't." Thirty years later he founded the United Farm Workers of America, the first union of migratory workers in the country.

The Chavezes resembled the Joads in every way but one: they were Mexican-Americans. The Joads had found a few sympathetic store owners on their way west. When the Chavezes entered a roadside restaurant, a young waitress greeted them coldly: "We don't serve Mexicans here. Get out." In an America still strictly segregated, she never thought twice about refusing service to outsiders, whether they were brown or black. "White trade only" read the sign out front. "Every time we thought of it," said Cesar, "it hurt us."

The Spanish had inhabited the Southwest for nearly 400 years, producing a rich culture that mixed Old World and Indian civilizations. By the turn of the twentieth century there were nearly 300,000 Mexican-Americans in the United States, largely in the Southwest. In the following decade Mexicans fleeing poverty

962

and revolution nearly doubled the Latino population of Texas and New Mexico. In Arizona this group more than doubled; in California it quadrupled. During the war labor shortages led Washington to sponsor a bracero (day laborer) program, and in the 1920s American farmers opened a campaign to attract Mexican farm workers, who would accept low wages. By 1930 the census listed nearly 1.5 million Mexicans living in the United States.

A deep ambivalence had always characterized American attitudes toward Mexicans, but the onset of the Great Depression turned most communities against them. Fearful of being burdened with their relief, cities like Los Angeles found it cheaper to ship them back to Mexico. Some migrants left voluntarily, but others were forced out. Beginning in 1931 the federal government launched a series of deportations, or "repatriations," of Mexicans, including their American-born children (who by law were citizens of the United States).

During the decade the Latino population of the country declined by 500,000. Most of those who remained lived in poverty. The average income of Mexican-American families in Crystal City, Texas, in the Rio Grande valley was $506 a year, a sum that represented the combined income of parents and children. Fewer than two Mexican-American children in ten completed five years of school.

Hard times were nothing new for African-Americans. "The Negro was born in depression," one black man said. "It only became official when it hit the white man." Depressed agricultural prices and rampant discrimination had spurred a great African-American migration from the Deep South on the eve of World War I. It continued through the 1920s, when over 800,000 moved to northern cities. Like their rural counterparts, these new urbanites found prosperity elusive, and as the Depression deepened black unemployment skyrocketed. By 1932 it reached 50 percent, twice the national level. Unemployed whites demanded that blacks be fired from their jobs as garbage collectors, street cleaners, elevator operators, and bellhops. A white clerk in Marianna, Florida, no different from millions of Americans, reasoned that "a nigger hasn't got no right to have a job when there are white men who can do the work and are out of work." By 1933 several cities reported between 25 and 40 percent of their black residents with no support but relief payments. Even skilled blacks who retained their jobs had their wages cut by half, according to one study of Harlem in 1935.

African-Americans made do as they had for years. "We had one big advantage," attested one black man. "Our wives could go to the store and get a bag of beans or a sack of flour and a piece of fat meat, and they could cook this. And we could eat it. . . . Now you take the white fella, he couldn't do this. His wife would tell him: Look, if you can't do any better than this, I'm gonna leave you." Migration from the rural South dropped to half of what it had been a decade earlier. As late as 1940 three of four African-Americans lived in rural areas; yet conditions there were just as bad as in cities. Forty percent of all black workers in the United States were farm laborers or tenants. In 1934 one study estimated the average income for black cotton farmers at under $200 a year.

The Depression aggravated racial prejudice. "Dust has been blown from the shotgun, the whip, and the noose," reported The New Republic in 1931, "and Ku Klux Klan practices were being resumed in the certainty that dead men not only tell no tales but create vacancies." Lynchings tripled between 1932 and 1933. In 1932 the Supreme Court ordered a retrial in the most celebrated racial case of the decade. In 1931 nine black teenagers had been accused of raping two white women on a train bound for Scottsboro, Alabama. Within weeks all-white juries had found the boys guilty and sentenced eight of them to death. The convictions rested on the testimony of the women, one of whom later admitted the boys had been framed. Appeals kept the case alive for most of the decade. In the end charges against four of the "Scottsboro boys" were dropped, while the other five received substantial prison sentences. One fled to Michigan, where the governor rejected demands to extradite him to Alabama.

Like many African-Americans, George Baker refused to be victimized by the Depression. In 1915 he had moved from Georgia to Harlem, changed his name to M. J. Divine, and founded a religious cult that promised followers an afterlife of full equality. In the 1930s "Father Divine" stressed economic cooperation and opened shelters, or "heavens," for regenerate "angels," black and white alike. His soup kitchens and missions fed 3000 hungry souls a day in Harlem, and soon the cult spread to other American cities and even abroad. Urban blacks had found a new messiah.

Some rural blacks joined the Southern Tenant Farmers Union, organized in 1934 by black and white tenants in Arkansas. "The landlord is always betwixt us, beatin' us and starvin' us and makin' us fight each other," an old black man advised the founders. "There ain't but one way for us to get him where he can't help himself and that's for us to get together and stay together." The union published its own newspaper, the *Sharecropper's Voice*, and attracted national support from Socialists and other radicals. Landlords became uneasy with union demands for a greater share of federal subsidies and an end to arbitrary evictions. Planters and riding bosses broke up union meetings and horsewhipped organizers. Although they won few concessions, union members hung together. Elsewhere the Depression divided black and white Americans, but in the Arkansas delta hard times drew them closer.

THE TRAGEDY OF HERBERT HOOVER

A cold, gray morning sent shivers through the crowd huddled in front of the Capitol on March 4, 1929. Herbert Hoover had just been sworn in as the thirty-first president of the United States. His voice, always a monotone, came booming over the loudspeakers: "I have no fears for the future of our country. It is bright with hope." Engineer, businessman, secretary of commerce for eight years, Herbert Hoover embodied executive competence and efficiency. No one seemed better suited to anticipate trouble or resolve it. "We were in a mood for magic," recalled journalist Anne McCormick of the inauguration. "We had summoned a great engineer to solve our problems for us; now we sat back comfortably and confidently to watch the problems being solved."

Within seven months a "depression" (a term coined by Hoover to minimize the crisis) had struck. Try as he might, he could not beat it. The magic failed, and the nation turned against him. "People were starving because of Herbert Hoover," one angry mother told her son in 1932. "Men were killing themselves because of Herbert Hoover, and their fatherless children were being packed away to orphanages . . . because of Herbert Hoover." The charge was unfair, but it stuck. Hoover's presidency, begun with such promise, became the worst ordeal of his life. Near the end of his term in 1932 he moaned that "all the money in the world could not induce me to live over the last nine months. The conditions we have experienced make this office a compound hell." He nonetheless felt duty-bound to accept his party's renomination for the presidency. His ordeal soon turned into a tragic and humiliating rejection.

The Failure of Relief

By the winter of 1931–1932 the story was the same everywhere: too little money, too many destitute. Private charities, the traditional sources of aid, had long since dried up. In 1932 Hull House, once a model of progressive benevolence, stood in "proud irrelevance." It was flooded, continued the critic Edmund Wilson, with a "sea of misery." In New York, city employees had been donating 1 percent of their salaries to feed the needy since 1930; yet New Yorkers were starving to death. The Red Cross furnished free vegetable seeds when the city council of Midland, Texas, gave land to the unemployed. There was not enough money to supply free food. "Compared to the size of the problem," wrote one historian, "it was like using a peashooter to stop a rhinoceros." By 1932 private charity had dwindled to 6 percent of all relief funds.

City resources were quickly depleted by an estimated 30 million destitute people. In 1930 the Emergency Work Bureau of New York City provided temporary jobs, or "work relief," for 37,000 people a week. The city had at least 300,000 unemployed. In Philadelphia relief payments to a family of four totaled $5.50 a week, the highest in the country. In New York the total was $2.39. The dimensions of the crisis sharpened the problems of discrimination as well. Houston and Dallas refused to grant any relief to African-Americans and Mexicans, and some cities gave nothing to unmarried people or childless couples, no matter how needy they were.

As property values fell and businesses failed, nearly 30 percent of taxes owed went unpaid. Deprived of revenue, cities stopped paving roads, repairing sidewalks, and plowing snow. Relief was expendable too. In 1931 New Orleans refused all new applications for aid. Oklahoma City began arresting unemployed men, charging them with vagrancy, and ordering them out of town. By the end of 1931, Detroit, Boston, Buffalo, and scores of other cities were bankrupt. When mayors sought loans, banks required them to cut relief rolls. The mayor of Detroit, which provided welfare for 50,000 families, dropped one-third of them so he could borrow money from automakers to keep the city running. By 1932 more than 100 cities had no relief appropriations at all.

Cities clamored for help from state capitals, but after a decade of extravagant spending and sloppy bookkeeping, many of the states were already running in the red. As businesses folded and property values tumbled, tax bases shrank and with them state revenues. Michigan, one of the few states to provide any relief, sliced funds from over $2 million in 1931 to $860,000 in 1932. Until New York established its Temporary Emergency Relief Administration in 1931, no state even had an agency to handle the problem.

Some people refused to accept help. By 1932 only one eligible family in four was receiving public assistance in cities. Contrary to popular stereotypes, recipients were reluctant to take aid. The "right people," said the wife of an unemployed railroad worker, never took "something for nothing." Like most Americans she regarded accepting cash or food as a sign of personal failure. When her husband told her they would have to go on relief, she gasped. To go on relief, said one man, was to endure a "crucifixion." Before applications could even be considered, all property had to be sold, all credit exhausted, all relatives declared flat broke. After a half-hour grilling about his family, home, and friends, one applicant left, "feeling I didn't have any business living any more." Hostile to the idea of public assistance, officials attached every possible stigma to aid. In 1932 residents of Lewiston, Maine, voted to bar all welfare recipients from the polls. Ten states had already written property requirements for voting into their constitutions. The destitute were being disfranchised.

The Hoover Depression Program

Every night he stayed at the White House during the Great Depression President Hoover dined in regal splendor. He had thought about economizing but decided it would be bad for the morale of the country. If he changed his habits one bit, it might be taken as a sign of lost confidence. So each evening Hoover entered the dining room in black tie, ready to consume seven full courses. Uniformed buglers heralded his arrival and departure with glittering trumpets, even when the only guest was his wife.

It was not that Herbert Hoover was insensitive—far from it. He never visited a bread line or a relief shelter because he could not bear to see suffering. When the press criticized him he withdrew, wounded and hurt. The cruel rumors that circulated about him—that dogs instinctively disliked him; that he had masterminded the kidnaping and murder of Charles Lindbergh's infant son in 1932; that roses wilted in his hands—were as painful as they were ridiculous. Hoover was doing all he could to promote recovery, more than any of his predecessors, and still he was scorned. His natural sullenness turned to self-pity. "You can't expect to see calves running in the field the day after you put the bull to the cows," Calvin Coolidge reassured him. "No," said an exasperated Hoover, "but I would expect to see contented cows."

Hoover's frustration was understandable. He had never failed before. Orphaned into poverty at nine, he became one of the first graduates of Stanford University in 1895, an expert engineer, and the owner of one of the most successful mining firms in the world. Before he turned 40, he was a millionaire. As a good Quaker he balanced private gain with public service. Saving starving refugees in war-torn Europe and flood victims at home, he became known as the greatest humanitarian of his generation. Finns added a new word to their vocabulary: to "hoover" meant to help.

From the fall of 1930 onward, Hoover assumed full responsibility for ending the crisis—and as humanely as possible. Treasury Secretary Andrew Mellon urged him to "liquidate labor, liquidate stocks, liquidate the farmers, liquidate real estate." Hoover ignored the advice and eased Mellon out of the administration. When Democratic leaders in Congress demanded all federal employment and salaries be cut by 10 percent, Hoover called the idea "heartless and medieval." Instead he worked 18 hours a day, cut his own salary, and developed a program to actively fight the Depression. His unprecedented strategy was grounded in Hoover's longstanding commitment to voluntarism, his faith in the power of capitalism to revive itself, and his conviction that too much government action would create an intrusive federal bureaucracy that threatened public freedoms and private initiative. Unfortunately the strategy was based on two widely held but faulty assumptions: the Depression was temporary and it had originated in the faltering economies of Europe.

Herbert Hoover.

Hoover understood the vicious cycle of rising unemployment and falling demand and knew the necessity for investment. So he invited business leaders to the White House and secured their pledges to maintain employment, wages, and prices. To further bolster public confidence, he not only decided to maintain his dining habits but also varied the rest of his routine as little as possible and minimized the seriousness of the collapse. Again and again he reassured Americans that "conditions are fundamentally sound" and that the "depression is over." When recovery proved elusive, Hoover's credibility vanished (so thoroughly that journalist Edward Angley published all of the president's sunny forecasts in 1931 and called the book *Oh Yeah!*).

Hoover tried to stimulate the economy indirectly to encourage private and local initiative. Right after the crash he demanded a tax cut to put more money into people's hands. In 1930 Congress happily complied. Toward the end of the year, he created the President's Emergency Committee on Employment (PECE) under Colonel Arthur Woods to encourage local relief programs. The Federal Farm Board, created in 1929 to stabilize agriculture, promoted the sale of farm commodities through cooperatives. In 1931 Hoover prompted Congress to expand the lending powers of the Federal Land Banks by $125 million and later urged the establishment of home-loan banks to discount mortgages. He endorsed and signed the Hawley–Smoot Tariff (1930), raising tariff walls to new heights to protect the United States from cheap foreign goods. He declared a one-year moratorium on payments of reparations and war debts in 1931 to give Europeans economic breathing space. At home he increased spending on public works to prime the economic pump. Before he was done, his public building program overshadowed those of all of his predecessors.

The program was in keeping with Hoover's associational philosophy, developed during his years as Commerce secretary (see pp. 931–932), of using government to promote private and local action. But nothing worked. Employers tried to keep their pledges; yet within months they were forced to reduce wages and lay off workers. Tax cuts were followed by tax increases when government spending and reduced revenues threw the federal budget out of balance. In 1932 Congress passed the largest peacetime tax increase in American history in order to make up the difference. The Revenue Act of 1932, supported by the president, brought added funds into the Treasury but stymied recovery by undermining investment and consumption. More trouble followed. In April 1931 Colonel Woods resigned as head of PECE after the president had rejected his recommendation for greater federal involvement in relief. Late in 1931 Hoover appointed the Organization on Unemployment Relief under Walter Gifford, president of the American Telephone and Telegraph Company. Less than a year later Gifford, who counseled against federal participation, confessed that he did not know how many people were unemployed.

The Hawley–Smoot Tariff was the greatest disaster of all. Over a thousand of the nation's leading economists had petitioned Hoover not to sign it. It left American loans as the only prop for European exports, brought on a wave of retaliation, and choked world trade. The Federal Farm Board was innovative in 1929 but never designed to handle the collapse of agriculture that took place after the crash. Woefully undercapitalized, it also failed to attack the principal farm problem, overproduction. Even public works did not induce recovery. Spending, which ran to more than $1 billion by the end of Hoover's administration, scarcely approached what was needed. To give even half the estimated unemployed jobs on

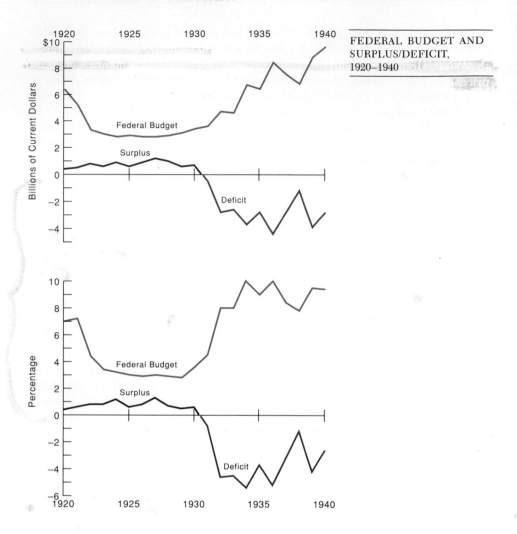

FEDERAL BUDGET AND
SURPLUS/DEFICIT,
1920–1940

public works would have cost $10 billion in 1932, when the entire federal budget amounted to only $3.2 billion.

Between 1930 and 1932 some 5100 banks failed in America as panicky depositors withdrew their funds. Losses amounted to over $3.2 billion. Yielding to pressure from congressmen and enlightened bankers, Hoover called for a revival of the War Finance Corporation of 1918. Early in 1932, the Reconstruction Finance Corporation (RFC) was mustered into service to fight the Depression. With a capital stock of $500 million (and the power to borrow four times that amount), the RFC could lend money to banks and their chief corporate debtors—insurance companies and railroads. Within three months bank failures dropped from 70 a week to 1 every two weeks. The Glass–Steagall Banking Act (1932) eased credit by allowing the Federal Reserve to use government bonds as a basis for $2 billion in new issues of currency.

From the start Hoover rejected the idea of direct federal relief for the unemployed. Critics pointed out that he had no compunctions about furnishing relief for banks, but Hoover did not budge. He feared that a dole or giveaway program (of the kind being used in Britain) would damage the character of recipients. "We are dealing with the intangibles of life and ideals," he reminded Americans. In particular, federal experiments with relief could have unhealthy results for the whole nation, perhaps even creating a permanently dependent underclass. Administration would be expensive and a bureaucracy would be needed to police the program. Not only would the state be meddling in the lives of its citizens, but also "direct relief from the Federal government would bring an inevitable train of corruption and waste." Hoover assumed neighborliness and cooperation would be enough. When Congress appropriated $45 million to save the livestock of drought-stricken Arkansas farmers in 1930, he vetoed an additional $25 million to feed farm families. Congress restored most of the cuts.

In 1930, as unemployment topped 4 million, Americans sent a new Congress to Washington. The off-year elections reduced the Republican majority to one in the Senate and gave Democrats a slim lead in the House. After rejecting Democratic proposals for federal public works and a federal employment service, Hoover slowly softened his stand on federal relief. In 1932 he dictated the terms of his own surrender in the Emergency Relief and Construction Act. It authorized the RFC to lend up to $1.5 billion for "reproductive" public works like toll bridges and slum clearance. The Treasury could lend an additional $350 million for public buildings such as post offices. Another $300 million was made available to states for direct relief of the unemployed. Neither Hoover nor Congress expected these loans to be repaid. Even so, they were woefully inadequate: when the governor of Pennsylvania requested funds to furnish the destitute with 13 cents a day for a year, the RFC sent him only enough for 3 cents a day.

Stirrings of Discontent

Hoover had given ground on relief, but like the rest of his Depression program it was too little and came too late. "The word revolution is heard at every hand," one writer noted in 1932. Three years into the Great Depression some observers wondered if capitalism had given out. Here and there bands of desperate people took matters into their own hands. In Wisconsin the Farm Holiday Association, under the leadership of Milo Reno, dumped thousands of gallons of milk on highways in a vain attempt to raise prices. Ten thousand striking miners formed a 48-mile motor car "Coal Caravan" that worked its way in protest across southern Illinois. In March a demonstration turned ugly when communist sympathizers led a hunger march on Henry Ford's Rouge Assembly Plant in Dearborn, Michigan. As 3000 protesters surged toward the gates, Ford police drenched them with hoses, then opened fire at point-blank range. Four marchers were killed and more than twenty wounded.

For all the stirrings of discontent, revolution was never a real danger. By 1932 the Communist party of the United States had 20,000 members, up from 6500 in 1929, but it was hardly a potent political force. Under the slogan "Starve or Fight!" the communists staged dozens of food, unemployment, and eviction protests. They led unionizing drives and courted intellectuals and the oppressed with their commitment to labor and civil rights. Deeply suspicious of Marxist doctrine, most Americans were unsympathetic. Fewer than 1000 African-Americans joined the party in the early 1930s, and in the election of 1932 the communist presidential candidate, William Z. Foster, polled just over 100,000 votes. At first belligerent and hostile to established politics, the communists adopted a more cooperative strategy to contain Adolf Hitler, whose Nazi party had won control of Germany in 1933. The Soviet Union ordered Communist parties in Europe and the United

States to join with liberal politicians in a "popular front" against Nazism. Thereafter party membership peaked in the mid-1930s at about 80,000.

Hoover was compassionate but only to a point. When 1600 communist-led hunger marchers came to Washington in December 1931, he was determined to protect their right to protest. The president ordered blankets, tents, a field kitchen, and medical aid for them. Washington police stood guard over their parade, and Hoover himself received their petitions at the White House. In January 1932 James Cox, a Catholic priest from Pittsburgh, led 10,000 unemployed men through Washington in a motorcade eight miles long. Hoover listened sympathetically as the priest pleaded for public works and a tax on the rich.

The veterans who descended on the capital half a year later received a different reception. In the summer of 1932 a ragtag army of World War I veterans came to Washington to cash in their Adjusted Compensation Certificates. In 1924 Congress had sent out about 3.5 million certificates for wartime service. Called "bonuses," they were due to mature at an average of $1000 each in 1945. Penniless and hungry, the veterans marched on Washington to press for immediate payment. Walter Waters, one of the leaders, was typical. He had served overseas with the 146th Field Artillery and had been discharged in June 1919. By 1930 he was married, assistant superintendent of a cannery in Portland, and happy. A year later he was destitute, his job and savings gone, possessions pawned, and his prospects bleak. The only thing of value he owned was his Adjusted Compensation Certificate.

In May 1932 Congressman Wright Patman from Texas introduced a bill for immediate payment of bonuses. Waters and 300 other veterans set out from Portland on a march to press their case in Washington. By the time they reached the capital in June, the "Bonus Expeditionary Force" had swelled to 15,000, the largest protest in the city's history. Bonus Army leaders met with congressional representatives, but the president refused to see them. For the first time since the armistice the gates of the Executive Mansion were chained shut.

Hoover dismissed the veterans as a special-interest lobby eager to feather an already soft nest. Veterans' benefits accounted for 25 percent of the federal budget, the largest single item. The cost of their bonuses—$2.3 billion—would have nearly doubled the deficit. Hoover was prepared to veto any bonus bill. When the House enacted one, the Senate spared him the trouble by blocking it. Some of the veterans went home, but about 10,000 stayed to dramatize their plight. Besides, they had nowhere else to go.

The Bonus Army conducted itself peaceably, drilling, parading, and policing its own. The few radicals in its ranks were quickly isolated. When two men were killed late in July as Washington police tried to evict some of the veterans from federal buildings, Hoover called in the army. He wanted nothing more than unarmed military support for the police; what he got was a bloody rout. Dressed in jodhpurs and all his medals, Army Chief of Staff General Douglas MacArthur personally led four troops of cavalry brandishing sabers, followed by six tanks and a column of infantry.

The operation commenced at dusk on July 28, 1932. First the soldiers cleared the Federal Triangle with bayonets and tear gas. A horrified Dwight Eisenhower, one of MacArthur's aides, watched helplessly as Major George S. Patton, Jr., rode down a crowd of Bonus marchers in the last mounted charge of the United States Cavalry. MacArthur then turned to the Bonus Expeditionary Force encampment on the Anacostia Flats across the Potomac River. Despite President Hoover's orders to halt, the general razed the camp that night. As the smoke drifted over the Capitol the next morning, the Bonus marchers had vanished. Among the routed veterans, who included some 300 casualties, was Joseph T. Agelino. In 1918 he had received the Distinguished Service Cross for saving the life of a young officer named George S. Patton, Jr.

Hoover took responsibility for everything but offered the lame excuse that Bonus marchers were "not veterans" but "Communists and persons with criminal records" bent on insurrection. An exhaustive survey of the Bonus Army conducted by the Veterans Administration belied the claim. More than 9 of 10 marchers had been veterans, nearly 7 of 10 had served overseas, and 1 in 5 was disabled. What they really wanted was food and jobs. Sadly, Hoover could provide neither. In Albany, New York, Governor Franklin Roosevelt, outraged by the bloodshed, exploded: "There is nothing inside the man but jelly." Like the hero of a classical tragedy, Herbert Hoover, prophet of the New Era, came tumbling down.

The tragedy was made all the more poignant by Hoover's considerable accomplishments. However cautiously he responded to the Depression, he had taken unprecedented federal action. Through the Reconstruction Finance Corporation the federal government intervened directly into the peacetime economy for the first time. With the Emergency Relief and Construction Act it assumed responsibility for relief, again for the first time. It underwrote the incomes of farmers through the Federal Farm Board and tried to save the homes of the middle class with mortgage loans. But nothing had been enough. Trapped by fears of big government and committed to the associational formula of private initiative and voluntary cooperation, Hoover could go no further.

The Election of 1932

Sensing the opportunity to recapture the White House for the first time since 1920, buoyant Democrats gathered in Chicago in June 1932 for their national convention. The platform blamed the Depression on the Republicans, called for a 25 percent cut in federal spending, and promised a balanced budget. It also vowed somehow to provide federal public works and unemployment relief. When the

THE ELECTION OF 1932

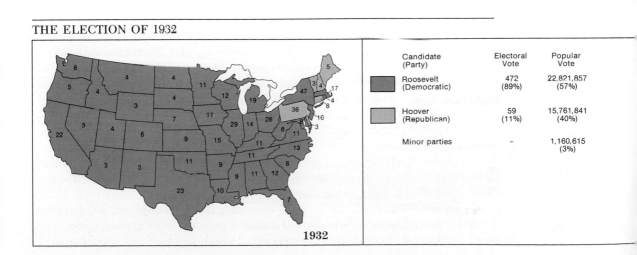

Candidate (Party)	Electoral Vote	Popular Vote
Roosevelt (Democratic)	472 (89%)	22,821,857 (57%)
Hoover (Republican)	59 (11%)	15,761,841 (40%)
Minor parties	–	1,160,615 (3%)

1932

convention heard the plank calling for repeal of Prohibition, pandemonium broke loose for 25 minutes. Uniting traditional supporters from the South and West with city dwellers from the Northeast, New York Governor Franklin D. Roosevelt swept all challengers aside on the fourth ballot. Effervescent and inspiriting, Roosevelt broke tradition by flying to Chicago to accept the nomination himself. "I pledge you," he told delegates, "I pledge myself, to a new deal for the American people." In that instant, Roosevelt found his campaign slogan—"the New Deal." Moments later, when an organ bellowed "Happy Days Are Here Again," he had a campaign song.

The Republicans refused to abandon the somber Hoover. In June 1932 their national convention opened in Chicago and endorsed his Depression program to the last detail. The party platform opposed government spending and direct federal relief and favored an extension of the tariff. On Prohibition, delegates waffled with a plank so ambiguous that neither side was pleased. Hoover was renominated by acclamation in a hall one-third empty. Thoughtlessly the band struck up "California, here I come/Right back where I started from." "I have seen many conventions," reported H. L. Mencken from the press gallery, "but this is the worst."

The campaign was over before it began. "I had little hope of re-election," Hoover later explained, "but it was incumbent on me to fight it out to the end." He believed the future was at stake. As he saw it, the contest was between more than two men or two parties. It was between two philosophies of government: the dangerous federal activism of Democrats against the voluntarism and prudent leadership of Republicans. Roosevelt, Hoover warned, would increase federal spending, inflate the currency, reduce the tariff, and "build a bureaucracy such as we have never seen in our history." Hoover called instead for balanced budgets, confident press releases, a cautious program of public works and government loans, and the mobilization of private resources.

Lacking a national following, Roosevelt tailored his appeal to as broad a constituency as possible. In Iowa he called himself a "farmer"; to the Commonwealth Club of San Francisco he prescribed a stiff dose of economic planning to ensure recovery. He demanded both a balanced budget and more federal relief for the unemployed. He attacked Hoover as a "profligate spender," then went on to describe his own costly program for expanding federal public works. Columnist Walter Lippmann called him a "balanced antithesis." "The country yearned for a Messiah," wrote one disappointed reporter. "Mr. Roosevelt did not look or sound like a Messiah," only "the one sure means of rebuking the party in power."

Election day brought a thundering rebuke of Hoover and the Republicans. Roosevelt received nearly 58 percent of the popular vote. Except for 1912, when the party was divided, no Republican presidential candidate had ever lost so badly. Norman Thomas, one of the few radicals in the race, won for the Socialists proportionately fewer votes than in 1912 or 1920. Democrats held majorities in both houses of Congress. As telling as their magnitude were the returns themselves. Roosevelt carried the South and West and almost all the industrial states. Immigrants, Catholics and Jews, farmers and industrial laborers, city dwellers and the rural poor—groups dissatisfied with Republican rule even before the Great Depression—were being galvanized into a vast coalition. With them the Democratic party would dominate politics for decades to come.

Early the next morning, returning to his town house from victory celebrations at the Biltmore Hotel in New York, Franklin Roosevelt experienced a rare moment of doubt. As his son James helped him to bed, he confessed, "I am afraid I may not have the strength to do this job. After you leave me tonight, Jimmy, I am going to pray. . . . I hope you will pray for me, too."

The challenge was daunting: over 12 million unemployed, an average of 30 banks failing every week, factories idle, farms on the auction block, prices plummeting. Hoover had recognized the need for action but failed to stop the terrible slide. People who had scorned government, including businessmen, were baffled and now looked to Washington. The nation awaited Roosevelt, but no one knew whether he would be equal to the job, not even the president-elect himself. All Roosevelt knew was that he would try anything to help. In one of his first acts as president, he ordered that no one telephoning the White House for aid be shut off. Someone in the administration would be found to answer every call.

SIGNIFICANT EVENTS

1926 — Miami real estate bust

1928 — Great Bull Market begins to peak

1929 — Herbert Hoover inaugurated; stock market crash; Federal Farm Board created

1930 — Hawley–Smoot Tariff raises rates; President's Emergency Committee on Employment created

1931 — Repatriation of Mexicans; Scottsboro boys arrested; New York establishes Temporary Emergency Relief Administration; President's Organization on Unemployment Relief created

1932 — Glass–Steagall Banking Act; Reconstruction Finance Corporation established; Emergency Relief and Construction Act; Farm Holiday Association formed; Bonus Army marches on Washington, D.C.; Franklin Roosevelt elected president

1933 — Walt Disney's *Three Little Pigs*; Legion of Decency formed; Motion Picture Production Code; "black blizzards" begin to create Dust Bowl

1934 — Southern Tenant Farmers Union organized

1935 — *Becky Sharp*, first color film; Communist party announces popular front

1936 — Margaret Mitchell's *Gone with the Wind* published

1937 — Marijuana Tax Act

1938 — Orson Welles' radio broadcast of *Invasion from Mars*

1939 — John Steinbeck's *The Grapes of Wrath* published

27

The New Deal

W inner, South Dakota, November 10, 1933. "Dammit, I don't WANT to write to you again tonight. It's been a long, long day, and I'm tired." All the days had been long since Lorena Hickok began her odyssey four months earlier. She often felt tired and sometimes out of sorts, especially when *Time* magazine had run that "damned article" about her. "I suppose I am 'a rotund lady with a husky voice' and 'baggy clothes,'" she admitted. But to call her "peremptory," to say that she had gotten her job as special investigator for the Roosevelt administration merely because she was a friend of the president's wife—that was too much!

True enough, when the new federal relief administrator had first come looking for an agent, Eleanor did recommend "Hick." Friendship had gone no further. Talent and experience put Hickok on the federal payroll. A hard-nosed reporter, she had been the first woman hired by the Associated Press. In the days when women were routinely handed delicate assignments, she covered politics, kidnapings, and worse. "One time I slept with a murderess," she recalled proudly of an interview. "There was only one bed, so she and I slept together."

Whatever *Time* wrote, Hickok knew she was doing an important job. Riding trains and airplanes, driving along roads so full of ruts you couldn't tell them from ploughed fields, traveling through "every man's land—and no man's land," she was reporting on Depression America. In three years she covered 7000 miles across 32 states—from the capital's notorious slums to a New England potato harvest to the Imperial Valley of California, where the thermometer in her car registered 126 degrees Fahrenheit.

Before she began her journey, she regarded the unemployed as most Americans did—a faceless legion of "muffled figures, backs curved against the wind, selling apples on the street corners." They were "chiselers" and "shovel-leaners" who lived on government handouts and make-work projects because they did not want regular jobs. The cross-country trek changed her. A national crisis became a series of personal crises, each with its own face and story, together adding up to a portrait of deprivation, anguish, and often courage.

Hickok found that the federal government's relief program, barely a year old, was making a difference. Half a billion dollars was being funneled into states, localities, and private charities. By the end of 1933 a million farm families were on relief. And more was needed. "Seems like we just keep goin' lower and lower," the 16-year-old daughter of a North Carolina sharecropper told Hickok. For two

Franklin Roosevelt was inaugurated on March 4, 1933. Skies were overcast, but the previous day's rain had stopped. Washington, wrote a reporter, "welcomes the 'new deal,' even though it is not sure what the new deal is going to be."

weeks, she, her sister, and their father had been living in a tobacco barn outside of Raleigh. Somehow hope still flickered in her determined blue eyes. Hickok couldn't explain it until she noticed that pinned to the girl's bosom, "as one wears a brooch," was a campaign button from the 1932 election—"a profile of the President." Hope sprang from the man in the White House.

Before Franklin D. Roosevelt and the New Deal, few Americans had any contact with the federal government. In 1932 the vast majority of them paid no federal income taxes. Federal welfare payments and public works projects had yet to be initiated. There were no government guarantees of minimum wages and maximum hours. Social Security did not exist, and federal deposit insurance, the sole protection for the funds of depositors, would not be enacted for another year. The old order was widely perceived to have failed, and nothing, least of all government, seemed capable of reviving it. The only federal institution people knew at all was the local post office, and these days it usually delivered bad news.

A change was perceptible, Hickok reported. In Pennsylvania, "The Federal government is hugely important." She found people all over America talking about federal programs. Perhaps it was Washington's long-awaited contributions to relief or maybe the new farm subsidies; just as likely it was Roosevelt. Wherever she went, Hickok seldom heard voters describe themselves as "Republicans"

Lorena Hickok (left) met Eleanor Roosevelt (right) in 1928 and thereafter served as her unofficial press adviser. She traveled with Eleanor during Franklin's campaign for the presidency in 1932, arranged her women-only press conferences, and became her closest friend. (In the center of this photograph is Paul Person, governor of the Virgin Islands.)

or "Democrats" any more. Instead they said they were "for the President." "This fellow Roosevelt is really trying to help us," one South Dakota farmer told her.

The mails carried other signs that plain people were looking to the president and the federal government as never before. During the first weekend after the inauguration nearly half a million letters and telegrams poured into the White House. For years the average remained between 5000 and 8000 a day, a new presidential record. It took a staff of 50 just to handle Roosevelt's public correspondence. In four years President Hoover had required only one.

Over half the letters came from those at the bottom of the economic heap. Most sought help, offered simple words of praise, or just expressed heartfelt gratitude. It seemed, wrote a Kansas man in 1932, "as though some Moses had come to alleviate us of our sufferings." Whatever the individual messages, their collective meaning was clear: Franklin D. Roosevelt and the New Deal had begun to restore hope and confidence. For the first time, Americans believed the federal government would help them through a great crisis. Here, if anywhere, is the true essence of what historians would call the "Roosevelt Revolution."

THE EARLY NEW DEAL (1933–1935)

On March 4, 1933, as the clocks struck noon, Eleanor Roosevelt wondered if it was possible to "do anything to save America now." One-fourth of the work force was unemployed; 30 million families had no means of support; there wasn't enough

money in the Treasury to meet the federal payroll. Eleanor looked at her husband, who had just been sworn in as thirty-second president of the United States. Franklin Roosevelt removed his hand from the 300-year-old family Bible, turned to the podium, and solemnly addressed the crowd, now over 100,000: "Let me assert my firm belief that the only thing we have to fear is fear itself—nameless, unreasoning, unjustified terror." Heeding the nation's call for action, he promised to convene Congress into special session and exercise "broad Executive power to wage a war against the emergency." The crowd broke into thunderous applause. Eleanor was terrified. "One has the feeling of going it blindly," she explained a few hours later, "because we're in a tremendous stream, and none of us know where we're going to land."

The New Deal unfolded in two legislative bursts, one in the hundred days after the inauguration, another in the hundred days at the end of 1935. Often chaotic and sometimes contradictory, the program pursued three broad goals: recovery, relief, and reform. Though recovery remained elusive, there were notable achievements in relief and reform. Above all the New Deal created a limited "welfare state." It never reached all Americans, but for the first time government was committed to maintaining minimum standards of well-being for those in need. Despite his dominating presence Franklin Roosevelt was not the New Deal. It was also the product of Congress, the Supreme Court, and ordinary Americans. Sometimes they pushed the New Deal further than Roosevelt wanted to take it; sometimes they set limits he disliked. Regardless, the New Deal reshaped America.

The Democratic Roosevelts

Franklin Delano Roosevelt understood the gravity of the crisis better than anyone. A friend told him that if he succeeded, he would go down as the greatest president in history. "If I fail," he replied, "I shall be the last one." Roosevelt had no intention of failing, but he was not quite sure how he was going to succeed. "Take a method and try it," he instructed his staff. "If it fails, try another. But above all try something." He had no master blueprint, no "economic panaceas or fancy plans." He was a pragmatist who improvised, he told reporters, like a football quarterback calling a play only when he had seen how the last one turned out.

One thing he did know beforehand: Americans were ready for change. Together he and Eleanor gave it to them, beginning with the White House itself. No more footmen; no more buglers; and above all, no more seven-course meals as Hoover had served. Instead visitors got fare fit for a boardinghouse, capped by a desert of a pineapple slice with two cherries and a walnut swimming in watery whipped cream. Roosevelt's lunches—hash and one poached egg—cost 19 cents. With millions of Americans on the edge of starvation, anything more would have been unseemly.

Almost nothing Roosevelt did was unseemly. Born of an old Dutch patrician family in New York, he had been pampered as a boy by an overbearing mother and an elderly, indulgent father. He grew up idolizing his cousin Theodore Roosevelt and mimicked his path to the presidency, except that Franklin was a Democrat. Like Theodore, he was graduated from Harvard University (in 1904), won a seat in the New York State legislature (in 1910), secured an appointment as assistant secretary of the navy (in 1913), and ran for the vice presidency (in 1920). Along the way he even married Theodore's niece Eleanor, a shy girl with a toothy grin, fantastic energy, and an unshakable commitment to social justice.

Though the Democrats lost the election of 1920, party bosses agreed that Franklin Roosevelt, barely 38 years old, had a bright future. Then disaster struck. On vacation at the family retreat in Nova Scotia in the summer of 1921, he returned from sailing only to succumb to a numbing fatigue. Normally vigorous, he could barely move. Doctors diagnosed the illness as poliomyelitis, a dreaded crippler when it did not kill. It paralyzed Roosevelt from the waist down. Confined to a wheelchair for the rest of his life, he could walk only with the aid of crutches and heavy steel braces.

Roosevelt seemed to emerge from the ordeal with greater patience, deeper conviction, and more empathy for the unfortunates of the world. The disease probably enhanced his appeal to Depression America. When they saw Roosevelt, voters imagined not a spoon-fed aristocrat but a man who had triumphed over personal adversity. In 1928, the year of Al Smith's disastrous presidential race, Roosevelt won the governorship of New York. A progressive like cousin Theodore, he stressed conservation of human as well as physical resources. As governor he pressed for old-age pensions and endorsed unemployment insurance in New York. In the wake of the stock market crash, he was the first governor to provide unemployment relief. Aid to the jobless, said Roosevelt, "must be extended by Government, not as a matter of charity, but as a matter of social duty." In 1931 New York's Temporary Emergency Relief Administration became the first state relief agency.

In the governor's mansion or the White House, Roosevelt was a natural leader. He loved power. "Wouldn't you be President, if you could?" he asked a visitor. "Wouldn't anybody?" He bubbled with enthusiasm. Meeting Franklin Roosevelt, said Winston Churchill, was like "uncorking a bottle of champagne!" His mind was "quick," observed editor William Allen White, but "superficial." Common sense ruled him, and he made no decisions that could be put off. Everything was on a "24-hour basis" so that all his options could be preserved until the last instant. A conventional budget balancer, he could be bold when it came to social reform. He adopted no single ideology. He cared little about political principles. What he wanted were results.

Two traits made Roosevelt a peerless politician—an unshakable faith in himself and the ability to persuade others. Radiating charm, he delighted in manipu-

Most photographers acceded to White House wishes that President Roosevelt never be shot from the waist down. After coming down with polio, Roosevelt helped to transform the ramshackle resort at Warm Springs, Georgia (where this picture was taken), into a treatment center for victims of the disease.

lating those around him. His deep voice and infectious smile were irresistible. And for all his high breeding he never lost the common touch. Roosevelt could take a difficult subject like banking, said humorist Will Rogers, and explain it so that anyone understood it, even bankers. Roosevelt could be ruthless and deceitful (for years he carried on a secret affair with Lucy Mercer Rutherford, his wife's former social secretary); yet he found it nearly impossible to fire anybody. It did not matter, for Roosevelt retained power by scattering it among competing agencies. Only the president had the authority to resolve their differences. "Bring it to Poppa," he told his staff, and time after time they did.

Regularly he reached out to the American people. Almost single-handedly he shifted the locus of newsmaking from New York to Washington. He held an unequaled number of press conferences (998) and became the first president to hire a press secretary. During Roosevelt's administration the United Press wire service tripled its Washington staff. His famous "fireside chats" brought Roosevelt into the homes of his countrymen. "My friends," he said in the first of 16 radio broadcasts, "I want to tell you what has been done in the last few days, why it was done, and what the next steps are going to be." During the campaign he had promised to remember the "forgotten man," and when he spoke Americans felt as if he had each of them in mind. "It was a sacred time," recalled one women of the fireside chats, "as if a father was talking to his children who were afraid."

Roosevelt relied on his wife, more than any president before him had, and Eleanor redefined what it meant to be First Lady. After the inauguration he sent her to visit the second encampment of the Bonus marchers. She ended up leading them in a sing-along. "Hoover sent the army, but Roosevelt sent his wife!" said one of them. Never had a president's wife been so visible. She was the first one to hold weekly press conferences. Her column, "My Day," appeared in 135 newspapers, and her twice-weekly broadcasts made her a radio personality second only to her husband. She became his eyes, ears, and legs, traveling 40,000 miles a year on behalf of the downtrodden. Secret Service men gave her the code name "Rover."

Eleanor claimed modestly that she was nothing more than a "spur" to action. Her husband used her, she said, as he did everyone because she "served his purposes." He served hers as well. She pressed him to hire more women and blacks, supported antilynching and anti–poll tax measures when he would not, and transformed the First Lady's office into a lobby for the underdog. By 1939 public opinion polls showed that more Americans approved of her than of her husband. Her modesty aside, the Democratic Roosevelts formed the most potent political team in American history.

The First Hundred Days

In his first hundred days in office Roosevelt orchestrated the enactment of 15 major pieces of legislation—a record that stood until Lyndon Johnson's Great Society of the 1960s. Congress shaped the programs, but with a sense of urgency and speed rarely seen on Capitol Hill. So rapidly were bills sent from the White House to Congress and back again that even the president confessed to being "a bit shell-shocked." Government began to dominate American economic life so much that conservatives feared the end of capitalism. But Roosevelt's aim was to save capitalism, though that did mean modifying it.

Before the election Roosevelt had gathered a group of economic advisers called the "Brains Trust." Headed by Columbia University professors Raymond

Moley, Rexford G. Tugwell, and Adolf Berle, the Brains Trust disagreed with Hoover's conclusion that the Depression was spawned overseas. Like Roosevelt they saw the Depression as the home-grown product of corporate greed, Republican mismanagement, and a massive failure of consumer purchasing power. Blending progressive New Nationalism with the more recent associationism of the 1920s, the Brains Trusters prescribed a multifaceted program under federal direction: experimentation to achieve recovery, reforms to end abuses and restore confidence, limits on production to boost prices, and centralized economic planning.

The first step toward recovery was saving the banks. When Roosevelt arrived in Washington he already had a draft of new banking legislation in hand. Since the crash 5500 banks had failed. The country's 18,569 banks had only about $6 billion on hand in cash to cover $41 billion in deposits. Even the soundest banks held most of their deposits in mortgages, securities, and other investments, all of which had fallen to a fraction of their former value. More currency was needed. Yet at the very time the Treasury was being called on to expand the money supply investors were squirreling away the gold on which it was based. By the eve of the inauguration governors in 38 states had temporarily closed their banks to stem the tide. Reflecting popular resentment, *Time* magazine coined a new word, "bankster," by combining "banker" with "gangster."

On March 5, the day after the inauguration, Roosevelt issued a decree halting all transactions in gold and proclaiming a four-day bank "holiday." The euphemism snapped the tension of the previous winter. Instead of panicking, Americans responded as if it were a holiday. They devised ingenious ways of conducting business—from using local currencies called "scrip" to bartering services for goods. (One Wisconsin wrestler signed a contract for a can of tomatoes and a peck of potatoes.) Roosevelt called Congress into special session on March 9 and introduced emergency banking legislation to shore up the system. By unanimous shout, the House passed the measure, sight unseen. The Senate, with a handful of dissents, followed later in the day. A haggard Roosevelt signed it that night.

The Emergency Banking Act was scarcely a radical measure. Instead of nationalizing banks it simply extended federal assistance to them. Sound banks would be reopened immediately with government support; troubled banks would be handed over to federal "conservators," who would help reorganize their assets. Federal loans would be available to keep them afloat. On Sunday, March 12, Roosevelt explained what was happening in the first of his fireside chats. Half the people in America had radios; nearly one in three tuned in. In calm, uncluttered language the president reassured the public that the banks were safe again. The next day deposits exceeded withdrawals, and two days later the stock market had its largest one-day increase in history. "Capitalism was saved in eight days," said one Roosevelt adviser.

Other financial measures buoyed public confidence in government and the economy. On March 10 Roosevelt requested sweeping powers to cut the federal budget by $400 million in veterans' payments and $100 million in salaries. Congress passed the Economy Act after only two days' debate. Later that spring a second Glass–Steagall Banking Act separated investment from commercial banking to limit speculation by bankers. Tucked into the statute was one of the most important achievements of the New Deal: federal insurance of bank deposits. Roosevelt opposed it on the grounds that it would underwrite weak banks, but Congress enacted it anyway. Soon the Federal Deposit Insurance Corporation was guaranteeing bank deposits up to $2500. Fewer banks failed during the rest of the decade than in the best year of the twenties. To clean up Wall Street, the Securities Act of 1933 reduced the advantage of insiders by requiring advance disclosure of information about new stocks. In 1934 the Securities Exchange Act established a new federal agency, the Securities and Exchange Commission, to police the stock market. Stricter regulation of banking and investment laid the groundwork for recovery.

The relief of human suffering was a second goal of the first hundred days. Middle-class Americans were a primary target. In 1932 a quarter of a million families lost their homes. During the first half of 1933 more than 1000 homes were foreclosed every day. The Home Owners' Loan Act helped one out of every five homeowners refinance their mortgages. To keep people from starving until recovery took hold, Congress created the Federal Emergency Relief Administration (FERA) in May 1933. Sitting amid unpacked boxes, gulping coffee and chain-smoking, former social worker Harry Hopkins began disbursing its $500 million appropriation as if, said a colleague, he were "turning on a fireplug." Hopkins spent $5 million in his first two hours on the job. To avoid charges of "federal dictatorship," the money came in matching grants to states, which then administered them as a dole, or giveaway program. In its two-year existence, FERA furnished over $1 billion in direct assistance to states, localities, and private charities. The system had its flaws. It left critical decisions over eligibility and dispersal in local hands, where local prejudices sometimes ruled. Poorer states, able to put up less, received less.

Like Hoover, Roosevelt feared that any public assistance might become a "narcotic," but he recognized the need for temporary aid in the depths of the Depression. Of the two possibilities he preferred work relief to cash allotments. Giving a person a job in exchange for a paycheck "preserves a man's morale," Hopkins explained. "It saves his skill. It gives him a chance to do something socially useful." As the winter of 1933–1934 approached, Hopkins persuaded Roosevelt to expand relief with a program to tide the unemployed over the chilly season. The Civil Works Administration (CWA) gave jobs, some of them useful, others makeshift and shoddy, to some 4 million Americans. Wages averaged $15 a week, hardly adequate but more than twice FERA payments. The work itself was as important as the money. "When I got that [CWA identification] card it was the biggest day of my whole life," an unemployed insurance man told Lorena Hickok. "At last I could say, 'I've got a job.'" Alarmed at the high cost of the program, Roosevelt disbanded the CWA in the spring of 1934. For the next year and a half, the FERA remained the principal source of public aid.

Another work relief program established during the hundred days proved to be more creative. The Civilian Conservation Corps (CCC) was Roosevelt's pet project, combining his concern for conservation with a compassion for youth. The CCC took unmarried 18- to 25-year-olds from relief rolls and sent them into the woods and fields of America. They protected and restored forests, beaches, rivers, and parks at wages of $1 a day. During its 10-year lifetime, the CCC provided 2.5 million jobs, all of them for men (which prompted some critics to chant, "Where's the she, she, she?").

The cause of conservation received a more powerful boost in May 1933, when Roosevelt signed an act creating the Tennessee Valley Authority (TVA). Long a dream of Nebraska senator George Norris, this experiment in regional development and social engineering aimed at transforming one of the poorest regions of the country. The TVA, still functioning today, began with the construction of a series of dams in seven states on the Tennessee River to control flooding, improve navigation, and generate cheap electric power. Soon, for the first time, thousands of rural families could flip a switch to get light or turn a knob to hear the latest news on the radio. TVA-generated electricity also served as a "yardstick" for measuring the prices of private utilities. In an effort to encourage "grassroots democracy," the TVA cooperated with state and local officials in social programs, from controlling malaria to furnishing library bookmobiles and constructing recreational lakes. Like many New Deal programs, the TVA has a mixed legacy. It saved 3 million acres from erosion, multiplied the average income in the valley tenfold, and repaid its original investment in federal taxes. It also pushed thousands of families from their land and became one of the worst polluters in the country.

The Riddle of Recovery

After years of Hoover paralysis, Roosevelt's first hundred days finally broke national despair. The economic depression proved more resistant. Though Roosevelt regarded recovery as his primary goal, the New Deal never reached it. Conditions did improve, but the Depression persisted. As late as 1939 industrial production had yet to reach 1929 levels. Nearly 10 million Americans walked the streets in search of work, and displaced farm families still huddled around campfires on western highways. Perhaps no one could have solved the riddle of recovery, but Roosevelt tried.

At first the president experimented with quick monetary fixes. In 1933 he took the nation off the gold standard by prohibiting banks from redeeming currency in gold coin and outlawing the export of gold. Then he reduced the value of the dollar by buying gold on the open market. Devaluation, he hoped, would make American goods cheaper for foreign buyers and raise commodity prices at home. By November 1934 the program had failed. Yielding to pressure from western farmers and miners, he began buying silver to inflate the currency and raise prices. This scheme also ended in failure. Investment, not artificially inflated prices, was the key to recovery.

In June 1933 Roosevelt launched a two-pronged attack on the many ills of industry: sagging prices and purchasing power, overproduction, "cut-throat" competition, unemployment, and declining wages. The National Industrial Recovery Act created two new agencies, the Public Works Administration (PWA) and the National Recovery Administration (NRA). Originally designed to work in tandem, they soon went separate ways. Harold Ickes, the irascible secretary of the interior, took over the PWA. Its purpose was to prime the economic pump by stimulating heavy industry and providing jobs with $3.3 billion in public works. Fearing waste and corruption, "Honest Harold" oversaw each project personally. He spent money so slowly that the PWA never achieved its goal. But it did make spectacular additions to the national inventory of public structures, including the Triborough Bridge and Lincoln Tunnel in New York, the port city of Brownsville in Texas, and the aircraft carriers *Yorktown* and *Enterprise*.

The National Recovery Administration took on the gargantuan tasks of maintaining prices, wages, and employment while controlling production and competi-

An NRA blue eagle decal.

THE TENNESSEE VALLEY AUTHORITY

The Tennessee River basin encompassed parts of seven states. Rivers honeycombed the area, which received some of the heaviest rainfall in the nation. A long-time dream of Senator George Norris, the Tennessee Valley Authority, created in 1933, constructed some twenty dams and improved five others over the next twenty years to control chronic flooding and erosion and to produce cheap hydroelectric power and fertilizers.

tion. Building on Hoover initiatives in the associational movement, Roosevelt cast the NRA as "a partnership in planning" between government and industry. NRA administrator Hugh Johnson had his doubts about chances for success: "This is just like mounting the guillotine on the infinitesimal gamble that the ax won't work." Johnson, a rough-hewn veteran of the cavalry, had served with the War Industries Board during World War I. He hoped to rekindle the wartime spirit of unity by calling on businessmen, laborers, and consumers to cooperate again.

Under the watchful eye of government, industries developed "codes of fair practices" to limit production, divide it among the various companies, and stabilize prices. In return government suspended antitrust laws to allow for business cooperation. Each code also promised labor improved working conditions, outlawing such practices as child labor and sweatshops. Section 7a of the original legislation, modeled on the War Labor Board, further protected workers by guaranteeing union rights to bargain with management and requiring codes to set minimum wages and maximum hours. To guard their interests consumers were promised a voice in making and administering codes.

Eventually more than 600 codes governed industries ranging from major ones like steel, oil, and construction to minor ones such as horse hair dressing and the

manufacture of shoulder pads. No business was forced to comply. Instead Johnson, a superb showman, relied on voluntary participation, promoted through patriotic campaigns. Casting about for a symbol of compliance, he hit on a blue eagle
with the legend "We Do Our Part." Soon Blue Eagle decals appeared all over the
country—in storefronts, in factories, even on the backs of chorus girls' costumes.
On the Boston Common Mayor James Curley led 100,000 children in a pledge to
"buy only where the Blue Eagle flies." For 10 hours New Yorkers watched a
quarter of a million people march down Fifth Avenue for the Blue Eagle. More
than 2 million employers pledged to abide by the codes.

The NRA leavened national spirits but failed to bring about recovery. Big
businesses dominated code-making. To guarantee profits they restricted production and raised prices, usually enough to cover forced increases in wages. "This
was scarcity economics," wrote one historian, "and it meant reduced purchasing
power." Businesses could survive, but without increasing production there would
be no incentive for expansion and new investment. Under such conditions hard
times could last indefinitely.

Disillusioned, owners of smaller businesses refused to comply with the codes.
Even participating firms found ways to avoid labor reforms and wage increases.
Company-sponsored unions competed with independent unions; collective bargaining often became a sham. Labor leaders began to refer to the NRA as the
"National Run Around." Consumers, promised representation in the NRA, had no
real power. Soon they started complaining about "NRA prices and Hoover
wages." On May 27, 1935, in *Schecter Poultry Corp. v. United States*, the Supreme Court struck down the NRA. The justices unanimously ruled that the NRA
exceeded federal power over interstate commerce and that its codes represented
"an unconstitutional delegation of legislative power" to an executive agency. Publicly distressed over the grounds of the decision, Roosevelt was privately relieved
to be rid of this "awful headache."

New Deal efforts to revive agriculture turned out better. Agriculture secretary Henry A. Wallace planned to increase farm prices by attacking the age-old
problem of overproduction. Under the Agricultural Adjustment Act of 1933 farmers would be paid for *not* planting crops. A tax on processors—millers, cotton
ginners, and the like—would finance the government subsidies under this program of "domestic allotments." In theory surpluses would be reduced, commodity
prices would rise, and agriculture would recover. In practice the Agricultural
Adjustment Administration (AAA) did help to increase prices of the seven major
commodities it covered: cotton, corn, tobacco, rice, wheat, hogs, and dairy products. For the first time in more than a decade farm income grew (from $5.5 billion
in 1932 to $8.7 billion in 1935). The Commodity Credit Corporation extended
loans on crops kept in storage, a revival of the Populists' old subtreasury plan (see
page 775). Loans were pegged slightly higher than market value as an additional
spur to prices.

Not all of the gains were attributable to government. In 1934 and 1935 dust
storms, droughts, and floods, particularly in the Great Plains and in the South,
helped to reduce harvests and boost prices. The AAA, moreover, failed to distribute its benefits equally. Like the NRA, the AAA favored big producers. To preserve democratic procedure, Roosevelt insisted that the program be voluntary and
that local farmers themselves choose the plots to be left fallow. Large farmers
controlled decision-making. In the South this frequently meant cutting the acreage of tenants and sharecroppers or forcing them from the land. Even when they
reduced their own acreage, large farmers often increased yields since they had the

money and equipment to cultivate more intensively. The New Deal stabilized the farm economy and set the pattern of future farm programs, but it also accelerated the trend toward large-scale, corporate "agribusiness."

In 1936 the Supreme Court declared the processing tax of the AAA unconstitutional in *Butler v. U.S.* A hastily drawn replacement, the Soil Conservation and Domestic Allotment Act of 1936, subsidized farmers for practicing "conservation" but paid them from general revenues instead of a special tax on processors. Farmers received benefit payments for taking soil-depleting staples off the land, thereby achieving reduction indirectly. Agents from the new Soil Conservation Service were so successful in educating farmers about scientific land use that production still increased. A second Agricultural Adjustment Act in 1938 returned production quotas.

Other agencies tried to help impoverished farmers. The Farm Credit Administration refinanced about a fifth of all farm mortgages. In 1935 the Resettlement Administration gave marginal farmers a fresh start by moving them to better land, and beginning in 1937 the Farm Security Administration furnished low-interest, long-term loans to help tenants buy family-size farms. In neither case did the rural poor have much political clout, and appropriations from Congress were never enough. In the end fewer than 5000 families (of a projected 500,000) were resettled, and less than 2 percent of tenant farmers got loans.

A SECOND NEW DEAL (1935–1936)

The early New Deal had tried to satisfy as many people as possible. Without a clear following, Roosevelt had catered to a variety of interests, acting as a broker who responded first to one group, then to another. The result was a makeshift concoction of "alphabet agencies." Organized groups—bankers, large farmers, big businesses—benefited most; unorganized groups— sharecroppers, tenants, the downtrodden—scarcely at all. Yet the focus remained broad, and all the activity, even when it was contradictory, had rekindled hope. In 1934 voters gave the Democrats an unprecedented endorsement by strengthening their majorities in Congress and handing them all but seven governorships. Never before had a party in power increased its popular vote in an off-year election. The "broker state," as it came to be called, made for good politics, whatever its economic shortcomings.

In 1935 politics helped to shift the course of the New Deal. Pressed by the persistence of unemployment and depression, worried about the 1936 presidential election, and stung by the hostility of many businesses, Roosevelt began to respond to calls for deeper change. Neither a radical nor a conservative, he moved in the direction he always wanted to go, "slightly to the left of center." A "second New Deal" emerged. It abandoned the partnership with business, addressed more directly the needs of the dispossessed, and stressed liberal reform. Even more than the early New Deal, this second New Deal brought the federal government into the lives of ordinary Americans.

Voices of Protest

"The revolutionary spirit burgeons," wrote historian William Leuchtenburg, "not when conditions are at their worst but as they begin to improve." The early successes of the New Deal invigorated its critics as well as its friends. One April day in 1934 a mob of 6000 stormed the Minneapolis city hall, tossing sticks, stones, and lumps of coal through the windows during a meeting of the city council. The rioters demanded government work at a living wage and greater relief. That summer in San Francisco longshoremen walked off the job and ignited a general strike that paralyzed the city. In the fall 1000 relief workers in Denver struck, infuriated by a cut in relief payments. All told, 1.5 million workers took part in some 1800 strikes in 1934. Conditions were improving but not quickly enough. Across the country voices of protest gathered strength.

A few angry voices came from the right, as businessmen accused Roosevelt of favoring labor and farmers. Some charged him with amassing enough power to become an American Hitler. The embattled rich were most nervous of all. "Five Negroes on my place in South Carolina refused work this Spring . . . saying they had easy jobs with the government," reported a retired Du Pont executive. Moved by his predicament, a group of corporate leaders and conservative Democrats founded the American Liberty League in August 1934 to protect the rights of property and the people who held most of it. Despite spending over $1 million in publicity, the League inflicted no serious wounds on Roosevelt or the New Deal. Few considered the plight of the wealthy a problem.

Louder voices came from the left. In Minnesota, Governor Floyd B. Olson of the Farmer–Labor party demanded more aid for farmers and workers. "I hope," he said in 1932, "that the present system of government goes right down to Hell." By 1934 he was calling himself a "radical" and soon toying with a third-party presidential campaign for 1936. In California discontented voters took over the Democratic party and nominated novelist Upton Sinclair, a Socialist, for the governorship. Running under the slogan "End Poverty in California" (EPIC), Sinclair proposed the distribution of surpluses through a production-for-use plan. Under his administration the state would confiscate idle factories and land and permit the unemployed to work for their own benefit. Republicans, anxious about the threat to private property, mounted a devastating counterattack. Hollywood tycoons contributed fake newsreels depicting Sinclair as a Bolshevik, atheist, and free-lover. Sinclair lost the election but won nearly 1 million votes.

Huey P. Long represented a greater threat. The flamboyant senator from Louisiana had ridden to power on a wave of rural discontent. Born on a family farm in the Louisiana hill country, Long was reared on the rhetoric of radical Populism. "There wants to be a revolution," his father once told him. Huey decided to make one happen by redistributing wealth in America. Comical and ruthless, he called himself the "Kingfish" (after a character in the popular "Amos 'n' Andy" radio show) and promised to make "every man a king" by "sharing our wealth." His plan was simple: the government would limit the size of all fortunes and incomes so that every family could be given an estate of $5000, enough to buy a house, an automobile, and a radio. There would be a guaranteed annual income of $2500. The young would get scholarships, the old pensions. By 1935, one year after its founding, the Share Our Wealth organization boasted 27,000 clubs and files containing nearly 8 million names.

Louisiana Governor and Senator Huey Long promised to make "every man a king," but critics predicted that only Long would wear the crown. Power-hungry and charismatic, the "Kingfish" made no secret of his presidential aspirations.

In the early years of the Depression, demonstrations of the unemployed, some organized by Communists and other radicals, broke out all over the country. On March 6, 1930, a Communist-led protest at Union Square in New York turned into an ugly riot. In 1935 Communist parties, under orders from Moscow, adopted the more cooperative strategy of allying with democratic and socialist groups against facism, proclaiming in the United States that "Communism is twentieth century Americanism."

Despite his gross underestimates of what it would take to subsidize the have-nots, Long was addressing a real problem, the uneven distribution of wealth in America. As governor of Louisiana (some called him "dictator"), he had attacked wealthy corporations, built bridges and roads in the poorest sections of the state, and given free schoolbooks to children, black and white alike. So when Long told the Louisiana legislature which bills to enact, when his private police force kidnaped political opponents, when he feathered his own financial nest, the downtrodden of Louisiana looked the other way. Democratic National Committee members shuddered at polls showing that the Kingfish might capture 3 million to 4 million votes in 1936, enough to put a Republican in the White House. The Kingfish himself might even make it there in 1940. But late in 1935, as he strode through the corridors of the Louisiana capitol, Long was shot to death by a disgruntled constituent whose father-in-law had been wronged by the Long political machine.

Father Charles Coughlin was Long's urban counterpart. As urban middle- and working-class people slipped into poverty, the Detroit "Radio Priest" grew in popularity. In weekly broadcasts from the Shrine of the Little Flower he offered bewildered followers—mainly ethnic Catholics from the lower middle class of the urban North—a simple explanation for their plight. A conspiracy of international bankers had toppled the world economy by manipulating currencies based on gold.

Like Long, Coughlin also touched on a real problem, the inadequate supply of money. And like the Kingfish, Coughlin exploited rather than solved it. He promised to end the Depression by such simple strokes as nationalizing banks, spreading work, and using silver to inflate the currency. (None would have

987

worked, since they would have dampened investment, one key to recovery.) Drawing on old Populist suspicions of eastern bankers and later spewing an ugly anti-Semitism, his radio sermons were soon drawing 30 million to 40 million listeners, the largest audiences in the world. At first Coughlin supported the New Deal, but when the president refused to adopt his schemes, he broke with the administration and Franklin "Double-Crossing" Roosevelt. In 1934 he created the National Union for Social Justice to rally his supporters. As the election of 1936 approached, it loomed as an ominous specter on the political horizon.

A more kindly challenge came from Dr. Francis Townsend, a 67-year-old physician who had retired from the public health service. One morning he looked out of his bathroom window to see three old women scavenging for food in an alley. Across the country aged Americans on shrinking incomes faced unemployment and illness without pension plans or medical insurance. Townsend vowed to bring their humiliation and suffering to an end. In 1934 he set up Old Age Revolving Pensions, Limited, to promote his plan for furnishing aid to the elderly and at the same time promoting recovery. Townsend proposed to pay citizens 60 years or older $200 a month provided they quit their jobs, surrender all other income, and spend the money within 30 days. The program would be financed by a 2 percent tax on commercial transactions.

As much as the elderly needed assistance, the Townsend plan was economic hokum. Townsendites expected to spend over half the national income to compensate less than one-tenth of the population. The plan would create no new jobs, and its 2 percent sales tax would fall on everyone, including impoverished American consumers. Yet the allure of the Townsend movement was undeniable. In 1935 almost 9 in 10 Americans believed that some form of government old-age pensions was necessary. By 1936 Townsend clubs counted 3.5 million members, most of them small businessmen and farmers at or beyond retirement age. The clubs gave them more than hope for added income: they provided a place where the elderly could socialize with people their own age, who saw things as they did, who believed they could save the economy and return the nation to old truths. Members brought Bibles to Townsend club meetings, sang hymns, and harrangued against alcohol, necking, wild youth, and big-city ways. Most of all they believed in Townsend and his plan. Under his leadership, the elderly became a new force in politics.

The Second Hundred Days

Reporting on the state of the Union to the new Congress in January 1935, the president struck a moderate tone as he looked to the coming year, "a genuine period of good feeling, sustained by a sense of purposeful progress." Even as he spoke, the forces of discontent—from businessmen on the right to demagogues on the left—were pushing him to bolder action, and so was Congress. Democrats, who controlled more than two-thirds of both houses, were prepared to outspend Roosevelt in extending the New Deal to more of their constituents. His advisers were pushing too. "Boys—this is our hour," crowed Harry Hopkins. "We've got to get everything we want—a works program, social security, wages and hours, everything—now or never." The result was a new flurry of legislation in 1935— "the second hundred days"—stressing longer term relief and more sweeping reform.

To ease the plight of the jobless Roosevelt first proposed a massive program of work relief. Despite a decline of 2 million from the ranks of the unemployed, millions more remained jobless at the end of 1934. "The forgotten man is still forgotten," a Pennsylvania worker wrote to Eleanor Roosevelt in 1935. In April 1935 Congress enacted the Emergency Relief Appropriation Act. Its $4.8 billion allocation (the largest to date in peacetime) was designed to put people to work. Some of the money went to the new National Youth Administration (NYA). It gave part-time employment to more than 4.5 million young people, almost half of them students. The Public Works Administration and the Civilian Conservation Corps also received funds, but the largest share went to the new Works Progress Administration (WPA) with super-relief administrator Hopkins at the helm.

Since the WPA aimed at disbursing most of its money in wages, its projects were usually of the pick-and-shovel variety. Constrained by rules against competing with private industry, WPA workers were sometimes forced into "boondoggles" like raking leaves or digging and filling holes. Critics called the program "We Piddle Around," yet Hopkins showed remarkable ingenuity in finding useful work. The WPA built or improved 20,000 hospitals, schools, airports, and playgrounds. WPA workers taught art classes to the mentally disturbed in a Cincinnati hospital; drafted a Braille map for the blind in Watertown, Massachusetts; and rode a packhorse pulling a library through the hills of Kentucky. Though pay averaged only $55 a month (barely half the annual subsistence level), 80 percent of the WPA budget went to wages. In 1935 alone, the agency employed over 3 million people, and before it was ended in 1943, it gave work to over 8.5 million. The WPA was a bold experiment, but it never reached Roosevelt's goal of giving jobs to all who could work.

The Social Security Act (1935) was intended to help the aged, infirm, and other "forgotten" men and women. Roosevelt favored what he called a "cradle-to-grave" system, an all-embracing social insurance program. Reflecting the limits of political feasibility, the Social Security Act was something less. It created a national system of old-age insurance funded by payroll taxes on employers and workers; state and federal funds for the care of the destitute over the age of 65; a federal–state system of unemployment insurance; and national aid to the states, on a matching basis, for care of dependent mothers and children, the crippled, and the blind, and for public health services.

For all its coverage, Social Security had defects. Compared to social insurance in Europe, the program was conservative and skimpy. Pension payments were not scheduled to begin until 1942 and would be no more than $10 to $85 a month, with subsidies to dependent children and the handicapped usually averaging less—and all inadequate even by Depression standards. Contrary to Roosevelt's wishes, Social Security also failed to cover everyone. To win the votes of southerners worried about its effect on race relations, the legislation excluded farmers and domestic servants, doubtless the neediest but often black. The payroll tax was another problem. It took money from workers and thereby reduced demand for goods at a time when mass purchasing power was already too low. Roosevelt had nonetheless insisted on the tax. Bad economics again made good politics, since retiring citizens would have a right to pensions because they had paid for them. "With those taxes in there," Roosevelt slyly observed, "no damn politician can ever scrap my social security program."

Social Security marked a historic reversal. The gospel of self-help was counterbalanced by a new social contract, however narrow. For the first time the federal government acknowledged the social rights of citizens and its responsibility to protect them. The welfare state, foreshadowed in the temporary relief measures of the early New Deal, was made permanent.

Congress may not have gone as far as Roosevelt wished on Social Security, but its labor legislation pushed him beyond his natural limits. A symbolic father to so many of his countrymen, Roosevelt regarded labor with similar paternalism. He wanted things done for workers, not by them. He had chosen a social worker, Frances Perkins, rather than a labor leader as secretary of labor. She agreed that enactment of Social Security, along with provisions for maximum hours and minimum wages, was what the New Deal needed to do for working men and women.

Robert F. Wagner, the liberal senator from New York, believed such government paternalism was not enough. The son of a janitor, Wagner was the strongest friend of labor in Congress. He wanted workers to be able to fight their own battles. In 1933 he pressed for the inclusion of Section 7a in the NRA to protect the rights of labor to organize and bargain collectively. When the agency was invalidated by the Supreme Court, Wagner sought to protect organized labor directly. Enacted in the summer of 1935 (with only the belated blessings of the president), the National Labor Relations Act, known as the "Wagner Act," created a National Labor Relations Board to supervise elections in plants and factories where workers wanted to organize. Once workers decided to join a union and selected their representatives by secret ballot, management had to negotiate with them. No company could engage in "unfair labor practices" such as firing employees for union activity or fostering company-controlled unions. The Wagner Act forced unions on no one but did guarantee the right of workers to band together and bargain collectively. It was, said admirers, "labor's Magna Carta." By 1941 the number of unionized workers had doubled.

Roosevelt responded to growing business hostility by turning openly against the wealthy and powerful. The Banking Act of 1935 centralized control of the money market in the Federal Reserve Board. By coordinated manipulation of interest rates and money supply government could influence the economy more than ever. The nation's financial capital moved from Wall Street to Washington. The Public Utilities Holding Company Act (1935) ordered the breakup of utility empires, long the target of progressive reformers. The giant holding companies produced nothing but inflated profits for speculators and high prices for consumers. Roosevelt wanted to dissolve them. The legislation, weakened by the powerful utilities lobby, ended up limiting their size. The Revenue Act of 1935 (called the "Wealth Tax Act") threatened to "soak the rich" but in the end brought only moderate taxes on high incomes and inheritances. Diluted like the holding company act, it was still a political victory for New Dealers, though mostly a symbolic one. "I am now on your bandwagon again, having slipped off," a Philadelphian told the president.

The second hundred days, like the first, wrought no fundamental changes in American life. The country was still capitalist, still democratic, still opposed to extremism. But there had been important shifts. Orthodox but practical, Roosevelt moved slowly to the left, in part to ward off the challenges of Long, Coughlin, and Townsend, in part to catch up with his own constituents. The price was business hostility, which surely inhibited recovery. As his partnership with business ended, he directed innovations more toward reform than the constant goal of recovery. No longer seeking to please everyone, Roosevelt turned to his natural allies, the down-and-out, the working and middle classes, liberal reformers, and rank-and-file Democrats. In 1935 his motives had been a mixture of instinctive decency and cold-blooded politics. His success would be measured in the election of 1936.

The Election of 1936

A June rain drenched the crowd of over 100,000 packed into the Franklin Field stadium in Philadelphia. No one minded. Loyal Democrats, they were there to see the president accept his nomination for a second term. As Roosevelt moved stiff-legged up the ramp, he reached down to shake the hand of a friend and suddenly pitched forward, falling to the ground. "Clean me up!" he snapped, his famous composure momentarily broken. Seconds later the curtain hiding the stage parted, and the president, now calm and unsoiled, flashed a smile at the cheering throng. "This generation of Americans," he told them, "has a rendezvous with destiny." It was a virtuoso performance because Roosevelt expected the coming election to turn on a single issue. "It's myself," he told one staffer, "and people must be either for me or against me."

The Republicans nominated Alfred M. "Alf" Landon of Kansas, the only Republican governor elected in 1932 who still survived in office. A former Bull Moose Progressive, Landon favored the regulation of business, the preservation of civil liberties, and several New Deal measures. Republicans outspent Democrats $14 million to $9 million in one of the first big-money advertising campaigns that would mark later presidential races. Yet despite his bulging war chest, Landon lacked luster as well as issues. Even his theme song (the old Oregon Trail ballad "Oh, Susanna") was out of tune with an electorate uninterested in reviving a bygone era. Landon and his running mate, Chicago publisher Frank Knox, were reduced to rebutting the New Deal with promises of retrenchment, a balanced budget, and a return to the gold standard.

Roosevelt ignored his opponents. He even ignored his own party. Instead he depicted himself as the leader of a great liberal crusade that knew no partisan lines. He turned the election into a contest between haves and have-nots. His most blistering attacks were launched at big business, already lost to him. The forces of "organized money are unanimous in their hate for me," he told a roaring crowd at New York's Madison Square Garden, "and I welcome their hatred." When the wealthy returned fire at Liberty League confabs and Chamber of Com-

THE ELECTION OF 1936

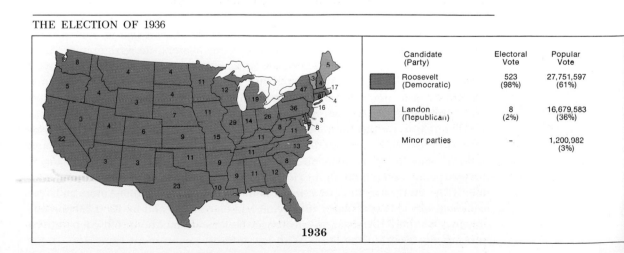

Candidate (Party)	Electoral Vote	Popular Vote
Roosevelt (Democratic)	523 (98%)	27,751,597 (61%)
Landon (Republican)	8 (2%)	16,679,583 (36%)
Minor parties	–	1,200,982 (3%)

1936

merce dinners, they only strengthened Roosevelt's hand. "At last we have a Man in the White House," wrote an Oregon woman, "and not a puppet of organized Wealth."

The strategy deflated the Republicans, discredited the right, and coopted the newly formed Union Party of Townsendites, Coughlinites, and the remnants of Huey Long's movement. The returns shocked even experienced political observers. Roosevelt won the largest electoral victory ever recorded—523 to 8. He received a whopping 60.8 percent of the popular vote and beat Landon by over 11 million votes. The Republican challenger won only two states, Maine and Vermont. "If Landon had given one more speech," quipped veteran reporter Dorothy Thompson, "Roosevelt would have carried Canada, too." Union party candidate William "Liberty Bill" Lemke of North Dakota polled only 882,000 votes; Socialist Norman Thomas recorded just 187,000. After the election, Father Coughlin, recalling the persecution of Christ, announced his retirement from politics.

Roosevelt's margin of victory came from those near the bottom of the economic ladder. Approximately 6 million more people cast ballots in 1936 than in 1932; 5 million of them voted for Roosevelt. Most were members of the poor and working classes expressing their support for the New Deal. More than 8 out of 10 trade union members, unskilled workers, and relief recipients voted for Roosevelt. Class replaced region as the dominant element in American politics.

A dramatic realignment took place, as important as the Republican rise to power in 1896. The Democrats reigned as the new majority party for the next 30 years. The "Roosevelt coalition" rested on three main pillars: traditional Democratic support in the South; the big cities, particularly ethnics and African-Americans; and labor, both organized and unorganized. The minority Republicans became the party of big business and small towns.

THE NEW DEAL AND THE AMERICAN PEOPLE

The lights did not go on in the Hill Country of Texas until 1939. Before then, local farmers read books after dusk and milked cows before dawn by the light of 25-watt kerosene lamps. Hill Country wives washed eight loads of laundry a week, all by hand. They hauled 200 gallons of water a day from wells and heated seven-pound "sadirons" on wood-burning stoves to press clothing. Farms had no milking machines, no washers, no automatic pumps or water heaters, no refrigerators. After sundown people could barely see each other. While other Americans enjoyed evenings listening to Jack Benny and the Lone Ranger on radio, Hill Country farmers sat in a silence broken only by their own voices. "Living—just living—was a problem," recalled one woman.

The reason for this limited life was simple: the Hill Country had no electricity. Utility companies resisted electrifying rural America because more money could be made in cities. Thus no agency of the Roosevelt administration changed the way people lived more dramatically than the Rural Electrification Administration (REA), created in 1935, at a time when less than 10 percent of American farms had electricity. Six years later 40 percent had electricity, and by 1950, 90 percent did. In 1935 the REA began to encourage the formation of nonprofit cooperatives to bring electricity to the farm. With low-interest government loans, the co-ops strung thousands of miles of power lines into the countryside. In the Smoky Mountains, along the Upper Peninsula of Michigan, on the slopes of the Continental Divide, and in the Hill Country of central Texas, communities saw their churches, stores, schools, and homes set aglow with a dazzling new light. Electric machines eased the drudgery of rural people; radios cut their isolation; light bulbs reduced the strain on their eyes and even improved the school grades of their children, who could now study at night. The New Deal did not always have such a marked impact; its overall record was mixed. But time and again it changed the lives of ordinary people as government never had before.

Outsiders Under the New Deal

In 1932 most African-Americans voted as they had since Reconstruction—for Republicans, the party of Abraham Lincoln and emancipation. But disenchantment with decades of broken promises of equality was spreading. "Go turn Lincoln's picture to the wall," publisher Robert Vann of the Pittsburgh *Courier* told black readers. "That debt has been paid in full." Not only did African-Americans turn Lincoln's picture to the wall; they replaced it with Roosevelt's. By 1934 they were voting for Democrats, and in 1936 they mounted a full-blown revolution in politics. "Let Jesus lead you and Roosevelt feed you," a black preacher told his congregation on the eve of the election. Three of four black voters cast their ballots for Roosevelt in 1936. By 1938 nearly 85 percent of black respondents in one poll counted themselves as Roosevelt Democrats.

The New Deal accounted for the dramatic change. Roosevelt's indifferent record on civil rights as governor of New York gave way to greater concern once he entered the White House. Never an open advocate of complete equality, he regarded African-Americans as one of many groups whose interests he brokered. Even that was an improvement over his predecessors. The federal government had been racially segregated since the days of Woodrow Wilson, and in the late 1920s black leaders referred to Hoover as "the man in the lily-White House."

Under Roosevelt government began once again to be racially integrated. Passionate partisans of civil rights like Eleanor Roosevelt and Secretary of the Interior Harold Ickes brought blacks into the administration. Political scientist Clark Foreman and economist Robert C. Weaver became advisers on racial affairs and later on black economic problems. Mary McLeod Bethune, who had risen from a sharecropper's shack to found Bethune–Cookman College, ran a division of the National Youth Administration. In May 1935, as the second New Deal began, Roosevelt issued Executive Order 7046 banning discrimination in the new Works Progress Administration.

African-Americans also pressed for such changes. Important as both symbols and contributers, black administrators formed the "Black Cabinet" to help shape federal policy. Outside of government the Urban League continued to lobby for economic advancement, and the NAACP drafted legislation to make lynching a federal crime. (Though publicly against lynching and privately in favor of the bill, Roosevelt refused to make the outlawing of lynching "must" legislation. He feared losing the support of southern congressmen he needed "to save America.") When NRA wage differentials ended up reducing the salaries of black workers in the

Mary McLeod Bethune.

South or NRA codes resulted the loss of their jobs to whites, black newspapers were quick to rename the agency "Negroes Ruined Again." In New York's Harlem the Reverend John H. Johnson organized the Citizens' League for Fair Play in 1933 to persuade white merchants to hire black clerks. After picketers blocked storefronts, hundreds of African-Americans got jobs with Harlem retailers and utility companies. Racial tension over employment and housing continued to run high, and in 1935 Harlem exploded in the only race riot of the decade.

Discrimination persisted under the New Deal. Government efforts to promote "grassroots democracy" often gave control of federal programs to localities, where prejudice produced inequalities. Relief payments to black clients in Atlanta, Georgia, averaged $19.29 a month; whites received $32.66. When local farm committees decided to retire acreage under the AAA, black sharecroppers and tenants were often the ones put out of production. New Deal showplaces like the TVA's model town of Norris, Tennessee, and the subsistence homestead village of Arthurdale, West Virginia, were closed entirely to blacks. Officials feared integration would promote trouble in these communal paradises.

African-Americans did benefit from the New Deal, but more as dispossessed citizens than as a disadvantaged race. The federally run WPA, whose employment practices were based on need, hired blacks for almost 20 percent of its jobs, even though they comprised less than 10 percent of the population. The minimum WPA wage of $12 a week was twice what many of them had earned before. Public Works Administrator Ickes established the first quota system for hiring blacks (based on their percentage of the local work force). By 1941 the number of African-Americans working for the government exceeded their percentage of the population.

Training programs, including Mary McLeod Bethune's enormously successful Office of Minority Affairs, helped to reduce black illiteracy from 16.4 percent to 11.5 percent by the end of the decade. Life expectancy jumped from 49 to 55 years for black women and from 47 to 52 years for black men in the 1930s. (Among whites it rose from 63 to 67 for women and from 60 to 62 for men.) Countless blacks shared the sentiments of a Washington cab driver who explained that he had voted for Roosevelt and the Democrats because they "favor the little man, and I've been a little man all my life."

The nearly 1 million Mexican-Americans in the United States received little assistance from the New Deal. Hispanic culture sometimes impeded relief efforts. The Mexican folk tradition of self-help inhibited some from seeking aid, while others remained unfamiliar with claim procedures. Still others failed to meet residency requirements. Low voter turnout and a high proportion of aliens among Mexican-Americans reduced their political power and the attention paid to their interests. Uneducated and unskilled, they often toiled as migrant farm workers outside the reach of many New Deal programs, including Social Security.

Throughout the Southwest and California, the Civilian Conservation Corps and the Works Progress Administration did help with jobs on the land and in construction. On Capitol Hill Dennis Chavez of New Mexico, the only United States senator of Hispanic descent, succeeded in channeling relief and other federal funds into Spanish-speaking communities. During the decade Hispanics, like blacks, were mired in poverty but developed enough faith in Roosevelt to switch from the Republican to the Democratic party.

After decades of neglect Indians found themselves the subjects of new federal interest. Indian families on reservations rarely earned more than $100 a year.

Their infant mortality rate was the highest in the country; their life expectancy the shortest; their education—usually no more than five years—the lowest. Their rate of unemployment was three times the national average. The Dawes Severalty Act of 1887 had sought to make Indians independent landowners, but poverty forced many to sell their federal allotments to white farmers and ranchers. By the 1930s Indian landholding had shrunk from 138 million to 48 million acres, most of it desert.

Commissioner of Indian Affairs John Collier, a social worker who had long fought for Indian rights, reversed the trend by acquiring land for Indians through federal and state grants. Indian Bureau agents tried to improve soil conservation by discouraging overgrazing and encouraging economic independence. Federal credit unions were organized on reservations, and federal funds underwrote Indian business ventures. Collier began to end years of assimilationist policies by promoting cultural pluralism and racial pride among the tribes. The Indian Bureau hired so many Indians that they made up more than a fourth of its employees by the end of the decade.

The Indian Reorganization Act of 1934 tried to revive traditional life and resurrect the tribal system. A special Court of Indian Affairs removed Indians from the jurisdiction of states. Tribes gained control of Indian lands. Elders were urged to celebrate festivals, artists to work in native styles, children to learn the old languages. Indians themselves were divided over Collier's policies. The Pueblos, with a strong communal spirit and already functioning communal societies, favored them. The tribes of Oklahoma and the Great Plains tended to oppose them. Individualism, the profit motive, and an unwillingness to share property with other tribe members fed resistance. So did age-old suspicion of all government programs, along with the genuine Indian desire for assimilation. The Navajos, under the leadership of J. C. Morgan, rejected the Indian Reorganization Act in 1935. Morgan saw tribal government as a step backward, and his people bitterly opposed Collier's efforts to discourage overgrazing by reducing the number of sheep. To the Navajos sheep had deep cultural meaning.

A New Deal for Women

The broker government of the New Deal was sensitive to a wide range of interests, and women quickly took advantage of the situation. Led by Eleanor Roosevelt and Secretary of Labor Frances Perkins, women invaded government. They headed the Women's and Children's bureaus of the Labor Department, directed the Mint, and served as assistant secretary in the Treasury Department. They found their greatest opportunities in the newly created agencies of the New Deal, where their appointments encroached less on the traditional preserves of men. Women worked on the consumers' advisory board of the NRA, helped to administer the relief program, and won appointments to the Social Security Board. Florence Jaffrey Harriman and Ruth Bryan Owen became the first women diplomats and Ohio judge Florence Allen the first woman on the Federal Court of Appeals. Many of them were friends, often with professional ties, and they formed a network of activists who informally promoted women's interests and liberal reform.

The New Deal achieved a mixed record in helping women. Three-fourths of the NRA codes included provisions for equal pay to women workers. The remaining quarter, covering industries like cloakmaking, electronics, and commercial laundries, which employed a high percentage of women, set lower minimum wages for them. The Works Progress Administration hired nearly half a million women in 1936, roughly 15 percent of all WPA workers. At the time, almost a quarter of the work force was composed of women. Men on WPA projects were paid $5 a day, women only $3. Social Security aided women with dependent children but excluded domestic servants, most of them women. The Federal Emergency Relief Administration built 17 camps for women in 11 states, while the National Youth Administration and the WPA created projects to train women and put them to work. On the other hand, the Civilian Conservation Corps employed no women at all.

Women became part of the Democratic party machinery as never before. At the 1936 Democratic National Convention in Philadelphia 219 women served as delegates, and over 300 stood by as alternates. (Only 60 were delegates at the Republican convention.) Eight women made seconding speeches. Under the leadership of social worker Mary W. "Molly" Dewson, the Women's Division of the Democratic National Committee played a critical role in the election. Thousands of women mounted a "mouth-to-mouth" campaign, literally traveling from door to door to drum up support for Roosevelt and other Democrats. When the ballots were finally tallied, women formed an important part of the new Roosevelt coalition.

The Rise of Organized Labor

The New Deal boosted the fortunes of organized labor by creating a hospitable environment for unionization. At the outset of the Depression under 3 million of the 48 million workers in America belonged to labor organizations. The nation's premier union, the American Federation of Labor (AFL), paid little attention to industrial workers. Historically bound to skilled labor, notoriously uncomfortable with the ethnics and African-Americans who worked in mass-production factories, and downright hostile to women, the AFL ignored major industries like rubber, automobiles, and steel. Under the protection of Section 7a of the National Recovery Administration the AFL increased its membership, but its cautious president, William Green, sought cooperation with management.

The thundering, barrel-chested John L. Lewis, head of the United Mine Workers (UMW) since 1919, led the drive to unionize the mass of unskilled laborers. Tough, charismatic, egotistical, and ambitious, Lewis voted for Hoover in 1932, then promptly called on Roosevelt at the White House in 1933. When the new president offered nothing but consolation for the sagging UMW, Lewis returned to the coal fields with a message he had somehow divined: "The President wants you to join a union." Within a year the UMW had 400,000 members. Raising his sights, Lewis called for the creation of a Steel Workers' Organizing Committee (SWOC) and for the admission of the United Auto Workers into the AFL. AFL leaders accepted the proposals, only to ignore them.

At the annual AFL convention in Atlantic City in 1935, Lewis demanded a commitment to the "industrial organization of mass production workers." The delegates, mostly from craft unions, voted down the proposal. "I was seduced," Lewis growled, "I am enraged, and I am ready to rend my seducers limb from limb." Near the end of the convention he made good on his threat. As he passed "Big Bill" Hutcheson of the carpenters union, angry words passed between the two. Lewis spun and with a single punch sent Hutcheson sprawling in a bloody heap. The blow signaled the determination of industrial unions to break the AFL's domination of organized labor. Three weeks later, on November 10, 1935, Lewis and the heads of seven other AFL unions announced the formation of the Committee for Industrial Organization (CIO). Charging the CIO with "dual organization" and "fomenting insurrection," the AFL suspended the rogue unions in 1936. The CIO, later rechristened the Congress of Industrial Organizations, turned to the unskilled.

CIO representatives concentrated on the mighty steel industry, which had clung tenaciously to the "open" or nonunion shop since the great strike of 1919. In other industries, the rank and file did not wait. Emboldened by the recent passage of the Wagner Act, a group of rubber workers at three companies in Akron, Ohio, spontaneously sat down on the job in early 1936. The new strategy worked at two of the companies. Since the strikers occupied the plants, managers could not replace them with strikebreakers. Nor could the rubber companies call in the military or police without the possibility of destroying their own property. The leaders of the United Rubber Workers Union opposed the "sit-downs," but when the Goodyear Tire & Rubber Company laid off 70 workers, 1400 workers struck on their own. A picket line, running some 11 miles around the facility, sprang up outside. Eventually Goodyear settled by recognizing the union and accepting its demands on wages and hours.

The biggest strikes erupted in the automobile industry. Automobile production had developed the assembly line to a fine art. "Where you used to be a man," complained one Chevrolet worker, "now you are less than their cheapest tool." Periodic speed-ups left laborers without a moment's rest. "When I get home I'm so tired I can't even sleep with my wife," said one of them. The new United Auto Workers (UAW) wanted to move cautiously, so workers took things into their own hands. The General Motors Company had exploited employees for years. Its 20 top executives earned $200,000 a year; its line workers barely $1000. A series of spontaneous strikes at General Motors plants in Atlanta, Kansas City, and Cleveland spread to Fisher Body No. 2 in Flint, Michigan, late in December 1936. Singing the unionists' anthem, "Solidarity Forever," workers took over the plant while wives, friends, and fellow union members handed food and clothing through the windows. When local police tried to break up supply lines, they were driven off in a hail of nuts, bolts, coffee mugs, and bottles.

In the wake of this "Battle of Running Bulls" (a reference to the retreating police), Governor Frank Murphy called out the National Guard, this time not to arrest but to protect strikers. Faced with the prospect of class warfare and little support from authorities, General Motors surrendered in February 1937. Less than a month later U.S. Steel capitulated without a strike, granting recognition to SWOC, a wage boost, and a 40-hour work week. By the end of the year every automobile manufacturer except Henry Ford had negotiated with the UAW. Bloody violence accompanied some drives, most notably in the effort to unionize the Republic Steel Company in Chicago. Police killed 10 strikers there on Memorial Day, 1937. Yet sooner or later much of industrial America was unionized. Rubber, electronics, and heavy metals all succumbed. In 1941, under the pressure of an impending war, even Henry Ford gave in.

Middle-class Americans, generally sympathetic to the union drives of the thirties, were horrified by sit-down strikes. The lack of respect for private property smacked of radicalism. In 1939 the Supreme Court outlawed the tactic. A momentous transfer of power had nonetheless taken place, and with relatively little bloodshed. By 1940 nearly one worker in three belonged to a union. The unskilled developed a powerful voice in the CIO (though the craft unions of the AFL still outnumbered them by more than a million). Women's membership in unions tripled between 1930 and 1940, and blacks made impressive gains. Millions of workers in the domestic and service trades, not to mention millions more on the farm, remained unorganized, but independent unions were at last a permanent feature of industrial America.

Through it all government played an important but secondary role. Roosevelt stood aside, favoring neither labor nor management. "A plague o' both your houses," he declared when the CIO tried to unionize the steel industry. The Wagner Act afforded laborers nothing more than the opportunity to organize and protection if they chose to. The workers themselves, galvanized by leaders like John L. Lewis, Walter Reuther of the United Auto Workers, and Philip Murray of the Steel Workers' Organizing Committee, won their own victories.

"Art for the Millions"

Under the influence of the New Deal the fine arts—from writing to painting, music, theater, and the new "art" form of photography—became a government project for the first time. Like everyone else, artists needed help. It made no sense, believed Harry Hopkins, to give a concert pianist or a Shakespearean actor a job digging ditches. Here was an opportunity to blend decency, culture, and democracy. Paid by the federal government, trained professionals would get financial assistance and preserve their talents. At the same time the government could bring art to the masses by employing skilled artists on public programs. Americans would taste high culture, some for the first time. "Art for the millions," as one administrator called it, was the dream of the New Deal.

"Federal One" was the bureaucratic umbrella of the Works Progress Administration that covered the arts programs. The Federal Writers Project (FWP) was perhaps the least controversial program. Under the direction of journalist Henry Alsberg, the FWP produced about a thousand publications. Its 81 state, territorial, and city guides were so popular that commercial publishers happily printed them. Reflecting the renewed interest in Americana, the FWP collected folklore, studied ethnic groups, and recorded the reminiscences of 200 former slaves.

The FWP employed established writers like Conrad Aiken, new ones including John Cheever, Jack Conroy, and Saul Bellow (later to win the Nobel Prize for literature), and black writers Richard Wright, Arna Bontemps, Zora Neale Hurston, Ralph Ellison, and others. "Actually to be paid for writing," Ellison exulted, "why that was a wonderful thing!" Little time was reserved for creative writing on the job, but work weeks averaged only about 30 hours. Richard Wright completed his acclaimed *Native Son*, a stinging novel of racial discrimination, in his spare time.

Nicolai Sokoloff, conductor of the Cleveland Symphony Orchestra, headed the Federal Music Project (FMP). At its peak it employed some 15,000 out-of-work musicians. For a token charge, Americans could hear the music of Bach and Beethoven. Touring orchestras brought FMP-commissioned compositions like those of Aaron Copland to people across the country, and professional musicians gave lessons for free. Musicologist Charles Seeger collected American folk songs, while the Composers Forum Laboratory gave creative talents like William Schuman their first serious hearings.

Holger Cahill, an authority on folk art, ran the Federal Art Project (FAP).

Watercolorists and draftsmen painstakingly prepared the *Index of American Design*, which offered elaborate illustrations of American material culture—andirons, skillets, figureheads from ships, even cigar-store Indians. At night hundreds of artists taught sculpture, painting, clay modeling, and carving in country churches, settlement houses, and schools. Jackson Pollock, Willem de Kooning, Anton Refregier—all destined to become important artists—made it through the Depression by painting for the government.

The most notable contribution of the FAP came in the form of murals. Under the influence of Mexican muralists Diego Rivera and José Clemente Orozco, American artists covered the walls of post offices and airports with huge murals glorifying American life and work. Frank treatments of class conflict often alienated conservatives and opened the FAP to charges of "communist infiltration" at the end of the decade. By then Americans (most of whom Roosevelt believed never had seen a "fine picture") could walk into San Francisco's Coit Tower and gaze at Victor Arnautoff's magnificent *City Life*. When the FAP held an exhibition at the New York World's Fair in 1940, over 2 million people filed through. Despite variations in quality Roosevelt was pleased. "Some of it good," he said, "some of it not so good, but all of it native, human, eager, and alive."

The Federal Theater Project (FTP) aroused the most controversy and probably reached the greatest number of people. As head of the FTP, Hallie Flanagan made government-supported theater vital, daring, and relevant. *Living Newspapers* dramatized headlines of the day; under the direction of Orson Welles and John Houseman an all-black company (one of 16 "Negro Units") set Shakespeare's *Macbeth* in Haiti, complete with voodoo priestesses and a corps of African drummers. Touring companies took classics to small towns, and on summer nights city children watched *Punch and Judy* and *Jack and the Beanstalk* from park benches. All told some 30 million people saw Federal Theater productions in its four-year history. Most of them had never seen stage actors before.

Some productions raised the eyebrows of congressional conservatives. *The Revolt of the Beavers*, a thinly veiled attack on capitalism, depicted a revolution of exploited, working-class beavers. *Triple-A Plowed Under*, a success with critics and ticket-buyers alike, exhorted farmers and consumers to band together against greedy middlemen. In 1938 and 1939 the House Committee to Investigate Un-American Activities under Martin Dies of Texas examined the FTP as "a branch of the Communistic organization." When Hallie Flanagan quoted sixteenth-century playwright Christopher Marlowe during her testimony, committee members asked whether he was a Communist. The WPA budget of 1939 cut the FTP, bringing government-sponsored theater to a quick end.

The documentary impulse to record life permeated the arts in the 1930s. Novels such as Erskine Caldwell's *Tobacco Road*, feature films like John Ford's *The Grapes of Wrath* and *How Green Was My Valley*, and government-sponsored documentaries by Pare Lorentz, *The River* and *The Plow That Broke the Plains*, stirred the social conscience of the country. Word and image were masterfully wed in the collaborative work of writer James Agee and photographer Walker Evans. *Let Us Now Praise Famous Men*, the chronicle of three tenant farm families, sold only 600 copies when it was published in 1941 but remains an unforgettable portrait of the 1930s.

New Dealers had more practical motives for promoting documentary realism. They wanted to undercut criticism of New Deal relief measures. In 1937 Rexford Tugwell established an Information Division in his Resettlement Administration.

Daily Lives

PUBLIC SPACE / PRIVATE SPACE

Post Office Murals

"How can a finished citizen be made in an artless town?" asked the postmaster of Pleasant Hill, Missouri, in 1939. Such weighty matters as citizenship and art might have seemed beyond an ordinary postmaster, but he did not think so—and neither did the New Dealers in Washington. They had just made his post office the recipient of a new painting entitled *Back Home: April 1865*, and in the eyes of the postmaster, they had performed a commendable service. His town, like so many others scattered across America, had been "wholly without objects of art." Now it had one that showed common people at an epic moment in history, the end of the Civil War. Townsfolk saw it every day, and every day it made them a bit more aware of their history, more comfortable with art, and more appreciative of the heritage of democracy.

The Fine Arts Section (FAS) of the Treasury Department, which sponsored the artwork for Pleasant Hill, was but one of the programs for artists underwritten by the New Deal. The largest and most famous, the Works Progress Administration's Federal Art Project (1935–1943), produced 18,000 easel paintings, 17,000 sculptures, and 2500 murals. It employed thousands of needy artists, mostly in the large cities where they lived, and placed their work in state and municipal institutions.

The Treasury Department had a similar mission but a different focus. Beginning in 1934, it commissioned artwork for federal buildings, over which it enjoyed jurisdiction. During its nine-year existence, the FAS hired 850 artists (one-sixth of whom were women) and commissioned nearly 1400 works. Unlike relief agencies, which handed out work on the basis of financial need, FAS artists competed for contracts on particular jobs. Most were for the 1100 new post offices built during the New Deal.

Post offices were an ideal medium for democratizing art. Often at the center of town, the rectangular brick buildings bespoke solidity, permanence, and service. They linked the community with a wider world and served as the junction of local and national interests. They were tangible symbols of the federal government, perhaps the only contact many citizens had with Washington. Yet rather than emphasizing government might with portraits of national heroes or friezes of eagles and flags, post office murals depicted the daily routines of common citizens, usually from the community or the region. Local committees helped to select both the artists and the subjects, and whenever possible local artists did the work. Here, as elsewhere in the New Deal, regard for community participation was meant to temper the sense that people were surrendering control to an intrusive central government.

From the artists' point of view the post office was hardly an ideal setting. Muralists required space and light, but most post office buildings were small and dark. The available walls, often no more than 6 by 12 feet, were usually above the postmaster's door at the end of a long, cramped lobby with hanging light fixtures and vestibules that obstructed vision. The giant murals of Diego Rivera, whose work had glorified the Mexican Revolution in the 1920s, were inspirational but also controversial. Post office muralists painted on a smaller scale and avoided controversy. They drew fewer figures and arranged them in the foreground to draw the atten-

Daily Lives

Back Home: April 1865, presented to the Pleasant Hill, Missouri, post office in 1939, was commissioned by the Fine Arts Section of the Treasury Department as part of its program to democratize American art by adorning public buildings with it.

tion of viewers. Sometimes they used geometric designs that carried the eye across the disruptive door or vertical lines that broke the painting into three parts.

In a decade of fear and insecurity, the murals stressed the continuity of past and present, suggesting old virtues that had made the country great would help it to overcome the current crisis. Grand themes were distilled to simple essences and timeless symbols embodied in plain experiences: a family enjoying a Sunday picnic; friends picking fruit; skaters gliding across a frozen pond; workers stringing electric wire; children waiting for the postman. Family, work, community—the enduring qualities of American life, at once ordinary and ideal, local and national—bound the country together in good times and bad.

More often than not, regionalism influenced subject matter: colonial and urban scenes in New England and the Mid-Atlantic states; agriculture and country life in the South; the frontier and Indian and Spanish culture in the West.

Rarely were artists permitted to deal with inflammatory subjects like war, radicalism, or poverty. And when locals did not like the results, they made their displeasure known. In Watonga, Oklahoma, Cheyennes gathered at the post office to protest as unfair and inaccurate a mural depicting Indians. Asked by a reporter if he were going to scalp the artist, Chief Red Bird replied that was "bow-and-arrow, horse-and-buggy-day business." The Cheyenne were "streamlined," he said. "We picket post office."

The quality of the murals varied greatly, but in the end they achieved their aim of reaching common folks by combining the ordinary and the aesthetic. Almost always they communicated a harmonious vision of America, inspiring viewers with faith in progress and faith in themselves. "How important it is," said Supreme Court Justice Harlan Stone, after seeing a mural in Big Spring, Texas, "that the humble people of this country should be impressed with the fact that the artist finds beauty and dignity in their life."

He placed Roy Stryker, his former Columbia University teaching assistant, in charge of its Historical Section. Stryker hired a cadre of talented photographers, not so much to furnish them with relief but to have an unvarnished record of the Great Depression to blunt anti–New Deal journalists and politicians. Later transferred to the Farm Securities Administration, the group included Russell Lee, Dorothea Lange, Ben Shahn, Walker Evans, and Marion Post Wolcott. Raw and haunting, their photographs turned history into art.

THE END OF THE NEW DEAL (1937–1940)

Signs of recovery were visible everywhere by the end of 1936. Apple vendors vanished from street corners, breadlines from cities. In Detroit more automobiles came rolling off assembly lines than at any time since 1929. Utility companies were billing more kilowatt-hours of electricity than ever. Industrial output had doubled since 1932. From the winter of 1932 to the fall of 1936 farm income had almost quadrupled.

Roosevelt and the New Deal had made a difference. The Farm Credit Administration prevented an average of 300 farm foreclosures a day. A loan from the Federal Housing Authority helped Pueblo chief Albert Looking Elk Martinez replace his adobe hearth with a gas stove and put linoleum over his dirt floor. "Your work saved our humble little home from the Deed Trust sharks," wrote a California real estate broker. "Life is 1000% better since you took Charge of our United States."

Still, full recovery remained elusive. National income was only half again as large as it had been in 1933. "I see one-third of a nation ill-housed, ill-clad, ill-nourished," Roosevelt told the crowd at his second inauguration on January 20, 1937 (the first January inauguration under new federal legislation). One dark cloud drifted toward the White House from the Supreme Court, whose recent rulings threatened to nullify the New Deal. Sensing the full depth of his power, with unprecedented popularity and bulging majorities in Congress, Roosevelt vowed to reform the federal judiciary. It was the biggest mistake of his presidential career. The move stunned the nation and marked the beginning of the end of the New Deal.

"Packing" the Courts

In its first 76 years the Supreme Court had invalidated only two acts of Congress; between 1920 and 1933 it struck down portions of 22 laws. This new judicial activism, spearheaded by a conservative majority, rested on a narrow view of the constitutional powers of Congress and the president. As the New Deal broadened those powers it came under judicial attack.

In 1935 the Court wiped out the NRA on the grounds that manufacturing was not interstate commerce and thus lay beyond federal regulation. In 1936 it canceled the AAA, reducing federal authority under the taxing power and the general welfare clause of the Constitution. In *Moorehead v. Tipaldo* (1936) the Court ruled that a New York minimum-wage law was invalid because it interfered with the right of workers to negotiate a contract. A frustrated Roosevelt complained that the Court had thereby created a "'no-man's land,' where no government—

Roosevelt's plan to "pack" the courts came under furious attack as a naked power grab and vindictive assault on the Supreme Court itself. Here cartoonist John Berryman lampoons the president as Roosevelt asks Interior Secretary and Public Works Administrator Harold Ickes if he would construct a new, bigger Supreme Court building flying FDR's flag.

State or Federal" could act. It seemed that no law would be safe, not the Wagner Act, not wages and hours legislation, not even Social Security.

Roosevelt knew he was the first president since James Monroe to serve four years without making a Supreme Court appointment. He had little more luck with federal judgeships, where Republicans outnumbered Democrats by more than two to one in 1933. By adding new judges to the federal benches Roosevelt planned to redress the balance. Masking his true intentions, he announced early in February 1937 that the federal courts were overburdened. Sitting judges were often too "aged or infirm" to keep up. In the interests of efficiency Roosevelt proposed to "vitalize" the judiciary with new members. When a 70-year-old judge who had served at least 10 years failed to retire, the president would add another. He wanted to appoint as many as six new justices to the Supreme Court and 44 new judges to the lower federal courts.

Roosevelt took such electrifying action because he regarded courts as political, not sacred, institutions. He had ample precedent for altering even the Supreme Court. Only in 1869 did Congress set its size at 9 (there had been as few as 5 and as many as 10 justices). Most Americans, however, still clung to such cherished symbols of stability. Few accepted Roosevelt's efficiency argument, and no one on Capitol Hill (which abounded with 70-year-olds) believed that seven decades of life necessarily made one incompetent. Worse still, Roosevelt unveiled the proposal without warning. Conservative–liberal antagonisms within Congress, even within his own party, fed the fight. "Boys," said the angry Democratic chairman of the House Judiciary Committee, "here's where I cash in my chips."

Suddenly, as if by judicial magic, the Court began reversing itself. By a vote of five to four in *N.L.R.B. v. Jones and Laughlin Steel Corporation*, the justices upheld the Wagner Act in April 1937. A month later they sustained the Social Security Act as a legitimate exercise of the commerce power. And when Justice Willis Van Devanter, a staunch conservative born before the Civil War, retired in 1937, Roosevelt at last could make a Supreme Court appointment. He nonetheless pressed ahead with court reform. When Democrat after Democrat abandoned him, Roosevelt finally accepted a substitute measure that ignored his proposal to appoint new judges. He later claimed to have won the war over the Court (eventually he named five justices), but victory came at a high price. The momentum of the 1936 election was squandered; the unity of the Democratic party was destroyed; and opponents learned that Roosevelt could be beaten. A conservative coalition of Republicans and rural Democrats had found the first of several common causes.

More Troubles

As early as 1936 Secretary of the Treasury Henry Morgenthau, Roosevelt's closest friend in the cabinet, began to plead for fiscal restraint. The economic omens were good, he argued, so the administration should reduce spending, balance the budget, and let business lead the way to full recovery. "The patient might scream a bit when he was taken off narcotics," Morgenthau reasoned, but the time had come "to strip off the bandages, throw away the crutches," and allow the economy to "stand on its own feet."

In the case of Roosevelt, Morgenthau was preaching to the converted. The president had never been comfortable with the alarming deficits prescribed by theorists like John Maynard Keynes. The British economist had developed a startling new theory that called on government to spend its way out of depression. When good times returned, government could pay off its debts through taxes. Such "countercyclical" activity (spending in bad times, taxing in good) should take place only in the absence of private investment, Keynes cautioned. Many Americans, including Federal Reserve Board chairman Marriner Eccles, had come independently to similar conclusions, but not Roosevelt. Even after meeting with Keynes in 1934, the president dismissed his "rigmarole of figures," later confessing that he had not understood a word of the economist's most important work, *The General Theory of Employment, Interest, and Money.*

As stock prices crept up and unemployment dipped, Roosevelt ordered cuts in federal spending. Early in 1937 he slashed WPA relief rolls by half and virtually halted PWA operations; the Federal Reserve Board tightened credit; the government began to collect $2 billion in new social security taxes. In the fall of 1937 the economy collapsed. Industrial activity plummeted, eliminating all the gains made since 1935. In three months the Dow Jones stock averages fell by 75 points. At the end of the year unemployment stood at 10.5 million. The president, sounding strangely like Hoover, told his cabinet to "sit tight and keep quiet," but the "Roosevelt recession" only deepened. Finally the spenders in this administration convinced him to propose a $3.75 billion omnibus measure in April 1938. Facing an election, Congress happily restored WPA cuts, quadrupled farm subsidies, and embarked on a new shipbuilding program. The economy revived but never recovered. Keynesian economics was vindicated, though for years after not generally accepted.

With Roosevelt vulnerable, the conservative coalition in Congress began to block the New Deal. Conservatives gutted a public housing law, wrote regional differentials into the minimum wage provision of the Fair Labor Standards Act (which also established maximum hours), and limited a presidential bill to reorganize the executive branch. Roosevelt's principal success came in a renewed attack on business. The Anti-Trust Division of the Justice Department under Thurman Arnold launched a campaign against big business, while Congress created the Temporary National Economic Committee to investigate corporate abuses. These were small consolations. The president, wrote Harold Ickes in August, "is punch drunk from the punishment that he has suffered recently."

Roosevelt struck back in the off-year elections of 1938. Across the West and

South he tried to purge Democrats who had deserted him, but every one of the five senators he targeted for defeat won reelection. Only in his home state of New York did he succeed, unseating Representative John J. O'Connor, the unfriendly chairman of the House Rules Committee. Republicans gained 13 governorships, 8 Senate seats, and 81 House seats. Democrats still held majorities in both houses, but the impetus was gone. For all intents and purposes the New Deal had passed into history.

The Legacy of the New Deal

As an active reform movement, the New Deal lasted only five years, from 1933 to 1938. It failed in its primary mission to end the Depression. Although the federal budget grew from $3.2 billion in 1932 to $9 billion in 1939, New Dealers never spent enough to make up for lost private investment. It was World War II that proved to be the agent of recovery. By 1945, after four years of war, federal expenditures stood at an astounding $100 billion, and only in 1943 did unemployment finally dip below its 1929 level.

Furthermore, New Dealers never achieved any fundamental change in the distribution of wealth and income. They never intended to, but in the end the wealthy received such a large proportion of all income that not enough mass purchasing power existed to sustain consumption and employment. Without consumption and employment, there was little incentive for businesses to mount further investment. The equation was simple, said Brains Truster Adolf Berle. "Unless the national income was pretty widely diffused there were not enough customers to keep the plants going."

Though it was a response to an immediate crisis, the New Deal fell within the progressive tradition. Like progressivism it sought to conserve capitalism by ending its abuses, regulating its excesses, and softening its impact. In doing so the New Deal relied, again like progressivism, on government activism, moderate reform, expertise, and new executive agencies. Despite its ultimate failure to bring about recovery, it left a lasting legacy. It placed responsibility for prosperity squarely with government, as a shaper and regulator of the economy. No administration would ever be able to escape this responsibility. In its securities and banking regulations, unemployment compensation, and maximum hours and minimum wage requirements the New Deal created stabilizers to forestall another breakdown. Strengthening the Federal Reserve system and enhancing control over credit made Washington, not Wall Street, the financial center of the nation.

Roosevelt modernized the presidency. He turned the White House into the heart of government, setting the public agenda, spreading new ideas, initiating legislation, and assuming responsibility for the whole nation. It became the place where decisions were made. A clerk calculated that Roosevelt made 35 decisions for every decision made by Calvin Coolidge. The power of Congress and of local and state governments diminished as a result, while the federal bureaucracy grew. In 1932 there were 605,000 federal employees; by 1939 there were nearly a million. Though later critics would charge the New Deal with creating an unwieldy, expensive, and dangerous bureaucracy, conversion to a war economy would have been perilously slowed without it. It is also important to remember that the size of government exploded during World War II, not the New Deal. By 1945 the number of federal employees had soared to 3.5 million.

The manifest failures of the private economy and private charity and of local and state governments promoted the expansion of federal authority. When mayors

What the New Deal Did . . .

	RELIEF	RECOVERY	REFORM
FOR THE FARMER:	Rural Electrification Administration (1936) Farm Security Administration (1937)	Agriculture Adjustment Act (1933)	
FOR THE WORKER:		National Industrial Recovery Act (1933)	National Labor Relations Act (1935) Fair Labor Standards Act (1938)
FOR THE MIDDLE CLASS:	Home Owners' Loan Act (1934)		Revenue ("Wealth Tax") Act (1935) Public Utilities Holding Company Act (1935)
FOR THE NEEDY:	Federal Emergency Relief Act (1933) Civilian Conservation Corps (1933) Civil Works Administration (1933) National Public Housing Act (1937) Emergency Relief Appropriation Act (1935)		
FOR PROTECTION AGAINST FUTURE DEPRESSIONS:			Federal Deposit Insurance Corporation (1933) Securities Exchange Act (1934) Social Security Act (1935)

and governors could not feed the people of their cities and states, Americans looked to Washington as the court of last resort. People came to feel that the federal government was concerned with their welfare. Roosevelt embodied the state as protector. "My mother looks upon the President as someone so immediately concerned with her problems and difficulties," wrote an insurance man, "that she would not be greatly surprised were he to come to her house some evening and stay to dinner." Home loans, farm subsidies, bank deposit insurance, relief payments and jobs, pension programs, unemployment insurance, aid to mothers with dependent children, guarantees of minimum wages and maximum hours—all touched the lives of ordinary Americans and made them more secure.

Never enough to furnish complete security, these programs were never intended to. The welfare state had limits. Most of its relief measures were designed to last no longer than the crisis itself. Millions of sharecroppers, migrants, domestic servants, and minorities fell through even its more nearly permanent safety nets. The commitment of the New Deal to furnishing minimum standards of subsistence for every American, not its failure to do so, won Roosevelt their support. He was, after all, almost the first to try.

At a time when dictators and militarists had taken hold in Germany, Italy, Japan, and Russia, the New Deal strengthened democracy in America. Roosevelt's "broker state" invigorated interest groups that had previously been unrepresented. It broadened access to government for unions, farm organizations, ethnic minorities, and some women. Under the AAA and the Wagner Act, for example, staple farmers and industrial workers actually voted to determine which crops to cut and whether to join a union. Like the welfare state, Roosevelt's broker state had its limits. The administration never developed ways to protect people who belonged to no organizations. The unorganized, like slum dwellers and most blacks, often found themselves ignored.

Under Roosevelt's leadership the Democratic party, divided and crippled for decades, became a mighty force in American politics. In a quiet but profound revolution, African-Americans were brought rapidly into the party's fold and its constituencies were further widened to include labor and farmers. Political attention shifted from the cultural divisions of the 1920s to bread-and-butter issues. In 1932 people had argued about Prohibition and European war debts. By 1935 they were debating Social Security, labor relations, tax reform, public housing, and the TVA. With remarkable speed, the New Deal had become part of American life.

During the 1930s the United States found a middle way between the extremes of communism and fascism. Blending public and private controls, the New Deal attempted to humanize industrial society and generate prosperity without sacrificing capitalism and democracy. Government—particularly the executive branch—took the lead. Yet New Dealers from the president down recognized that they could not do everything. "I never believed that the Federal government could solve the whole problem," Eleanor Roosevelt told the National Youth Congress in February 1939. "It bought us time to think. . . . Is it going to be worth while?" Only future generations could say.

SIGNIFICANT EVENTS

1933 — Franklin Roosevelt inaugurated as president; bank "holiday"; "hundred days" legislation passed; repeal of Eighteenth Amendment (Prohibition); Townsend movement begins

1934 — Securities and Exchange Commission; American Liberty League; Indian Reorganization Act

1935 — Emergency Relief Appropriation Act; Rural Electrification Administration authorized; *Schecter Poultry Corp. v. United States* invalidates National Recovery Administration; Huey Long organizes Share Our Wealth Society; "second hundred days" legislation passed; Father Charles Coughlin creates National Union for Social Justice; Huey Long assassinated

1936 — *Butler v. U.S.* invalidates Agricultural Adjustment Administration; Soil Conservation and Domestic Allotment Act; Congress of Industrial Organizations formed; Roosevelt reelected; United Auto Workers union begins sit-down strikes; John Maynard Keynes' *The General Theory of Employment, Interest, and Money* published

1937 — Roosevelt announces court "packing" plan; Roosevelt recession

1938 — Fair Labor Standards Act sets minimum wages/maximum hours; Congress establishes Temporary National Economic Committee

1939 — Marian Anderson gives a concert at the Lincoln Memorial; Executive Reorganization Act

28

America's Rise to Globalism

John Garcia, a native Hawaiian, worked as a pipe-fitter's apprentice at the Pearl Harbor Navy Yard in Hawaii. On Sunday, December 7, 1941, he was enjoying a lazy day off. By the time his grandmother came rushing in to wake him at eight that morning, it was already too late. "The Japanese were bombing Pearl Harbor," he recalled her yelling to him. John listened in disbelief. "I said, 'They're just practicing.'" "No," his grandmother replied. It was real. He catapulted his huge frame from bed, ran to the front porch, and caught sight of the antiaircraft fire in the sky. "Oh boy" were his only words.

Hopping on his motorcycle, he sped the four miles to the harbor in 10 minutes. "It was a mess," he remembered. The U.S.S. *Shaw* was in flames. The battleship *Pennsylvania*, a bomb nesting one deck above the powder and ammunition, was about to blow. When ordered to put out its fires, he refused. "There ain't no way I'm gonna go down there," he told the navy officer. Instead, he spent the rest of the day pulling bodies from the water. There were so many he lost count. He couldn't tell "how many were alive and how many were dead."

Surveying the wreckage the following morning, he noted that the battleship *Arizona* "was a total washout." So was the *West Virginia*. The *Oklahoma* had "turned turtle, totally upside down." It took two weeks to get all the fires out. John and his fellow workers spent the next month cutting through the *West Virginia*'s superstructure, trying to save the men trapped inside. "About three hundred men we cut out of there were still alive by the eighteenth day." John's girlfriend was not. She had been killed by an errant American shell as she prepared for church on Sunday morning.

The world had been at war since 1939, but Americans had largely been spared. Two vast oceans had seemed to protect the United States—until now. The surprise attack at Pearl Harbor suddenly transformed the Pacific into an avenue of potential assault. All along the West Coast panic spread as radio reports carried the news that America was on the verge of war. Dennis Keegan, a young college student at the University of San Francisco, could not believe it, even though his younger brother Bill was training in Canada to fly with the Royal Air Force. "These places were so far away from us," Dennis said after hearing about Pearl Harbor. "It just didn't seem possible that we were at war."

Images of its battleships in flames sent the United States into global war, although the losses at Pearl Harbor were more shocking than disabling. The West Virginia, *shown here, settled to the shallow bottom with guns still firing and was later repaired.*

That night Keegan drove into downtown San Francisco. Market Street was "bedlam." "The United Artists Theater had a huge marquee with those dancing lights, going on and off," he recalled. "People were throwing everything they could to put those lights out, screaming Blackout! Blackout!" The next day a false army report of 30 Japanese planes flying toward the coast triggered air raid sirens throughout the city. Unsubstantiated rumors put Japanese aircraft carriers off the mouth of the Columbia River. Blackouts were declared as far inland as Boise, Idaho.

Los Angeles turned trigger-happy. A young policeman named Tom Bradley (who later served as mayor of the city) heard "sirens going off, aircraft guns firing." "Here we are in the middle of the night," he said, "there was no enemy in sight, but somebody thought they saw the enemy." In January 1942 the Rose Bowl was moved from Pasadena, California, to Durham, North Carolina. Early that same year submarines shelled Santa Barbara. The Japanese also floated balloons carrying incendiary devices from ships off the coast. One reached Iowa without doing any damage.

The Japanese attack on Pearl Harbor created a sense of panic along the West Coast of the United States. Hasty defenses like these sandbags stacked in front of the telephone company in San Francisco were thrown up to ward off an attack that never came.

Although the Japanese never came any closer, in a world with long-range bombers and submarines, no place seemed safe: this was global war, the first of its kind. Arrayed against the Axis powers of Germany, Italy, and Japan were the Allies—Great Britain, the Soviet Union, the United States, China, and the Free French. Their armies fought from the Arctic to the southwestern Pacific, in the great cities of Europe and Asia and the small villages of North Africa and Indochina, in malarial jungles and scorching deserts, on six continents and across four oceans. Perhaps as many as 100 million people took up arms; some 40 million to 50 million lost their lives.

Tragedy on such a scale taught the generation of Americans who fought the war that they could no longer isolate themselves from any part of the world, no matter how remote it might seem. Manchuria, Ethiopia, and Poland had once seemed far away, yet the road to war had led from those distant places to the United States. Retreat into isolation had not cured the worldwide depression or preserved the peace. Most Americans now came to believe that to avoid other such disasters once this war was ended, the United States must assume far wider responsibility for managing the world's geopolitical and economic systems.

THE UNITED STATES AND THE COLLAPSE OF THE VERSAILLES SYSTEM

The outbreak of World War II had its roots in the devastation of World War I, when almost an entire generation of young men had been killed or maimed in five years of carnage. War debts eroded economic health. The political disorganization of central Europe and Asia produced vacuums of power soon filled by the forces of fascism. The nations dissatisfied with the terms of the peace—Germany, the Soviet Union, Italy, Poland, Japan—sought to achieve unilaterally what the victors had denied them at Versailles. Faced with an unstable world economy, the United States turned away from collective action. In one of his final speeches Warren Harding declared that American participation in the League of Nations was an issue as "dead as slavery." That did not mean the United States would simply isolate itself from world affairs. Bankers and businessmen eagerly pursued markets abroad. Sometimes they worked under government auspices, sometimes independently. In general, though, little consensus existed about how the United States could work with other nations to ensure peace and prosperity.

Economic Diplomacy

The World War I victors saddled Germany with $33 billion in war costs, partly to repay their own war debts to the United States. When Germany defaulted on reparations in 1923, French forces occupied the Ruhr valley, the industrial heartland of Germany. Germany struck back by inflating its currency, a move that dramatized the crushing burden of debt. In 1923 Germans carried bushels of money to pay for food. Runaway inflation wiped out the savings of the middle class, shook confidence in the new German Weimar Republic, and soon threatened the economic structure of all Europe.

Emerging from the war as the leading creditor nation of the world, the United States, more than any nation, had some capacity to bring order to the world's economic systems. Congress instead acted first to protect American prosperity by adopting the highly restrictive Fordney–McCumber Tariff in 1922. Only then did the Harding administration respond to the growing crisis in Europe. To temper German inflation American business leaders Charles G. Dawes and Owen D. Young persuaded the victorious Europeans to adopt a plan to scale down reparations. In return the United States promised to help stabilize the German economy. Encouraged by the State Department, American bankers made large loans to Germany, which the Germans used to pay their reparations. The European victors then used the money to repay their war debts to the United States, which amounted to taking money out of one American vault and depositing it in another. In 1926 the United States also reduced European war debts. Canceling them altogether would have made more sense, but few Americans were that forgiving. As President Coolidge remarked, "They hired the money, didn't they?"

The United States sought to maintain world trade by promoting American business overseas. Multinational corporations eager to develop markets and facilities abroad made use of a new consular service that provided them with business information, while the Departments of State and Commerce pressed to keep open markets Europeans and Japanese threatened to close. In the Middle East, the United States pressured the British to allow American oil companies to participate in major oil operations in Iraq, Kuwait, and Bahrain Island. American capital constructed branch factories in Scandinavia, mined tin in Bolivia, developed rubber plantations in the Dutch East Indies. With high tariffs restricting the American market, the nations of Europe had difficulty expanding economies burdened by reparations and war debts. The Dawes Plan helped to stabilize Germany but did nothing to calm European fears that German militarism might revive.

Avoiding War

The end of World War I failed to halt an arms race among the great powers. The United States vied with Britain, France with Italy, and Japan with nearly everyone for naval supremacy. Within the United States two factions sought to end military escalation, but for different reasons. A variety of pacifists and peace activists blamed the arms race between Germany and England for having brought the world to war in 1914. They believed disarmament would secure peace forever.

Republicans in the tradition of Theodore Roosevelt had few qualms about military rivalry but worried about spiraling costs. With a small single-ocean fleet, for example, Japan could threaten British and American interests in the Pacific basin. Yet both Great Britain and the United States chose to maintain navies in two oceans.

In an effort to cut the budget and still protect China and the Philippines, Secretary of State Charles Evans Hughes invited eight nations to a naval disarmament conference in Washington, D.C., in November 1921. Barely had the delegates taken their seats when Hughes offered an electrifying proposal. Scrap 2 million tons of capital ships (battleships and battle cruisers), he said, and cancel those under construction. The plan would sink more tonnage than had been destroyed in the history of naval warfare. A "tornado of cheering" welled up, as delegates whooped, waved their hats, and embraced each other. Hughes proposed to save their treasuries from bankruptcy.

Three major treaties emerged from the Washington Naval Conference. A Five-Power Agreement froze capital ship construction for 10 years and limited maximum capital tonnage to 500,000 tons for the United States and Great Britain, 300,000 for Japan, and 167,000 each for France and Italy. It was the first disarmament treaty in modern history. Britain, the United States, France, and Japan also signed a Four-Power Agreement to respect one another's holdings in the Pacific. Finally, a Nine-Power Pact guaranteed the independence and territorial integrity of China. Political restraint would substitute for naval strength.

What seemed so bold on paper proved ineffective in practice. French resentment over low ratios tied to Italy rather than Japan led France to refuse limits on land armaments and smaller warships such as submarines, cruisers, and destroyers. Soon the arms race concentrated on these areas. The Soviet Union and Germany had been completely excluded. In 1922 the two outcast nations met at Rapallo, Italy, where they agreed on a secret plan for German remilitarization, in violation of the Treaty of Versailles.

Peace advocates continued to seek some way to prevent war. At the same time the French sought some means to prevent any revival of German military strength. French Foreign Minister Aristide Briand in 1928 proposed a bilateral Franco-American treaty outlawing war. Under pressure from both pacifists and isolationists at home, American Secretary of State Frank Kellogg transformed Briand's proposal into an international treaty against war. Every major nation except the Soviet Union joined the Kellogg–Briand Pact of 1928. "Peace is proclaimed," said Kellogg as he signed the document with a foot-long pen made of gold. In fact most people recognized the pact as a harmless gesture, at best a sign of hope. Whatever hope it did represent proved forlorn.

Neither the Kellogg–Briand Pact nor the Washington Conference treaties directly addressed the upheavals in China. For years rival factions had warred ruthlessly among themselves, agreeing only that foreign powers should leave. In 1927 the Nationalists, led by Chiang Kai-shek, consolidated power by massacring thousands of their Communist party allies. Civil war flared intermittently for the next 20 years. Meanwhile Japanese nationalists, eager to secure raw materials and markets for their resource-poor island nation, moved to control the Shantung peninsula and Manchuria, two regions they believed vital to Japan's future as a world power. In 1931 the Japanese Military Command in Manchuria used an explosion on the rail lines near Mukden as a pretext to justify military occupation of the whole province. A year later the Japanese converted Manchuria into a puppet state and named it Manchukuo.

The Western powers faced a quandary. Japanese moderates wanted to restrain their military adventurists in China, but the military factions in Japan would probably be strengthened if the United States and Europe imposed sanctions. President Herbert Hoover had cautiously supported investigation by the League of Nations; then, when the Japanese took over Manchuria in 1932, he instructed Secretary of State Henry Stimson to announce that the United States refused to recognize any violation of open-door principles, infringement of American rights, dismembering of China, or breaches of the Kellogg–Briand Pact. Even though Stimson had wanted to do more, this policy of nonrecognition became known as the Stimson Doctrine. The principle, no matter how sound, failed to restrain Japan. Within a month Japanese cruisers were shelling Shanghai, a port city in China. When the League of Nations condemned Japan in 1933, the Japanese simply withdrew from the League. The seeds of war in Asia had been sown.

Becoming a Good Neighbor

The history of American restraint in Europe and Asia had no counterpart in Latin America. By 1924 the United States was running the financial affairs of 10 nations south of the border. Harding had landed troops in Honduras, and in 1927 the Coolidge administration used marines in Nicaragua to keep Mexican-supported rebels from gaining power. When rebel leader César Augusto Sandino (who would later inspire the "Sandinista" rebels of the 1970s) refused to participate in American-supervised elections, Coolidge ordered the marines to stay.

By the late 1920s interventionism under the Roosevelt Corollary (page 865) had become both an embarrassment and a potential liability. No European state was likely to violate the Monroe Doctrine. A few Latin American states, moreover, had grown strong enough to resist direct interference by the United States in defense of North American interests. Even Coolidge relented and in 1927, rather than confront Mexico over the confiscation of American-owned properties, he sent Ambassador Dwight Morrow to ease tensions. The Depression gave the United States added incentive to improve hemispheric relations. In 1933, when critics compared the American position in Nicaragua to Japan's in Manchuria, Secretary Stimson ordered the marines to withdraw. In those gestures and President Hoover's efforts to cultivate goodwill south of the border lay the roots of a "Good Neighbor" policy.

Under Franklin Roosevelt being a good neighbor meant correcting the political (but not the economic) inequities between the United States and Latin America. At the seventh Pan-American Conference in 1933, his administration accepted a resolution denying any country "the right to intervene in the internal or external affairs of another." Roosevelt completed the withdrawal of marines from Nicaragua and Haiti. In 1934 he negotiated a treaty with Cuba that renounced the American right to intervene under the Platt Amendment (page 864). Henceforth the United States would replace direct military influence with indirect economic influence. Secretary of State Cordell Hull embarked on a crusade to lower tariffs under the new Trade Agreements Act (1934), which led to agreements with six Latin American (and seven European) nations. In 1936 Roosevelt crowned the Good Neighbor policy by opening the Pan-American Conference in Buenos Aires with a speech declaring that outside aggressors "will find a Hemisphere wholly prepared to consult together for our mutual safety and our mutual good."

The greatest test of the Good Neighbor policy came in 1937 and 1938, when

Bolivia and Mexico expropriated the properties of American oil companies. Roosevelt's desire to protect American interests was compromised by his fear that intervention would drive Mexico into arrangements with Japan, Germany, or Italy. When an arbitration committee awarded the oil companies $24 million rather than the $450 million they demanded, Roosevelt accepted the decision.

With the threat of war approaching in Europe, the Roosevelt administration found a new Latin willingness to cooperate over hemispheric protection. At the Havana Conference in 1940 all the ministers agreed to treat an attack on one nation as an attack on all. By the end of the year Roosevelt had worked out defense agreements with every Latin American country but one. The United States could now face war with the American hemisphere largely secured.

THE DIPLOMACY OF ISOLATIONISM

During the 1920s Benito Mussolini had capitalized on appeals to Italian nationalism and fears of communism to assume power in Italy. Having destroyed all political opposition, he declared himself the leader, *Il Duce*, and adopted a program of national solidarity and state management of the economy while spinning dreams of a new Roman empire. Mussolini embodied the rising force of fascism. Then on March 5, 1933, one day after the inauguration of Franklin Roosevelt, the German Reichstag (Parliament) gave Adolf Hitler control of Germany. Magnetic and mystical, Hitler headed the National Socialist, or "Nazi," party. Riding a wave of anti-communism and anti-Semitism, the Nazis promised to unite all Germans in a Greater Third Reich that would last a thousand years. Just over a week earlier, Yosuke Matsuoka had led the Japanese withdrawal from the League of Nations. Under the lead of militarists, Japan began to carve out its own Greater East Asia Co-Prosperity Sphere. By the end of the decade the rise of fascism and militarism in Europe and Asia brought the world to war.

Neutrality and Appeasement

"It's a terrible thing," Franklin Roosevelt said in the mid-1930s, "to look over your shoulder when you are trying to lead—and to find no one there." As much as he wanted the United States to play a leading role in bringing order to world affairs, Roosevelt often found the nation reluctant to follow. Though the Depression was international in scope, most politicians clamored for national solutions. Only when a potential economic interest was involved could Roosevelt command wide support for foreign initiatives. For example, businessmen welcomed his decision in 1933 to recognize the communist regime in Russia. Not only did Roosevelt hope recognition would increase Russian–American trade, but he also thought the Soviet Union would help contain Japanese expansion in Asia and fascism in Europe.

For every step Roosevelt took toward internationalism abroad, the Great Depression forced him home again. In 1933 he sent a delegation under Secretary of State Cordell Hull to participate in the London Economic Conference. Europeans were seeking to reduce war debts, lower American tariff barriers, and stabilize the value of currency. Roosevelt refused to allow Hull even to discuss war debts or tariff reduction. After dramatically dispatching White House adviser Raymond Moley with a message for the Conference, he rejected a proposal on currency stabilization. With the United States mired in the Depression he wanted no foreign entanglements to inhibit his attempts to revive the economy.

Roosevelt's rejection of an international policy was politically shrewd. Programs to combat the Depression at home gained broad support; efforts to resolve crises abroad provoked controversy. In 1935 Senate hearings conducted by Gerald P. Nye of North Dakota revealed that bankers and munitions makers, so-called "merchants of death," had made enormous profits during World War I. The committee report implied, but could not prove, that business interests had even steered the United States into war. "When Americans went into the fray," declared Senator Nye, "they little thought that they were there and fighting to save the skins of American bankers who had bet too boldly on the outcome of the war and had two billions of dollars of loans to the Allies in jeopardy."

Nye's charges fed the debate over the growing threat to peace. By 1935 leading public figures agreed war was imminent; they agreed, too, that the United States should stay out. But on the question of what policy to follow the divisions were profound. Internationalists like the League of Women Voters and former secretary of state Henry Stimson favored collective security. "The only certain way to keep out of a great war is to prevent war," Stimson declared; "the only hope of preventing war . . . is by the earnest, intelligent, and unselfish cooperation of the nations of the world towards that end."

Isolationists opposed the collective security formula. Yet the simple isolationist or internationalist tag does not adequately describe the range of people and opinions in this debate. The isolationists themselves were deeply divided. Their camp included liberal reformers like George W. Norris and conservatives like Robert A. Taft of Ohio, a concentration of midwesterners as well as major leaders from both coasts like Senator Hiram W. Johnson of California and Representative Hamilton Fish of New York, and a number of Democrats as well as leading

A flag company of Hitler youth parade past their *Fuhrer*, Adolf Hitler (centered in the balcony doorway). Hitler's shrewd use of patriotic and party symbols, massed rallies, and marches exploited the possibilities for mass politics and propaganda.

Republicans. What united the isolationists was not party, ideology, or region, but a shared opposition to war and a belief that the United States should avoid alliances or political commitments to other nations. Pacifists added yet another element to the debate. Powerful groups like the Women's International League for Peace and Freedom insisted that disarmament, not the League of Nations or other collective security schemes, was the only road to peace.

It was internationalist Charles Warren who gave the isolationists a strategy to avoid war. If bankers' loans, arms shipments, and American travel on belligerent ships had pulled the United States into World War I, Warren proposed laws to prohibit these activities when another conflict broke out. Debate in Congress centered on a proposal to prohibit the sale of arms to all belligerents in time of war. Internationalists opposed the idea, arguing that the embargo should apply only to aggressor nations to prevent the aggressors from striking when they were ready, leaving their unprepared victims without access to arms. The president, internationalists suggested, should use the embargo selectively. Isolationists, however, did not want to give Roosevelt that power and they had the votes they needed. The Neutrality Act of 1935 required an impartial embargo of arms to all belligerents. The president had authority only to determine when a state of war existed.

Roosevelt had wavered throughout this debate, seeming at times to favor legislation and at times to oppose it. He had threatened to veto the bill but accepted it when it was limited to six months. Even so, he warned, it might "drag us into war rather than keeping us out." The isolationists were reluctant to grant what Roosevelt wanted: discretionary power to respond flexibly to crises.

The limitations of congressional neutrality became immediately apparent. In October 1935 Benito Mussolini ordered Italian forces into the North African country of Ethiopia. Against tanks and planes, the troops of Emperor Haile Selassie fought with spears and flintlock rifles. Roosevelt immediately invoked the Neutrality Act in hopes of depriving Italy of war goods. Italy needed not arms, but oil, steel, and copper, none of which fell under the Neutrality Act. When Secretary Hull called for a "moral embargo" on such goods, hard-pressed American businesses shipped them anyway. With no effective opposition from the League of Nations or the United States, Mussolini quickly completed his conquest. Congress then extended neutrality into 1936, adding a prohibition on loans or credits to belligerents.

Neutrality legislation also benefited Nazi dictator Adolf Hitler. On March 7, 1936, two weeks after Congress renewed the Neutrality Act, German troops thrust into the demilitarized area west of the Rhine. In the face of this flagrant violation of the Treaty of Versailles, Britain and France did nothing, while the League of Nations sputtered out a worthless condemnation. Roosevelt remained aloof. The Soviet Union's lonely call for collective action fell on deaf ears.

In 1931 the Spanish monarchy had been replaced by a democratic republic. In July 1936 Generalissimo Francisco Franco, emboldened by Hitler's success, led a rebellion against the newly elected Popular Front government. When civil war erupted, Spain became a staging ground for World War II. Hitler and Mussolini sent supplies, weapons, and troops to Franco's fascists, while the Soviet Union and Mexico aided the left-leaning government. The war divided opinion in Europe and America. Catholics supported the anticommunist Franco forces. Leftists embraced the Loyalists, who backed the democratic government. Some 3200 American citizens, the "Abraham Lincoln Brigade," joined the Spanish Loyalists' fight against fascism. Over half this rag-tag force of soldiers, nurses, and ambulance drivers died in the struggle. In the face of domestic political divisions Roosevelt stood by, even though until 1937 the neutrality laws did not apply to civil wars. By 1939 the Spanish republic had fallen to Franco.

As the world edged toward war, Congress struggled to keep America safe. Immediately after the outbreak of the Spanish Civil War, financier Bernard Baruch suggested a way to permit American trade (and thus to promote recovery at home) without risking war. Belligerents could buy supplies other than munitions but would have to pay beforehand and carry the supplies on their own ships. "Cash-and-carry" was adopted in the Neutrality Act of 1937. If war spread, the British navy would ensure that supplies reached England.

Cash-and-carry worked well in Europe but not in Asia. Japan, after provoking a clash with Chinese forces at the Marco Polo Bridge south of Beijing, invaded southern China in 1937. In a thinly veiled effort to give China continued access to American goods, Roosevelt refused to invoke neutrality. This policy benefited Japan, which had conducted a greater volume of trade with the United States. Without the discretion to impose embargoes selectively, Roosevelt could do little else.

By 1937 war seemed inevitable in both Europe and Asia, especially after Germany, Japan, and Italy signed the Anti-Comintern Pact. Ostensibly a pledge of mutual support against the Soviet Union, the agreement created a Rome–Berlin–Tokyo axis that paralyzed Europe with fear. Roosevelt groped for some way to contain these "bandit nations." In 1937 he joined with the French and British to condemn Japan's war against China. That October he gave his first foreign policy speech in 14 months. Seeming to favor collective action, he called for an international "quarantine" of aggressor nations. The isolationist press was quick to condemn the president. The large majority of editorial opinion, however, applauded the president's remarks. For reasons that are unclear, Roosevelt retreated from the position he had boldly staked out. When Japanese planes sank the American gunboat *Panay* on China's Yangtze River that December, he meekly accepted an apology for the unprovoked attack.

The president was simply too beleaguered on the domestic front to risk confrontation with powerful isolationists over foreign policy. His "court-packing" plan in 1937 (page 1002) had emboldened his opposition among both conservative Democrats and Republicans. When Roosevelt again asked Congress to give him discretionary authority over the arms embargo in 1939, he suffered a discouraging defeat. "Well, Captain," Vice President John Nance Garner told him, "we may as well face the facts. You haven't got the votes, and that's all there is to it."

What made Roosevelt's impotence so frustrating was the growing menace of Nazism in Europe. In 1938 German troops entered Austria in yet another violation of the Treaty of Versailles. Hitler then insisted that the 3.5 million ethnic Germans in the Sudetenland of Czechoslovakia be brought into the Reich. With Germany threatening to invade Czechoslovakia, in September 1938 Britain's prime minister Neville Chamberlain and French premier Edouard Daladier flew to Munich, where they struck a deal to appease Hitler. Czechoslovakia would give up the Sudetenland in return for German pledges to seek no more territory in Europe. The Munich Pact, Chamberlain announced to cheering English crowds, would bring "peace in our time." Six months later, in open contempt for the European democracies, Hitler took over the remainder of Czechoslovakia. "Appeasement" became synonymous with betrayal, weakness, and surrender.

War in Europe

By 1939 Hitler made little secret of his intentions to recapture territory lost to
Poland after World War I. Russia was the key to his success. If Soviet leader
Joseph Stalin joined the Western powers, Hitler might be blunted. But Stalin,
who coveted eastern Poland, suspected the West of seeking to turn Hitler against
him. On August 24, 1939, the foreign ministers of Russia and Germany signed a

WORLD WAR II IN EUROPE AND NORTH AFRICA
Coordination of Allied strategy was crucial to victory. As Soviet forces engaged the bulk of
the Axis armies across a huge front, the defense of Stalingrad prevented Hitler from reinforcing Rommel against the British in North Africa. After winning North Africa, the Allies
turned north to knock Italy out of the war. The final key to defeating the Nazis was the
invasion of Western Europe at Normandy. D-Day would not have been possible had the
Allies been unable to use England as a base to gather their forces. (1939 boundaries are
shown.)

nonaggression pact, shocking the rest of the world. The secret protocols (revealed after World War II) of the Molotov–Ribbentrop Agreement freed Hitler to invade Poland without having to fight a two-front war. Stalin could extend his western borders by bringing the Baltic states (Latvia, Estonia, and Lithuania), eastern Poland, and parts of Romania and Finland into the Soviet sphere.

On the hot Saturday of September 1, 1939, German tanks and troops lunged into Poland. "It's come at last," Roosevelt sighed. "God help us all." Within days France and England declared war on Germany. Stalin quickly moved into eastern Poland, where German and Russian armor took just three weeks to crush the Polish cavalry. As Hitler consolidated his hold on eastern Europe, Stalin turned to Finland. Many Americans were eager to support the Finnish cause, especially since the Finns alone had paid their war debts. But isolationists in Congress gutted a Finnish aid bill.

As spring arrived in 1940, Hitler moved to protect his sea lanes by capturing Denmark and Norway. The French retreated behind their Maginot Line, a steel and concrete fortification at the German border, while German panzer divisions supported by airpower knifed through Belgium and Holland in a *blitzkrieg*—a "lightning war." The Low Countries fell in 23 days, giving the Germans a route into France. By May 1940 a third of a million British and French troops lay pinned on the beaches of Dunkirk. Only a strenuous rescue effort, staged by the Royal Navy and a flotilla of English pleasure craft, saved them—clearing the way for the German march to Paris. On June 22, less than six weeks after the German invasion, France capitulated—in the very railway car where Germany had surrendered in 1918.

Suddenly, only Britain stood between Hitler and the United States. If the Nazis got control of the British fleet, the Atlantic Ocean could easily become a gateway to America. Isolationists mobilized in the America First Committee to keep the country out of war. Ohio Senator Robert Taft, aviator Charles Lindbergh, and Socialist party presidential candidate Norman Thomas endorsed the idea of a "Fortress America." They believed that hemispheric defenses alone could protect the nation from any onslaught. At the other end of the spectrum, in 1940 internationalists formed the Committee to Defend America by Aiding the Allies. Headed by editor William Allen White, it boasted some 600 chapters and supported aid to England short of war. Anyone who thought the Nazis would wait until the United States was ready, claimed one of its advertisements, was "either an imbecile or a traitor."

By the spring of 1940 Roosevelt had abandoned impartiality in favor of outright aid to the Allies. In May he requested funds to motorize the army (it had only 350 tanks) and build 50,000 airplanes a year (fewer than 3000 planes existed, most of them outmoded). Despite isolationist opposition he had persuaded Congress to adopt a bill for the first peacetime draft in history. Congress, earlier planning to slash the military budget, voted over $17 billion for defense.

Then came summer and the onslaught of thousands of German fighter planes and heavy bombers to soften Great Britain for a German invasion from occupied France. In addition, German submarines were sinking British convoys at an alarming rate. As radio reporters relayed graphic descriptions of London in flames and Royal Air Force pilots putting up a heroic defense, a majority of Americans became convinced that the United States should help Britain win the war, though few favored military involvement. So Roosevelt adopted policies designed to help the British help themselves. In September 1940 he agreed to give Britain 50 old destroyers in return for leases on British bases in the Western Hemisphere and a pledge not to let the Germans capture their navy. The destroyers-for-bases deal, Roosevelt told the nation, was the most important "reinforcement of our national defenses that has been taken since the Louisiana Purchase."

In the 1940 election campaign isolation was no longer the issue. Both Roosevelt and his Republican opponent, Wendell Willkie, favored an internationalist course short of war. In defeating Willkie, Roosevelt promised voters that "your boys are not going to be sent into any foreign wars." He portrayed the United States, instead, as "the great arsenal of democracy." Since the British no longer could pay for arms under the provisions of cash-and-carry, Roosevelt proposed a scheme to "lease, lend, or otherwise dispose of" arms and supplies to countries whose defense was vital to the United States. That meant sending supplies to England on the dubious premise that they would be returned when the war ended. Roosevelt likened "lend-lease" to loaning a garden hose to a neighbor whose house was on fire. Isolationists saw that lend-lease was a way to tie the United States more closely to the Allied cause. Senator Robert Taft thought "chewing gum" made a better comparison than a garden hose. After a neighbor used it, "you don't want it back." In March 1941, over the angry cries of isolationists, a large majority in Congress voted to pass the Lend-Lease Act.

By the summer of 1941 the United States and Germany were on the verge of war. For two months American destroyers had been escorting British ships as far as Iceland (though Roosevelt insisted it was a "patrol," not a convoy). The United States extended its defensive sphere to include Greenland and Iceland. Then Hitler, as audacious as ever, broke his alliance with the Soviet Union and in June 1941 launched a surprise invasion. The Allies expected a swift Russian collapse. Soviet armies had fought poorly in the Finnish War, and Stalin's purges three years earlier had decimated the officer corps. But the Russians threw up a heroic resistance, and Roosevelt extended lend-lease to the Soviet Union in August 1941.

That month Roosevelt also held secret meetings with the new British prime minister, Winston Churchill, on warships on Argentia Bay, off the coast of Newfoundland. Both leaders recognized the value of cooperation. Almost every day since England and Germany had gone to war, the two men had exchanged phone calls, letters, or cables. Churchill wanted Roosevelt to save Britain from bankruptcy and defeat. Roosevelt believed that if England collapsed, the United States would confront Germany and Japan alone. The Argentia meetings cemented the friendship between Roosevelt and Churchill—one key to Allied victory. The two leaders also issued the Atlantic Charter to define Allied war aims. The Charter condemned aggression and embraced the "Four Freedoms"—freedom of speech and expression, freedom of worship, freedom from want, and freedom from fear—which Roosevelt had proposed in a January speech. When talk turned to a postwar international organization, Roosevelt hedged. He wanted to avoid any commitment that might mire him, like Woodrow Wilson, in domestic controversy.

By the time Churchill and Roosevelt met at Argentia Bay, American destroyers in the North Atlantic were already stalking German U-boats and reporting their whereabouts to British commanders. Despite Hitler's orders to avoid engaging American patrols, several incidents occurred, including the sinking in October of the destroyer *Reuben James* with the loss of over 100 American sailors. Although public support for efforts to assist the Allied cause was growing, Roosevelt's policies still provoked angry debate. Interventionists criticized Roosevelt for being too cautious; isolationists attacked him for being too provocative and for

During World War II Franklin Roosevelt and British Prime Minister Winston Churchill developed the closest relationship ever between an American president and the head of another government. The two distant cousins shared a sense of the continuities of Anglo-American culture and of the global strategy of the war.

deceiving the American people. As late as September 1941 eight of ten Americans were against going to war. Roosevelt believed only an unprovoked attack would unite public opinion behind a declaration of war. He did not suspect that Japan, not Germany, would solve the problem for him.

Disaster in the Pacific

Preoccupied by the fear of German victory in Europe, Roosevelt sought to avoid a showdown with Japan. Hitler seemed the more dangerous enemy, who needed to be dealt with first. The navy, Roosevelt told his cabinet, had "not got enough ships to go round, and every little episode in the Pacific means fewer ships in the Atlantic." But precisely because American as well as European attention was centered on the conflict in Europe, Japan was emboldened to expand militarily into Southeast Asia.

Living on a string of crowded islands, possessing few resources, the Japanese nationalists envisioned a new order in the western Pacific. Through the "Greater East Asia Co-Prosperity Sphere," Japan would replace the European powers in Asian markets and promote just enough development to nurture local support for Japanese domination. To Japanese leaders, the Co-Prosperity Sphere was simply an Asian Monroe Doctrine. To American leaders, it threatened the principles of the open door and the survival of Chinese independence. Japan had been waging

The Geography of Global War

the region with the outline of the United States overlaid, in scale. The war had to be fought over an area which, in terms of the Western Hemisphere, was like placing the U.S. Army's Australian center of operations somewhere in South America. On the same scale, Tokyo would lie far up in northern Canada, Iwo Jima somewhere in Hudson Bay, Guam in Quebec, Tarawa and Guadalcanal in the mid-Atlantic, Singapore in Utah, Manila in North Dakota, central Java in Texas, Midway Island near Iceland, and Hawaii off the coast of Scotland.

Such extraordinary distances spurred the United States to devise a two-front strategy to defeat Japan (map, right). MacArthur's army forces used Australia as a base of operations in the southwest Pacific, aiming for the Philippines and the southeast coast of China. Once those areas were secured, forces could then launch air attacks and finally, if necessary, a full-scale invasion of Japan. The navy, under command of Admiral Nimitz, set out to destroy the Japanese fleet and to conduct a series of amphibious landings on island chains in the central Pacific. Once Japan's

In the world's first truly global war, the need to coordinate and supply troops and materiel became paramount. During World War II U.S. factories produced more goods than the three Axis powers combined. But as German U-boats took a heavy toll on Allied shipping in the North Atlantic, the problem became delivering those goods where they were needed. The solution was a logistical nightmare: send supplies to Russia on a 12,000-mile odyssey around Africa to the Persian Gulf and then across Iran by land. The elimination of German submarines and the recapture of the Mediterranean area greatly eased the shipping problem and, as much as any single battle, ensured victory.

In the Pacific the problem was one of sheer distance. To impress upon newly arrived officers the vastness of the war theater, General MacArthur showed them a map of

SOVIET UNION

MONGOLIA

MANCHURIA
• Harbin

• Vladivostok

KOREA

CHINA

Peking •

JAPAN
• Tokyo

Nagasaki
Aug. 9, 1945
Hiroshima
Aug. 6, 1945

Nanking •
Shanghai •

Chungking •

NDIA
(Br.)

BURMA

Rangoon •

THAILAND

Bangkok •

FRENCH
INDOCHINA

Saigon •

Canton •

Hong
Kong

Formosa

PHILIPPINES

Manila •

Okinawa
Apr.-June 1945

Iwo Jima
Feb.-Mar. 1945

Wake
Dec. 23, 1941

Leyte Gulf
Oct. 23-26, 1944

Guam
July 21, 1944

Tinian
July 24, 1944

MALAYA

Singapore •

Palau
Sept. 15, 1944

Eniwetok
Feb. 17, 1944

Kwajalein
Jan. 31, 1944

Marshall
Islands

Borneo
May-July 1945
Borneo

Caroline Islands

Tarawa
Nov. 20, 1943

Java Sea
Feb.-Mar. 1942

Java

DUTCH EAST INDIES

Sumatra

New Guinea

Solomon
Islands

Guadalcanal
Aug. 1942-Feb. 1943

Gilbert
Islands

Port
Moresby

Coral Sea
May 7-8, 1942

CORAL
SEA

AUSTRALIA

Sakhalin
Island

Kuril Islands

Attu

Kiska

Aleutian Islands (U.S.)

PACIFIC OCEAN

Midway
June 3-6, 1942

Hawaiian Islands (U.S.)

Pearl Harbor
Dec. 7, 1941

Mariana
Islands

Atomic bomb

Major battles

Farthest extent of
Japanese control

U.S. forces (Nimitz)

U.S. forces (MacArthur)

Soviet forces

British forces

Other Allied forces

navy had been destroyed and Okinawa captured, U.S. bombers devastated Japanese
cities from the air. British forces launched
separate operations in Burma, forces under
Chiang Kai-shek occasionally engaged Japanese forces on China's mainland, and in August 1945, Soviet troops attacked northern
China.

war on China since 1937 and by the summer of 1941 its forces controlled the China coast and all major cities. By occupying French Indochina (now Vietnam) in July, Japan stood ready to conquer all of the Southeast Asian peninsula and the oil-rich Dutch East Indies.

Japan's thrust into Indochina forced Roosevelt into action. He embargoed trade, froze Japanese assets in American banks, and barred shipments of vital scrap iron and petroleum. His actions divided the Japanese cabinet. Military leaders were willing to risk war to achieve security, but Prime Minister Fumimaro Konoye proposed instead a summit meeting with Roosevelt to iron out major differences. In fact, the two nations' goals were so at odds that no diplomatic resolution was possible. The Japanese military demanded that Konoye win recognition of recent conquests and Japanese dominance of Asia. At a meeting in Washington, Secretary of State Cordell Hull told Ambassador Kichisaburo Nomura that Japan must renounce the Tripartite Pact with Italy and Germany and withdraw from China before summit talks could begin. Even as Hull and Nomura talked, the Japanese military were planning to capture the East Indies. In October General Hideki Tojo, leader of the militants, replaced the more moderate Konoye; the war party had complete control of the government. Secretly the Japanese began preparing to attack American positions in Guam, the Philippines, and Hawaii. They planned one final round of diplomacy before striking. When Japanese Ambassador Nomura learned from Secretary Hull in late November that the United States still insisted on complete withdrawal from China, Japanese militarists decided on war.

As the Hull–Nomura talks collapsed, American military leaders urged Roosevelt to avoid direct conflict until the United States had built up its national defenses. Massive Japanese troop movements southward indicated an assault on British and Dutch holdings. If the Japanese attacked American possessions, most expected the blow to fall on Guam or the Philippines. In late November a Japanese armada slipped from Hitokappu Bay in the remote Kuril Islands, then part of Japan. Observing strict radio silence, the six carriers and their escorts steamed across the North Pacific toward the American base at Pearl Harbor in Hawaii. On Sunday morning, December 7, 1941, as a Western Union messenger pedaled to deliver an alert to the base commander, the first sortie of Japanese planes roared down on the Pacific Fleet lying at anchor. For over an hour the Japanese pounded the harbor and adjacent airfields. Altogether 19 ships—the heart of the Pacific Fleet—were sunk or battered. Practically all of the 200 American aircraft were damaged or destroyed. More than 2400 men died. Only the aircraft carriers, by chance on maneuvers, escaped the worst naval defeat in American history.

In Washington, Secretary of War Henry Stimson could not believe the news as it was relayed to his office. "My God! This can't be true, this must mean the Philippines." Later that day the Japanese did attack the Philippines, along with Guam, Midway, and British forces in Hong Kong and the Malay peninsula. On December 8, Franklin Roosevelt told a stunned and grieving nation that "yesterday, December 7, 1941" was "a date which will live in infamy." America, the "reluctant belligerent," was in the war at last.

The Japanese had given Adolf Hitler no warning about the attack, but on December 11, 1941, Germany and Italy honored their treaty with Japan by declaring war on the United States. Hitler apparently thought he had little to lose, since Germany and America were already fighting an undeclared war in the Atlantic. He certainly miscalculated the willingness and capacity of Americans to fight. Such errors in judgment ultimately doomed his dream of a thousand-year Reich.

Had Roosevelt known the attack on Pearl Harbor was coming, as some of his critics and enemies have charged? After all, American intelligence had cracked Japan's secret codes. Much information indicated that Pearl Harbor was at risk. Yet Roosevelt not only refused diplomatic compromise but also left the fleet exposed, seeming almost to provoke an attack to bring the United States into the war. Was it mere coincidence that the vital aircraft carriers were at sea, leaving obsolete battleships to bear the brunt of the attack? Since the attack on Pearl Harbor so neatly served Roosevelt's purposes, many critics argue that he must have contrived to bring it about. This argument is circumstantial, not factual. Roosevelt, wanting to fight Germany more than Japan, would have preferred an incident in the Atlantic rather than the Pacific. More important, the intelligence signals were confusing and analysts lost track of the Japanese fleet as it moved toward Hawaii. Evidence pointed more to an attack on Guam or the Philippines.

No one in Japan believed a surprise attack would bring victory against the United States—only time to consolidate a defensive perimeter that would prove impenetrable to the weak-willed Westerners. And no one in America thought the Japanese audacious or sophisticated enough to raid Pearl Harbor, some 4000 miles from Japan. Such cultural misperceptions had deadly consequences for both sides. They explain the coming of war better than any conspiracy theory.

MISFORTUNES OF WAR

On December 8, 1941, few Americans could have found much cause for hope in the smoking wreckage of ships and planes that had once been the heart of the United States' forces in the Pacific. Over the next four years one of history's great ironies unfolded. Uniting the American people as nothing else, the stunning defeat at Pearl Harbor doomed the Axis. To the Allies' resolve to defeat militarism and fascism were now added the enormous material and human resources of the United States. Victory would not come easily, nor would the alliance of the British-American democracies with the Soviet communist dictatorship be easy to sustain. The Allies needed to forge a strategy that would win both the war and the peace to follow.

Strategies for War

Two world leaders sensed better than most what Pearl Harbor meant. One was Admiral Yamamoto Isoruku, head of the Japanese navy and the man who planned the attack. The other was Winston Churchill, prime minister of England. Yamamoto had mixed feelings about the United States, where he had served several tours of duty as a young officer. He dismissed its navy as a "social organization of golfers and bridge players," yet he admired its capacity for industrial organization and production. He had warned of the folly of making war on the United States, but if Japan insisted on war, Yamamoto urged a paralyzing opening blow. He promised victory at Pearl Harbor and a free hand in the Pacific for six months, no more. As it turned out six months was not quite enough.

Winston Churchill greeted the news of Pearl Harbor with elation and shock. "We have won the war," he thought and that night slept "the sleep of the saved and thankful." Great Britain would no longer stand alone in the North Atlantic and the Pacific wars. Two weeks later Churchill headed to Washington to coordinate strategy with Franklin Roosevelt. At the meeting (code-named ARCADIA) the two leaders announced production schedules for ships, planes, and armaments that were so large some critics openly laughed—at first. A year later combined British, Canadian, and American production boards not only met but exceeded the schedules.

Roosevelt and Churchill also planned grand strategy. Outraged by the attack on Pearl Harbor, many Americans thought the United States should concentrate on Japan. The two leaders reaffirmed an earlier decision to defeat Germany first. The Pacific war would be fought as a holding action. To assure effective cooperation the two established the Combined Chiefs of Staff, a unified British-American military command based in Washington. The Arcadia Conference also led to a definition of war aims—sufficiently idealistic to rally support for the war and broad enough to avoid specific commitments. The Declaration of the United Nations (the countries at war with the Axis), made on January 1, 1942, called for easing restrictions on trade among nations, demanded disarmament of aggressors, and hinted at participation in some future security system—ultimately the United Nations.

Gloomy Prospects

In 1942 the Allies could plan for victory only on faith. German armies controlled almost all of Europe. Having narrowly survived the Battle of Britain, the British had forestalled a German invasion from France, but no counterattack to liberate France or the Low Countries seemed remotely possible. By the end of the summer the Nazis stood before the Soviet Union's three major cities—Leningrad, Moscow, and Stalingrad. British and American leaders doubted the Russians could long survive the Nazi onslaught. In North Africa General Erwin Rommel's Afrika Korps swept into Egypt and stood within striking distance of the Suez Canal—a crucial link to the resources of the British Empire.

The critical battle for the North Atlantic appeared equally precarious. As soon as prowling German U-boats spotted a convoy, they would attack in groups called "Wolfpacks." So deadly were they that merchant sailors developed a grim humor about sleeping. Those on freighters carrying iron ore slept above decks, since the heavily laden ships could sink in less than a minute. On a ship with general cargo seamen slept with clothes on and doors open to ease their escape. On oil tankers, however, sailors closed their doors, undressed, and slept soundly. If a torpedo hit, no one would survive. U-boat sailors called the first six months of 1942 "the American hunting season," as they sank 400 Allied ships in United States' territorial waters. All of America's productive capacity would mean nothing if supplies never reached Europe.

In the Far East the situation was desperate. After Pearl Harbor Japanese forces invaded the Philippines, British Malaya, and the Dutch East Indies. The British bastion of Singapore fell in just one week, and in March, at the Battle of Java Sea, the Japanese navy destroyed almost the entire remaining Allied naval force in the western Pacific. In April 1942 General Douglas MacArthur, commander of American forces in the Philippines, fled to Australia with his family in a small patrol boat. In what appeared to be an empty pledge, he vowed, "I shall return." The closest thing to success was the heroic but doomed fight of American and Philippine troops on Bataan and Corregidor. Unprepared for a mass surrender, the victorious Japanese led some 76,000 survivors on a "death march" that cost 10,000 lives. By the summer no significant Allied forces stood between the Japanese and India or Australia. The Japanese even captured two undefended islands in the Aleutian chain off the coast of Alaska. Americans feared that the West Coast of the United States might be next.

The chain of spectacular victories disguised fatal weaknesses within the Axis alliance. Japan and Germany were fighting separate wars on two fronts. They never coordinated strategies. Vast armies in China and Russia drained them of both manpower and supplies. Fearful of alienating domestic support, Hitler had not placed German industry on a full war footing before 1942. Japanese industry depended on a steady flow of materials from conquered territories. Disrupted shipping could cripple the war economy. Most important, the Axis had conquered too much territory too quickly. Brutal occupation policies alienated subject populations and forced Axis armies to leave large occupying forces to maintain control and move supplies. The Nazis diverted precious resources into the extermination of Europe's Jews, Slavs, and Gypsies. Resistance movements grew as the victims of Axis aggression fought back.

A Grand Alliance

Defeat at first obscured the Allies' strengths. Chief among these were the manpower of the Soviet Union and the productive capacity of the United States. Relatively safe from the fighting, Americans could concentrate their efforts on producing enough food and war materials to supply two separate wars at once. By the end of the war American factories had turned out 300,000 airplanes, 87,000 warships, 400,000 artillery pieces, 102,000 tanks and self-propelled guns, and 47 million tons of ammunition.

The Allies benefited too from exceptional leadership. The "Big Three"— Joseph Stalin, Winston Churchill, and Franklin Roosevelt—all had shortcomings but were able to maintain a unity of purpose that eluded Axis leaders. All three understood the global nature of the war. To a remarkable degree they managed to set aside their differences in pursuit of a common goal—the defeat of Nazi Germany. The arch-anticommunist Churchill pledged Britain's resources to assist the defense of the world's largest communist state. The anti-imperialist Roosevelt poured American resources into the war effort of two of Europe's major imperial powers.

Whenever differences of ideology, national interest, or military objectives threatened to split the alliance, the Big Three managed a compromise. In 1942 Stalin made three demands on his allies: recognition of his territorial ambitions in eastern Europe, including the former Baltic states and parts of Poland, Finland, and Romania; huge shipments of war materiel; and the opening of a second front in western Europe. The last demand was the most vital. By the end of the year the Soviets were facing 3.5 million Axis troops along a 1600-mile front in eastern Europe. One diplomat remarked that Stalin's foreign minister knew only four words in English: "yes," "no," and "second front."

Churchill and Roosevelt refused all three of Stalin's demands. In 1942 the Western Allies did not have enough supplies for their own forces, much less for Stalin's. Even if they could assemble the materiel, they did not have enough ships to carry it. Nor were Churchill and Roosevelt willing to jeopardize Allied harmony by discussing postwar Russian territorial ambitions. And in 1942 the Allies simply lacked sufficient trained soldiers, landing craft, and air support for a successful invasion of Europe.

Churchill himself flew to Moscow in August 1942 to give Stalin the bad news: no second front in Europe until 1943. Postponed again until mid-1944, the second front became a source of festering Russian suspicion. But after an initial surge of anger over the postponement, Stalin accepted Churchill's rationale for a substitute action, a British–American invasion of North Africa set for the end of 1942. Code-named Operation Torch, the North African campaign could be mounted quickly, would bring British and American troops into direct combat with the Germans, and stood an excellent chance of succeeding. Here was an example of the personal contact that assured Allied cooperation. The alliance sometimes bent but never broke.

The Naval War in the Pacific

Despite the Allied decision to concentrate on defeating Germany first, the earliest signs of success came in the Pacific. At the Battle of Coral Sea in May 1942 planes from the aircraft carriers *Yorktown* and *Lexington* stopped a large Japanese invading force headed for Port Moresby in New Guinea. For the first time in history two fleets fought without seeing each other. The age of naval aviation had arrived. The Japanese fleet actually inflicted greater damage but decided to turn back to nurse its wounds. Had they captured Port Moresby, the Japanese could have severed Allied shipping routes to Australia.

A daring bit of Allied showmanship led the Japanese High Command into the decisive battle of the Pacific war. Desperate for some good war news, President Roosevelt had urged the Joint Chiefs to bomb the Japanese home islands as soon as possible. On April 18, 1942, sixteen Army B-25 bombers rolled off the deck of the navy aircraft carrier *Hornet*. All of them bombed Tokyo before crash landing along the China coast. The "Doolittle raid," named for its commander, Colonel James Doolittle, inflicted only slight physical damage but humiliated the Japanese army and navy. To extend Japan's defenses, Admiral Yamamoto ordered the capture of Midway, a small island guarding the approach to Hawaii.

The Americans, in possession of decoded Japanese transmissions, were ready. On June 3, as the Japanese main fleet bore down on Midway, a patrol plane from the American carrier task force spotted smoke from the ships. Caught between attacks on Midway, the Japanese were not fully prepared to defend themselves. Planes from the carriers *Hornet*, *Enterprise*, and *Yorktown* sank four enemy carriers, a cruiser, and three destroyers. The United States lost only the *Yorktown*. More important, the Japanese lost many of their best carrier pilots, who were more difficult to replace than planes. The Battle of Midway broke Japanese naval supremacy in the Pacific and stalled Japan's offensive. In August 1942 American forces launched their first offensive—on the Solomon Islands, east of New Guinea. With the landing of American marines on the key island of Guadalcanal, the Allies started on the bloody road to Japan and victory.

Turning Points in Europe

By the fall of 1942 the Allies were seeing successes in the European war. Erwin Rommel's Afrika Korps had pushed as far east as El Alamein, 75 miles from the port of Alexandria, by July 1, 1942, but the Germans were too exhausted to move

U.S. marines stage an amphibious landing at Tarawa. On this 300-acre island in the Gilberts, west of Hawaii, 4700 Japanese troops had built a complex chain of fortifications. Just reaching the beach and crossing it, the marines suffered 1500 deaths or injuries. By the time the Japanese surrendered, all but 17 Japanese and almost 1000 Americans had died, with over 2000 wounded.

farther. Rather than follow up Rommel's successes, Hitler sent reinforcements to the Russian front to buoy a collapsing situation. On October 24 British forces under General Bernard Montgomery counterattacked. With bagpipes skirling in the night, Montgomery's forces broke through Rommel's lines. Weeks later, the Allies' Operation Torch, Churchill's second-front invasion of North Africa, began, under the command of General Dwight D. Eisenhower, with attacks at Oran and Algiers in Algeria and Casablanca in Morocco. An American defeat in February 1943 at the Kasserine Pass in Tunisia was followed by a string of victories under General George S. Patton. By May 1943 Rommel had fled from North Africa, abandoning 300,000 German troops.

Success in North Africa provided a stirring complement to the dogged Russian stand at Stalingrad. From August 1942 until February 1943 Axis and Soviet armies, each with over a million troops, fought one of the bloodiest engagements in history. Each side suffered more casualties than the Americans did during the entire war. When it was over, the Russian lines had held. The Germans lost an army and their momentum; Stalin's forces went on the offensive, moving south and west through the Ukraine toward Poland and Romania. By the fall of 1942 the Allies had also gained the edge in the war for the Atlantic. Boatyards launched record tonnages of new ships. Improved air patrols, new convoy systems, and better antisubmarine weapons—such as improved depth charges and sonar, which located submerged vessels by bouncing sound waves off them—helped sink 785 out of the nearly 1200 U-boats the Germans built. Success in the North Atlantic allowed troops and supplies to reach Europe and Stalin's beleaguered forces.

THOSE WHO FOUGHT

World War II opened a new world to its combatants. Nineteen-year-olds who had never left home found themselves swept off to Europe or the South Pacific. Many of them looked forward to combat. "I was going to gain my manhood," recalled one soldier. But combat soon hardened such troops. The same soldier, after taking part in an assault on the French coast, concluded that war was "a nightmare." Looking at newly arrived troops, he now had but one thought: "You poor innocents." Only a feeling of camaraderie sustained him, a "special sense of kinship," he called it. "The reason you storm the beaches," he said, "is not patriotism or bravery. It's that sense of not wanting to fail your buddies."

War brought together Americans from all regions, social classes, and ethnic backgrounds. It afforded women and minorities a chance to dispel many stereotypes. Soldiers were subjected to regimentation, hierarchy, and obedience—all unnatural to civilians living in a democracy. The regimentation was necessary because a successful global war required coordination from the platoon on the battlefield to the high commands in Washington, from the farms and shop floors to the executive offices of large corporations and government bureaucracies. Mobilization for war had its benefits. For one, rapid expansion of the economy finally brought an end to the Depression.

The Wartime Military Branches

The military services had been out of favor during the interwar years. Congress denied the military enough funds even to maintain adequate supplies and modern equipment. Generals and admirals spent most of their time in bitter interservice rivalry for greater shares of restricted budgets. With low pay and little chance for advancement, many able officers left. Leadership became stagnant. Success often resulted from skill at bridge or golf rather than military command.

With the outbreak of war in Europe, military spending in the United States rose rapidly. The president mobilized the National Guard and won approval of a peacetime draft. When Pearl Harbor came, the army had 1.6 million men in uniform. By 1945 it had over 7 million, the navy 3.9 million, the army air corps 2.3 million, and the marines 600,000. Increases in size and equipment transformed the services into huge organizations. The navy, for example, opened the war with 4500 vessels, including 17 battleships, 7 large carriers, and 18 heavy cruisers. By the time peace came, there were 91,000 vessels of various sizes. The army air corps had 9000 planes in 1941 but only 1100 fit for combat. By 1945 its pilots flew over 72,000 planes.

A revised draft law enabled the military to take men between the ages of 20 and 44 for a term that lasted until the war ended. A later amendment limited the

As the United States prepared for war the military found itself desperately short of equipment. Here a plank laid over a wooden tripod served trainees as a substitute field gun. Such shortages lasted until the nation converted its industry to full-time war production.

upper age to 38 and reduced the lower to 18. By 1945 some 31 million American males had registered for the draft. Out of that pool nearly 10 million were inducted. Another 5.3 million men and women volunteered. Over 200,000 women joined the auxiliary branches of the services. Minorities enlisted in unusually large numbers because the military offered training and opportunities unavailable in civilian life.

Once drafted or enlisted, many Americans traveled far from home for the first time. One young soldier who had never been outside of the Midwest wrote, "I was absolutely bowled over by Europe, the castles, the cathedrals, the Alps. It was wonderment." By 1943 the army provided temporary housing for 5 million people in all parts of the country. The average soldier had about a year's worth of training: 13 weeks of "basic," 26 weeks of advanced training with an assigned division, and a final 13 weeks under simulated combat conditions. Even if they had worked in factories, young Americans were unprepared for the regimentation, limits on their personal freedom, and loss of individual identity imposed by military life. They had to adopt new habits: regular hours, three meals a day, and personal hygiene, including the army haircut.

Griping about shared indignities and incompetent leaders became a reflex. Many boys grew homesick, yet for most young men the military opened new regional, social, and ethnic horizons. "The first time I ever heard a New England accent," said a midwesterner, "was at Fort Benning. The southerner was an exotic creature to me. The people from the farms. The New York street smarts." More than any other social institution the military acted as a melting pot. It also offered educational opportunities and job skills or suggested the need for them. "I could be a technical sergeant only I haven't had enough school," reported one Navaho soldier in a letter home to New Mexico. "Make my little brother go to school even if you have to lasso him." Not all that soldiers and sailors learned was of redeeming

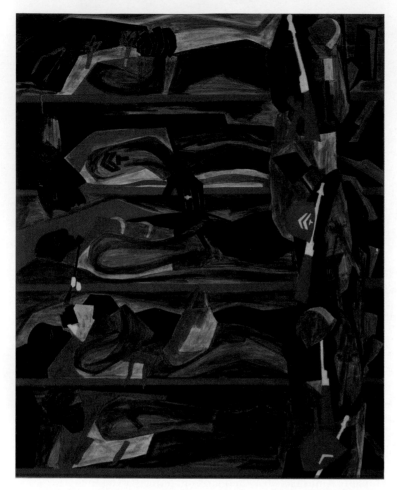

In *Shipping Out* black artist Jacob Lawrence, a veteran of the New Deal's Federal Arts Project, commemorated black troops heading overseas in the crowded confines of a troop ship. African-Americans served in segregated units more often in service roles than in combat. It was ironic that, in a war against Nazi racism, race remained a central issue among Americans.

value. Gambling, prostitution, drinking, and thievery were as much a part of military life as spit and polish and close-order drill.

Prejudice against blacks and other minorities carried over from civilian life. The army was strictly segregated and generally assigned blacks to noncombatant roles as cargo handlers, laborers, or mess personnel. The navy accepted them only as cooks and servants. At first the air corps and marines would not take them at all. In time leaders of the black community pressured the military to ease segregation and allow black soldiers to play a more active role. The army did form some black combat units, usually with white officers, and a black air corps unit. It even promoted Colonel Benjamin O. Davis to brigadier general. The marines enlisted some blacks and found that given adequate training, effective leadership, and an opportunity, black units fought with heroism. Segregation still remained the rule. The American Red Cross even kept "black" and "white" blood plasma separated, as if there were a difference.

Sometimes racial tensions led to open fighting between black and white troops. More common was the anguish suffered by a group of blacks stationed in Salina, Kansas. One day the owner of a restaurant blocked their entrance: "You boys know we don't serve colored here." They knew, of course; no place in town served blacks. But from the doorway, they stared in disbelief as lunch was served to German prisoners of war. "If we were *Untermenschen* in Nazi Germany," said one of the black soldiers, "they would break our bones. As 'colored' men in Salina, they only break our hearts." Despite the persistence of such prejudices, over a million black men and women served during the war.

Women at War

World War II brought an end to the military as an exclusive male enclave that women entered only as nurses. During the prewar mobilization, Eleanor Roosevelt and other women leaders had campaigned for a regular military organization for women. The War Department came up with a compromise that allowed women to be "in the army but not of it," as one observer noted. The Women's Army Auxiliary Corps (WAAC) brought women into the army but with inferior status and lower pay. By 1943 the "Auxiliary" had dropped out of the title: WAACs became WACs, with full army status, equal ranks, and equal pay. (The navy had a similar force called the WAVEs.)

Women could look with a mixture of pride and resentment on their wartime military service. Thousands served close to the battlefields, where they labored as technicians, mechanics, radio operators, postal clerks, and secretaries. While filling a vital need, these were largely traditional female jobs that implied a separate and inferior status. Until 1944 women were prevented by law from serving in war zones, even as noncombatants. There were women flyers, but they were restricted to shuttling planes behind the lines. WAVEs and WACs had limited social opportunities. While on duty their lives were heavily regulated. At many posts they lived behind barbed wire and could move about only in groups under armed escort.

Over There

Service in the military did not necessarily mean fighting in the war. The army used almost 2 million soldiers just to move supplies. In the Pacific theater only one enlisted man in three and two of five officers actually saw combat. Most battles were reasonably short, followed by long periods of waiting and preparation. One army division was in action for only one month in a year and a half. Soldiers in the European theater stayed longer on the front lines, often several months in a row. On the other hand, they usually spent less time overseas and had safer rear-area bases and healthier recreational facilities than those elsewhere.

In the Pacific conditions barely improved when soldiers left the front lines. Enemies stalked them everywhere. Dysentery, typhus, and even plague were as dangerous as the Japanese. On many days the thermometer rose over 110 degrees Fahrenheit. Most personnel lived in dirt-floored tents without screens, and disease-bearing insects took a heavy toll. Over 40 percent of all infantry soldiers in the Pacific were treated at least once for malaria. Showers were rare; fresh food was rarer still. The average soldier ate canned foods, called "K-rations," which were long on calories and short on flavor. One marine claimed that during his two years in the Pacific he had seen fresh eggs less than five times.

Wherever they fought, American soldiers usually lived in foxholes dug by hand with small shovels. Whenever possible they turned a hole in the ground into a home. "The American soldier is a born housewife," observed war correspondent Ernie Pyle. No sooner did a soldier settle in than he tried to tidy his makeshift home for visitors. Between battles, movies were about the only entertainment many troops had. Each film was a tenuous link to a more comfortable world at home, a place American soldiers yearned for with special intensity. It was not a country or an idea for which they fought so much as a set of memories—a house with a green lawn, a car, Mom and Pop, and a slice of pie.

As with most wars, the infantry bore the brunt of the fighting and dying. They suffered 90 percent of the battlefield casualties. World War II at least brought great advances in the treatment of wounds. Innovations such as the Mobile Auxiliary Surgical Hospital (MASH) and air evacuation saved countless lives. The use of antibiotics and improved treatment of the wounded saved many who would have died. Yet war is ultimately a bloody business. Almost 400,000 Americans died and over 600,000 were wounded before the war ended.

Science Goes to War

Before American entry into the war, British and American cryptographers, using advanced communications technologies, had cracked both the German and Japanese secret codes, gaining access to war plans and enabling the Allies to anticipate Axis troop movements. That was just one way in which scientists demonstrated their importance to the war effort. Some American scientists warned that failure to keep pace with enemy advances could prove fatal. In June 1941 Roosevelt appointed Vannevar Bush head of the Office of Scientific Research and Development (OSRD). Its mission was to organize the scientific community for war. Bush brought together scientists and engineers from private industry, universities, and the military as well as émigré scientists who had fled to the United States to escape fascism. For the first time America became an international center of scientific research.

Early reversals in the war revealed defects in the equipment and strategic thinking of Allied forces. The success of aircraft against battleships spelled the end of an era in naval warfare. The aircraft carrier and the submarine would become the keys to naval supremacy. The Battle of Britain and the European air war spurred the development of a new generation of fighter planes and long-range bombers. To combat enemy bombers and submarines, English and American scientists rushed to perfect electronic detection devices such as radar and sonar.

While sonar was helping to win the submarine war in the North Atlantic, American submarines were wreaking their own devastation on Japanese shipping in the Pacific. By 1944 the home islands faced serious shortages of vital raw materials. Of the 8 million tons of shipping with which Japan entered the war, American submarines sent 5 million to the bottom of the sea by late 1944. Above the water, the newly developed techniques of radar-controlled naval and antiaircraft gunnery gave American ships a decided edge in crucial sea battles. It was possible to hit targets obscured by darkness, fog, or smoke. One of the most crucial technical advances was also one of the best kept secrets of the war, the proximity fuse. By placing a small radio device in a warhead, scientists created a shell that did not need to hit a target to destroy it. Use of the proximity fuse accounted for the success of American antiaircraft guns against Japanese planes and German V-1 bombs.

Scientific advances saved lives as well as destroying them. New techniques for using blood plasma and whole blood meant that more wounded soldiers could survive. Insecticides, pesticides, and drugs limited the spread of infectious diseases like malaria and syphilis, which are often more deadly than bullets. Penicillin had its first widespread use in World War II. The health of the nation actually improved during the war. Life expectancy rose by three years overall (five years for blacks). Infant mortality was cut by more than a third, and in 1942 the nation recorded its lowest death rate in history.

Science sometimes proved a two-edged sword. The pesticide DDT helped to control malaria and other diseases that are spread by insects. Only later did DDT's dangerous ecological consequences become apparent. Some advances had long-term benefits not fully clear until after the war. In figuring out how to break codes, find submarines, or hit targets from high altitudes, mathematicians often had to deal with complex calculations. To speed their work, engineers designed new machines to manipulate numbers at great speed. Thus the war ushered in the Computer Age.

So, too, did it bring on the Atomic Age. In 1938 German scientists discovered the process of atomic fission: when bombarded by atomic particles, atoms of uranium-235 split, releasing an enormous amount of energy. If properly harnessed, fission could furnish the power to run great cities or the bombs to destroy them. Emigré scientists like Enrico Fermi, Albert Einstein, and Leo Szilard understood all too well the military potential of the German discovery. In 1939 they had alerted President Roosevelt to the possibility that the Nazis were developing atomic weapons. He ordered OSRD to make atomic fission research a top priority. Within a few years over 100,000 scientists, engineers, technicians, and support workers from the United States, Canada, and England at 37 installations across the country were engaged in the largest research and development effort in history, code-named the Manhattan Project.

Atomic bomb development was one of the most tightly guarded secrets of the war. Security was designed to keep the Russians as much as the Germans or Japanese in the dark. Roosevelt and Churchill did not intend to share their atomic monopoly with friend or foe, despite the urging of the respected Danish physicist Niels Bohr, who feared that a lack of international agreement would lead to an arms race. The key to success was not so much secret discoveries, but money (the project cost $2 billion) and industrial, scientific, and technical resources to produce nuclear fuels and a bomb design.

Total War

Under the new conditions of war, air power became crucial to many battles. Control of the air was necessary for amphibious operations as well as for traditional land warfare. Planes could disrupt troop movements, break supply lines, spot enemy formations, and attack defensive fortifications. Air-power strategists had a more aggressive vision for heavy bombers. Large waves of planes could attack industrial and military targets deep in enemy territory, devastate the home front, and cripple the enemy war effort. The first test of such "strategic bombing" came in 1942, when 1134 planes of the British Royal Air Force (RAF) destroyed some

20,000 homes, 1500 stores and offices, and about 60 factories around Cologne, Germany. Horrific as that sounds, the attack did not level the city, as RAF planners had predicted. Indeed, later studies indicated that for all the damage done, strategic bombing did not substantially reduce Axis productivity, which actually increased until the last months of the war. Still, it disrupted Japanese and German industry, brought the war home to the civilian population, and diverted enemy forces from the front to home defense.

Raids on Dresden and on Tokyo symbolized the horrors of the new technology. Dresden, a charming German city almost untouched by the twentieth century, had been largely ignored until February 1945. The RAF hit it first; then, with fires still raging, the American bombing wave struck. A huge inferno drew all the oxygen out of the center city, so that victims who did not burn suffocated. The city and its 60,000 people died. In March 340 American bombers hit Tokyo with incendiary bombs. The resulting "firestorms," whipped by strong winds, leveled 16 square miles, destroyed 267,000 homes, left 83,000 dead, and injured 41,000. The heat was so intense that the water in canals boiled. With long-range air power the traditional "front line" vanished. Everyone became a potential combatant, every village a potential target in a total war.

D-Day and the Fall of the Third Reich

After driving the Germans from North Africa in May 1943, Allied strategists yielded to Churchill's plan to slice into the "soft underbelly of the Axis" by invading Italy through Sicily. Late in July, two weeks after a quarter of a million British and American troops had landed on Sicily, Mussolini fled to German-held northern Italy. Although Italy surrendered early in September, Germany continued to pour in reinforcements. It took the Allies almost a year of bloody fighting to get to Rome, and at the end of the war they had yet to break German lines. Along the eastern front, Soviet armies steadily pushed the Germans out of Russia and back toward Berlin.

In January 1944 General Dwight D. Eisenhower, fresh from battle in North Africa and the Mediterranean, took command of the massive Allied preparations for Operation Overlord, the cross-Channel invasion of the continent. By June all attention focused on the coast of France, for Hitler, of course, knew the Allies were approaching. He suspected they would hit Calais, the French port city closest to the British Isles. Allied planners did their best to convince the Germans that was their plan, even placing fake armaments across the English Channel. On the morning of June 6, 1944, the invasion began—not at Calais but on the less well-fortified beaches of Normandy. Almost 3 million men, 11,000 aircraft, and over 2000 vessels took part in the D-Day operation.

As Allied forces hit the beaches, luck and Eisenhower's meticulous planning favored their cause. German attempts to defeat airborne troops, dropped by parachute behind coastal defenses, left Utah beach lightly defended. Persuaded the Allies still wanted Calais, Hitler delayed the movement of two reserve divisions. His indecision allowed the Allied forces to secure a foothold. Over the next few days more than 1.5 million soldiers landed on the beaches—but they still had to move inland. The hedgerows that separated the fields of frugal Norman farmers provided the Germans with effective barriers against troops and tanks. The Allied advance from Normandy took almost two months, not several weeks as expected.

The complicated logistics of maintaining supply lines were as important as the heroics of troops during the D-Day invasion. Like Ulysses Grant during the Civil War, Dwight Eisenhower was a master of such details.

Once Allied tanks broke through German lines their progress was spectacular. In August Paris was liberated, and by mid-September the Allies had driven the Germans from France and Belgium.

All went well until December 1944, when Allied forces under General Omar N. Bradley stalled in the Ardennes Forest because of fuel shortages. Hitler, risking one last, desperate gamble, threw in his reserves on December 16, 1944. The Germans succeeded in pushing back the Allied lines along a 50-mile bulge toward Bastogne. There the Germans trapped the 101st Airborne Division. When asked to surrender, General Tony MacAuliffe sent back a one-word reply: "Nuts!" His troops held, General George Patton raced to the rescue, and the last German offensive collapsed. The Battle of the Bulge, as it was called, delayed the Allied invasion of Germany by six weeks, but Hitler lost 200,000 men and 600 tanks he could not replace. Little stood between the Allies and Berlin.

Two Roads to Tokyo

In the Pacific, American forces defied the conventional military wisdom. Instead of concentrating military force against a weak point in enemy lines, the American forces were split into two campaigns. The navy favored the tactic of leapfrogging from island to enemy-held island, using amphibious warfare conducted by naval forces and marines. Army General Douglas MacArthur argued for recapturing the Philippines as a staging area for the liberation of China and the invasion of Japan. In the bleak days of 1942 MacArthur—flamboyant and jaunty with his dark sunglasses and corncob pipe—had emerged (with the help of his public relations

Daily Lives

TIME AND TRAVEL

Air Power Shrinks the Globe

War has always been a great accelerator of social change, often in unanticipated ways. So World War II advances in air power and strategic bombing eventually changed the international order. In the short term, both the Allied and Axis powers hoped to use aircraft to damage enemy resources and morale in order to bring about surrender. But the new tactics for accomplishing this goal led to the development of missiles and long-range bombers, whose ultimate consequences included shrinking the effective distances between nations and even realigning international relations.

During World War I, airplanes had played only a secondary role in military strategy. While the popular imagination thrilled to the stories of dogfights and "flying aces," relatively primitive airplanes were hampered by short flying ranges and an inability to carry heavy loads. Between the two wars, airframes grew stronger, engines more powerful, and payloads greater. Air-power strategists began to suggest that concerted waves of planes could attack industrial and military targets deep in enemy territory, which before had remained safe unless ground troops had fought their way overland to reach them. Hitler grasped the strategic possibilities and insisted that Germany's air force as well as its army rearm and modernize.

Once Hitler's bold offensive had subdued France in the opening moves of the war, Air Marshal Herman Goering predicted that bombers from the German *Luftwaffe* would soon bring England to its knees. The Battle of Britain, fought during the winter of 1940–1941, signaled the start of the age of modern air warfare. For the first time in history, one nation tried to conquer another from the skies. Goering's boast failed; England continued doggedly to resist, demonstrating that air-power theorists had exaggerated the potentials of strategic bombing. And while Allied bombing contributed to victory, it succeeded largely through the sustained pattern of destructiveness, not from any startling technological innovation. In the last year of the war heavy bombers dropped almost 2 million tons of bombs on Germany alone, three times as much as in the previous four years.

To ensure the success of aerial warfare, aircraft designers on both sides had to make their planes bigger and faster. On the first major raid the English launched, they used the Wellington bomber, a plane 65 feet long with a wing span of 86 feet and a bomb load of 1500 pounds. By contrast, the B-29s that bombed Hiroshima and Nagasaki only three years later were some 99 feet long, with a wing span of 141 feet and a capacity of up to 10 tons. The Wellington flew 255 miles an hour and cruised as high as 12,000 feet, with a range of 2200 miles, whereas the new B-29s could travel over 350 miles an hour, at altitudes up to 30,000 feet, with a range of up to 5000 miles—more than double the Wellington's. During these same years, German scientists looked to increase the speed and range of their weaponry with a new V-1 pilotless "buzz bomb" (named for the sound of its jet engine) and the V-2 rocket, the first true missile used as a weapon. Launched from bases in Europe, V-1's and V-2's easily reached targets in England. For all the terror they inspired, however, they were not accurate and the Germans could not launch them in sufficient quantities to mount a decisive threat.

Germany and Britain also rushed to produce the first fighter planes with jet

Daily Lives

The Boeing Stratocruiser was a modified version of the B-29 that carried atomic bombs to Hiroshima and Nagasaki. As a commercial airliner, it made transatlantic travel a practical reality by virtue of its range and carrying capacity.

engines. Hitler foolishly insisted on using Germany's jets as bombers—where sheer speed was not essential—rather than as fast interceptors, which would have given German pilots an edge in air combat. Too few were produced to make a real difference, and technical problems made the new "rocket" planes as dangerous to their pilots as the enemy. Similarly, the Japanese had designed a piloted "rocket bomb" that could race on its suicidal mission at over 500 miles an hour. None ever hit an Allied ship.

Although these technologies proved indecisive in the war, the competition to create longer range aircraft capable of carrying heavier payloads led to far-reaching changes in the postwar world. With some modifications the B-29 bomber was reborn as the Boeing Stratocruiser, capable of carrying over 80 passengers from the United States to Europe without stopping to refuel. The British, having pioneered jet propulsion, introduced by 1952 the first commercial jet airliner, the De Havilland Comet. By 1955, when Boeing introduced its 707 jet, 200 passengers could be carried up to 4000 miles at 550 miles an hour. It was now possible to work in both New York and Los Angeles on the same day. Cheap flights from Puerto Rico to New York encouraged hundreds of thousands of Hispanic immigrants to come to the continental United States. Travel to Europe, Hawaii, or the Orient was no longer restricted to the very rich.

Equally significant, the technology of air power encouraged a fundamental change in most Americans' perception of the world. In 1919, at the end of World War I, Americans were determined not to become involved again in the affairs of Europe. Between the wars Arthur Vandenberg, a Republican senator from Michigan, was one of the nation's leading isolationists. That was before Pearl Harbor and before Vandenberg visited London during the war. As German V-1 and V-2 missiles brought terror from the skies, the senator came to believe that an isolationist policy no longer made sense. Physical distance would never again be a safeguard from attack, because air power had reshaped the strategic map of the world. The United States was now a matter of hours, not days, away from both friends and potential enemies.

officers) as America's only military hero. To refuse him command would erode public faith in the war effort. For that reason the Combined Chiefs of Staff had given him control of the southwestern Pacific. MacArthur believed the future of America lay in the Far East and that the Pacific theater, not the European, should have top priority. He warred constantly with his superiors in Washington, complaining that they were scheming to deny him troops and supplies. In March 1943 the military chiefs agreed to his plan for a westward advance along the northern coast of New Guinea toward the Philippines and Tokyo.

By July 1944 the navy's leapfrogging campaign had reached the Marianas, east of the Philippines. From there B-29 bombers could reach the Japanese home islands. As a result, Admiral Chester W. Nimitz, commander of the Pacific Fleet, proposed bypassing the Philippines in favor of a direct attack on Formosa (now Taiwan). MacArthur, outraged, accused the U.S. Joint Chiefs of Staff and the president of breaking a promise he had made "to eighteen million Christian Filipinos that the Americans would return." President Roosevelt himself came to Hawaii to resolve the impasse between Nimitz and MacArthur, giving MacArthur the green light. Backed by over 100 ships of the Pacific Fleet, MacArthur splashed ashore on the island of Leyte in October 1944 to announce his return.

The decision to invade the Philippines led to savage fighting until the war ended. As the retreating Japanese armies left Manila, they tortured and slaughtered tens of thousands of Filipino civilians. The United States suffered 62,000 casualties redeeming MacArthur's pledge to return. A spectacular U.S. Navy victory at the Battle of Leyte Gulf spelled the end of the Japanese Imperial Navy as a fighting force.

WAR AND DIPLOMACY

The coordination of Russian, British, and American efforts in far-flung theaters of war went beyond military strategy. The Allies had to negotiate constantly in order to set supply priorities, choose commanders in combined operations, and divide and administer conquered territories. Inevitably, the questions of war slid into questions about the peace that would follow. What would happen to occupied territories? How would the Axis powers be punished? After World War I the powers of Europe met at Versailles to mete out justice, peace, and a stable world order. Those dreams had collapsed in a mere 20 years; now millions more were dead. The peace had to be won as well as the war. If not, the cycle of violence might never end.

War Aims

Although Roosevelt and Churchill had spelled out their war aims in the Atlantic Charter of 1941, the Allies did not necessarily accept all its provisions. Churchill himself had reservations about the principle of self-determination. It was all very well for restive colonials to be given a greater voice in their own affairs, he argued, but he had "not become the King's First Minister to preside over the liquidation of the British Empire." Churchill also believed that only a stable European balance of power, not an international agency, could preserve peace. In his view the

Soviet Union was the greatest threat to postwar peace, and so he courted the United States as a counterweight.

Suspicious of the capitalist powers, Premier Joseph Stalin seemed unwilling to trust Russian security to their goodwill or to an international body. He left no doubt that the Soviet Union would ignore the Atlantic Charter whenever it conflicted with Soviet interests. An expansive notion of Russian security defined his war aims. Twice in the last 20 years Germany had marched through eastern Europe to invade Russia, and expelling them during this latest drive cost the Soviet Union some 20 million people—nearly 8 percent of its population. (By contrast the United States lost less than 0.5 percent of its population.) For future protection Stalin expected to annex the Baltic states, once Russian provinces, along with bits of Finland and Romania and about half of prewar Poland. In eastern Europe and other border areas such as Iran, Korea, and Turkey, he wanted "friendly" neighbors. It soon became apparent that "friendly" meant regimes subservient to Moscow. As for Asia, Stalin hoped to drive Japan off the mainland and return Russia to the position it had held under the czars.

The kind of peace Franklin Roosevelt sought was unclear. He opposed Churchill's balance of power plan and did not share his almost obsessive distrust of Russia. At the same time, he wished to allay Stalin's suspicions and bring the Soviet Union into an international peacekeeping system. Early on, Roosevelt promoted his own balance of power, which he called the "Four Policemen." The Soviet Union, Great Britain, the United States, and China would guarantee peace through military cooperation. The concept was badly flawed. China was hardly a great power and could not keep peace in Asia; Roosevelt had included it only because he wanted an international order, not an exclusively Western one. Furthermore, the Four Policemen did not involve a major continental power aside from the Soviet Union. The security of Europe would rest on Stalin's cooperation. Finally, smaller countries, largely pawns in this system, might not take kindly to the four cops patrolling the beat.

By 1944 Roosevelt had discarded the Four Policemen in favor of an international organization based on a new League of Nations. Having served under Woodrow Wilson in World War I, Roosevelt shared his internationalism and particularly his faith in collective security. Equally important, a broad spectrum of influential Americans wanted to resurrect the League. This time, however, all the great powers would participate, including the United States. Whether Churchill and Stalin—or the American people as a whole—would accept the idea was not yet clear.

The Road to Yalta

The outlines of a postwar settlement—and the sticking points where a settlement was most unlikely—were worked out in a series of summit conferences of the Allied leaders. In January 1943, with Rommel on the defensive in North Africa and Morocco newly liberated, President Roosevelt met Winston Churchill at Casablanca. Stalin had not come; he never left Soviet-occupied territory. He was angry about the delay of a second front in the west and worried that the Americans and British might make a separate peace with Germany, leaving the Soviet Union alone to continue the war. To reassure him, Roosevelt announced with Churchill's blessings that the war would end only with the "unconditional surrender" of all enemies. Just what that meant was not always clear, even to Roosevelt.

By November Italy's surrender was in hand, the war against Germany was going well, and Churchill and Roosevelt agreed to make the hazardous trip to Teheran, Iran, so the Big Three could meet for the first time. Here each leader had a chance to take the personal measure of the other. ("Seems very confident," Roosevelt said of Stalin, "very sure of himself, moves slowly—altogether quite impressive.") The president used the occasion to work his considerable charm on Stalin, teasing Churchill for Stalin's benefit, keeping it up "until Stalin was laughing with me, and it was then that I called him 'Uncle Joe.'" Stalin finally won the commitment to the D-Day operation he had so long been seeking; in return he promised to launch a spring offensive to prevent the transfer of German troops to the west. He also reaffirmed the earlier Russian pledge to join the war against Japan once Germany was beaten. In the matter of winning the war, the Allies hammered together a united front. Teheran was the high point of cooperation among the Big Three.

There had been differences, however, most significantly over the postwar peace rather than the conduct of the war. How large these differences were became clearer in February 1945, at the final meeting of the Big Three, at the Russian resort city of Yalta, located on the Black Sea. By then, Russian, British, and American troops were all closing in on Germany. Roosevelt arrived tired, ashen. The trip to Yalta would have taxed the resources of a robust young man, and Roosevelt was neither youthful nor healthy. At 62, limited by his paralysis, he also suffered from heart disease, hypertension, and hardening of the arteries. His doctors had urged him to follow a less demanding schedule and he listened patiently, then ignored their advice, keeping to his busy schedule without reducing his consumption of cigarettes and cocktails. And he was mindful that although Germany was all but beaten, Japan still held out in the Pacific. Under no circumstances did he want Stalin to withdraw his promises to enter the fight against Japan or to join a postwar international organization.

Churchill, for his part, arrived at Yalta profoundly mistrustful of Soviet intentions. As Germany and Japan disintegrated, he saw vacuums of power opening up in Europe and Asia, which the Russians appeared only too eager and able to fill. Most diplomats in the American State Department and a growing number of military officers and politicians agreed. It seemed to them that Britain and the United States needed to work together to rein in Soviet ambitions. The problem was particularly evident in the disagreements over Poland, raised at first during the Teheran Conference. Hitler's invasion of Poland had touched off the war, and Britain fought in part to ensure the survival of an independent Polish state.

Stalin, on the other hand, saw Poland as the historic corridor of invasion for Russia's enemies. As Soviet troops reentered Poland, he insisted he would recognize only the Communist-controlled government at Lublin, whereas Britain and the United States backed an exile government in London. Stalin also demanded that Russia receive territory in eastern Poland, for which the Poles would be compensated with German lands. That was hardly the "self-determination" called for in the Atlantic Charter. Roosevelt saw that he could not force Stalin's hand, since Soviet troops occupied all of Poland. So he proposed a compromise. Poland would have a coalition government, including representatives from both Lublin and London. Free elections held after the war would settle the question of who should rule. The Soviets would also receive the territory they demanded in eastern Poland, and the western boundary would be established later.

Similarly, the Allies remained at odds about Germany's position in the postwar era. Stalin was determined that Germany would never invade Russia again. Many Americans shared his desire to have Germany punished and its war-making capacity eliminated. At the Teheran Conference, Roosevelt and Stalin proposed that the Third Reich be drastically dismembered, split into five powerless parts. In the following months Secretary of the Treasury Henry Morgenthau had even come up with a plan to dismantle German industry and limit Germany to an agrarian economy. Churchill briefly accepted the idea but then reconsidered, fearful of repeating the economic disaster that followed World War I. A healthy European economy required an industrialized Germany. And Churchill was much less eager to bring low the nation that was the most natural barrier to Russian expansion.

As with Poland, the Big Three avoided a clear definition of terms for Germany. It would be divided into separate occupation zones (France would receive a zone carved from British and American territory). Four powers would jointly occupy Berlin, while an Allied Control Council supervised the national government. Reparations became the final sticking point. Stalin insisted on $20 billion to compensate Russia for its wartime losses. He needed German resources to rebuild his own shattered economy. Churchill and Roosevelt accepted that figure only as a "basis for discussion" at a later date.

When the Big Three turned their attention to the Far East, Stalin held a trump card. Fierce Japanese resistance on Okinawa and Iwo Jima, where American casualties exceeded 70,000, plus the horror of kamikaze attacks, persuaded Roosevelt that only a bloody invasion of the home islands could force Japan to surrender. He came to Yalta determined to win Stalin's agreement to enter the Pacific war at the earliest date. Many British and Americans feared Stalin would wait until the invasion of Japan before sending his troops into Manchuria to reap the fruits of victory. Instead Stalin agreed to declare war within three months of Germany's defeat, but his price was high. Stalin wanted to reclaim Russia's losses in the Russo-Japanese War of 1904–1906: renewed control of the Kuril Islands and the island of Sakhalin, the port of Darien, and control over the Chinese Eastern and South Manchurian railroads. Although Stalin had been supporting the Communist forces under Mao Tse-tung, in return for the Allied concessions in Asia he was willing to sign a friendship pact with Chiang Kai-shek's nationalist government.

The agreement on China, like all the agreements reached at Yalta, depended on Stalin's willingness to cooperate, in this case with Chiang. In public Roosevelt put the best possible face on what Allied leaders had achieved. A new world organization would "provide the greatest opportunity in all history" to secure the peace. And as if to lay to rest the specter of isolation that had destroyed Wilson's dream, Roosevelt told Congress, "We shall take responsibility for world collaboration, or we shall have to bear the responsibility for another world conflict." Privately Roosevelt was less sanguine. He told his friend Sam Rosenman as they worked on his speech to Congress that he doubted, "when the chips were down, Stalin would be able to carry out and deliver what he had agreed to."

The Fallen Leader

The Yalta Conference marked one of the last and most controversial chapters of Franklin Roosevelt's presidency. Critics charged that the concessions to Stalin had been too generous—a violation of Atlantic Charter principles and a threat to

American national interests. Poland had been betrayed; China sold out; the United Nations crippled at birth. Those critics offered various explanations for the president's failures: his ill health, his naiveté, his hubris, even communist infiltration of his entourage.

Yalta was no "sellout"; it was a diplomatic success for Russia based on its military role in Europe. Roosevelt conceded little that Stalin could not have taken for himself. By 1945, after four years of bloody sacrifice, Soviet troops controlled most of eastern Europe. The president had come to Yalta with two goals. Above all he wanted to guarantee Soviet entry into the Pacific war. That he achieved (though the successful development of the atom bomb would change the significance of Stalin's declaration of war). Second, Roosevelt hoped that Stalin would honor the spirit of the Yalta pledges by holding free elections and promoting self-determination in areas liberated by Russian armies. Even Winston Churchill, an outspoken critic of Soviet ambitions, concluded that although "our hopeful assumptions were soon to be falsified . . . they were the only ones possible at the time."

Roosevelt himself sensed the hollowness of Stalin's vows. On March 23, 1945, he told a friend, "We can't do business with Stalin. He has broken every one of the promises he made at Yalta." That did not mean that Roosevelt had lost his faith in postwar cooperation. Rather, he seemed to have decided that future deals with the Russians must involve a quid pro quo, or trade-off. In that spirit, the president had already refused to share atomic secrets or to commit the United States to financing postwar reconstruction without political concessions.

What peace Roosevelt would have achieved we can never know. He returned from Yalta visibly ill. On April 12, 1945, while sitting for his portrait at his vacation home in Warm Springs, Georgia, he complained of a "terrific headache," then suddenly fell unconscious. Two hours later Roosevelt was dead, the victim of a cerebral hemorrhage that deprived many Americans of the only president they had ever known. Not since the assassination of Lincoln had the nation been so grieved by a loss. Under Roosevelt's leadership government had become a protector, the president a father and friend, and the United States the leader in the struggle against Axis tyranny. Eleanor recalled how many Americans later told her that "they missed the way the President used to talk to them. . . . There was a real dialogue between Franklin and the people."

Franklin Roosevelt guided the nation through the deepest depression in its history and then to the verge of global greatness. The man who replaced him was Harry S. Truman. "Who the hell is Harry Truman?" the chief of staff had asked when Truman was nominated for the vice presidency in 1944. Into his untested hands now fell the awesome responsibility for victory in war and peace.

SIGNIFICANT EVENTS

1921–1922	Washington Naval Disarmament Conference
1922	Fordney–McCumber Tariff
1923	German inflation
1924	Dawes Plan
1926–1933	United States involvement in Nicaragua's internal affairs
1928	Kellogg–Briand Pact
1929	Crash signals onset of worldwide economic crisis
1930	Hawley–Smoot Tariff
1931–1932	Japan invades Manchuria; Stimson Doctrine
1933	London Economic Conference; Roosevelt recognizes the Soviet Union
1935	Nye Committee hearings; first Neutrality Act
1936	Second Neutrality Act; Buenos Aires Conference
1937	Third Neutrality Act (cash-and-carry); Roosevelt's quarantine speech; *Panay* incident
1938	Munich meeting; settlement of Mexican appropriation crisis
1939	Fall of Czechoslovakia; Molotov–Ribbentrop Pact; World War II begins in Europe
1940	Germany launches blitzkrieg against Low Countries and France; America-First Committee and Committee to Defend America by Aiding the Allies formed; Roosevelt supports preparedness and peacetime draft; destroyers-for-bases deal; Roosevelt wins third term
1941	Congress adopts Lend-Lease Act; Germany invades Soviet Union; Roosevelt and Churchill sign Atlantic Charter; Japan occupies Indochina; Roosevelt imposes embargo against Japan; Pearl Harbor attacked; Hitler and Mussolini declare war on the United States
1942	Declaration of the United Nations; submarine war in the Atlantic; Bataan and Corregidor fall; battles of Guadalcanal, Coral Sea, and Midway fought; American and British troops invade North Africa; WACs receive full status; Manhattan Project begins
1943	Churchill and Roosevelt announce unconditional surrender at Casablanca; British-American forces invade Italy; Big Three meet at Teheran
1944	D-Day invasion of France; Battle of the Bulge; U.S. forces return to Philippines; island-hopping campaign reaches Guam and Saipan; Allies invade Germany
1945	Yalta Conference; Roosevelt dies; Truman becomes president

29

War on the Home Front

I n 1940 Washington was still a sleepy provincial southern city with but one function, the operation of a national government. Unlike Paris, London, or Rome, it had no cosmopolitan glitter. It had just one legitimate theater and a hopelessly inept professional baseball team. Haute cuisine ran to the deep-fat fried. Washington's summers were so hot and steamy the British ambassadors were entitled to wear the same outfits, including pith helmets, that diplomats wore in Southeast Asia and tropical Africa. A third of the city was black, rigidly and completely segregated and except for a small middle class forced to live in slum shacks without plumbing or electricity. Young Americans eager to make their mark in the world avoided Washington. The 200,000 people with government jobs were clerks, secretaries, and bureaucrats paid to move paper, not to worry about politics and public policy.

Ten years of the New Deal had done little to shake the city out of its provincial ways. The city's small southern social elite largely ignored the army of social workers, economists, labor specialists, and lawyers who had come to town eager to heal the nation's sick economy. By 1940 New Deal efforts had shown mixed results. Some 10 million workers and about a third of all blacks were still unemployed. New Deal agencies by 1940 took little initiative beyond doling out public monies to their various constituents of poor farmers, unemployed workers, and special interest groups. Many New Dealers had left Washington once it was clear that the conservatives had frustrated the spirit of reform.

Leon Henderson was not among them. He believed that the war engulfing Europe and Asia offered an opportunity to bring new vitality to New Deal programs. As foreign war orders heated up the economy, critical raw materials needed for planes, ships, and guns went to make automobiles, radios, and toasters. Shortages, black marketeering, and inflation threatened to disrupt the recovery from 10 years of depression. Henderson had a plan to turn a motley collection of bureaucracies into an efficient government capable of managing a vast wartime economy. Even a year before Pearl Harbor, he understood that the capacity of the United States to produce war goods could spell the difference between victory and defeat. The economy needed more central direction, more planning, if it was to produce on the scale required for a global effort to defeat fascism.

Henderson's friends were not surprised that he thought in such broad terms. They considered him a brilliant, if decidedly eccentric economist. He had a volcanic temper, a midriff that overflowed his waistline, and a way of stepping on

With war industries depending so heavily on the labor of women and minorities, patriotic posters exhorted them to support the troops overseas. "WOW," ordinarily a slang term for an attractive woman, here stands for Women Ordnance Workers.

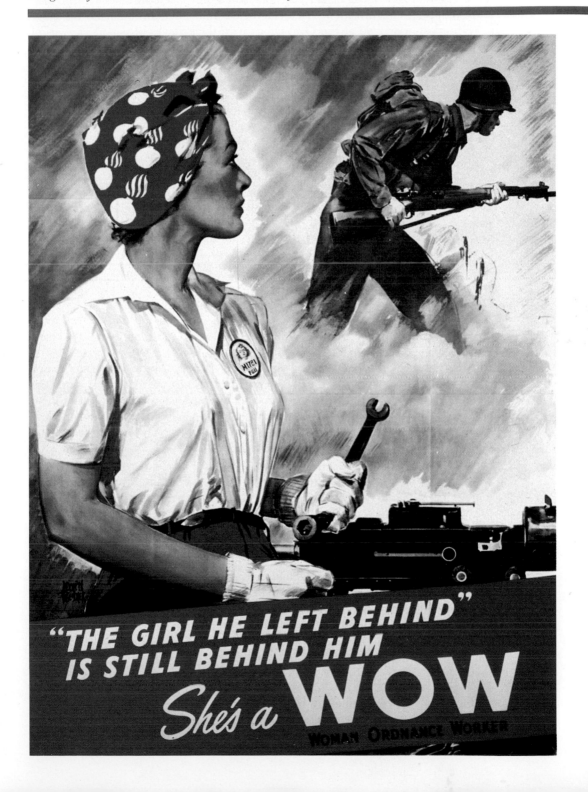

political toes that ought to have been avoided. When angered he had been known to punch taxi drivers and slam his fist through a table. Now his anger was directed at government inefficiency. To lead his attack he needed Roosevelt's full support. So he did what New Dealers had long done when they had a big headache; he took it to "Poppa." The president's secretary gave him an hour to make his case.

Henderson arrived at the Oval Office with thick stacks of papers, a swirl of graphs and charts, and a young lawyer, David Ginsburg, to help explain it all. Roosevelt took one look at the armada of paper and must have sensed the magnitude of what Henderson had in mind. So he did what he always did when confronting issues he hoped to avoid; he launched a diversionary counterattack. From his desk he produced papers of his own. These were blueprints for temporary office buildings that the president had agreed must be built along the Mall that stretched between Capitol Hill and the Washington Monument. The various defense agencies had grown so fast that the government had run out of space to house them.

Long years in government had taught Roosevelt that temporary structures, whether buildings or agencies, had a way of becoming permanent. Some of the hideous buildings thrown up during World War I were still in use. That would not happen this time, the president insisted. The "tempos" would be so ugly that nobody could want to keep them and so flimsy they would collapse in less than 10 years. What did Henderson and Ginsburg think of them, he wanted to know. For an hour the three discussed the blueprints—where the doors would go, how many floors the buildings should have, and just how ugly they might be. Henderson fidgeted as his precious hour frittered away. By the time he left, nothing had been decided, none of his questions heard or answered, and nothing done to prepare the government or the nation for war.

Roosevelt, like the nation, was simply not yet prepared to face the complex task of coordinating so vast an undertaking. He knew little and cared less about the details of copper shortages that disrupted munitions manufacturing, of railroad bottlenecks that slowed the shipment of Allied war goods, or a thousand and one other components of the emerging war economy. Only when matters became critical would he find some way to deal with them. Thus when war came, the nation had yet to transform itself into the arsenal of democracy.

The war condensed into four years social, economic, and political changes that might ordinarily take decades to achieve. With 12 million men and women in uniform, labor-hungry war factories gobbled up the jobless. Women, blacks, and Hispanics found unprecedented opportunity. Unemployment virtually disappeared. After years of depression-spawned penny-pinching, people had money again. Where war industries located, boom towns sprang up overnight. The West Coast, for example, had less than 10 percent of the population in 1940 yet it produced 20 percent of all war goods. Experts estimated that 25 to 50 years of economic growth had been squeezed into 3 years. Prefabricated houses, much like Roosevelt's tempos, appeared all over the country to contain the workers as small towns turned into cities overnight. Federal authorities ordered 42,000 units at the start of 1942 alone. Within a year they had ordered tens of thousands more. Most communities expected to tear them down once the war ended and the workers moved on.

Like other cities throughout the nation, Washington too became a boom town with prefabricated offices and housing. In the year after Pearl Harbor 70,000 people arrived; government employment grew by over 5000 people each month.

The population of the metropolitan area soared to over a million. Traffic congested the city streets at all hours of the day. New government war agencies proliferated. To the TVA and SEC were added the WPB, OPA, WMC, BEW, NWLB, FEA, and worst of all an agency that issued regulations for plumbers—the PWPGSJSISIACWPB. No one in Washington could have identified what all those initials stood for.

These agencies would not all simply disappear when the war ended. Some were reborn as postwar agencies; thus the OSS (Office of Strategic Services) became the CIA (Central Intelligence Agency). Others shifted their functions and many of their war workers to permanent agencies like the War and Navy departments. Power became more centralized in the federal government. Like government, big business, big labor, and big agriculture grew bigger still and sent their representatives to Washington to lobby for government support.

None of this happened with the kind of planning that Henderson had hoped to achieve. His own efforts to impose rationing and fight inflation as director of the Office of Price Administration mired him in endless controversy. Roosevelt dumped him in 1943. Henderson had his measure of vindication because the tempos, like so much of the largely unplanned expansion of government and big business, survived the end of the war. No matter how ugly, no matter how flimsy, they defied Roosevelt's careful attempt at planned obsolescence. Most remained in use until the 1960s, housing all those offices necessary in a government that had assumed responsibilities on a global scale. World War II had transformed Washington from a provincial southern city into the capital of the free world.

THE SINEWS OF WAR

In December 1941, within weeks of Pearl Harbor, Franklin Roosevelt announced production schedules so ambitious that few Americans believed they were possible. The president's goals staggered the imagination: 60,000 airplanes, 45,000 tanks, 20,000 antiaircraft guns, and 8 million tons of merchant shipping by the end of 1942. The figures were so astonishing partly because the shortages facing the United States were so severe. At some training bases, recruits drilled with broomsticks rather than rifles. Pilots flew training planes made of plywood. Unless the American economy expanded quickly and efficiently, the war might be lost in the factories before it could be won on the battlefields.

War Production

The process of gearing up was far from smooth. Scarred by the Depression, manufacturers resisted expanding plant capacity. Revived consumer spending encouraged production of civilian rather than military goods. Roosevelt was reluctant to make enemies of business leaders whose support he needed for war conversion. Thus he initially gave federal war agencies few of the powers Henderson envisioned. Severe bottlenecks had resulted. Electric power, steel, aluminum, railroad equipment, and skilled workers were all in short supply. The military agencies allocated scarce resources to favored producers so generously that parts, raw materials, and labor were in short supply. The key to successful conversion lay with the automobile industry, which consumed some 80 percent of the nation's rubber, 18 percent of its steel, and 14 percent of its copper. Domestic automobile sales had grown in 1941, so automakers were reluctant to convert to war production. Until they began to make badly needed tanks and planes, industrial output would lag far behind growing war demand.

In early 1942 President Roosevelt recognized the need for more direct control. He established the War Production Board (WPB) under the direction of former Sears, Roebuck president Donald M. Nelson. On paper, Nelson's powers were impressive. He was charged with responsibility for nothing less than administering the war economy. Under the Second War Powers Act of 1942 Congress gave the WPB authority to allocate resources and organize factories in whatever way promoted national defense. In one of its first acts, the WPB ordered an end to all car and truck production. Once accustomed to new models every year, the American people would now drive their present cars until the end of the war.

In practice, Nelson was scarcely the dictator the economy needed. Other federal agencies with their own czars controlled petroleum, rubber, and labor resources. Nelson also allowed the military agencies to continue their own procurement. They placed most of their orders with the largest industrial firms, with whom they had long done business. Not only did small businesses suffer, but the concentration of economic power in the hands of large corporations increased significantly. Rather than exercise controversial authority over industry, Nelson offered lucrative inducements to encourage voluntary compliance. Even then, it was not until the late spring of 1942 that the auto industry actually ceased producing cars.

By 1943 President Roosevelt realized that Nelson could not bring order out of chaos. Bottlenecks still hampered production. The president created the new Office of War Mobilization (OWM) and installed Supreme Court Justice James F. Byrnes as director. Widely respected as a political facilitator, Byrnes became the dictator the economy needed. His authority was so great and his access to Roosevelt so direct that he became known as the "assistant president." By assuming control over vital materials such as steel, aluminum, and copper, OWM allocated them on a more systematic basis. The logjams disappeared.

The Story of Rubber

The history of industrial mobilization is too complicated to tell in a short space. Every industry from transportation to petroleum to metals to agriculture had its special problems meeting the needs of war. The story of rubber is representative.

Rubber may not seem as vital as steel or gasoline, but jeeps, trucks, tanks, planes, and a host of other machines cannot function without it. Each tank required about a ton of rubber; each battleship as many as 75 tons. By 1942 war planners realized that the United States faced a crippling shortage. Before Pearl Harbor, 90 percent of raw rubber was imported from Southeast Asia. War with Japan cut off the source of supply. Prewar imports from South America amounted to only a trickle. Synthetic rubber was a possible substitute, but the United States produced only 40,000 tons in 1941, when almost a million were needed.

What had caused this shortfall, and, more important, what could be done to remedy it? Assistant Attorney General Thurman Arnold offered a shocking answer to the first question. The Standard Oil Company of New Jersey (later Exxon) had developed methods for producing a synthetic rubber called Buna-S. Standard had then entered a cartel agreement with a German chemical company, I. G. Farben, which gave Farben control over the patents. Worse yet, Standard had maintained the cartel even after Germany declared war! Once Arnold began an antitrust suit in 1942 Standard agreed to turn over the patents to the government. The delay cost crucial months in launching the synthetic rubber industry in America.

Standard Oil was not the only company exposed. Senator Harry S. Truman, head of the watchdog committee for defense industries, opened hearings on corporate collusion, while Arnold prepared antitrust cases against General Electric, Du Pont, and other major corporations with similar patent-pooling agreements. The War and Navy departments overruled him. They feared that businesses would concentrate on fighting the suits rather than producing war goods. After 1943 antitrust enforcement took a holiday.

Whatever the antitrust policies of the government, synthetic rubber would take time to produce. To supplement supplies, Roosevelt launched a drive to collect scrap rubber. He urged Americans to turn in their "old tires, old rubber raincoats, old garden hose, rubber shoes, bathing caps, [and] gloves." The president was after more than rubber. His appeal stoked the volunteer spirit that kept the nation behind the war. Whenever possible, the president preferred voluntarism to the compulsion of law. It worked. Americans surrendered over 450,000 tons of scrap in just four weeks. Even though most of it was never actually used, the drive allowed people to contribute to the war effort.

Conservation turned out to be more productive. If people drove less, they could keep their tires longer. Gasoline rationing was one way to limit auto use. But like so many good ideas, rationing offended special interests. Oil companies resisted any limit to consumption and state governors worried about the loss of revenues with reduced gasoline taxes. Unhappier still were the motorists for whom unlimited driving was linked to freedom. One party leader eager to avoid retribution from angry drivers in the 1942 congressional elections suggested that "an appeal by the President for voluntary cooperation will get patriotic support and will be politically safer." So Roosevelt created a nonpartisan committee that proposed mandatory gasoline rationing and a crash program for manufacturing synthetic rubber, which Roosevelt imposed only after the elections.

When war cut off the United States from its rubber supply in Malaysia, old tires were recycled to help meet the shortage. Most Americans were unable to replace their car tires during the four years the United States was at war. The manufacturers of synthetic rubber eventually eased the crisis.

Synthetic rubber rather than rationing finally resolved the crisis. To create this new industry, the administration made several decisions that illustrate how the war accelerated industrial consolidation. Roosevelt appointed William M. Jeffers, a business executive, as rubber director in late 1942. Jeffers, in turn, staffed his agency with executives from the rubber industry. The government then spent over $700 million to build new plants around the country. For a token fee it leased the plants to established companies, which ran them for a guaranteed profit. In addition, the industry chose to use a petroleum process for Buna-S rather than one based on grain alcohol, which American farmers supported.

By 1944 Jeffers' agency had ended the rubber shortage. The synthetic process produced some 800,000 tons of rubber, roughly 87 percent of annual need. One plant in West Virginia produced as much rubber as 20 million trees. There would be a price to pay. Synthetic production caused far more pollution than conventional methods. And after the war, the large rubber companies bought the war factories for about one-tenth of the actual cost. Companies like Goodyear and Firestone became even larger and more entrenched. The story of rubber, with both its successes and hidden costs, could be repeated for most industries.

The Miracle of Production

During World War II America worked a miracle of production as important to victory as any battle. Two years after Pearl Harbor American factories doubled the output of Germany, Italy, and Japan combined. From 1939 to 1945 the gross national product grew from $91 billion to $166 billion. (In World War I it had not changed significantly.) Manufacturing rose by 96 percent and transportation volume by 109 percent. Shipbuilding increased by almost 2000 percent. What made this possible was not only centralized planning but also massive conversion of industries, large and small. While the "Big Three"—Ford, General Motors, and Chrysler—generated some 20 percent of all war goods, small business also played a vital role. A manufacturer of model trains, for example, made bomb fuses.

Henry J. Kaiser, a California industrialist, symbolized the creative financing and management that made such an accomplishment possible. His lobbyists in Washington found him generous government loans for building factories. He also circumvented restrictions to find the steel he needed. By offering extravagant wages and benefits, including day care for the children of working mothers, he lured workers to his new shipyards, most of which were located on the West Coast. By applying assembly line techniques he reduced the time required to build cargo vessels (known as Liberty ships) from almost a year to 56 days. His yards finished one in a record 14 days. Speed had its price: Liberty ships were slow and barely seaworthy. (One of them actually split in half at its launching.) Despite an occasional misstep, Kaiser built ships in the quantity the war effort demanded.

The aircraft industry also transformed the industrial landscape of the West Coast. In 1939 aircraft factories employed about 46,000 workers and built almost 6000 planes. When production peaked in 1944, the industry had 2.1 million workers producing almost 100,000 planes. Most of the new factories were located around Los Angeles, San Diego, and Seattle, where large labor pools, temperate climates, and available land made the locations attractive.

The military relied on large, established firms in part because they had more experience producing in large volume. At the same time lucrative war contracts helped large corporations increase their dominance over the economy. In 1939 firms with over 500 employees produced just under half the nation's goods. This total had risen to 62 percent in 1944. Workers in companies with over 10,000 employees amounted to just 13 percent of the work force in 1939; by 1944 they comprised over 30 percent.

In agriculture a similar phenomenon occurred. The number of sharecroppers and tenants dropped by a third, the farm population in general by almost a fifth. Yet farm productivity increased by 30 percent. This was achieved by consolidating small farms into large ones, using more tractors, and spreading more artificial fertilizers. Large commercial farming by corporations rather than individuals (later called "agribusiness") came to dominate the agricultural sector. Its political agents in the Farm Bureau Federation guaranteed high commodity prices and a powerful voice in Washington after the war.

Almost as important as the benefits of rising wages, increased savings, and higher status were less tangible gains that came from new pride in work done for a common cause. Civilians volunteered for civil defense, hospitals, or the many scrap drives. Tiny "victory" gardens added 8 million tons of food to the harvest in 1943; car pooling conserved millions of tires; deferred consumption limited inflation. Children became "Uncle Sam's Scrappers" and "Tin-Can Colonels" as they scoured vacant lots for valuable trash. One 13-year-old in Maywood, Illinois, collected over 100 tons of paper between Pearl Harbor and D-Day. Movie stars donated their talents to sell war bonds. Morale ran high because people believed that every contribution, no matter how small, helped defeat the Axis.

WAR WORK

War production brought back prosperity, but not without stresses. Unemployment, which stood at almost 7 million in 1940, virtually disappeared by 1944. Jeff Davies, president of Hoboes of America, reported in 1942 that 2 million of his members were "off the road." In retirement communities like San Diego nearly 4 retirees in 10 returned to work. Employers, eager to overcome the labor shortage, welcomed handicapped workers. The hearing impaired found jobs in deafening factories; dwarfs became aircraft inspectors because they were able to crawl inside wings and other cramped quarters. By the summer of 1943 nearly 3 million children aged 12 to 17 were working. Mail deliverers were in such short supply that the Post Office began to zone and number the nation's cities.

By 1945 average income had jumped to nearly $3000 a year, twice what it had been in 1939. Farm income rose by 250 percent. The distribution of wealth shifted in favor of those with lower incomes. The top 5 percent, who had received about a quarter of all income in 1940, dropped to 16 percent in 1944 (though their real income actually rose). Personal savings tripled. Demands for loans dropped so dramatically that banks were charging interest rates of only 2.5 percent.

War and Consumption

Newly affluent Americans often discovered that store shelves were empty of the goods they wanted most. Whether essentials such as food and clothing or luxuries

Daily Lives

CLOTHING AND FASHION

Dress on the Home Front

World War II dislocated American lives in endless ways. Millions went into the armed services; tens of millions moved to new areas to work in war industries. For most of those who left home, high war wages and the exposure to new opportunities compensated for the disruption of leaving familiar ways behind. Frankie Cooper, for one, decided the time had come to leave the family chicken farm in rural Kentucky, where she had lived for all her 21 years. Together with her husband and two small children she headed to East St. Louis, an industrial city on the Illinois bank of the Mississippi River.

In Kentucky Cooper had lived without indoor plumbing, electricity, a telephone, or department stores. She had never driven a car and made most of her dresses from chicken-feed sacks. In East St. Louis Cooper discovered a new world. War work brought her and her husband a prosperity they had never known. Now she could afford to buy clothes off the rack, ready made. Having never worn stockings, Cooper did not mind that silks and nylons were in short supply. A woman could always resort to painted-on stockings, or leg makeup, so long as she was careful to paint the seam straight.

Newfound prosperity made it much easier to live with wartime restrictions. The War Production Board designed rules to save on scarce materials and promote efficiency in the workplace. By 1942 it had banned full skirts, pleats, patch pockets (rule L-85, "no fabric over fabric"), and zippers. Order M-217 sought to conserve leather by limiting shoes to six colors. In an effort to save wool, the government forbade the manufacture of suits with two pairs of pants (which wore out faster than coats), vests, double-breasted lapels, and cuffs. Most of the changes were intended to be so subtle that old suits would not seem out of style. A new look might stimulate "a buying rush for 'victory suits,' which would defeat the conservation aim of the order."

Shortages forced the WPB to order a reduction in the fabric for women's bathing suits as well. Gone were the single-piece suits with billowing skirts. In came the two-piece look featuring a bare midriff. The *Wall Street Journal* concluded that "the two-piece bathing suit now is tied in with the war as closely as the zipperless dress and the pleatless skirt." After surveying women to find out which cosmetics were essential to morale, the War Production Board ruled that bath oil was in, bath salts out, and that face powder, lipstick, rouge, and deodorant were crucial.

Many changes came without any government coercion. The military cut of women's coats, low-cut shoes for comfort on the job, shorter hair less likely to catch in machinery, and simple jumpers or pinafores made to look like uniforms were all practical adjustments to wartime necessity. Freed from the domination of Parisian styles, American designers developed their own look. Wide, padded shoulders in both men's and women's suits gave way to a more natural shoulder and, for women, bare arms. Ballerina-length gowns replaced floor-length evening dresses. Smaller hats that complemented the natural styles displaced the large, frilly ones popular during the 1930s. Interchangeable skirts and blouses, coupled with hats, gloves, purses, and other accessories, allowed women to create a large wardrobe with fewer clothes.

Daily Lives

Having waited so long in line, this woman decided she could not wait to return home before putting on her strictly rationed nylon stockings.

And the shortage of rubber encouraged the redefinition of women's ideal body shape. Girdles were no longer available to rein in unsightly bulges. *McCall's*, a popular women's magazine, advised its readers to "stay slim for healthy beauty and morale. . . . Go slow on fats and sweets. And take exercise." In fact, *McCall's* was defining not simply new fashion, but a new lifestyle. Both women and men would now lead more active lives. To accommodate this new pattern, clothing became more casual. Women and men were far more likely to wear slacks, light blouses, and open-collared shirts in public.

The war had left the United States on the verge of a sexual revolution that was reflected in the new fashions but went far beyond clothing. Sleeveless blouses and dresses, two-piece bathing suits, and shorts exposed far more of the female body than had ever before been acceptable. That look was not only more revealing, but also softer and more feminine. Feminists would later charge that it reflected a male preoccupation with women as sex objects. As the nation turned from war work to postwar domesticity, advice columns urged women to assume more feminine roles, especially since returning veterans yearned for "admiration, or at least submissiveness." While a career might yield social prestige, only through marriage and child rearing, roles that were "protective or nurturing, passive and receptive," could women realize their biological destiny. Such warnings were far from the last word. Over the course of the next 40 years Americans would choose clothing styles that reflected a continual redefinition of gender roles, sexual practices, marital relationships, and the image of how the human body ideally should look.

like liquor and cigarettes, consumers found their desires restricted by shortages and rationing. Problems were most severe in cities like Los Angeles, Detroit, New Orleans, and Washington, D.C., which boomed with new war workers. Schools, public transportation, and other municipal services could not keep pace. Even people with the money had difficulty finding a house or an apartment at any price.

The public reaction hardly suggested a nation tightening its belt for war. "Americans are finding fun," noted one report, "—and lots of it." Liquor consumption increased by 30 percent. The city of Minneapolis ran out of whiskey. Attendance at movie theaters and night clubs reached new peaks. In 1944 wagering at race tracks was two and a half times greater than it had been in 1940. The average sale in department stores was $2 before the war; by 1944 it had soared to $10. Scarcity of cloth inspired new fashions like the women's two-piece bathing suit and men's pants without cuffs. Pocket book sales skyrocketed from several hundred thousand to 40 million by the end of the war. The demand for Bibles was so great that they had to be rationed.

Rationing and price controls were imposed by the Office of Price Administration (OPA) to restrain consumers with bulging wallets. Under Leon Henderson OPA established a system to allot such goods as sugar, gasoline, meats, butter, and shoes. Consumers received coupons that allowed them to buy set amounts at fixed prices. To restock their shelves, merchants had to return the coupons to the government. Local boards determined the coupon quota for each family. Abuses were unavoidable. People with connections could receive additional allotments by pleading special hardships. Meanwhile merchants complained that OPA had set prices too low.

Henderson lacked the weapons to halt inflation. The OPA had no way to limit wages or farm prices. Increased income left consumers with billions to spend. He did try to impose a maximum price ceiling ("General Max"), but wholesalers and retailers found ways to avoid its restrictions. They substituted inferior goods or sold on the black market instead. Public hostility to OPA reached such a crescendo in 1943 that Henderson resigned. Eager consumers snapped up goods in quantities that often defeated the purpose of government restrictions. Though most Americans abided by the rationing program, those willing to pay the price could find almost anything on the illegal "black market." On the black market in Philadelphia a $5 pair of shoes could be purchased for $7, while in Washington, D.C., boneless ham sold for $1.25 a pound, almost twice the legal price.

Resourceful entrepreneurs discovered a gold mine in the war. Robert Woodruff of Coca-Cola demonstrated shrewdness that made patriotism pay dividends. He avoided the restrictions of sugar rationing by persuading the military that Coke was vital to the morale of soldiers and sailors. Everywhere American forces went, Coke went with them. One dismayed doctor on a malaria-infested South Pacific island opened a shipment of quinine only to discover he had been sent Coke instead. Woodruff did not make unusual profits from his wartime operations. Rather, he managed to make the American thirst for Coke a global phenomenon. Coca-Cola's reward came after the war when it sold its product worldwide. Similarly, Philip Wrigley convinced the army that soldiers would fight better if each K ration package contained a stick of Wrigley Spearmint gum. War workers could ward off boredom and fatigue with timely chewing. The combined appeal to patriotism and wartime necessity made gum, like Coke, an essential product.

Slower speeds conserved gas and rubber.

Willow Run

In every city swollen with new workers the war boom created similar strains. Old residents resented the disruption of their communities. Pressures on housing aggravated already simmering racial tensions. Families suffered as they moved into new communities where living space and schools were crowded; parents were away at work or at war; and local government could not meet the demand for services.

Perhaps more than any other town or city, Willow Run, Michigan, came to symbolize wartime dislocations. In 1941 Henry Ford picked this site 27 miles west of Detroit for his new bomber factory. At its height in 1944 the main plant covered 67 acres and employed 42,000 workers, about 40 percent of whom were women. Willow Run also attracted many poor southerners unaccustomed to life in an industrial community. The population of the county around Willow Run grew by almost 50 percent within two years.

Available housing did not increase to accommodate the newcomers. Federal plans to build the community ran afoul of a variety of interests. Realtors and property owners feared a glut of housing after the war when the factory shut down. Republican politicians assumed they would lose control, as new residents swelled the ranks of the Democratic party. If taxes rose and property values fell, the old residents would suffer. Faced with stiff local opposition, the government reduced the scale of its proposed housing project. Voters rejected a plan to build new schools.

Willow Run nearly buckled under the weight of the war boom. In one two-story house, five men slept in the basement, a family of five lived on the first floor, four people rented the second floor, nine men had cots in the garage, and four families parked trailers in the yard. Sewage polluted water supplies and led to periodic outbreaks of dysentery. Medical facilities could not provide most people with basic care. The schools had to run double sessions to meet demand. Many workers quit rather than abide the indignities of such a life. For others, particularly newcomers from the South, conditions were little worse and often better than those they had left behind.

Women Workers

World War II improved the economic status of women, but it did not alter conventional views about gender roles. Women's work was acceptable so long as it was seen as temporary and not as the beginning of a sexual revolution. World War I had had little long-term impact on women. By 1920 women faced layoffs, renewed job discrimination, and segregation into traditionally female jobs. Until World War II employment for women rose only in domestic service and clerical work, significantly the lowest paying jobs.

Real gains for women came after 1941 as the military and war industries absorbed the reserve pool of male workers. With as many as 12 million men in uniform, women (especially married women) became the largest untapped source of labor. Suddenly the popular media, which had discouraged them from competing with men for jobs, now urged them to enlist in the work force. Labor shortages forced traditionalists to stifle complaints that working at jobs considered masculine would create a nation of "Amazon women." What faithful wife or sister could sit at home when the media warned that shortages of war goods threatened the lives of American soldiers? A former schoolteacher recalled listening to a conversation at a

Between 1940 and 1945 the female labor force increased over 50 percent. Many women performed jobs that once were considered exclusively male. Lionized with nicknames such as "Rosie the Riveter," women like this airplane factory worker proved that many gender stereotypes had no basis in reality.

friend's house: "She and her sister at the dinner table were talking about the best way to keep their drill sharp in the factory. I never heard anything like this in my life. It was just marvelous." "Rosie the Riveter" and "Commando Mary" symbolized the flood of women workers who heeded their country's call.

These women were not mostly young and single, as women workers of the past had been. From 1940 to 1945, some 6.5 million women entered the work force, over half for the first time. A majority were either married or between 55 and 64 years old. Having accounted for just one worker in four in 1940, women amounted to more than one in three by 1945. Patriotism alone could not explain their willingness to leave families and homes for the factories. Rising war wages were a powerful inducement. Indeed, with husbands who earned low military pay many families could not get by without additional income. Other families discovered that dual incomes allowed a rapid improvement in standards of living.

Many women preferred the relative freedom of work and wages to the confines of home. With husbands off at war, millions of women had more free time as the demand for household services declined. Wartime restrictions limited leisure activities. Work provided a satisfying outlet for the unutilized energy of women. In part this satisfaction reflected an improvement in the quality as well as quantity of jobs. Black women in particular realized dramatic gains. Once concentrated in low-paying domestic and farm jobs with erratic hours and tedious labor, some 300,000 rushed into factories that offered higher pay and more regular hours. Given the chance to learn such skills as welding, aircraft assembly, and electronics, women shattered many stereotypes about their capabilities.

Most Americans assumed that when the war ended veterans would pick up their old jobs and women would return home. "We were sold a bill of goods," remembered one woman. "They were hammering away that the woman who went to work did it to help her man, and when he came back, she cheerfully leaped back to the home." Surveys showed that the vast majority of Americans, whether male or female, continued to believe that child rearing was a woman's primary responsibility. The birth rate, which had fallen during the Depression, began to rise in 1943 as prosperity returned.

The war thus led to few structural changes to accommodate the new circumstances of women as both mothers and workers. Women with young children needed day care. The government was slow to provide even minimal facilities. And where they did exist, many mothers were reluctant to use them. They or other family members continued to care for children. Working mothers thus tended to have higher absentee rates and work shorter hours. For them, the demands of the job remained secondary to those of the home.

Other traditional barriers blocked women from altering economic structures. Most professions restricted the entry of women into graduate programs or other career paths. As women flooded into government bureaucracies, factory production lines, and corporate offices few received managerial status. Supervision remained man's work. Many employers found ways to circumvent government regulations ordering equal pay for men and women. General Motors, for one, simply changed its old job classification from overtly discriminatory male–female designations to equally restrictive "heavy–light" categories. Women, of course, were left in "light," lower paying jobs. Even when the government discovered such practices, it was reluctant to enforce its own rules. Economists feared that raising wages for women would spur inflation.

Social trends acted as another brake on advances for women. Wartime statistics revealed stresses undermining the family and threatening public morality. Alcohol abuse, teenage prostitution, divorce, and juvenile delinquency all were on the rise. Some observers blamed such trends on working mothers, who were said to neglect their families. In fact, there was no clear evidence that the families of mothers who stayed home fared any better than those where mothers held outside jobs. The real problem lay with extraordinary mobility during the war. Crowded into new communities with inadequate schools and recreational facilities, young people had few outlets for their energies. Some towns tried to occupy them with roller skating, dancing, and bowling. When trouble came, the children of newcomers were more likely to be arrested than were children familiar to local police. Rather than build new recreational facilities, concerned public agencies were just as likely to recommend compulsory rules restricting mothers from work. Only labor shortages prevented the acceptance of such rules. The war inspired a change in economic roles for women without fomenting a revolution in attitudes about gender. That would come later.

A QUESTION OF RIGHTS

Franklin Roosevelt and his administrators saw national unity as vital to victory. That meant minimizing tensions across lines of race, ethnicity, and social class. Roosevelt condemned the assaults on civil liberties committed during the frenzy of World War I. There would be no repetition of the raids on dissident groups, of mobs menacing immigrants, or of appeals to spy on one's neighbors. Americans in general were horrified by Japanese and Nazi atrocities, especially toward the "lesser breeds" of Asia and Europe. It was difficult to practice racism at home while fighting it abroad, but it was not impossible. The war sometimes aggravated intolerance, raising serious questions of minority rights.

Little Italy

Aliens from enemy countries fared far better in World War II than in World War I. Immigration restriction had greatly reduced the numbers of foreigners who had not yet become citizens. When war came there were about 600,000 Italian aliens and 5 million Italian-Americans in the United States. Whether aliens or citizens, all had struggled during the Depression. Most still lived in Italian neighborhoods centered around churches, fraternal organizations, and clubs. Some had been proud of Mussolini and supported *Fascismo*. "Mussolini was a hero," recalled one Italian-American, "a superhero. He made us feel special," especially with anti-Italian prejudices so strong. All that stopped after Pearl Harbor. During the war, Italian-Americans unquestioningly pledged their loyalties to the United States.

At first the government treated Italians without citizenship (along with Japanese and Germans) as "aliens of enemy nationality." They could not travel without permission, enter strategic areas, or possess shortwave radios, guns, or maps. By 1942 few Americans believed that German- or Italian-Americans posed any kind of danger. Eager to keep the support of Italian voters in the 1942 congressional elections, Roosevelt chose Columbus Day, 1942, to lift restrictions on Italian aliens. The segregation of Italian-Americans ended. Henceforth they would maintain their ethnic unity as a matter of choice, not necessity.

Concentration Camps

Japanese-Americans, whether aliens or citizens, did not find similar tolerance. Far more than the Italians, the 127,000 Japanese in the United States had remained separated, often because state laws and local custom created complex barriers to assimilation. In the western states where they were concentrated around urban areas, most Japanese could not vote, own land, or live in decent neighborhoods. The 1924 Immigration Act had permanently barred 47,000 Japanese aliens, known as "Issei," from becoming American citizens.

This near-apartheid system forced most Japanese-Americans to remain isolated from the mainstream of American life. Despite such restrictions, some Japanese achieved success in farming and small businesses like landscaping. Their accomplishments sometimes added to the hostility of white neighbors. Pearl Harbor intensified ugly racial prejudice. One California undertaker captured popular sentiment when he announced, "I'd rather do business with a Jap than with an American."

By February 1942 West Coast politicians began to press the Roosevelt administration to evacuate the Japanese from their communities. It did not seem to matter that about 80,000 were American citizens, called "Nisei," and that no evidence indicated they posed any threat whatsoever. To some politicians, lack of evidence seemed proof in itself. California Attorney General Earl Warren thought it significant that no sabotage had been reported. "It looks very much to me," he stated, "as though it is a studied effort not to have any until the zero hour arrives.

American propaganda during World War II was not as hysterical as it had been during World War I. Still, hostile images of the enemy stirred popular fears. While Germans were sometimes shown as brutal, it was more common to associate the Japanese with racism, brutality, and savagery.

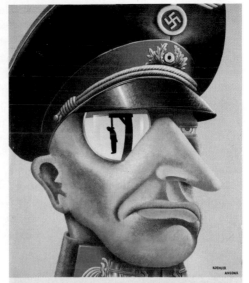

This is the Enemy

. . . That was the history of Pearl Harbor. I can't believe the same thing isn't planned for California." General John De Witt, commander of West Coast defenses, was more blunt: "A Jap's a Jap. . . . It makes no difference whether he is an American citizen or not." In response, the War Department in February 1942 drew up Executive Order 9066, which allowed the exclusion of any person from designated military areas. Under De Witt's authority, the order was applied only on the West Coast against Japanese-Americans.

Even that violation of Nisei rights did not satisfy more racist elements. Forty percent of the people on the West Coast believed that all Japanese were loyal to another government. To the north, Canada had already ordered all Japanese males between 18 and 65 to work camps away from the Pacific coast. In the United States vigilante violence soon broke out against the Japanese and their property. Pressure for removal mounted. "Put them all into concentration camps," one man was quoted as saying, "and work it out after the war's over!" By late February Roosevelt had agreed that both Issei and Nisei would be evacuated from the West Coast. But where would they go? When some 9000 moved on their own initiative, politicians from other states complained loudly. The army thus began in March to ship the entire Japanese community to "assembly centers."

Sudden removal imposed numerous hardships, many of them unnecessary. Few Japanese had time to arrange for the care or sale of property left behind. Most incurred heavy financial losses as they sold out far below market value. Their distress became a windfall for people who had long resented their economic competition. Once the Japanese reached the assembly centers at race tracks, fair grounds, and other temporary sites they encountered other indignities. The army had not prepared the sites to offer basic sanitation, comfort, or privacy. "We lived in a horse stable," remembered one young girl. "We filled our cheesecloth with straw—for our mattress." The authorities at least had the decency to keep families together.

The question of where to send the detainees was not resolved until September 1942. Milton Eisenhower, who headed the War Relocation Authority (WRA), had hoped to distribute people in small numbers to CCC-style work camps. That plan ran into opposition from state officials. Instead, most of the Japanese were interned in 10 camps in remote areas of seven western states. Notions that the camps might become self-sufficient communities proved wishful thinking. Even resourceful farmers could not raise food in arid desert soil.

No claim of humane intent could change the reality—these were concentration camps. Internees were held in wire-enclosed compounds by armed guards. Temporary tar-papered barracks housed families or small groups in single rooms. Each room had a few cots, some blankets, and a single light bulb. That was home. Bathing, meals, laundry, and recreation all took place in communal facilities. Attempts to introduce community self-government failed. Relocation had undermined the prestige of traditional elder leaders. The younger Nisei, who usually spoke English, were better able to deal with the authorities but were often more hostile.

Some Japanese within the camps protested, and rioting occasionally erupted. That only hardened opposition to a WRA plan that had permitted some 17,000 Nisei to leave the camps during 1943. In response, over 18,000 Japanese designated as disloyal were sent to a special camp at Tule Lake in California. About 8000 of these asked to go to Japan rather than suffer further indignities. Yet when given the chance to enlist, thousands of Nisei distinguished themselves in combat. Despite all they had suffered they accepted the one right left them—to die for their country.

Having created the camps, the government eventually found them hard to close. As late as 1944 the War Department warned that the West Coast would not tolerate rapid release of the Japanese. Many of the internees were now afraid to leave the relative safety of camps for life in hostile communities, but there was no reason to keep the camps open. Roosevelt finally decided after his reelection in 1944 that the time had come to let the Japanese go. As of January 1945 all Japanese had permission to leave at will. In late 1945 the WRA closed the last of the camps and one of the sorriest chapters in American history.

Even the Supreme Court lent its authority to the policy. In the case of *Hirabayashi v. United States* (1943) the Court upheld the discriminatory military curfew aimed at Japanese citizens. The majority opinion stated baldly that "residents having ethnic affiliations with an invading enemy may be a greater source of danger than those of different ancestry," even though the army had never demonstrated that any danger existed. The unanimous decision masked a divided Court. Justice Frank Murphy, who had wanted to dissent, got his chance in *Korematsu v. United States* (1944). The Court this time ruled that exclusion of Japanese-American citizens in wartime was legal. With the support of Justices Owen Roberts and Robert Jackson, Murphy criticized his colleagues for their automatic deference to a military decision and the "legalization of racism." Such an opinion had influence. On the same day in *Ex parte Endo* the Court declared it illegal to detain loyal citizens more than temporarily. That did little to help Mitsue Endo. She had spent over two years in a relocation camp waiting for the Court to decide her case.

Concentration camps in America did not perpetuate the horror of Nazi death camps, but they were built on racism and fear. Worse, they violated the traditions of civil rights and liberties for which Americans believed they were fighting.

Minorities on the Job

The war gave minority leaders an opportunity to press for broader civil rights. "A jim crow army cannot fight for a free world," the NAACP declared. The Pittsburgh *Courier*, a major black newspaper, advocated the "Double V"—"victory over our enemies at home and victory over our enemies on the battlefields abroad." Such ideas of racial justice had been the driving force in the life of A. Philip Randolph, long an advocate of greater black militancy. Randolph had demonstrated his gifts as an organizer and leader of the Brotherhood of Sleeping Car Porters, the most powerful black labor organization. He was determined to secure for blacks their rights in defense industries and the armed forces. "The Administration leaders in Washington will never give the Negro justice," Randolph argued, "until they see masses—ten, twenty, fifty thousand Negroes on the White House lawn." In 1941 he began to organize a march on Washington.

By using executive orders, President Roosevelt could have granted almost all of Randolph's demands aimed to end segregation in the government, defense industries, unions, and the armed forces. Only Randolph's insistence that the government refuse collective bargaining rights to unions closed to blacks required congressional action. The president, however, had never been a stalwart opponent of racial discrimination. He would have preferred to placate Randolph with a few kind words and gestures, but Randolph refused to be charmed. He predicted that 100,000 blacks would march on Washington in mid-1941 if Roosevelt did not act.

Under pressure from Randolph, the president in June 1941 finally issued Executive Order 8802. Federal policy now banned racial discrimination in the employment of workers in government or defense industries. To carry out that policy, the order established the Fair Employment Practices Commission (FEPC). In some ways that was the boldest step toward racial justice since the Civil War era. But the FEPC had only marginal success in breaking down barriers against blacks and Hispanics. It was one thing to ban discrimination, quite another to enforce that ban in a society still deeply divided by racial prejudice.

Mexican farm workers offer a case in point. During the Depression western farmers paid them below-subsistence wages, offered squalid housing, and sometimes left them stranded in the countryside between picking seasons. As unemployed white workers sought farm jobs, pressure mounted to reverse the flow of Mexican immigration. Traditional discrimination in education, housing, and jobs grew more severe. Local authorities discovered that it was cheaper to deport Mexicans, even some who were citizens or in the United States legally, than to provide relief to which they were entitled.

The war reversed that pattern. Efforts by the FEPC opened industrial jobs in California's shipyards and aircraft factories, which had previously refused to hire Hispanics. Thousands migrated from Texas, where job discrimination was most severe, to California, where war work created new opportunities. Labor shortages led the southwestern states to join with the Mexican government under the bracero (contract labor) program to recruit Mexican labor.

In Texas, by contrast, antagonism to braceros ran so deep that the Mexican government tried to prevent workers from going there. In 1942 the FEPC began to investigate systematic discrimination in the oil and mining industries. With support from labor unions company officials blocked Hispanics from training programs and job advancement. In this case, the State Department stymied the inquiry because Assistant Secretary Sumner Welles claimed that hemispheric relations might suffer. Disclosures would also afford Axis agents a wealth of propaganda with which to embarrass the United States. Not until late 1943 was the FEPC able to proceed.

Black Americans experienced similar frustrations. Early wartime prosperity bypassed them almost entirely. In 1941 half a million blacks were still unemployed while another two million worked at marginal, low-paying jobs. Over half of all defense jobs were closed to minorities. For example, with 100,000 skilled and high-paying jobs in the aircraft industry, blacks held about 200 janitorial positions. The federal agency charged with placing workers honored local employment practices. Generally that meant "whites only." The Office of Production Management refused to introduce antidiscrimination clauses into defense contracts. Unions segregated black workers or excluded them entirely. One person wrote to the president with a telling complaint: "Hitler has not done anything to the colored people— it's people right here in the United States who are keeping us out of work and keeping us down." Discrimination in housing, restaurants, transportation, and hotels added to the sense of grievance.

Eventually the combination of labor shortages, pressures from black leaders, and initiative from government agencies opened the door to more skilled jobs and higher pay. The federal government increased its employment of blacks from 60,000 to over 200,000. Beginning in 1943 the United States Employment Service rejected requests with racial stipulations. The National Labor Relations Board announced it would no longer certify unions that barred minorities. Faced with a dwindling labor pool, many employers finally opened their doors. By 1944 blacks, who accounted for almost 10 percent of the population, held 8 percent of the jobs. The wage gap narrowed so that black men (and white women) earned about 65 percent as much as white males. The lure of industrial jobs drew some 400,000 blacks from southern farms where they had eked out livings in sharecropping and tenant farming. About half went to the West Coast, half to the Northeast and Upper Midwest.

White hostility to blacks was never far from the surface. In Philadelphia in 1943 the local streetcar company claimed its union contract prevented the hiring of blacks as motormen (drivers) or conductors. Nonetheless, the FEPC ordered the company to upgrade some blacks. After considerable foot-dragging eight blacks received promotions by July 1944. On August 1 several hundred white workers struck to protest the upgrading of blacks. The city's 1600 streetcars, 600 buses, and 500 railway cars stopped. Since Philadelphia was one of the nation's most vital industrial centers, the government moved quickly to crush the strike. Eight thousand army troops manned the streetcars and kept the peace. FBI agents arrested strike leaders. Two days after it began, the strike was ended.

The victory in Philadelphia was an exceptional case. When the government confronted a more powerful union, like the Brotherhood of Locomotive Firemen and Engineers, it was not as forceful. A railroad strike could have brought the entire economy to a halt. In the large majority of cases, employers and unions defied FEPC orders for equal treatment of minorities. As the war ended, the old practice of "last-hired, first-fired" resumed. Even in postwar boom industries like car making, minorities were quickly downgraded to lower paying jobs.

At War with Jim Crow

At the beginning of World War II three-fourths of the 12 million black Americans lived in the South. Hispanic Americans, whose population exceeded a million, were concentrated in a belt along the United States–Mexican border. When jobs for minorities opened in war centers, blacks and Hispanics became increasingly urban. Whether rural or urban, both groups suffered from deeply entrenched systems of segregation that denied them basic rights to decent housing, jobs, and political participation. The explosiveness of that prejudice became clear in 1942. Competition for housing and the use of public facilities like parks, beaches, and transportation between whites and rapidly expanding minority populations became fierce.

In some cities government funds created new housing. One such project built in Detroit was named to honor the black poet and abolitionist Sojourner Truth. It included 200 units for black families. Federal authorities had picked a site for the houses along the edge of a Polish neighborhood. When the first black families tried to move in, they faced an angry mob of whites. Finally, local officials had to send several hundred National Guardsmen to protect the newcomers, as Ku Klux Klan members looked on menacingly.

The incident only provoked Detroit blacks and whites into greater confrontations. On a hot evening in June 1943, the simmering hatreds boiled over. At first scattered fighting broke out among blacks and whites returning from a local park. Suddenly, widespread gunfire, looting, and mob violence broke out. Angry blacks assaulted white workers leaving night shifts. White mobs dragged blacks off streetcars and buses. Police and snipers exchanged rifle fire. Six thousand soldiers from nearby bases finally imposed a troubled calm, but not before the riot had claimed 34 lives and property damage was widespread. Refusing to take black grievances seriously, local officials accused the NAACP and the "militant" Negro press for stirring up trouble. The black community charged that the police, shooting indiscriminately at blacks, did nothing to stop white rioters.

Detroit was not the only racially divided city, and blacks were not the only victims. Hispanics in southern California suffered the same indignities as black Americans. By 1943 overt Anglo hostility had come to focus on the *pachucos*, or "zoot suiters." These were young Hispanic men and boys who had adopted the outrageous style of Harlem hipsters: greased hair, swept back into a ducktail; broad-shouldered, long-waisted suit coats; baggy pants, pegged at the ankles, polished off with a swashbuckling keychain. The Los Angeles city council passed an ordinance making it a crime even to wear a zoot suit. For most "zooters" this style was a modest form of rebellion; for a few it was a badge of criminal behavior; for white servicemen it was a target for racism.

In June 1943 taunting turned to violence. Sailors from the local navy base invaded Hispanic neighborhoods in search of zooters who had allegedly attacked

The loose fit and pegged ankles of the zoot suit made it ideal for the jitterbug, a dance craze that swept the country in the era of big jazz bands. When the fashion became especially popular with urban Hispanic and black minorities, "zoot suiters" found themselves the targets of local officials and angry servicemen who resented the outrageous look of this teen subculture.

servicemen. The self-appointed vigilantes grabbed innocent victims, tore their clothes, cut their hair, and beat them bloody. When Hispanics retaliated, the police arrested them, all the while ignoring the actions of white servicemen. Irresponsible newspaper coverage made matters worse. "ZOOTERS THREATEN L.A. POLICE," charged one Hearst paper.

Accusations against zooters could not long mask the cause of the violence. Los Angeles in 1943 had limited recreational facilities for servicemen. Living outside American society, Hispanics offered convenient targets for servicemen's unfocused energies and irrepressible prejudices. Soon after the "zoot-suit riots," a citizens committee created at the urging of California Governor Earl Warren placed the blame where it belonged—on both sides. Underlying Hispanic anger were the grim realities of filthy housing, unemployment, disease, and white racism. All that added up to a level of poverty that wartime prosperity eased but in no way resolved.

Minority leaders realized some legal gains during the war. The Congress of Racial Equality (CORE), a nonviolent civil rights group inspired by the Indian leader Mohandas K. Gandhi, used sit-ins and other peaceful tactics to desegregate some restaurants and movie theaters. In 1944 the Supreme Court outlawed the "all-white primary," an infamous device used by southerners to exclude blacks from voting in primary elections within the Democratic party. Because Democratic candidates in the South often ran unopposed in the general elections, the primary elections were usually the only true political contests. In *Smith v. Allwright* the Court ruled that since political parties were integral parts of public elections, they could not deny minorities the right to vote in primaries. In so ruling the Court opened a legal door to further assaults on the Jim Crow system. "I see World War II as having been a step on the first rung of the ladder," concluded one black soldier. "But I wouldn't want to wish it on anybody else." With race as with gender, the war sowed the seeds of future upheaval. Hispanic, black, and Indian veterans would play leading roles in the postwar struggle for equality.

POLITICS AS USUAL

Politics did not go into eclipse after Pearl Harbor. As Roosevelt told reporters, "Dr. New Deal" had retired so that "Dr. Win-the-War" could go about his business. Politics nonetheless proceeded as usual. The increasingly powerful anti–New Deal coalition of Republicans and rural Democrats saw in the war an opportunity to attack liberal programs they had long resented. The president, for his part, was a politician who never lost sight of election returns. Without an electoral mandate (whether a Democratic Congress in 1942 or a fourth presidential term in 1944) Roosevelt could not achieve the victory he sought in war and peace.

Paying the Piper

One of the most difficult questions Roosevelt faced was how to pay the enormous cost of fighting the war. The federal budget, only about $9 billion in 1939, jumped to $100 billion by 1945. The national debt soared from $49 billion in 1941 to $259 billion by the end of the war. The money came from three major sources: taxes,

THE IMPACT OF WORLD WAR
II ON GOVERNMENT
SPENDING
Note that after both world wars
nonmilitary government spending
was greater than in the prewar
eras.

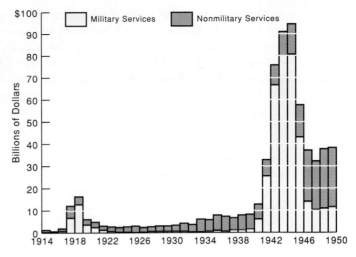

borrowing, and inflation (which amounts to a hidden tax). Tax receipts accounted
for about 41 percent; borrowing provided the remainder. As personal income
rose, inflation threatened to eat away higher earnings.

Americans agreed on little beyond controlling the war profits of individuals
and corporations. Liberal New Dealers urged Roosevelt to pursue the tax and
fiscal policies recommended by British economist John Maynard Keynes. Steeply
graduated individual and corporate taxes would restrict inflation while falling on
those best able to pay. Compulsory war bond purchases could further check prices
through forced savings. The progressive tax structure would also lead to a more
equitable distribution of wealth. Conservatives viewed such proposals as socialis-
tic schemes to "soak the rich." They believed, quite correctly, that the liberal
revenue program was designed to achieve social reform. They proposed voluntary
war bond drives and sales taxes that would ease inflation by limiting consumption.
In this case low- and middle-income taxpayers would shoulder most of the burden.

The Roosevelt approach mixed conservative and liberal elements: it was voluntary and compulsory, regressive and progressive. The Treasury Department
sold war bonds through advertising campaigns rather than enforced savings. A
volunteer group, the War Advertising Council, organized publicity for bond
drives. Manufacturers without products to sell paid instead for war bond advertisements. Their motives were not entirely patriotic. The advertisements kept the
names of companies like General Electric and General Motors in the public eye,
while much of their cost could be written off company taxes.

The Treasury Department had concluded that higher taxes were the best way
to limit inflation and generate needed revenue. Vote-conscious politicians winced,
but the Treasury recommended a highly progressive tax bill anyway. Secretary
Morgenthau proposed surtaxes on personal and corporate incomes and higher
taxes on excess profits (to limit war profiteering), estates and gifts, luxury items,
and scarce war goods. The most innovative feature of Morgenthau's bill was the
new payroll deductions. No longer would taxpayers have to set aside money to pay
the Internal Revenue Service (IRS) at the end of the year.

Conservatives in Congress balked at such sweeping reforms. They continued
to press for sales taxes. After six months of wrangling, in which Roosevelt gave no

support to Morgenthau's bill, the Revenue Act of 1942 emerged, in the president's words, as "the greatest tax bill in American history." It was something less. Gone were most of the progressive features. To placate supporters of the sales tax, the administration agreed to a 5 percent tax on incomes over $624 a year. That provision struck hardest at low-income workers, most of whom would pay federal taxes for the first time. Some 13 million people paid in 1941; under the Revenue Act almost 50 million would fall into the IRS net. A 1943 bill required employers to collect taxes through payroll deductions.

Future tax bills ran into similar opposition. In 1944 Congress passed a bill so laced with favors to business and empty of new revenue provisions that Roosevelt vetoed it. He charged Congress had provided "relief not for the needy but for the greedy." House Majority Leader Alben Barkley of Kentucky, a staunch New Dealer, resigned in outrage at the presidential slight of Congress. Both houses overrode Roosevelt's veto. Even though the president and Barkley patched up their quarrel, equitable taxation had suffered an irreversible defeat.

1942: A Farewell to Reform

The fight over taxes reflected deeper political currents running against the New Deal. New Deal foes moved quickly to eliminate the Civilian Conservation Corps, the National Youth Administration, and the largely ineffectual National Resources Planning Board. They gutted the Farm Security Administration and blocked moves to extend Social Security and unemployment benefits. They also thwarted Thurman Arnold's antitrust crusade. Conservatives masked their ambition to dismantle much of the New Deal behind the argument that such programs impeded war mobilization.

In the election of 1942 Roosevelt avoided Woodrow Wilson's error of making an off-year election a referendum on war policies; still the Republicans gained 44 seats in the House and 9 in the Senate. New York elected Thomas E. Dewey as governor, the first Republican since 1920. Republicans won 26 governorships in states that held 342 out of 531 electoral votes. More striking was the character of New Deal losses and conservative gains. Progressives like Senator George Norris of Nebraska lost, while diehard isolationists like Hamilton Fish (from Roosevelt's home county), won handily. The GOP began eyeing the White House.

Organized Labor

Wartime labor politics introduced a disruptive factor into Roosevelt's New Deal coalition. Though the president had never fully embraced organized labor, unions had become an important element in the Democratic party as well as a rich source of campaign funds. More conservative elements in the party wanted to curb union power. Wartime prosperity brought unprecedented gains for unions, though not without a continuation of the sometime violent struggles of the 1930s. Even as surging employment brought 1.5 million new members into the union fold, skilled workers of the American Federation of Labor and industrial workers of the Congress of Industrial Organizations vied for dominance. Just as divisive was the failure of labor leaders to agree to support Roosevelt's policies. And most workers had grievances with management. In 1941 alone more than 2 million workers walked off their jobs over wages and access to unions.

In 1942 Roosevelt moved to end labor strife. He established the War Labor Board (WLB), modeled on the old World War I agency, with the authority to impose arbitration in any labor dispute. To protect major interests, the WLB included equal representation for labor, management, and consumers. If the parties rejected the final decision, the president could seize the plants in question. In its most far-reaching decision the WLB adopted a "maintenance of membership" policy. Employers had always fought for the "open shop" where workers were free to be union members or not. Labor leaders demanded the "closed shop," which forced all workers in a plant to join a single union. The WLB formulated a compromise that gave workers 15 days to leave the union after a contract was signed. Any worker who remained a member had to pay union dues for the life of the contract. That policy led to an almost 40 percent growth in union membership between 1941 and 1945, when a record 14.75 million workers had union cards.

Labor's ability to redress its grievances was restricted by a "no-strike" pledge adopted shortly after Pearl Harbor. By 1943 workers saw the pledge as a burden. They pressed for repudiation even if it provoked a backlash in Congress and the press. A rash of new strikes threatened to disrupt war production. In 1943 some 3.1 million workers walked off their jobs. Railroad workers threatened to block the war effort when they tied up the rail lines just before Christmas. General George C. Marshall cursed it as the "damnedest crime ever committed against America." Finally the government seized the railroads and then granted wage increases. Between 1941 and 1945, almost 15,000 work stoppages took some 6.75 million workers off the job. All told, nearly 40 million work days were lost.

Such an account creates the impression that wartime labor policy was a failure. In reality the Roosevelt administration managed to limit the impact of quarrels between labor and management. Put another way, statistics reveal worker dedication to the war effort. Stoppages actually accounted for only about one-tenth of a percent of total work time during the war. Workers most often struck in defiance of their union leadership and left their jobs for just a few days.

One union, the United Mine Workers (UMW), and its leader, John L. Lewis, were responsible for a disproportionate share of disruptions. Wartime inflation affected coal miners more severely than most other workers. Wage scales were low. As Lewis angrily charged, "The coal miners of America are hungry. They are ill-fed and undernourished." Much of the animosity toward unions was provoked by Lewis' tactics in 1943, when he authorized a series of short strikes. Finally Roosevelt seized the mines and ran them for a time. Roosevelt had no love for Lewis, who had fought him in 1940 and whose militancy caused him nothing but political headaches. At times the president considered arresting UMW leaders and drafting striking miners, but as Secretary of the Interior Harold Ickes reminded him, a "jailed miner produces no more coal than a striking miner." The president, moreover, did not wish to antagonize more moderate labor leaders. With his blessings Ickes negotiated a settlement giving the miners generous benefits.

In helping the UMW, Lewis hurt the cause of labor. A huge coal shortage along the East Coast had left homes dark and cold. Most Americans thought of Lewis as public enemy number one. "John L. Lewis—Damn your coal black soul," wrote the military newspaper *Stars and Stripes*. In the fall of 1943 antiunion elements in Congress pushed through the Smith–Connolly Anti-Strike, or War Labor Disputes Act. It gave the president more authority to seize vital war plants shut by strikes and required union leaders to observe a 30-day "cooling-off" period before striking. Roosevelt wanted even more power, but he recognized the anti-

John L. Lewis.

union goals of Smith–Connolly supporters. He vetoed the bill, only to be overridden in both houses by large margins. In the end Roosevelt gained the authority he sought but maintained labor's support for the difficult 1944 presidential campaign.

1944: A Fourth Term

In the spring of 1944 no one knew whether Roosevelt would seek an unprecedented fourth term. The president's health had declined noticeably. Pallid skin, sagging shoulders, and shaking hands seemed open signs that he had aged too much to run. In July, one week before the Democratic convention, Roosevelt announced his decision: "All that is within me cries out to go back to my home on the Hudson River. . . . But as a good soldier . . . I will accept and serve."

Conservative Democrats wanted to rid the ticket of Vice President Henry A. Wallace, leader of the most progressive wing of the party and an outspoken internationalist. The CIO warmly endorsed him. Roosevelt left the public impression that he wanted Wallace on the ticket but before the convention tried to replace him with James Byrnes of South Carolina, the head of the Office of War Mobilization. The president had not reckoned on CIO leader Sidney Hillman, who supported Wallace and opposed Byrnes as an enemy of labor and of civil rights. At the convention the divided delegates settled on Harry S. Truman of Missouri, a loyal New Dealer who had distinguished himself during the war as head of the Senate committee monitoring defense expenditures.

The Republican ticket rejected the liberal internationalist Wendell Willkie in favor of the moderate governor of New York, Thomas E. Dewey. Dewey never had a chance. Countless reports of victory in Europe and the Pacific undermined his charges that Roosevelt had mismanaged the war. Both candidates warmly endorsed postwar American participation in international affairs. On domestic issues Dewey often sounded like a New Dealer. The GOP platform had so few criticisms of actual programs that one historian called it "the most significant endorsement of Roosevelt's policies yet written." Republicans fell back on old strategies of attack, condemning inefficiency and waste in government, excessive centralization of political power, and the destruction of free enterprise.

Roosevelt's campaign championed two reforms popular with liberals and soldiers. In his January State of the Union message the president outlined a bill aimed to ensure economic security and prosperity after the war. It was, he suggested, "a second Bill of Rights" that would guarantee jobs, decent living standards, greater opportunities for small businesses, better housing, and more protection against unemployment, old age, sickness, and injury. It was an agenda for a good society, not a plan to revive the New Deal, and once reelected Roosevelt did little to achieve it.

By contrast the "GI Bill of Rights" of 1944 was perhaps the most significant social legislation of the war years. Sociologists have identified occupation, place of residence, and level of education as three crucial determinants of social class. The GI Bill granted veterans the means to improve their status in these areas and more. It gave them occupational guidance, priority for jobs, loans to establish small businesses and farms, educational benefits and technical training, and mortgage assistance to buy homes. Later amendments added health care, particularly for those disabled by the war. Since the bill applied to soldiers only, it gained support even among those who normally opposed such social programs. Seeing the legislation as an opportunity to win the gratitude of veterans, the normally conservative American Legion gave its wholehearted endorsement.

By late summer Dewey's campaign had failed to excite many voters. Alice Roosevelt Longworth, the daughter of Theodore Roosevelt, compared Dewey to the little man on a wedding cake. Eventually Dewey and other frustrated GOP candidates resorted to "red baiting." Victory for Roosevelt would bring Communist labor leaders like Sidney Hillman into the White House, they charged. Latent anti-Semitism and nativism made Hillman and other ethnic labor leaders favorite targets. Voters turned away from such extremism. They gave Roosevelt and the Democrats 25.6 million popular votes to Dewey's 22 million. Roosevelt swamped his rival in the electoral college by a count of 432 to 99. The Democrats lost just one seat in the Senate, picked up 20 in the House, and captured 5 new governorships. In defeat, many frustrated GOP leaders decided to make "red baiting" their focus in future elections.

VICTORY

As he was sworn in on April 12, 1945, Harry Truman recognized the awesome task of replacing Franklin Roosevelt. In the brief period he had served as vice president, Truman had met with Roosevelt fewer than 10 times. He knew almost nothing about the president's postwar plans and promises. When a newspaperman addressed him as "Mr. President," he winced. "I wish you didn't have to call me that," he said. He asked the press corps to pray for him, but prayers would not prevent foreign leaders from taking advantage of his inexperience, so Truman adopted a tough pose and made his mind up quickly. People welcomed the new president's decisiveness as a relief from Roosevelt's evasions. Too often, though, he acted before the issues were clear.

As Truman assumed the presidency, the Allies had already launched the final blows against the Axis. The victory in the Pacific promised to be bloody. At Okinawa, just 370 miles south of Japan, American amphibious forces ran into fierce resistance. Over 3500 kamikaze pilots targeted the invasion fleet, inflicting serious damage. Japanese defenders threw nightly human wave assaults against Allied troops. The Americans suffered 50,000 casualties and the Japanese 100,000 deaths before the island fell in late June. Victory in Europe was much closer. By spring an army of 150 Russian divisions had reached the Oder River just to the east of Berlin. In March American troops commanded by General Omar Bradley had captured Cologne on the west bank of the Rhine and by a great stroke of luck captured an undamaged bridge at Remagen. By April Bradley's forces were sweeping into central Germany as British forces under General Bernard Montgomery moved to the north.

The Holocaust

The invading armies were not prepared for the horror of the concentration camps they discovered. As part of a plan to implement "the final solution" to Germany's problems, Hitler had ordered in areas under Nazi rule the systematic extermination of all European Jews as well as Gypsies, homosexuals, and others considered deviant. The SS, Hitler's security force, had established six extermination centers in Poland at Chelmno, Belzec, Majdanek, Sobibór, Treblinka, and Auschwitz. By rail from all over Europe they shipped Jews to die in the gas chambers.

In April 1945, at the concentration camp in Buchenwald, Germany, Senator Alben Barkley of Kentucky viewed a grisly reminder of the horrors of the Nazis' "final solution." As vice president under Harry Truman, Barkley urged the administration to support an independent homeland for Jews in Israel.

No issue of World War II more starkly raised questions of human good and evil than the Holocaust. And tragically, the United States could have done more to save at least some of the 6 million Jews the Nazis killed. Until the fall of 1941 the Nazis permitted Jews to leave Europe, but few countries, including the United States, would accept them. American restrictions, which had been lowered slightly in 1938, became progressively tighter. There are three factors explaining the exclusionary policy. First and foremost was the Depression. Many Americans feared that any rise in immigration would make joblessness worse. That concern coincided with a second impulse to tighten rather than loosen the restriction system established under the Immigration Act of 1924. Opinion polls showed that in 1938, as Nazi persecution of Jews increased, 71 to 85 percent of all Americans opposed easing quotas to help refugees. In 1939 some 66 percent objected to a one-time exception that would have admitted 10,000 children. The war in no way eased opposition to the admission of European refugees.

A third factor was an ugly strain of anti-Semitism that peaked in 1944 when pollster Elmo Roper warned that it "had spread all over the nation and is particularly virulent in urban centers." According to the polls Americans mistrusted Jews more than any European people except Italians. With the exception of a few bitter cranks, anti-Semites refrained from advocating outright persecution. More common was a kind of passive anti-Semitism that nurtured negative feelings but no overt hostilities. Jewish leaders feared, probably with cause, that pressure to ease immigration restrictions would make anti-Semitism worse. "I see in the papers that 200,000 Refugee Jews in Hungary will not live through the week," a typical letter to Congress began. "Thats too Damn Bad what in the Hell do we care about Jews in Hungary."

What was more tragic was the anti-Semitism of senior State Department officials who systematically frustrated Jewish efforts to emigrate to the United States. Immigration policy fell under the authority of Assistant Secretary of State Breckinridge Long, who embraced the upper-class American tradition of unmodulated anti-Semitism. President Roosevelt could have used an executive order to clear the obstacles Long and his officials created, but for several reasons he did not. For one, he was no stranger to gentlemanly anti-Semitism and thus discounted the virulence with which Long enforced his prejudices.

The president also received mixed signals from the American Jewish community. Jews wanted to help refugees, especially after 1942 as news of the death camps leaked from Europe, but they were not sure how to do so without aggravating anti-Semitism. Until the last year of the war polls showed that most Americans thought that only about 100,000 Jews had been killed. Jews were also split on the question of Zionism and the pressures to establish a Jewish homeland in Palestine. The British had blocked Jewish emigration to Palestine and opposed Zionism to avoid alienating the Arabs. Roosevelt and his advisers ultimately decided that the best way to save Jews was to win the war quickly. That still does not explain why the Allies did not do more: they could have bombed the rail lines to the camps, sent commando forces, or tried to destroy the death factories.

Treasury Secretary Henry Morgenthau, the one Jew in Roosevelt's cabinet, had at first gone along with the president and the British on the questions of Palestine and refugees. Then his staff informed him that the State Department at Breckenridge Long's insistence had since 1942 prevented information on the "final solution" from reaching the United States. In 1943 Long also blocked a plan Morgenthau and Roosevelt both approved to ransom Jews in Romania and 6000 Jewish children in France. By January 1944 Morganthau became so exasperated with the State Department that he sent Roosevelt a report entitled "The Acquiesence of this Government in the Murder of the Jews." Roosevelt stripped Long of his authority and appointed a War Refugee Board charged with saving as many Jews as possible. In the 1944 election both parties adopted pro-Zionist planks, and Roosevelt promised to seek the establishment of a Jewish commonwealth in Palestine. But some 18 precious "long and heartbreaking" months had been lost and with them an untold number of lives.

At Yalta, the Big Three did not discuss, much less resolve the issue of Palestine. Returning home in February 1945, Roosevelt stopped for talks with King Ibn Saud of Saudi Arabia. He impressed Roosevelt with Arab determination to end further Jewish immigration to Palestine. To many American Jews, the president now seemed to waver on his election promises, but it was Harry Truman who would face the survivors and their dreams of a Jewish homeland.

The United Nations

Truman also inherited responsibility for establishment of the United Nations Organization (UNO). The breakdown of the world economy during the 1930s followed by the horrors of World War II led the Allies to seek a new framework for the international system. That system, many Americans believed, required an end to economic nationalism, trade barriers, and currency problems that had led to depression and war. Most postwar planners defended the "open door" to trade. At the Chicago Aviation Conference in 1944 they had insisted on ready access for American airlines to routes and airports around the globe. At a 1944 meeting at Bretton Woods, a resort in New Hampshire, the Americans had created two new economic organizations: the International Monetary Fund (IMF) and the International Bank for Reconstruction and Development (the World Bank). The IMF would promote trade by stabilizing national currencies while the World Bank would invest in economic growth. Since the United States supplied most of the capital for both organizations, it would also dictate policy.

In late summer 1944 the Allies met at Dumbarton Oaks, a Washington estate, to lay out the structure for the UNO. An 11-member Security Council would oversee a General Assembly composed of all members. At Yalta, Roosevelt had won Stalin's support for the UNO but the price was high. Fearful that the Western powers would control the General Assembly, Stalin extracted three seats for the Soviet Union by arguing the fiction that the Ukrainian, Belorussian, and Lithuanian republics were independent states. Roosevelt at first resisted but gave in under pressure from Churchill.

Although Truman had no intention of altering Roosevelt's course on the UNO or other wartime agreements, he almost immediately adopted a more hostile approach to Stalin and the Soviet Union. Truman had heard the same message from many sources: the Soviets could not be trusted. They had already begun to violate agreements on eastern Europe made at Yalta. Only if the United States stood firm, advisers counseled, could the Soviets be forced to keep their word. When Foreign Commissar V. M. Molotov stopped in Washington on his way to the organizational meeting of the UNO in San Francisco on April 25, Truman delivered a severe tongue-lashing to the startled Soviet leader. When Molotov objected, Truman retorted, "Keep your agreements and you won't be talked to that way."

Truman soon discovered that tough talk did not easily solve Allied differences. The April 1945 meeting in San Francisco to establish the new United Nations Organization revealed deep divisions between the Soviets and Americans. When United States delegates urged the admission of Argentina, the Soviets scoffed at permitting the entrance of a fascist regime. The United States prevailed, and it became clear that the UNO would favor the Western powers in most postwar disputes.

Ending the War

While the UNO convened, the Axis collapsed. As Mussolini attempted to escape to Germany antifascist mobs in Italy had captured and slaughtered him like a pig. Adolf Hitler committed suicide in his Berlin bunker on April 30. Two weeks later General Eisenhower accepted the German surrender. Allied leaders then planned to meet in July at Potsdam, just outside of Berlin, to consider the future of Europe and victory over Japan. With reports that Japan might fight for another five years, Truman wanted Stalin to enter the Pacific war. He was chagrined to learn that overzealous aides had abruptly canceled lend-lease shipments to Russia. Ships already at sea were ordered home. Truman countermanded the order, but not before he received a torrent of bitter complaints from the Soviet Union.

To repair the rifts, Truman asked Roosevelt's trusted adviser Harr
to see Stalin in Moscow. Though near death, Hopkins made the ardu
reached a series of important compromises. Stalin agreed to bring me
Polish government-in-exile in London into the Communist regim
land. That left the Communists in charge but saved face for Churchill a
Stalin also repeated his commitment to join the Pacific war, accepted an Ame
formula for voting in the Security Council of the UNO, and promised to meet
Truman in Germany.

Though Hopkins' trip improved the tone of Soviet–American relations, irreconcilable differences over postwar political settlements, especially in Germany
and eastern Europe, split the Allies. At Potsdam Truman met Churchill (who lost
office during the conference) and Stalin for the first time. Talks lasted for two and a
half weeks without substantial agreement. Two issues dominated the meeting.
Both sides agreed that Germany should be occupied and demilitarized. But
whereas the British and Americans did not want to burden Germany with excessive reparations as they had after World War I, Stalin insisted that Russia receive a
minimum of $10 billion regardless of the impact on the postwar German or Euro-
pean economy. A complicated compromise allowed Britain and the United States
to restrict reparations from their zones but eliminated prospects for a centralized
government in Germany.

Atomic Diplomacy

The most crucial issue never reached the bargaining table at Potsdam. On July 16,
1945, the first atomic fireball rose from the desert in Alamagordo, New Mexico.
The next day news of the successful test was flashed to Truman at Potsdam from
the Manhattan Project director, General Leslie Groves. Two questions loomed:
Should the United States warn Japan before using the bomb? And even more to
the point, should Truman tell Stalin? The possibility of not using the bomb or
offering a demonstration, as a number of concerned Manhattan Project scientists
urged, had been dismissed by a high-level committee of administrators, scientists,
and political and military leaders.

Truman seemed a changed man—firmer, more confident—after he received
the word from Alamagordo. He "told the Russians just where they got on and off
and generally bossed the whole meeting," observed Churchill. The president
chose not to tell Stalin about the bomb, only mentioning obliquely that the United
States possessed a weapon of "awesome destructiveness." Instead of being cowed,
Stalin smiled, remarking casually that he hoped the Americans would use their
new weapon to good effect against Japan. (Most likely, spies had already informed
Stalin about the atomic bomb, so Truman's reference came as no surprise.) Atomic
diplomacy had failed its first test. If, as some historians believe, Stalin immediately stepped up the Russian program to build an atomic bomb, then the decision
to keep the bomb secret helped launch the nuclear arms race.

Without consulting Stalin, Truman and Churchill decided to use the bomb
with only an implied warning to the Japanese. Along with Chiang Kai-shek of
China they issued an ominous ultimatum, threatening "prompt and utter destruction" if Japan did not surrender. On two points the Potsdam Declaration was
silent. It never mentioned the atom bomb and it gave no indication that the
vanquished could retain their emperor, a sacred institution to the Japanese. Tokyo
made no formal reply.

Moderates in Japan had been pressing for peace since April 1945. They needed only assurances on keeping the emperor to overcome military diehards. Truman and Churchill knew Japan was on the verge of defeat and were aware that peace feelers had been sent to the Russians. Why then did the Allies offer no compromise on the emperor and instead cling to their policy of unconditional surrender? Some historians have charged that Secretary of State James Byrnes, a staunch anticommunist, wanted a combat demonstration of the bomb as a dramatic warning to the Soviet Union. Aware of the bomb's potential, Stalin would have reason to resolve issues on British and American terms.

Most evidence indicates that Truman decided to drop the bomb to end the war quickly. In doing so he followed the recommendations of the high-level Interim Committee appointed to review bomb policy. Military leaders believed Japan would not surrender without an invasion. The estimated cost in Allied lives ran as high as half a million to a million casualties. The terror of kamikaze attacks and the fierce resistance encountered at Okinawa served as grim reminders of Japanese fanaticism. Byrnes, among others, thought the American public would accept no formula that departed from unconditional surrender. And most American officials did not think the Japanese peace feelers were serious. Late in July 1945 Truman ordered crews on Tinian Island in the South Pacific to drop the bomb as soon as weather permitted.

When the president left Potsdam on August 2, nothing of importance had been settled. Germany's future as well as the question of reparations remained clouded. The agenda for a peace conference had still to be decided. Allied leaders had not even agreed when, if ever, they would meet again. Truman hoped that James Byrnes would be able to negotiate at future meetings of Allied foreign ministers, and both believed that "the bomb assured ultimate success in negotiations."

Before Truman's ship reached the United States the world learned what atomic warfare might mean. On August 6, 1945, the *Enola Gay,* a B-29 bomber, dropped a uranium bomb called "Little Boy" on Hiroshima, an industrial and military center. The blast leveled four square miles of the city, killing nearly 80,000 people (including 20 American prisoners of war). A German priest came upon dazed soldiers who had looked up as the bomb exploded. Their eyeballs had melted from their sockets. Another eyewitness spoke of survivors "so broken and confused that they moved and behaved like automatons." Two days later the Soviet Union declared war on Japan, and on August 9 a second atomic bomb (a plutonium weapon nicknamed "Fat Man") exploded over the port of Nagasaki. Another 60,000 were killed instantly. In both cities people who lived through the horror began to sicken and die. Radiation poisoning, unexpected by many of the scientists who built the bomb, claimed tens of thousands of additional lives.

Truman told his cabinet he could not bear the thought of killing more women and children and ordered a halt to the bombing. No more bombs were necessary. Breaking all precedents, the emperor intervened and declared openly for peace. On September 3 a humiliated Japanese delegation boarded the battleship *Missouri* in Tokyo Bay and signed the document of surrender. World War II had ended.

Frozen forever at 8:16 a.m., Japanese time: the moment when an atomic bomb exploded over Hiroshima.

"World War II changed everything," observed a retired admiral long after the war. Before the war Americans seldom exerted leadership in world affairs. In its wake the world looked to the United States to rebuild the economies of Europe and Asia and to maintain peace. World War II not only had shown the global interdependence of economic and political systems, but also increased that interdependence. Out of the war developed a truly international economy.

At home the trends toward bigness and centralization vastly accelerated. Supported by government, old industries grew and new industries like synthetic rubber sprang up. Advances in electronics, communications, and aviation brought the world closer to every home. Government grew, too. The size of the national debt alone guaranteed that Washington would continue to dominate the economy. The military services might shrink, but never again would they starve as they had between the wars. Americans would learn that a strong defense required a large federal bureaucracy and a generous military budget.

Three fears loomed, even as victory parades snaked down the nation's main streets. First, cutbacks in military spending might bring on another depression. The middle classes, greatly expanded by wartime prosperity, increasingly looked to government not to extend New Deal reforms but to help them preserve and continue their recent gains. Second, Stalin's efforts to control eastern Europe threatened the liberal peace plans of Franklin Roosevelt. Finally, there was the atomic bomb. The United States might control it for the present, but what if it fell into unfriendly hands? In the atomic age no one in the world, not even the United States, was safe any more.

SIGNIFICANT EVENTS

1941   A. Philip Randolph plans march on Washington; Roosevelt creates Fair Employment Practices Commission

1942   War Production Board and War Labor Board created; rubber shortage; Office of Price Administration provokes controversy; Revenue Act; Roosevelt lifts restrictions on enemy aliens; internment of Japanese-Americans

1943   Office of War Mobilization replaces WPB; payroll deductions adopted; suspension of antitrust prosecutions; race riot in Detroit; zoot-suit riots; Smith–Connolly Act

1944   Strikes in Philadelphia; *Smith v. Allwright;* Dumbarton Oaks and Bretton Woods meetings; Roosevelt wins fourth term; G.I. Bill of Rights; War Refugee Board created

1945   Truman becomes president; Allied troops liberate extermination camps; first United Nations Organization meeting; Germany surrenders; Potsdam Conference; atom bombs dropped on Japan; World War II ends

PART 6

THE UNITED STATES
IN A
NUCLEAR AGE

At Los Alamos in July 1945, during the final feverish days of work on the first atomic bomb, a few scientists calculated the possible unexpected effects of an atomic blast. The strategic bombings at Dresden and Tokyo showed how a firestorm, once started, sucked oxygen from the surrounding atmosphere, feeding upon itself and enlarging the inferno. No one had ever set off an atomic explosion, and some scientists worried that an even greater chain reaction might follow, one that would not only ignite the atmosphere around it but would envelop the earth's atmosphere, leaving the planet in ashes. Members of the team checked and rechecked the calculations before deciding those fears were invalid.

In the half-century since Hiroshima, the atomic nightmare has returned repeatedly to haunt the world. The threat now appears to be not from the detonation of a single bomb but from an all-too-human chain reaction, in which escalating violence leads to atomic strike and counterstrike, followed by a decades-long radioactive "nuclear winter," from which intelligent life could never fully recover.

During the heady victory celebrations of 1945, the threat of nuclear annihilation seemed distant. Although President Truman and many other American leaders had become increasingly distrustful of Stalin, the United States preserved a clear atomic monopoly. The dangers from radioactive fallout had impressed only a handful of officials and even fewer of the public, who were treated to cheery fantasies of the peacetime use of atomics, including an article in the May 1947 *Collier's* magazine in which a recovered paraplegic emerged from the mushroom

cloud of his atomic treatment, his wheelchair almost miraculously left behind. By 1949, when fallout from Russian atomic tests indicated the U.S. monopoly had been broken, the grim global realignment was already well established. Two superpowers, the Soviet Union and the United States, had replaced the players in the old "balance of power" politics that had defined European politics for two centuries.

The polarization of the globe into two camps, each dominated by a superpower, would have seemed strange even 20 years earlier. But in the long view, the result was not surprising. Ever since the beginning of expansion in the sixteenth century, Europe's greatest growth came along its peripheries, both west and east. Along the continent's west-facing rim, the Portuguese, Spanish, Dutch, French, and English reached beyond themselves for commercial and colonial empires. By the late nineteenth century England's colonial offshoot, the United States, was coming into its own even farther west. Over these same centuries of expansion, Europe's eastern flank saw Russian settlers pushing across the steppes of Eurasia, turning more and more grasslands into cultivated fields. Farther north, Russian fur traders were bringing the forest and tundra of Siberia into the Russian orbit, just as French and English fur traders were encroaching on the forests of the Canadian shield.

In area and vastness of resources, the Soviet Union surpassed even the United States, its boundaries encompassing 12 time zones. Given the centuries-long tradition of authoritarian rule (*czar* is the Russian derivative of Caesar), the Russian Revolution of 1917 took a firmly centralized approach to modernization. At sometimes frightful cost (the attempt to collectivize its peasant farmers alone starved or killed 10 million) Stalin brought the Soviet Union to its position as superpower by the end of World War II. The peripheral powers of Europe—the United States and Russia—had become dominant. And by 1960 both were relying on large stockpiles of nuclear weapons as the ultimate guarantors of their security and power.

Able to annihilate each other many times over, the two superpowers hoped to guarantee the peace through a system of deterrence. The knowledge of "mutual assured destruction," nuclear strategists suggested, would prevent either side from being the first to launch a missile attack. Yet that strategy was a frightening one precisely because the globe could not be cut simply into two halves—communist and noncommunist—each with clearly unified political and economic interests. Just as the "federal union" of the United States had been often riven by ethnic, religious, or economic rivalries, conflicts worldwide were arising out of similar dynamics, threatening to widen into war where the prestige of either superpower became critically involved.

Both the Soviets and the Americans discovered the limits of projecting their power and prestige in regional conflicts. For more than a decade, the United States sought unsuccessfully to win a war against North Vietnam by conventional means, before withdrawing in defeat. For another decade, the Soviet Union waged a similarly unsuccessful war in Afghanistan. In both cases, though the rival superpowers justified their involvement in terms of a battle for democracy and liberty or for democratic socialism, regional rivalries clearly played a dominant role. In the Vietnam conflict, the Communist Ho Chi Minh was enough of a nationalist to prefer nearly any form of government, including French colonial rule, to domination by Vietnam's traditional enemy, China. It mattered not that China was ruled by a Communist "comrade," Mao Tse-tung. During their war in Afghanistan, the Soviets quickly discovered that their dogged rebel opposition was inspired by an Islamic faith. The 1979 revolution in Iran brought the Ayatollah Khomeini to power and further demonstrated that Islamic fundamentalism would play a crucial role in the Middle East and the Saharan subcontinent.

Thus the world of the 1980s and 1990s was shaping up to be less a bipolar world, divided between two superpowers, than multipolar, with a great many regional rivalries and interests. These regional strains and conflicts could not be ignored, for the technology of industrialization had created a truly global theater of markets, cultures, and politics. Beginning in the 1970s, even the natural limits of the globe were becoming apparent.

In America, the boom and development mentality of the 1950s and 1960s was tempered in the 1970s as the environmental costs of air and water pollutants, strip mining, pesticides, and a host of other abuses became obvious. Similarly, by the mid-1970s most major rivers in the Soviet Union had been polluted by industrial wastes, significant fish kills being reported in the Ural, Volga, and Dnieper rivers. China, whose coal reserves are as great as those of the United States and the Soviet Union combined, was boosting its coal-fired electric generating plants from a 35,000-megawatt output in 1980 to a projected 92,000 megawatts in the year 2000. Already northern Chinese cities are heavily polluted by the burning of coal, and damage from acid rain can be charted in neighboring regions. China, the United States, and the Soviet Union combined account for nearly half of all humanly produced emissions of carbon dioxide, whose addition to the atmosphere threatens to raise the earth's temperature, creating a greenhouse effect that could change the world drastically. In the late 1980s recurring drought ravaged sub-Saharan Africa, leading to thousands of deaths from famine. As heat waves and drought severely damaged American crops in 1988, some scientists warned that the global warming trend had begun.

A nuclear winter or a greenhouse summer? Both grim alternatives make it clear that, half a millennium after the civilizations of two hemispheres achieved sustained contact, their ultimate fates are indivisibly intertwined.

CHRONOLOGY

AMERICAN EVENT	YEAR		GLOBAL EVENT
First atomic weapon detonated	1945	TRUMAN	United Nations founded
Truman Doctrine proclaimed	1947		
Marshall Plan aids postwar Europe	1948		Czechoslovakia falls to the Communists
			State of Israel created
	1949		U.S.S.R. explodes atomic bomb
			Communists seize power in China
McCarthy begins anticommunist campaign	1950		Korean War begins
	1953	EISENHOWER	Armistice in Korea
Brown v. Board of Education	1954		French defeated in Indochina
Postwar baby boom peaks	1957		Soviet Union launches *Sputnik*
	1959		Castro wins power in Cuba
	1961	KENNEDY	First Soviet manned space flight
			Soviets erect Berlin Wall
	1962		Cuban missile crisis
Civil rights march on Washington	1963	JOHNSON	U.S.-U.S.S.R. nuclear test-ban treaty
Kennedy assassinated			
Johnson launches war on poverty; escalates war in Vietnam	1964		Beatles become international rock stars
Voting Rights Act passed	1965		Mao Tse-tung launches radical "Cultural Revolution"
Chavez leads farm workers campaign			
	1967		Israeli-Arab Six-Day War
Martin Luther King assassinated	1968		Viet Cong launch Tet Offensive
Robert Kennedy assassinated			
First human flight to the moon	1969	NIXON	
Watergate burglars arrested	1972		SALT I signed
Indians protest at Wounded Knee	1973		Vietnam peace accord signed
			Yom Kippur War
			OPEC oil boycott
Nixon resigns	1974	FORD	
	1977	CARTER	Panama Canal treaty signed
	1978		Camp David accords signed
			Islamic revolution in Iran
U.S. recognizes Communist China	1979		Soviet Union invades Afghanistan
Nuclear accident at Three Mile Island			
"Reagan Revolution" tax and budget cuts	1981	REAGAN	Japan is graduating more engineers per year than the United States
Gramm-Rudman Act passed	1985		Mikhail Gorbachev becomes Soviet premier
Arms-for-hostage deal with Iran	1986		Fire at Chernobyl nuclear reactor
	1989	BUSH	
More than half of U.S. city landfills exhausted	1990		
	2000		Three out of five cities with population greater than 15 million are in third world

30

Cold War America

The war had been over for almost five months and still troop ships steamed into New York and other ports, discharging soldiers eager to meet their wives or perhaps a little anxious if they happened to spend their last military hours in floating crap games where thousands of dollars changed hands. Timuel Black was packing his duffel below decks when he heard some of the white soldiers calling, "There she is! The Statue of Liberty!" Black felt a little bitter about the war. He'd been drafted in Chicago in 1943, just after the race riots, and his father, a strong supporter of civil rights, was angry. "What the hell are you goin' to fight in Europe for? The fight is here." He wanted to go off with his boy to demonstrate in Detroit—and he would have, except the roads were being blocked and the buses and trains screened to prevent Negroes' coming in to make trouble.

In any case, Black was soon off to fight the Nazis, in a segregated army, with separate mess halls, separate bunks, even separate towns in Britain to visit on weekends off. He'd gone ashore during the D-Day invasion, survived the Battle of the Bulge, and marched through one of the German concentration camps. "The first thing you get is the stench," he recalled. "Everybody knows that's human stench. You begin to realize something terrible had happened. There's quietness. You get closer and you begin to see what's happened to these creatures. And you get—I got more passionately angry than I guess I'd ever been." He thought: if it could happen here, to the Germans, it could happen anywhere. It could happen to black folk in America. So when the white soldiers called to come up and see the Statue of Liberty, Black's reaction was, "Hell, I'm not goin' up there. Damn that." But after all, he went up. "All of a sudden, I found myself with tears, cryin' and saying the same thing [the white soldiers] were saying. Glad to be home, proud of my country, as irregular as it is. Determined that it could be better. Just happy that I had survived and buoyed up by the enthusiasm of the moment."

Across the other side of the continent, Betty Basye was working as a nurse in a burn-and-blind center at Menlo Park, California. Soldiers from the Pacific were shipped back there: "Blind young men. Eyes gone, legs gone. Parts of the face. Burns—you'd land with a fire bomb and be up in flames." She'd joke with the men, trying to keep their spirits up, talking about times to come. And when word of V-J Day was broadcast, the hospital erupted in celebration. "Our superintendent of nurses led a conga line up and down the hospital, serpentine, up past

The mushroom-cloud image captured both the spectacle and potential horror of atomic warfare. With scant regard for the effects of radioactive fallout, the Defense Department conducted above-ground tests like this one near Las Vegas, Nevada, in 1953.

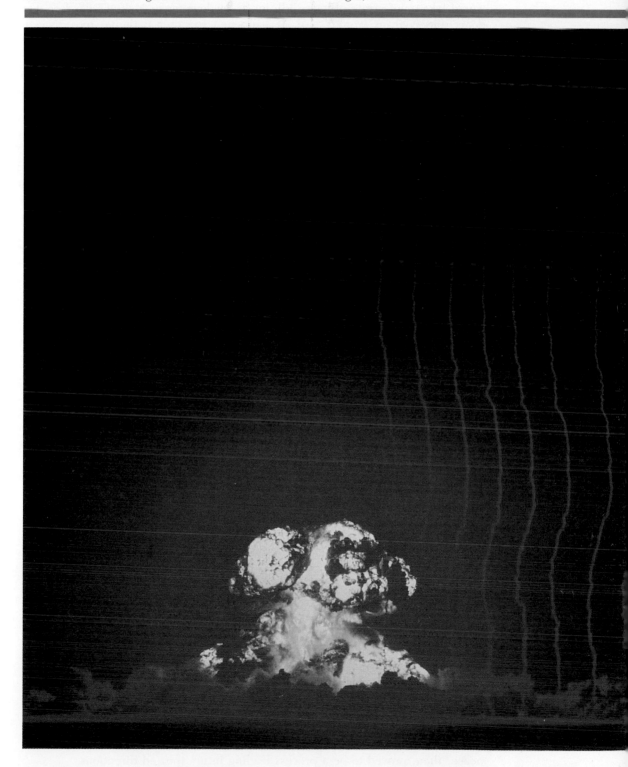

every bed. This took hours, because it was ward after ward. . . . Absolute bedlam." And then Basye had to think about her own future. She kept her job for a while and was transferred to Pasadena, along with many of her patients. She would take one favorite of hers, Bill, for walks downtown. Half of Bill's face was gone, and civilians would stare. It happened to other patients, too. "Nicely dressed women, absolutely staring, just standing there staring." Some people wrote the local paper, wondering why disfigured vets couldn't be kept on their own grounds and off the streets. Basye sensed an indignation welling up. The war was over—"and we're still here." After a time, she started dating a soldier back from the South Pacific. "I got busy after the war," she recalled, "getting married and having my four children. That's what you were supposed to do. And getting your house in suburbia."

When Joe Hanley returned home he wasn't thinking about a house in suburbia or even settling down. Getting off the streetcar in his old neighborhood, Chicago's North Side, the first thing he saw was a bar: "I'll have a shot and a beer," he said, and the bartender didn't take his money. "Welcome back, kid." Hanley didn't feel that welcome. He'd gone to war half convinced he'd be only "part of the cannon fodder. The sacrificial lamb. . . . It was a big surprise to everybody when you came home. What are you doing here? You know?" During the war, his foxhole buddy Kevin and he had been charging up a hill. "He went in one direction and I went in another, hit the ground," and the next thing Hanley knew, Kevin was dead. It got to him. Kevin had a wife and young daughter; Hanley, nobody. The wrong man had been killed. After the Allies swept through Germany, his unit was sent to guard POWs. The Germans kept telling them, "Within 10 years you'll be fighting the Russians." Crazy! A lot of Germans felt that way. Back in Chicago, Hanley got a job in a local tavern and became the neighborhood bookie. He felt life was a joke. "Why worry about anything if within a moment or two you might die? Why get serious about it?" When gambling didn't provide enough action, he joined the police, hoping for more danger. But it seemed like child's play next to war. He did feel an obligation to Kevin and looked up his widow to tell her how it had been at the end and to befriend the young daughter. The acquaintance turned into friendship, and in 1949 Hanley married Kevin's wife. Life was slowly returning to normal.

Yet as Hanley, Basye, and Black were soon to discover, what was "normal" in these first years of peace was not entirely clear. The first truly global war had left a large part of Europe in ruins and the old balance of power shattered. Even if most Americans and their leaders wished to return to their isolationist attitudes of the 1930s—and, by and large, they did not—the dramatic events occurring month after month during 1945 and 1946 made it clear that the affairs of the wider world would not go away. For in the end, the United States converted not so much to peace as to a "cold war" against its former ally, the Soviet Union.

This undeclared war came to affect not only American foreign affairs, but almost every aspect of American life. Abroad, it justified a far wider military and economic role for the United States in areas like the Middle East and the Pacific rim from Korea to Southeast Asia. At home it sent major and minor politicians scurrying across the land in a search for Communist spies and "subversives" that took them from the State Department to Hollywood and into college classrooms. It influenced the curriculum teachers felt free to teach and even dictated the kinds of movies Americans watched. It dramatically increased the role of the military–industrial–university complex formed during World War II. "Reconversion" to peace, then, proved to be a process leading in unexpected directions.

CONVERSION: "THE AMERICAN PEOPLE WANT A REST"

At war's end, many business leaders feared that a sudden drop in government purchases would bring back the hard times of the 1930s. Munitions and aircraft factories would stand idle, while once-booming war communities like Willow Run became ghost towns. Instead, Americans went on a buying spree. High war wages had piled up in savings accounts and war bonds. Eager consumers set off to find the new cars, appliances, and foods unavailable during the war. Despite a sharp drop in government spending (from $83 billion in 1945 to only $31 billion in 1946), the gross national product fell less than 1 percent and employment actually increased. Consumers had taken up the slack.

In fact, demand was so high that shortages were widespread. Consumers found the lines in stores long, prices rising, and goods scarce. By the time the Office of Price Administration (OPA) lifted wage and price controls in June 1946, the inflation rate had jumped from an average of 2 percent during the war years to over 16 percent. And with demand so high, the scramble for goods became feverish. A customer determined to have fresh meat might be inspired to tip the butcher for the difficult task of lifting an order across the counter. Fresh hundred-dollar bills dropped at a salesman's feet circumvented the long wait for a new car. Builders held lotteries to see which lucky few out of thousands of applicants could have a new house.

Postwar Work

The transition from war to peace also meant significant dislocations in the job market. With millions of veterans looking for peacetime jobs, workers on the home front, especially women and minorities, found themselves out of work. By 1946 some 2.25 million women had left their jobs and another million were laid off. Yet heavy postwar consumer demand allowed 2.75 million women to find jobs, so that by 1950 women constituted 28 percent of the work force, up from 24 percent in 1940.

More to the point, the status of women's work declined. Their employment in the professions and managerial roles fell. Most women who returned to jobs after being laid off lost their seniority and had to move into lower positions that paid less. Most were concentrated in jobs that mirrored their traditional family responsibilities for nurturing: they were nurses, not doctors; teachers, not principals; tellers, not bankers. Far more worked in service (as maids, waitresses, or secretaries) than in manufacturing. The combined demands of work and family forced many women into low-paying part-time and unskilled jobs. Most places of employment were heavily segregated by gender. About 75 percent of women worked at female-only jobs. In fact, gender segregation in the workplace was worse in 1950 than in 1900 and more complete than segregation by race.

Equally important was the shift in attitudes in the prevailing culture. War employment had given many women their first taste of economic independence. As peace came, almost 75 percent of the working women in one survey indicated that they hoped to continue their jobs. But with peace came pressure for women to return to their more traditional roles. Male social scientists stressed how important it was for women to accept "more than the wife's usual responsibility for her marriage" and offer "lavish—and undemanding—affection" to returning GIs. One marriage counselor urged women to let their husbands know "you are tired of living alone, that you want him now to take charge."

For minorities, the end of the war brought a return of an old labor practice, "last hired, first fired." At the height of the war over 200,000 blacks and Hispanics had found jobs in shipbuilding. By 1946 that number had dwindled to less than 10,000. The influx of Mexican laborers under the bracero program temporarily halted. In the South, where the large majority of blacks lived, wartime labor shortages had become surpluses. Returning black and Hispanic veterans discovered that for them conditions at home had hardly improved.

Those workers who were not union members had no way to protest being laid off, but organized labor was determined to preserve the gains made during the war. As reconversion brought an abrupt decline in hours and overtime, unions demanded pay increases of up to 30 percent to make up for lost wages. When management balked, strikes spread across the nation. Autoworkers walked off the job in the fall of 1945; steelworkers in January 1946; miners in April. Strikes in such key industries seriously threatened to impede peacetime production. In 1946 some 5 million workers struck, a rate triple that of any previous year. Antiunion sentiment soared.

Most labor–management confrontations came eventually to the White House, where negotiators generally settled on wage increases ranging between 18 and 22 percent. But the crisis peaked in May 1946 with a threatened national rail strike, which would have paralyzed the nation's transportation network. An outraged President Truman asked, "What decent American would pull a rail strike at a time like this?" On May 23 he announced that the government would seize the railroads, while he requested power to draft striking workers into the military. The strike was settled before the threat could be carried out, but Truman's action startled liberals and conservatives alike. Few people approved the idea of using the draft as a punitive tool. Labor leaders, for their part, became convinced they had lost their friend at the White House.

The New Deal at Bay

Inflation, shortages, and labor unrest spelled political trouble for Harry Truman. In September 1945 he had boldly claimed his intention to extend the New Deal into the postwar era, with legislation to guarantee full employment, subsidized public housing, national health insurance, and a peacetime version of the Fair Employment Practices Commission to fight job discrimination. But by 1946 the spirit of reform had given way to a more conservative agenda. Truman's political stock had fallen in and out of Washington. Most of Franklin Roosevelt's old advisers had left the administration to lead more peaceful and private lives. In Congress, a coalition of conservative Republicans and southern Democrats stymied the president's attempts at further reform. All he achieved was a watered-down full-employment bill, which created the Council of Economic Advisors to guide the president's policies and at least established the principle that the government rather than the private sector was responsible for maintaining full employment.

As the elections of 1946 approached, Republicans harped on the production shortages, the procession of strikes, the mismanagement of the economy. "To err is Truman," proclaimed the campaign buttoms—or, more simply, "Had Enough?" Evidently many voters had. The Republicans gained control of both houses of

Congress and 25 of 48 governorships. Not since 1928 had the Democrats fared so poorly.

Leading the rightward swing was Senator Robert A. Taft of Ohio, son of former president William Howard Taft. Bob Taft not only wanted to halt the spread of the New Deal—he wanted to dismantle it entirely, and especially limit the power of unions. "We have to get over the corrupting idea we can legislate prosperity, legislate equality, legislate opportunity," he said in dismissing the liberal agenda. In 1947 he led the fight to pass the Taft–Hartley Act, over Truman's veto. In the event of a strike, the bill allowed the president to order workers back on the job during a 90-day "cooling-off" period while collective bargaining continued. It also permitted states to adopt "right-to-work" laws, which banned the closed shop by eliminating union membership as a prerequisite for many jobs. Union leaders criticized the new law as a "slave-labor" act but discovered they could live with it, though it did hurt union efforts to organize, especially in the South.

Thus by 1947 the domestic conversion from war to peace was largely completed. In leaving behind the war and the Great Depression, most Americans did not repudiate the major accomplishments of the New Deal: Social Security, minimum wages, a more active role for government in reducing unemployment. But by and large they were not prepared to extend those reforms. As Truman himself conceded, "The American people have been through a lot of experiments and they want a rest."

Yet they were not to get one—at least not the sort they had been counting on. As the economy gradually shifted into a postwar boom, the rest of the world struggled to recover from years of devastation. Power had shifted from Europe to the periphery where in the new alignment the United States and the Soviet Union regarded each other as the world's two reigning superpowers—and as mortal enemies. Since this realignment had such serious and long-lasting consequences, it is worth looking in some detail at the pivotal events of 1945 and 1946. What happened that led the Western powers to split with their Soviet allies? How did the breach become irreparable?

THE RISE OF THE COLD WAR

In October 1944, with France recently liberated and the Allies on the offensive, Winston Churchill journeyed to Moscow to see Joseph Stalin. Getting down to work only at ten in the evening (Stalin loved to do business late at night), the two men discussed how the great powers might prevent conflicts from arising once the war was won. Churchill took out a sheet of paper and jotted down a number of smaller nations. Beside each he put a percentage indicating the amount of influence Britain or Russia might have. Romania—90 percent for the Russians. Greece—90 percent for the British, along with the Americans. Bulgaria—75 percent for the Russians. Hungary and Yugoslavia—50 percent each. Stalin read the list impassively, then handed it back to Churchill, who became a bit embarrassed at so baldly dividing the world into spheres of influence. He suggested burning the paper and also told Stalin that, as far as more public discussions went, it was "better to express these things in diplomatic terms and not to use the phrase 'dividing into spheres' because the Americans might be shocked. But as long as he and Marshal Stalin understood each other, he could explain matters to the President"—that is, of course, Roosevelt.

Roosevelt was not as naive about world affairs as this account might suggest. He too could speak matter-of-factly about the postwar world being managed by the "Four Policemen"—the United States, Russia, Britain, and China. And with Stalin as one of the policemen, Roosevelt was ready to concede that the Soviet Union could not be denied its own "sphere of influence." But he also knew that such big-power settlements went against long-cherished American ideals. Since the early Republic, Americans had championed, in principle at least, the right of small nations to determine their own fates, with their freedom guaranteed by treaties and international organizations. Such idealism inspired Woodrow Wilson's hopes for the League of Nations and Roosevelt's later support for the United Nations. In a sense, Roosevelt sought to balance two strands of thought: the traditional idealism of Wilson and the more practical recognition that the United States could not guarantee democracy in every nation and under every circumstance. Spheres of influence would inevitably continue to exist.

Truman was a different man. Lacking Roosevelt's experience or his easy confidence that he could manage "Uncle Joe," the new president approached the Sovi-

President Harry Truman and his Secretary of State James Byrnes relax on their return from the Potsdam Conference. At his first meeting with Stalin, Truman believed he needed to "stand up" to the Russians, and Byrnes consistently reinforced this approach as the cold war set in.

ets with a good deal more suspicion. "Stalin is an SOB, but of course he thinks I'm one, too," Truman commented after their meeting at Potsdam in July 1945. Behind all the diplomatic bowing and bluffing, what were the Soviets' real intentions? Stalin had spoken of adjusting Poland's borders, which could be chalked up as a matter of legitimate defensive security. But he had also asked that Russia assume joint control of the Dardanelles, Turkey's gateway to the Mediterranean. And he asked that the Soviet Union become trustee of Libya, Italy's former African colony. As one British diplomat at Potsdam aptly put it, the great debate was "whether Russia [is] peaceful and wants to join the Western Club but is suspicious of us, or whether she is out to dominate the world and is hoodwinking us." Truman and his advisers, like the diplomat, tended to opt for the same answer: "It always seems safer to go on the worse assumption."

With the war over, the Soviets resumed their claims to Libya and the Dardanelles. Furthermore, local Communists led the fighting to overturn the traditional monarchy in nearby Greece. And in November 1945 Soviet forces occupying part of Iran lent support to rebels seeking autonomy from the Iranian government. Asia, too, seemed a target for Soviet ambitions. Russian occupation forces in Manchuria were turning over captured Japanese arms to the Chinese Communist forces of Mao Tse-tung. Russian troops controlled the northern half of Korea. In other areas like Vietnam leftist nationalists were fighting against the return of colonial rule. To deal with this combination of menace and disorder Harry Truman and his advisers sought to frame a policy.

The View from West and East

Americans tended to suspect the worst of the Soviets, and for several reasons. To begin with, a deep ideological gulf had long separated the two nations. Since the October Revolution of 1917, most Americans viewed the Bolsheviks with a mixture of fear, suspicion, and loathing. Marxists, after all, had rejected both religion and the notion of private enterprise, two institutions central to the American dream. Further, Stalin's brutal purges during the late 1930s horrified the public and, even more important, left a lasting imprint on the American diplomatic corps. Finally, Soviet propagandists had made no secret of their intention to export revolution throughout the world, including the United States.

The most recent lesson of history—the war itself—seemed to dictate a stiff response to the Soviets. When Neville Chamberlain attempted a policy of appeasement with Hitler in 1938, it only emboldened German expansionism. After the war, Secretary of the Navy James Forrestal applied the Munich analogy when he argued that acceding to Russian demands would seem like an attempt "to buy their understanding and sympathy. We tried that once with Hitler. . . . There are no returns on appeasement." To many of Truman's advisers, the Soviet dictator seemed to be every bit as much bent on world conquest as Hitler had been.

Of course, Stalin's true intentions remain an open question, for historians have little information about the inner workings of the Soviet state. But the case can at least be made that after the war, Soviet attitudes did not center on a scheme for world domination. As they evaluated their situation, they saw the United States quite vigorously at work establishing its global influence. American occupation forces in Europe and Asia ringed the Soviet Union. American corporations owned or controlled vast oil fields in the Middle East and, along with the French and British, were a strong presence in Southeast Asia. In Latin America, the

United States had its own well-established sphere of influence. At the new United Nations, countries friendly to the United States far outnumbered those with links to the Soviet Union. And, of course, the United States alone possessed the atomic bomb. Stalin had reason to fear that the anticommunists in the American government would seek to exploit the weakness of his war-ravaged nation.

The Russians, too, had mastered their own lessons of history. Napoleon had invaded their nation in 1812; the "big powers" had forced Russia to give up territory after the Crimean War and at the Congress of Berlin. Germany had violated their land twice during the twentieth century. Given such precedents, Stalin might well have wished to protect the Soviet Union by controlling the nations surrounding him. Indeed, for a dictator accustomed to absolute power within his own territory, such an outlook was almost sheer habit. As one Yugoslav Communist leader remarked of Stalin, "Everything beyond the control of his police was a potential enemy."

The superiority of the American economy created another source of conflict. While Russia had been left devastated by Germany's invasion, the war had doubled the gross national product of the United States. The efficiency of American farms and factories, the quality of American consumer goods, along with technological innovation in the military and civilian sectors, gave Soviet leaders a feeling of inferiority. They realized that the Soviet Union could not compete successfully in the open world system the United States sought to establish after World War II. To make matters worse, the United States had quickly terminated its lend-lease program after V-J Day and refused a large loan that Stalin desperately needed to begin rebuilding his nation. As a final irritant, Americans were becoming increasingly reluctant to allow the Soviets to claim reparations from the Germans to help Russia back on its feet.

Toward Containment

The disagreements and mutual suspicion arising out of these conflicting points of view came to a head in the first months of 1946. For his part, Stalin announced in February that the Soviet Union would have to take unilateral steps to preserve its national security. In a world dominated by capitalism, he warned, future wars were inevitable. To assure against "any eventuality," the Russian people must be prepared to accept a new five-year plan for economic development.

Although some Americans thought Stalin was merely rallying Russian support for his domestic program, the speech confirmed the Truman administration's worst fears. "I'm tired of babying the Soviets," remarked the president, who in any case seldom wore kid gloves. Even Truman's mother passed along a message: "Tell Harry to be good, be honest, and behave himself, but I think it is now time for him to get tough with someone." *Time* magazine, an early voice for a "get tough" policy, called Stalin's speech "the most warlike pronouncement uttered by any top-rank statesman since V-J day" and was soon publishing maps showing the global threat of "Communist Contagion." In March Winston Churchill warned that the Soviets had dropped an "Iron Curtain" between their satellites and the free world.

Joseph Stalin.

As policymakers groped for an effective way to deal with these developments, the State Department received a diplomatic cable, extraordinary for both its 8000-word length and its impact on policy in Washington. The author, George Kennan, chargé d'affaires in Moscow and long a student of Soviet ways, argued that Russian leaders, including Stalin, were so paranoid that it was impossible to reach useful accommodations with them. "Nothing short of complete disarmament, delivery of our air and naval forces to Russia, and resigning of the powers of government to American Communists would even dent this problem," he wrote. Without the respectable cloak of Marxist ideology, Stalin "would stand before history, at best, as only the last in that succession of cruel and wasteful Russian rulers."

While Kennan's analysis was not particularly new, it did provide a clear framework for analyzing Soviet behavior and a strategic concept for responding to the Russians—"containment." By bringing to bear firm diplomatic, economic, and military counterpressure, the United States could block Soviet aggression wherever it occurred. Out of frustration the Soviets would be forced to drop their plans of conquest and alter their domestic institutions. Only then would an accommodation between East and West be possible. Hundreds of copies of Kennan's "long telegram" were made and sent to high officials in Washington as well as American diplomats abroad. Truman wholeheartedly adopted the doctrine of containment.

The Truman Doctrine

During the rest of 1946, the administration found few opportunities to apply the policy of containment. At first it seemed that Iran, with its strategic location and British-run oil fields, might serve the purpose. The Joint Chiefs of Staff, the combined American military command, had declared Iran's independence vital to the United States, for Iran held the key to secure oil fields in the Persian Gulf region. An oil mission sent to the area in 1943 had reported that vast Middle East oil fields would soon displace those in the United States as the center of world production. American oil companies had already established a major position in the region. During the war the U.S. government had taken a far more active role in the affairs

---

As American fears of Soviet intentions increased, journalists often described communism as though it were a disease, an inhuman force, or savage predator. In April 1946, *Time* magazine, a particularly outspoken source of anticommunist rhetoric, portrayed the spread of "infection" throughout Europe and Asia by the "Red Menace."

of Iran, Turkey, Saudi Arabia, and other Middle East states. Although Great Britain lost much of its regional influence to the United States, British diplomats welcomed the American presence as a safeguard against future Soviet expansion.

Iran seemed a likely Soviet target. British, American, and Russian troops occupied much of the country during the war. All three had negotiated unsuccessfully for oil concessions. By December 1945 the British and Americans had largely withdrawn, but the Soviet forces remained as part of a strategy to wrest economic and political concessions. In March 1946 Secretary of State James Byrnes went to the United Nations, determined to force a showdown over Soviet occupation of northern Iran. But before he could extract his pound of Russian flesh, the Soviets reached an agreement with Iran to withdraw their troops.

The critical cold war moment came in early 1947. As Europe reeled under severe winter storms and a depressed postwar economy, Great Britain announced it could no longer send aid to the beleaguered governments of Greece and Turkey. Truman decided to adopt a militant posture. Specifically, he wanted $400 million in military and economic aid for Greece and Turkey. The president went before Congress in March, determined to "scare hell out of the country." With the world divided into two hostile camps, he warned, the United States had to be prepared to step forward and help "free people" threatened by "totalitarian regimes." This position soon became known as the Truman Doctrine.

Critics were quick to point out that Truman had placed no limits on the American commitment. His was a proposal not simply to contain the communist threat to Greece and Turkey but also to resist Soviet expansion everywhere. Robert Taft thought it was a mistake to talk about a bipolar world divided into communist and anticommunist camps. Truman painted the alternatives in such strong colors, however, that Congress voted overwhelmingly to grant aid. In doing so, the nation took the critical step in entering the cold war. It linked Soviet communism with rebel movements all across the globe. It committed Americans to a relatively open-ended conflict. It expanded the president's powers to act in the face of a communist threat. All these actions would be debated in the decades to come, but by 1947 the die had been cast. Anticommunism had been established as a dominant theme in American policy, both foreign and domestic.

The Marshall Plan

For all its importance, the Truman Doctrine did not address the area of primary concern to Washington, Western Europe. Postwar economic collapse had left national treasuries empty, city streets dark, homes without heat, people starving, and factories closed. By 1947 American diplomats were warning that without American aid to revive the European economy, Communists would seize power in Germany, Italy, and France.

In June 1947 Secretary of State George C. Marshall stepped before a Harvard commencement audience to announce a New Deal–style recovery plan for Europe. He invited all European nations, East or West, to request assistance to rebuild their economies. Unlike the Truman Doctrine proposals, Marshall's speech made no mention of the communist menace, but his plan to provide Europe massive economic aid was designed to eliminate conditions that allowed Communists to take advantage of discontent. At the same time, generous credits would create far greater European demand for American goods, thus assuring markets and prosperity for the United States. And the secretary was gambling that fears of American economic penetration would lead the Soviets and their allies to reject his offer. At first neo-isolationists in Congress stymied aid under the guise of exercising fiscal conservatism. But when Communists expelled the non-Communists from Czechoslovakia's government, Congress approved the Marshall Plan, as it became known. And as the secretary anticipated, the Soviets blocked the efforts of Czechoslovakia and Poland to participate. The onus for dividing Europe fell, as Marshall guessed it would, on the Soviet Union, not the United States.

The Fall of Eastern Europe

Aggressive American efforts to stabilize Europe and the eastern Mediterranean placed Stalin on the defensive. At home he waged a battle against Western cultural influence. Even Russian soldiers and former prisoners of war were tainted, in his eyes, for allowing themselves to be captured or simply exposed to the West. Thousands were sent off to the Siberian labor camps, among them writer Alexander Solzhenitsyn, who later described the experience in *One Day in the Life of Ivan Denisovich.*

More shocking to the Western nations were Stalin's steps to consolidate Soviet political and military domination of Eastern Europe. In 1947 Stalin had moved even more forcefully against the moderate governments in Hungary and Czechoslovakia. Since 1945 Hungary had been ruled by a government chosen under relatively free elections. In June 1947 Soviet forces imposed a Communist regime subservient to Moscow. President Truman described that action as an "outrage." In February 1948 the duly elected government of Czechoslovakia was toppled and, shortly after, it was announced that the popular Czech foreign minister, Jan Masaryk, had fallen to his death from a small bathroom window. Suicide was the official explanation, but many suspected murder. In response to the Marshall Plan, Soviet foreign minister V. M. Molotov initiated a series of bilateral trade agreements tightly linking the Soviet and Eastern European economies in the COMECON (Council of Mutual Economic Assistance). In addition, he established the Cominform (Communist Information Bureau) to assert greater political control over foreign Communist parties.

Stalin's aggressive steps provoked further American efforts to win the cold war. By 1949 the United States and Canada had joined with Britain, France, Belgium, the Netherlands, and Luxembourg to establish the North Atlantic Treaty Organization (NATO) as a mutual defense pact. For the first time since Washington's Farewell Address in 1793 the United States during peacetime had entered into entangling alliances with European nations.

A crisis over Germany had precipitated that departure from tradition. In the process of forming NATO the Western powers had decided to transform their occupation zones into an independent West German state. The Western-controlled sectors of Berlin, however, lay over 100 miles to the east, well within the Soviet zone. On June 24 the Soviets reacted by blockading land access to Berlin. Truman's response was unequivocal: "We are going to stay, period." But he resisted the proposal of General Lucius Clay to shoot his way through the blockade. Instead, the United States began a massive airlift that lasted almost a year. In May 1949 Stalin lifted the blockade, conceding that he could not prevent the creation of West Germany.

Truman's firm handling of the Berlin crisis won him applause from both Dem-

COLD WAR EUROPE

By 1956 the postwar occupation of Europe had hardened into rigid cold war boundaries. The United States reacted to the presence of Soviet conventional forces in Eastern Europe by rearming West Germany and creating the NATO alliance (1949) for the defense of nations from the North Atlantic through the Mediterranean basin. The U.S.S.R. formed a counteralliance under the Warsaw Pact (1955). While Bonn became the de facto capital of West Germany, Berlin remained the official capital and into the 1960s the focus of the most severe cold war tensions.

ocrats and Republicans. They were equally enthusiastic about another bold presidential action, the recognition of Israel in May 1948, minutes after the Israelis announced their independence. Truman had previously supported the immigration of Jews into Palestine, despite the opposition of oil-rich Arab states and diplomats in the State Department. Though the president was sympathetic to the idea of a Jewish homeland, he was also sensitive to the advice of political advisers preparing for the 1948 presidential campaign. As British Prime Minister Clement

Atlee observed, "There's no Arab vote in America, but there's a heavy Jewish vote and the Americans are always having elections."

The Atomic Shield versus the Iron Curtain

During the first months of the Berlin blockade, Truman and his advisers considered the possibility of war and its new ultimate question: would the atom bomb be used? Truman said he prayed not, but if the need arose, he would not flinch. The Department of Defense, planning for every eventuality, initiated a request for the transfer of bombing authority. But Truman drew the line: he was not going to have "some dashing lieutenant colonel decide when would be the proper time to drop one."

Increasingly the bomb loomed like a shadow falling across the developments of the postwar world. Truman's dilemma pointed up a major question: who would control the use of such monumental power, American civil or military authorities? In the international arena, should there be any controls over its development? What should happen if the Soviets developed their own bomb? In 1946 Americans were shocked to discover that Russian spies had been caught stealing Canadian atomic secrets. It was naive to think similar efforts were not being made in the United States. Truman asked how soon the Soviets might get the bomb, and he was assured by General Leslie Groves, head of the wartime Manhattan Project, that it would be at least 20 years, although American atomic scientists warned that the day might come within 5 years.

For the time being, however, Americans had their monopoly. In August 1946 President Truman signed the McMahon Bill, which established the Atomic Energy Commission (AEC) as a civilian agency with control over all fissionable materials for both peacetime and military applications. But General Groves had been working behind the scenes to give the military a decisive voice. It was Groves who had leaked information to the press about the spy ring delivering secrets to the Soviet Union. He wanted Congress as well as the public to doubt that scientists and civilians could be trusted with key secrets (though privately Groves admitted that no vital information had been lost). His campaign succeeded in amending the McMahon Act to give the military review over many civilian decisions. It also imposed such severe restrictions that sharing of information with Britain and Canada became virtually impossible. Under its terms, the AEC could not even permit the export of radioactive isotopes for medical research to neutral Sweden and Norway.

The idea of international control of atomic energy through the United Nations proved similarly vulnerable to cold war fears. Undersecretary of State Dean Acheson, TVA Director David Lilienthal, and physicist Robert Oppenheimer headed a committee that proposed to give a United Nations agency authority over the mining, refining, and use of the world's atomic raw materials. They believed that the Acheson–Lilienthal plan would afford the United States more security in the long run than a short-lived nuclear monopoly. But Truman put his adviser Bernard Baruch in charge of presenting the recommendations to the United Nations in June 1946. Baruch, a staunch cold warrior, was determined the United States would not give up its nuclear monopoly. His revised proposal ensured that the United States would be able to use the international agency not only to protect its own atomic resources but also to monitor the industrial and military uses of atomic energy within the Soviet Union.

The Soviets, naturally, rejected Baruch's proposal and instead introduced their own plan calling first for destruction of all nuclear bombs, then for an agreement never to use them, and, finally, for discussions about controls. Baruch had no intention of bargaining. It was either his plan or nothing, he announced. And so it was nothing, as the last serious attempt to achieve international cooperation collapsed. And while the United Nations debated, the United States conducted a nuclear bomb test on Bikini Atoll in the Pacific Ocean. The Truman administration had never seriously intended to sacrifice the American nuclear monopoly.

Atomic Deterrence

Ironically, because of the strict secrecy in developing the bomb, many of the military planners in charge of integrating it into American strategic planning knew little about it. Even Truman, in 1946, had no idea how many bombs the United States actually possessed. (For the two years after Hiroshima, it was never more than two.) The chiefs of the armed forces had at first tended to dismiss the weapon, in part from ignorance and in part from fears that too great a reliance on it might encourage the public to believe that conventional forces had become obsolete. But the situation soon changed.

By 1947 a tight-fisted Congress had cut the size of America's army down to a million soldiers. At the same time, the cold war was heating up in earnest. George Marshall, who had commanded some 8 million soldiers during the war as Army Chief of Staff, was now under pressure as secretary of state "to give the Russians hell." But as he ruefully observed, "My facilities for giving them hell—and I am a soldier and know something about the ability to give hell—was $1\frac{1}{3}$ divisions over the entire United States. That is quite a proposition when you deal with someone who has over 260 [divisions] and you have $1\frac{1}{3}$." Thus military planners were almost forced to adopt a nuclear strategy as the only deterrent to the overwhelming superiority of conventional Soviet forces in Europe.

At first what passed for nuclear strategies were little more than doomsday scenarios to incinerate vast areas of the Soviet Union. A 1946 war plan, "Pincher," modestly projected the obliteration of 20 Soviet cities in response to an attack on Western Europe. But the Joint Chiefs of Staff kept pressing the civilian AEC to permit stockpiling of more and more bombs. In 1948 "Fleetwood" raised the tally of cities to 77, with 8 bombs aimed for Moscow, 7 for Leningrad. Not until "Dropshot," the following year, did planners correct a major flaw in Fleetwood. If Moscow and Leningrad disappeared, who would be left to surrender? Dropshot recommended sparing those two cities until the second week. As military use of atomic materials continued to mount, David Lilienthal, the demoralized head of the Atomic Energy Commission, confessed that rather than promoting peaceful applications of nuclear energy, his agency had become "nothing more than a defense contractor for the Defense Department."

By 1948, then, not only was the cold war in full swing, but many Americans had hopes that the United States would win it. The Joint Chiefs of Staff had committed themselves to nuclear deterrence based on an American nuclear monopoly. Western Europe was on its way to economic recovery, thanks to the Marshall Plan. Soviet pressures on Greece, Turkey, and Iran had abated. Yet in one sense, success brought little comfort. The ideology of the cold war portrayed the Soviet Union as more than simply a major power seeking to protect its interests and expand where opportunity permitted. The Soviets were bent on dominating the world, even overthrowing the United States either from without or within. This was a war being fought not only across the globe but right in America, by unseen agents using underhanded means. In this way, the cold war mentality soon came to shape the lives of Americans at home much as it did American policy abroad.

THE COLD WAR AT HOME

With the worries of subversion and espionage increasing, President Truman acted to protect his own administration from the disloyalty of "Reds, phonies, and 'parlor pinks'" on the one hand and from the attacks of the Republican right on the other. On March 22, 1947, ten days after proposing the Truman Doctrine with its aid to Greece and Turkey, he signed an executive order establishing a Federal Employee Loyalty Program. Since there were over 2 million people employed by the government, plus another half million applying for jobs every year, it would be impossible for the Federal Bureau of Investigation (FBI) to examine them all; the order required supervisors to review and certify the loyalties of those who worked below them, reporting to a system of federal loyalty review boards. The FBI was to follow up any "derogatory information" that was unearthed.

The system quickly got out of hand. The conservative head of the Loyalty Review Board, Seth Richardson, made it clear that, in his opinion, the government could "discharge any employee for reasons which seem sufficient to the Government, and without extending to such employee any hearing whatsoever." Those accused would have no right to confront their accusers. After several years the difficulty of proving that employees were actually disloyal became clear, and Truman allowed the boards to fire those who were "potentially" disloyal or "bad security risks," such as alcoholics, homosexuals, and debtors. Suspected employees, in other words, were assumed guilty until proven innocent. After some 5 million investigations, the program identified a few hundred employees who, though not Communists, had at one time been associated with suspect groups. Rather than calm public fears, the loyalty program gave credibility to the growing "red scare."

HUAC, Hollywood, and Hiss

About the same time, the House Committee on Un-American Activities (HUAC) joined the hunt. Established in the 1930s, it gained the national limelight in 1947 with an investigation of communist influence in the film industry. Hollywood, with its wealth, glamour, and highly visible Jewish and foreign celebrities, had long aroused a mixture of attraction and suspicion among traditional Americans. "Large numbers of moving pictures that come out of Hollywood carry the communist line," charged committee member John Rankin of Mississippi. Indeed, during the Depression some Hollywood figures had developed ties to the Communist party or had become sympathetic to party causes. To generate support for the Allied cause during the war, with Roosevelt's blessing, Hollywood produced films with a positive view of the Soviet Union like *Mission to Moscow* and *Song of Russia*.

In 1947 HUAC interrogated a parade of movie stars, screen writers, and

Daily Lives

POLITICAL CULTURE

Film Noir in an Uncertain Cold War

For many years film had been recognized as a powerful medium of communication, for political purposes as much as for entertainment. During World War I, American audiences were rallied to support the Liberty Loan program with movies like *Stake Uncle Sam to Play Your Hand*, in which evil Germans in pointed helmets ravished innocent Belgian women. During World War II, Hollywood willingly promoted the war effort, whether highlighting Nazi atrocities in *Hitler's Children* or promoting the virtues of America's new-found Soviet ally in *Song of Russia*.

Such films were overt propaganda. But commercial and artistic films could also reflect the political temper of an era, conveying more subtle nuances within American culture. Outwardly, the public mood following World War II seemed one of celebration and joy. In the face of both the Great Depression and the horrors of World War II the United States had won its way to economic prosperity and triumph abroad. Yet beneath the surface of public optimism flowed a surprising current of pessimism and alienation. That darker mood produced a distinctive style, especially in the movies of the postwar era.

The gangster and hard-boiled detective films of the 1930s had already introduced audiences to an urban world of violence and disorder. But many films of the 1940s were more disturbing. Called *film noir* (literally, black film) by French critics, the new genre was visually darker and more abstract, dealing in pessimistic themes and brutal, even pathological characters. Sinister forces from without menaced the heroes or heroines, who themselves had become psychologically more complex. Sexual and spiritual confusion replaced altruism and moral decency as motives. Gone were the prostitutes with hearts of gold, the stoic wives, and the sweet marriageable girls. The *femmes noires* tended to be sulky sirens, temptresses, or sinister black widows, who might double-cross their men or ensnare them in webs of suffocating domesticity.

What brought this dark mood into the traditionally upbeat Hollywood scene? Partially, it reflected a European influence on the home-grown film industry. Just as émigrés fleeing from Nazi regimes influenced the sciences and arts, European directors like Fritz Lang, Billy Wilder, and Otto Preminger brought their cosmopolitan tastes and a visually abstract style to the American cinema. They favored scenes with sharp contrasts of dark and light in which only a portion of the screen was lit and the rest left dark. When the war came, that style became a practical necessity. Shortages of lights, electricity, and technical crews forced directors to underlight their sets. Thematically, stark lighting was used to produce a bleaker image that emphasized the shadowy world of films dealing with urban crime, international intrigue, personal anxiety, and totalitarian evil. British director Alfred Hitchcock in *Suspicion* (1941) and *Shadow of a Doubt* (1943) introduced audiences to heroes—played by matinée idols like Cary Grant and Joseph Cotton—who seemed breezy and cheerful at first, but as the plot advanced, appeared more and more to be calculating murderers.

Even after wartime restrictions had ended, directors continued to use the same visual effects by choice, in part due

Daily Lives

Son John: A Communist so low, he lied with a hand on the family Bible.

to the change in the political climate. With the cold war in full swing and two atomic superpowers confronting each other, the attitudes of *film noir* had ample reason to flourish. Many Americans suspected that the masters of science and progress had unwittingly unleashed fundamentally destructive forces of nature. In friendly hands, such power promised safety; in alien hands, it threatened American survival. News that Soviet spies had stolen atomic secrets fed a national fear. How could America be safe from enemies it could neither see nor recognize, in a world where people of privilege betrayed society's trust? Such issues echoed *film noir*'s preoccupation with mistaken identity and misplaced loyalties.

Thus, the protagonist in the 1949 *film noir* classic *D.O.A.* (the abbreviation for "Dead on Arrival"), fleeing to the big city in search of liberation, discovers that he has been mysteriously poisoned by a fatal radioactive drug, prompting him to devote the remaining hours of his life to tracking down his murderer, killing him, and then giving himself up to the police. Similarly bleak films, focusing on corrupt police, fascistic authorities, or even invaders from outer space, allowed Americans to address new fears of dehumanizing communism and nuclear annihilation through stories that were old and familiar. Similar themes of distrust and betrayal were widespread in American culture, appearing in the writings of authors as varied in style, subject, and background as James Jones and Norman Mailer, who wrote about World War II (*From Here to Eternity* and *The Naked and the Dead*), the black novelist Ralph Ellison (*The Invisible Man*), and J. D. Salinger (*The Catcher in the Rye*).

The conviction that film had the power to shape as well as reflect public attitudes brought the House Un-American Activities Committee to Hollywood in order to drive "subversives" out of the film industry. Chastened producers soon jumped on the anticommunist bandwagon, producing a succession of staunchly patriotic films. In *My Son John* (1952), for example, two doting parents discover that their boy has become a Communist spy willing to lie even with his hand on the Holy Bible. Still, despite these pious pleas for conformity, congressional critics came to realize that the Hollywood "dream factory" could spin out *film noir* nightmares as easily as it manufactured patriotic fantasies.

producers about subversive influences in the film industry. Some witnesses were considered "friendly" because, like Gary Cooper, Robert Montgomery, and Ronald Reagan, they answered committee questions or supplied names of suspected leftists. But some refused to inform on others or to answer questions about prior ties to the Communist party. Eventually 10 uncooperative witnesses, known as the "Hollywood Ten," refused on First Amendment grounds to say whether they were or ever had been Communists. They served prison terms for contempt of Congress. Also serving time was Chairman J. Parnell Thomas, who was convicted of payroll fraud.

For all its probing, HUAC never offered any convincing evidence that filmmakers were spreading subversive propaganda. About the most damning evidence presented was that one eager left-leaning extra, when asked to "whistle something" during his walk-on part, hummed a few bars of the Communist anthem, the "Internationale." The investigations did, however, inspire Hollywood to produce such films as *The Iron Curtain* (1948), in which a Russian spy ring in the United States is exposed, as well as *Red Menace* (1949), *I Was a Communist for the FBI* (1950), and *My Son John* (1952). The studios also purged actors suspected of disloyalty, adopting a "blacklist" that prevented admitted or accused Communists from finding work. Since no judicial proceedings were involved, victims of false charges, rumors, or spiteful accusations found it nearly impossible to clear their names.

In addition to congressional hearings, the government employed a variety of legal, political, and investigatory strategies to harass suspected subversives. The Taft–Hartley Act required union officials, but not management, to sign affidavits pledging no Communist affiliation. Under such pressures, the CIO expelled 11 left-wing unions because the members had democratically elected Communists or suspected Communists to union posts. CIO leader Philip Murray defended the action as necessary to remove "the dirty, filthy traitors." The Justice Department undertook a direct attack on the small and largely ineffective American Communist party. It charged the leadership under the wartime Smith Act (1940) with conspiring to advocate the violent overthrow of the government. Prosecutors built their case largely on the testimony of FBI informers who had infiltrated the party, though it was not an illegal organization.

Suspicion of aliens and immigrants led finally to the passage, over Truman's veto, of the McCarran International Security Act (1950). It required all Communists to register with the attorney general, forbade the entry of anyone who had belonged to a totalitarian organization, and allowed the Justice Department to detain suspect aliens indefinitely during deportation hearings. It was supported overwhelmingly in Congress (three future presidents voted for it—Kennedy, Johnson, and Nixon). Among the handful of representatives who dared to criticize it was Senator William Langer, an independent Republican of North Dakota, who called it "one of the most vicious, most dangerous pieces of legislation against the people that has ever been passed."

The notion that subversives were undermining the government seemed confirmed in 1950 when a jury convicted former State Department official Alger Hiss of perjury. Hiss, an adviser to Roosevelt at the Yalta Conference, had been accused by former Communist Whittaker Chambers of passing secrets to the Soviet Union during the 1930s. The hunt for evidence, first led by the young Congressman Richard M. Nixon of HUAC, took the press and public on a dramatic journey, including a trip to Chambers' farm where three microfilms were extracted from a hollow pumpkin, said to be a drop for spy secrets. Though the evidence in the case was far from conclusive, the jury convicted Hiss, not of espionage, but for lying about his association with Chambers. While the trial was in progress, the nation was further shocked by news from Britain that a high-ranking physicist, Klaus Fuchs, had spied for the Russians while working on the Manhattan Project. Evidence in the Fuchs trial led to the 1951 prosecution of Ethel and Julius Rosenberg as part of an atomic spy ring. The Rosenbergs were convicted of espionage and then executed in 1953 despite appeals for clemency.

The Ambitions of Senator McCarthy

Into this climate of fear, where legitimate concerns mixed with irrational hysteria, stepped Joseph R. McCarthy, the junior senator from Wisconsin. McCarthy, a corrupt Senate mediocrity in search of an issue to get him reelected, settled on anticommunism. To an audience in Wheeling, West Virginia, in February 1950 he waved a sheaf of papers in the air and announced that he had a list of 205—or perhaps 81, 57, or "a lot" of—Communists in the State Department. (No one, including the senator, could remember the number, which he continually changed.) In the following months McCarthy announced charge after charge. He had penetrated the "iron curtain" of the State Department to discover "card-carrying Communists," the "top Russian espionage agent" in the United States, "egg-sucking phony liberals," and "Communists and queers" who wrote "perfumed notes."

It seemed not to matter that McCarthy never substantiated his charges. When examined, his lists proved to be of people who had left the State Department long before or who had been cleared by the FBI. When forced into a corner, McCarthy simply lied and went on to another accusation. No one seemed beyond reach. In the summer of 1950 a Senate committee headed by Millard F. Tydings of Maryland concluded that McCarthy's charges were "a fraud and a hoax," but few in government were bold enough to attack "Jolting Joe" from Wisconsin, especially after 1952 when he helped defeat Tydings and several other Senate critics.

McCarthy was in one sense a maverick who over time wreaked havoc on the political system and both parties. He may even have sincerely opposed communism. Certainly, his imagination for communist demonology was almost without bounds. But in another sense, McCarthyism was the bitter fruit Truman and the Democrats reaped from their own attempts to exploit the anticommunist mood. McCarthy, more than Truman, had tapped the fears and hatreds of a broad coalition of Catholic leaders, conservatives, and neo-isolationists who harbored suspicion of things foreign, liberal, internationalist, cosmopolitan, or vaguely intellectual. They saw McCarthy and his fellow witch hunters as the protectors of a vaguely defined but deeply felt spirit of Americanism. For them the notion that all Americans, including Communists, were entitled to free speech smacked of heresy. Those who criticized America or defended its enemies were not entitled to its freedoms, the McCarthyites and many cold war liberals had concluded.

By the time Truman stepped down as president, 32 states had laws requiring teachers to take loyalty oaths, government loyalty boards were asking employees what newspapers they subscribed to or phonograph records they collected, and a library in Indiana had banned *Robin Hood* because the idea of stealing from the rich to give to the poor seemed rather too leftish. As one historian commented, "Opening the valve of anticommunist hysteria was a good deal simpler than closing it."

THE CULTURE OF PROSPERITY

No matter how strident it might be, anticommunist hysteria could not dampen the simple joys of getting and spending. The postwar years opened an era of unprecedented prosperity. Two forces drove this economic boom. One was unbridled consumer and business spending that followed 16 years of depression and war. The other was a rapid expansion in government expenditures at the local, state, and federal levels. The three major growth industries since World War II—health care, education, and government—were spurred by public spending. Equally important was the federal government's expenditure in the military–industrial sector. The defense budget, which fell to $9 billion in 1947, reached $50 billion by the time Truman left office.

What this growth made clear was that Americans, despite their wish to avoid any more "experiments," did not abandon the basic premises of the New Deal. The government maintained its commitment to setting a minimum wage, raising it again in 1950 from 45 to 75 cents. Social Security coverage was broadened to cover an additional 10 million workers. Furthermore, a growing list of welfare programs benefited not only the poor, but veterans, middle-income families, the elderly, and students. The most striking of these was the GI Bill of 1944.

Soldiers as Civilians

For returning veterans, the GI Bill of Rights created unparalleled opportunity. Between 1945 and 1952 the federal government spent some $13.5 billion on education and training. Veterans with more than two years service received all tuition and fees plus $50 a month ($75 for married GIs) for three years of college education at any school. States like New York and California rapidly expanded their university systems to meet the demand from veterans. By 1948 the government was paying the college costs of almost 50 percent of all male students as over 2 million veterans went to college on the GI Bill.

Increased educational levels encouraged a shift from blue- to white-collar work and self-employment. Although available jobs in areas like mining and manufacturing increased little if at all, work in areas like insurance, teaching, state and local governments, construction, and retailing expanded rapidly. Veterans also received low-interest loans to start businesses or farms of their own and to buy homes. By the 1950s the Veterans Administration (VA), which doled out this federal largesse, funded the purchase of some 20 percent of all new houses.

The GI Bill accelerated trends that would transform American society into a prosperous, better educated, heavily middle class suburban nation. Between 1945 and 1970 veterans, especially those with college educations, earned over 40 percent more than nonveterans. The GI Bill also contributed to the economic advantages white males held over minorities and females. Few women received benefits under the bill. Many lost their jobs or seniority to returning veterans. Blacks and Hispanics, even those eligible for veterans' benefits, were hampered by Jim Crow restrictions in segregated universities and jobs in both the public and private sectors. The Federal Housing Administration even helped draw up "model" restrictive housing covenants neighborhoods could adopt in order to "retain stability" by segregating according to "social and racial classes."

The Baby Boom

For many Americans the Depression followed by the war had interrupted plans for beginning a family. The postwar era changed that dramatically. In 1946 Americans married in record numbers, twice as many as in 1932. The United States had in fact one of the highest marriage rates in the world. (The divorce rate peaked, too, in 1946, but most of those divorced promptly remarried.) The brides were younger, which translated into unusual fertility. During the Depression birth rates had been at an all-time low, about 18 to 19 per thousand. They began to rise during the war and by 1952 had passed 25, one of the highest fertility rates in the world. Americans also chose to have larger families, as the number with three children tripled and those with four or more quadrupled. "Just imagine how much these extra people, these new markets, will absorb—in food, in clothing, in gadgets, in housing, in services," one newspaper columnist predicted. Not only did the baby boom contribute to the expanding economy; the prosperity and newer attitudes that came with it also reshaped childrearing practices.

The new preoccupation with courtship and marriage focused attention on issues of sexuality. One controversial foray into this territory was *Sexual Behavior in the Human Male* (1948, followed by *Sexual Behavior in American Women*, 1952), written by social researcher Alfred Kinsey. Commentators called the *Kinsey Report* "the most talked about book of the twentieth century." Polls indicated that 20 percent of the nation had read it or knew about it. Kinsey revealed among other things that about a third of all males had experienced some form of homosex-

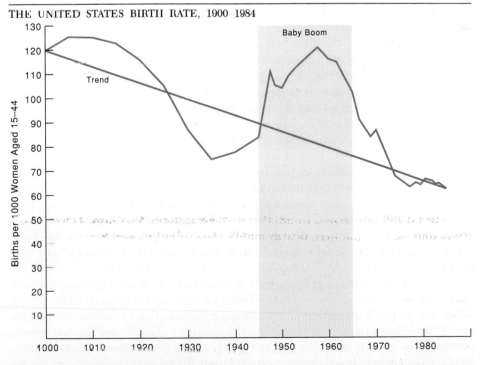

THE UNITED STATES BIRTH RATE, 1900–1984

Births per 1000 Women Aged 15–44

Baby Boom

Trend

Sources : U.S. Bureau of the Census, *Historical Statistics of the United States* and *Statistical Abstract of the United States*, various years.

ual activity, that extramarital sex was common for both men and women, and that women enjoyed sex in much the same way men did. Socioeconomic factors of race, class, ethnicity, and age often dictated sexual preferences. Middle-class whites avoided premarital intercourse more than lower class whites. At the same time, the middle class did more petting, kissing, and masturbating, while the lower classes were shy about kissing but less shy about intercourse.

It is difficult in more sexually liberated times to appreciate the impact of Kinsey's work. Perhaps most controversial was his claim that couples who had premarital sex tended to be better adjusted in marriage. Critics charged that Kinsey was a "menace to society" who would destroy the morals of the nation. Some accused him of abetting communism and called on Senator McCarthy's Permanent Investigating Subcommittee to investigate him. Other Americans found liberation in the discovery that behaviors once treated as sinful or perverse were widely accepted.

Hail, Suburbia

The boom in marriage and families created a need for housing; the growing prosperity, an intense desire for a home of one's own. At war's end, 5 million families were searching, eager to find anything, tired of living doubled up with other families, or in basements, or even in coal cellars. Housing was so scarce that one newspaper carried an advertisement offering a large icebox "which could be fixed up to live in." But with the help of the GI Bill and the rising prosperity, the chance to own, not merely rent, housing became a reality for over half of American families (up to 55 percent in 1950, from 43.6 in 1940).

In the postwar era a house was more often in a suburb than in a city. By the 1950s urban growth outside the South and West had virtually stopped, while the population in communities ringing central cities grew almost 50 percent. Urbanites wanting to escape the crowding and chaos of large cities were drawn to more pastoral communities with names like Park Forest, Briarcliff Manor, or Pacific Palisades. During the 1940s the increasing movement of the poor, Hispanics, and blacks into urban centers encouraged more affluent whites to move to the suburbs. Here families could find the detached single-family house with a lawn and garden idealized in American culture.

In the 1940s inexpensive suburban housing became synonymous with the name of William Levitt. From building houses for war workers, Levitt learned how to use mass production techniques. In 1947 he began construction of a 17,000-house community in the New York City suburb of Hempstead. All the materials for a Levittown house were precut and assembled at a factory, then moved to the site for assembly. If all went according to schedule, a new house was erected on a cement slab every 16 minutes. Buoyed by his success in Hempstead, Levitt later built other developments in Bucks County, Pennsylvania, and Willingboro, New Jersey.

The typical early Levitt house, a "Cape Codder," had a living room, kitchen, bath, and two bedrooms on the ground floor and an expansion attic, all for $7990. None had custom features, insulation, or any amenities that complicated construction. "The reason we have it so good in this country," Levitt said, "is that we can produce lots of things at low prices through mass production." Uniformity in house style extended to behavior as well. Levitt discouraged owners from changing colors or adding distinctive features to the house or yard. Buyers promised to cut the grass each week of the summer and not to hang out wash on weekends.

In the wake of the baby boom and a demand for new homes, mass-produced houses soon filled suburban developments all across the United States. By varying styles only slightly, developers were able to construct houses quickly at prices many young couples could afford.

Blacks were expressly excluded. Other suburban communities excluded Jews and ethnics in the restrictive covenants that dictated who could take up residence.

By 1950 some 5 million new housing units had been built, many in the new suburbs. But over 2.5 million families still lived doubled up. In California, a state with three cars registered for every four residents, suburbs bloomed across the landscape. By 1962 California had become the nation's most populous state. Growth was greatest around Los Angeles, once the center of the most extensive (1100 miles) urban electric railroad system in the world. In 1940 city planners launched construction of a freeway system to lure shoppers into downtown Los Angeles. Instead, white Angelinos saw the road network as an opportunity to migrate to the suburbs. Eventually one-third of the Los Angeles area was covered by highways, parking lots, and interchanges, increasing to two-thirds in the downtown areas. Los Angeles County developed a higher percentage of detached housing (about 67 percent) than other major cities like Chicago with 28 percent, New York with 20 percent, and Philadelphia with 15 percent.

Much of the white population that moved to the suburbs was replaced by blacks and Hispanics, who were part of larger migrations, especially of millions of southern black families leaving the South over the next two decades to search for work in urban centers. The majority headed for the Northeast and Upper Midwest. While central cities lost 3.6 million whites they gained 4.5 million blacks. Indeed, by 1960 half of all black Americans would live in central cities. Blacks and Hispanics were also drawn to California. In 1940 only 1.8 percent of California's population was black. By 1950 that percentage increased to 4.3 (and to 8 by 1970). As of 1945, only Mexico City had a larger Hispanic population than Los Angeles. And by the 1960s the 3 million Hispanic Californians made up 16 percent of the

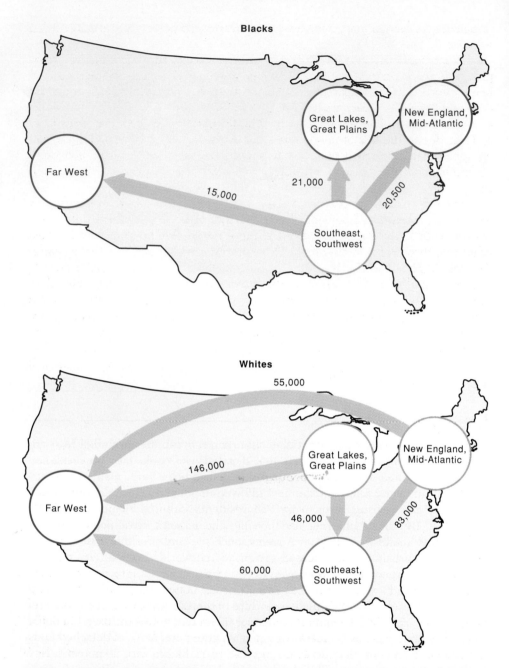

Blacks

Great Lakes, Great Plains

New England, Mid-Atlantic

Far West

15,000

21,000

20,500

Southeast, Southwest

Whites

55,000

Great Lakes, Great Plains

New England, Mid-Atlantic

146,000

Far West

46,000

83,000

60,000

Southeast, Southwest

Source: Frank Levy, *Dollars and Dreams: The Changing American Income Distribution* (New York: Russell Sage Foundation, 1987), p. 106.

AVERAGE ANNUAL REGIONAL MIGRATION, 1947–1960

While African-Americans were moving in significant numbers to urban centers in the Northeast, Midwest, and Far West, whites were being drawn to the increasingly diversified economy of the South as well as the new industries stimulated by the war in the Far West. By the 1970s, the trend became known as the "Sunbelt" phenomenon.

population. Although most came from rural Mexico, 85 percent eventually settled in cities.

When poor black and Hispanic migrants poured into cities after the war, their prospects were particularly bleak. Earlier waves of European immigrants had been absorbed by the expanding urban economy, but during the 1950s the flight of jobs and middle-class population to the suburbs made it impossible for blacks and Hispanics to follow the same path. With fewer jobs and declining educational systems due to the loss of middle-class taxpayers, the cities were no longer well equipped to acculturate the newcomers and integrate them into the economy. Unemployment for the most recently arrived was over 40 percent in the worst areas.

Since few blacks or Hispanics could afford the cost of suburban living, they accounted for less than 5 percent of the population there. Black suburbanites were poorer, held lower status jobs, lived in more ramshackle housing, and had less education than blacks in the cities. The pattern for whites was just the opposite. The few black suburbs that existed dated from before the war and had little in common with the newer white "bedroom communities." Blacks who could afford to move could not find suitable housing at any price. Real estate agents refused to show them houses; bankers would not provide mortgages. And many communities adopted either restrictive covenants or zoning regulations that kept blacks and other "undesirables" out. William Myers finally managed in 1957 to buy a house from a white family in Levittown, Pennsylvania, but the developers did not sell directly to blacks until 1960.

The Flickering Gray Screen

The move to the suburbs, combined with generally shorter working hours in white-collar jobs, influenced the way Americans spent leisure time. Nowhere can this better be seen than in the popularity of television.

Television was not new in the 1940s. The technology had existed since 1927, and in 1939 the National Broadcasting Company (NBC) and Columbia Broadcasting System (CBS) had begun regular broadcasting. Programs included bits of musicals, vaudeville acts, and sports, transmitted by some 23 stations around the country. The war halted broadcasting as skilled personnel and equipment were shifted to military work, but with the coming of peace television quickly realized its potential as a mass medium. The Radio Corporation of America (RCA) rushed to produce modestly priced black-and-white sets and to improve the quality of picture tubes. By 1949 Americans owned a million television sets tuned into 108 licensed stations. Just three years later 15 million sets had been sold and by 1960 there were 46 million sets. Indeed, more Americans had televisions than had bathrooms.

The networks offered sports, news (with film produced by movie studios), dramatic series, and puppet shows like "Kukla, Fran, and Ollie" and "The Howdy Doody Show" for children. In 1948 the networks assumed an important role in politics as they covered both the Democratic and Republican conventions. Two years later, the medium showed its ability to combine entertainment, politics, and news by televising a series of hearings on organized crime chaired by Senator Estes Kefauver. Some 30 million viewers watched the New York City hearings broadcast live. The star attraction was mobster Frank Costello, who headed a large interstate criminal organization with close ties to city governments. Forbidden to show the witness himself, the television cameras focused on his hands as he nervously tore up bits of paper before finally walking out. Senator Kefauver gained such widespread fame that he emerged as a leading presidential candidate in the 1952 elections.

The spread of television soon transformed traditional habits of entertainment. At war's end, Americans had been a nation of moviegoers. About 75 percent of the potential audience went to the movies three times a month. Radio satisfied the need for news and information in over 90 percent of all homes, with listeners tuning in an average of five hours a day. By the early 1950s both media had experienced a dramatic decline in popularity. Movie attendence dropped to half of its 1946 peak and over 4000 neighborhood theaters closed in cities around the country. Many of them were replaced in the suburbs by popular drive-ins, which allowed whole families to enjoy movies in the comfort of their cars. But even that novelty failed to attract people in the same numbers. Radio suffered, too, as television lured away established comedians like Jack Benny, George Burns and Gracie Allen, and "Amos 'n' Andy."

The move to the suburbs reinforced this pattern. The big theaters and sports stadiums were still in the cities, where attendance was dropping; the fans were increasingly in the suburbs. In the more decentralized environment, baby boom parents spent much of their free time at home with their children. They could watch sports and movies on television. Even restaurant owners felt the squeeze. When Sid Caesar and Imogene Coca appeared on Saturday nights in "Your Show of Shows," diners rushed home to their television sets.

Television was no less immune to the red scare than Hollywood had been. In 1950 broadcasters and advertisers received an ominous booklet with a red hand closing over a microphone. "The Cominform and the Communist Party U.S.A. now rely more on radio and TV than the press and motion pictures as 'belts' to transmit pro-Sovietism to the American public," announced the authors of *Red Channels: The Report of Communist Influence in Radio and Television*. Then followed a list of some 151 of the most widely admired and talented names in broadcasting. Many people thought at first the list was a joke, but the authors were dead earnest. And though most of the named celebrities had been unjustly accused, many suddenly found themselves "controversial" and their shows canceled.

THE POLITICS OF FRUSTRATION

Going into the 1948 elections, Harry Truman had two strong suits. The first was the economy, which was back on track. The second was the bipartisan support won for his anti-Soviet foreign policy. But for all that, Truman found himself in deep trouble. The conservative mood that gave the Republicans control of the 80th Congress seemed to guarantee them victory in 1948. A coalition of Republicans and southern Democrats had eviscerated the president's legislative program. Inflation threatened to erode economic gains. And there was the problem of Truman himself. He seemed to lack, as one newspaper observed, "the stature, the vision, the social and economic grasp, or sense of history required to lead the nation in time of crisis." As much as people might admire Truman's spunk, his feisty spirit, and his honesty, many Democratic politicians would have preferred war hero Dwight Eisenhower as their candidate.

As if that were not enough, the New Deal coalition which Franklin Roosevelt had held together for so long seemed to be coming apart. On the left stood Henry Wallace, a capable secretary of agriculture and vice president under Roosevelt, then secretary of commerce under Truman. But Wallace wanted to pursue New Deal reforms even more vigorously than did Truman, and he continually voiced his sympathy for the Soviets at a time when the rest of the administration was moving rightward. Truman had fired him in 1946. Two years later, disaffected liberals bolted the Democratic party to support Henry Wallace at the head of a third-party Progressive ticket.

At the same time, the southern conservative wing of the party bitterly opposed Truman's moderate civil rights programs, which included proposals for a voting rights bill and an antilynching law. Truman sincerely opposed discrimination and knew, as well, that it was good politics to hold on to the black vote, which Roosevelt had wooed away from the Republican party for the first time since Reconstruction. But Truman also hailed from the border state of Missouri and knew how strong the sentiment for segregation was. At the 1948 Democratic National Convention he hoped to soft-pedal civil rights in the party platform, but he was outvoted by the liberal wing of the party. At that point delegates from several Deep South states stalked out of the convention. Soon they banded together to create the States' Rights or "Dixiecrat" party, with J. Strom Thurmond, the segregationist governor of South Carolina, as their candidate.

With the Democrats seemingly hopelessly divided, the Republicans had turned confidently once again to New York Governor Thomas Dewey and, as his running mate, the popular liberal governor of California, Earl Warren. The aloof Dewey inspired little enthusiasm, but he also had few enemies. "You have to know Dewey well to really dislike him," one disgruntled supporter of Robert Taft quipped. Two months before the election political pollster Elmo Roper stopped canvassing the voters. It seemed clear that Dewey would walk away with the election.

Truman, however, would not roll over and play dead. He launched an all-out attack against the "reactionaries" in Congress: that "bunch of old mossbacks . . . gluttons of privilege . . . all set to do a hatchet job on the New Deal." Hiring a

ELECTION OF 1948

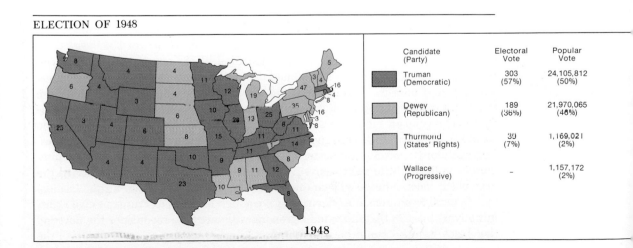

Candidate (Party)	Electoral Vote	Popular Vote
Truman (Democratic)	303 (57%)	24,105,812 (50%)
Dewey (Republican)	189 (36%)	21,970,065 (46%)
Thurmond (States' Rights)	39 (7%)	1,169,021 (2%)
Wallace (Progressive)	–	1,157,172 (2%)

1948

train, he whistle-stopped 30,000 miles across the country, making almost 400 speeches in eight weeks. Over and over he hammered away at the "do-nothing" 80th Congress, which, he told farmers, "had stuck a pitchfork" in their backs. As Truman pounded on the podium to emphasize his attack, someone would yell, "Give 'em hell, Harry!" "I'm a-doin' it," the president would shoot back. Still, on election day the odds makers were giving Dewey the edge by as much as 20 to 1. Hours before the polls closed the archconservative Chicago *Tribune* happily head-lined "Dewey Defeats Truman." Once again, the experts were wrong. Not only did the voters return Truman by over 2 million popular votes, but they also gave the Democrats commanding majorities in the House and Senate.

The defection of the liberal and conservative extremes had allowed Truman to hold the New Deal coalition together. He had been the first major presidential candidate to campaign in Harlem. Jews grateful for his stand on Israel, Catholics loyal to the Democratic party, and ethnics all supported him. Farmers hurt by falling prices had deserted the Republicans. An easing of inflation had reminded middle-income Americans that they had benefited enormously under Democratic leadership. "I have a new car and am much better off than my parents were. Why change?" one suburban voter remarked.

The Fair Deal

As Harry Truman assumed the presidency in his own right, he expressed his conviction that all Americans were entitled to a "Fair Deal" from their govern-ment. His agenda called for a vigorous revival of New Deal programs and, echoing an old Populist idea, an effort to forge stronger links between farmers and labor.

In reality New Deal liberalism was in a period of decline. The coalition of Democratic and Republican conservatives in Congress rejected plans for a St. Lawrence Seaway in the Northeast, a TVA-style project in the Missouri River Valley, and other regional projects. The American Medical Association lobbied strongly to block a program of national health insurance. The Catholic church opposed federal aid to education, since it did not authorize subsidies to parochial schools. Furthermore, Truman could not forge a working coalition between farm-ers and labor. The farm block would not support labor in its attempts to repeal the Taft–Hartley Act, nor would labor vote to help pass farm price supports designed to encourage family farms at the expense of larger agribusinesses.

Civil rights legislation proved even more frustrating. Truman's Committee on Civil Rights had published its report, *To Secure These Rights,* in 1947. The com-mittee exposed a racial caste system that denied blacks employment opportuni-ties, equal education, voting rights, and decent housing. But every time Truman appealed to Congress to implement the committee's recommendations southern senators threatened to filibuster. Truman was forced to resort to executive author-ity to achieve even modest results. In his most direct attack on segregation, he issued an executive order in July 1948 banning discrimination in the armed forces. Segregationists predicted disaster, but experience would soon show that inte-grated units had little racial tension and fought well. Truman also appointed the first black federal judge and another black as governor of the Virgin Islands.

Several Supreme Court decisions gave added impetus to Truman's civil rights initiatives. In cases that indicated a growing willingness to reconsider the doctrine that black facilities could be "separate but equal" (*Plessy v. Ferguson,* 1896) the Court in *McLaurin v. Oklahoma State Regents* and *Sweatt v. Painter* (1950) struck down state education laws clearly designed to create separate but inferior facilities. But even if the courts moved in Truman's direction, Congress did not. On the domestic front Truman remained largely the conservator of Franklin Roosevelt's legacy.

Beyond Containment

Leadership in foreign affairs had been a strong point in Truman's first term. In his second term, success deserted him. American scientists reported in August 1949 that rains monitored in the Pacific contained undeniable traces of hot nuclear waste. Only one conclusion seemed possible. The Soviet Union had exploded a bomb more powerful than either of those used on Hiroshima and Nagasaki. When Truman announced the news, Congress was debating whether to spend $1.5 billion for military aid to the newly formed NATO alliance. The House stopped debating and voted the bill through, while Truman directed that research into a newer, more powerful fusion or hydrogen bomb continue. Senator Arthur Vandenberg, a leading Republican spokesman on foreign policy, summed up the reaction of many to the end of the American nuclear monopoly: "This is now a different world."

Then in December came more bad news. The long embattled Nationalist government of Chiang Kai-shek fled mainland China to the offshore island of Formosa. Chiang's defeat at the hands of Communist forces led by Mao Tse-tung came as no surprise to the State Department, which had long been monitoring the situation. The Nationalists' corruption and inefficiency had bedeviled American efforts to bring stability to China both during and after World War II. In 1947 full-scale civil war broke out. By February 1949 almost half of Chiang's demoralized troops had defected to the Communists. So the December defeat was hardly unexpected.

But Republicans, who had up until 1949 supported the president's foreign policy, now broke ranks. For some time, a group of wealthy conservatives and Republican senators had resented the administration's preoccupation with Europe. Time–Life publisher Henry Luce used his magazines to campaign for a greater concern for Asian affairs, and especially more aid to defeat Mao Tse-tung. Luce and his associates, known as the "China Lobby," were supported in part with funds from the Chinese Embassy, and when Chiang at last collapsed, his American backers charged the Democrats with letting the Communists win. Secretary of State Dean Acheson published State Department documents showing that nothing short of direct American intervention would have saved Chiang's corrupt and unpopular regime. But the China Lobby charged that Acheson's defense was nothing more than a "whitewash." And it was soon after that Joseph McCarthy began his hunt for "traitors" in the State Department.

Though irritated by such charges, the Truman administration itself was moving to a more assertive foreign policy—one that would militarize containment. The new policy was developed by the National Security Council (NSC), formed in 1947 when Congress attempted to make the military services more efficient by unifying them into a single Department of Defense. (The Central Intelligence Agency was also created at this time.) From the beginning, the NSC had lobbied for an active policy to win the cold war, "in which our national security is a stake and from which we cannot withdraw short of eventual national suicide." In April 1950 it sent Truman a document, NSC-68, which came to serve as the framework for American policy over the next 20 years.

NSC-68 argued that rather than hold the Soviets at bay, the United States should "strive for victory." To that end NSC-68 called for an immediate increase in defense spending from $13 billion to $50 billion a year, to be paid for with a large tax increase. Most of the funds would go to rebuild conventional forces, but the NSC saw the need to develop the hydrogen bomb to offset the Soviets' nuclear capacity. At the same time the American people had to be mobilized to make the necessary sacrifices, while the United States worked (NSC-68 never explained how) to make "the Russian people our Allies" in undermining their totalitarian government. Once again, national defense planners assumed that American policy could force the Soviets to liberalize their society while creating conditions under which "our free society can flourish."

Efforts to implement the policy provisions of NSC-68 at first aroused widespread opposition. Critics like George Kennan, the "father of containment," argued that the Soviets had no immediate plans for domination outside the Communist bloc and that NSC-68 recommendations were too simplistic and militaristic. Fiscal conservatives, both Democrat and Republican, resisted any proposal for higher taxes. Truman's own secretary of defense, Louis Johnson, claimed the new military budget would bankrupt the country. But all such reservations were swept away on June 25, 1950. "Korea came along and saved us," Acheson later remarked.

Korea

In 1950 Korea was about the last place Americans could have imagined themselves fighting a war. Since World War II the country had been divided along the 38th parallel, the north controlled by the Communist government of Kim Il Sung, the south by the dictatorship of Syngman Rhee. Preoccupied with China and the rebuilding of Japan, the Truman administration's interest had dwindled steadily after the war. When Secretary of State Dean Acheson discussed American policy in Asia for the National Press Club in January 1950, he did not even mention Korea.

On June 24 Harry Truman was enjoying a leisurely break from politics at the family home in Independence, Missouri. In Korea it was already Sunday morning when Acheson called the president to report that North Korean troops had crossed the 38th parallel, possibly to fulfill Kim Il Sung's proclaimed intention to "liberate" the South. Soon Acheson confirmed that a full-scale invasion had taken place. The United Nations, meeting in emergency session, had already ordered a ceasefire, which the North Koreans were ignoring. With that, Truman flew back to Washington, convinced that Stalin and his Chinese Communist allies had ordered the invasion. Kim, Truman reasoned, would hardly have acted on his own. Thus the threat of a third world war, this one atomic, seemed agonizingly real. Truman and his advisers wanted to respond to the crisis firmly enough to deter aggression, but without provoking a larger war with the Soviet Union or China.

Truman did not hesitate; American troops would fight the North Koreans, though the United States would not declare war. The fighting in Korea would be a "police action" supervised by the United Nations. On June 27 the United States' delegate to the Security Council succeeded in passing a resolution to send United Nations forces to Korea. That move succeeded only because the Soviet delegate, who had veto power, had walked out six months earlier in protest over the Council's refusal to seat mainland China. (Indeed, his absence from the Security Coun-

THE KOREAN WAR
In their opening offensive North Korean troops almost pushed South Korean and American forces into the sea at Pusan, but MacArthur rallied United Nations forces, made a successful landing at Inchon behind North Korean lines, and then crossed the 38th parallel into North Korea. Red Chinese troops counterattacked, inflicting on U.S. troops one of the most humiliating defeats in American military history. Fighting continued for another two years.

cil vote undermines the idea that Stalin, rather than Kim Il Sung, had masterminded the North Korean attack.)

Truman's forceful response won immediate approval across America, while Congress quickly voted the huge increase in defense funds needed to carry out the recommendations of NSC-68. American allies were less committed to the action. Though 16 nations contributed to the war effort, the United States provided 50 percent of the ground troops, 86 percent of the naval units, and 93 percent of the air force. By the time the UN forces could be marshalled, North Korean forces had pinned the South Koreans within a small defensive perimeter centered around Pusan. Then Douglas MacArthur, commander of the UN forces, launched a daring amphibious attack behind North Korean lines at Inchon, near the western end of the 38th parallel. Fighting eastward, MacArthur's troops threatened to trap the invaders, who fled back to the North.

Now Truman made a fateful decision. With the South liberated, he gave MacArthur permission to cross the 38th parallel, drive the Communists from the North, and reunite the country under Syngman Rhee. With Senator Joe McCarthy on the attack at home, the 1950 elections nearing, and the McCarran Internal Security Act just passed, Truman was glad enough for the chance to vanquish a few North Koreans. By Thanksgiving American troops had roundly defeated northern forces and were advancing on several fronts toward the frozen Yalu River, the boundary between Korea and China. MacArthur, emboldened by success, promised that the boys would be home by Christmas.

China, however, had grown increasingly restive. Throughout the fall offensive, Premier Zhou Enlai had warned that his country would not tolerate an American presence on its border. Washington, knowing that Stalin had declared the Korean conflict to be merely a "civil war" and off limits, assumed that Mao Tsetung was essentially a Soviet puppet. Ignoring the Chinese warnings, MacArthur grandly launched his end-the-war offensive. On October 26 American troops captured a Chinese prisoner "so that you began to know at that point something was happening," Secretary of State Acheson recalled. On November 26 some 400,000 Chinese troops poured across the Yalu, smashing through the lightly defended UN lines. At Chosan they trapped 20,000 American and South Korean troops, inflicting one of the worst defeats in American military history. Within three weeks they had driven UN forces back behind the 38th parallel. So total was the rout that Truman wondered publicly about using the atom bomb. That remark sent a frightened British prime minister Clement Attlee flying to Washington to dissuade Truman. The president readily agreed that the war must remain limited and withdrew his nuclear threat.

Military stalemate in Korea brought into the open a simmering feud between MacArthur and Truman. The general had made no secret of his political ambitions or of his differences with Truman over American policy in Asia. He was eager to bomb Chinese and Russian supply bases across the Korean border, to blockade China's coast, and to unleash Chiang Kai-shek on mainland China. On March 23 he issued a personal ultimatum to Chinese military commanders demanding total surrender. To his Republican congressional supporters he sent a letter declaring, "We must win. There is no substitute for victory."

Truman saw MacArthur's public statements as a threat to the tradition of civilian leadership and his strategy as an open invitation to another world war. Outraged by such insubordination, he made plans to discipline the general. When Omar Bradley reported that the rumors of dismissal had reached the Far East and that MacArthur might try to resign, the irate Truman replied, "The son of a bitch isn't going to resign on me. I want him fired!" Military leaders agreed that MacArthur had to go. On April 11 a stunned nation learned that the celebrated military commander had been relieved of his duties. As cheering crowds greeted MacArthur in one of the largest ticker-tape parades in New York City's history, Truman's move seemed one of the great political mistakes of his career. MacArthur had the unprecedented opportunity to address a joint session of Congress before a national television audience. Rabid supporters tried to impeach Truman and Acheson.

Behind the personal feud raged an important debate over foreign policy. While MacArthur demanded an all-out effort in Asia, Acheson told Congress that Korea was but one link in a worldwide "collective security system." General war in Asia would threaten American interests in Europe. The Korean War had to be fought with Europe always foremost in American strategy. Or as General Omar Bradley argued, a showdown in Asia would lead to "the wrong war, at the wrong place, at the wrong time, and with the wrong enemy." Congressional leaders were thus persuaded of the need to accompany limited war in Korea with a military build-up in Europe. As for MacArthur, it was soon apparent that in his 14 years abroad he had lost touch with American political realities. His verbosity at congressional hearings bored even his own supporters. He soon retired to an expensive suite in a New York hotel to await the Republican presidential nomination, which, to his amazement, never came.

Korea took its toll on Truman's political fortunes as well. After July 1951, aimless peace talks dragged on along the border at Panmunjon. While the negotiators argued over the reunification of Korea and what to do with North Korean prisoners of war who refused to go home, the United States suffered another 32,000 casualties in an ugly war of attrition. There were no brilliant victories, only month after month of trench warfare, exhausted GIs, and sagging morale. Secretary of State Acheson spent much of his energy defending the Korean stalemate before hostile Republican senators like Richard Nixon of California, who inveighed against "Dean Acheson's cowardly college of Communist containment." In March 1952 Truman's popularity had sunk so low that he lost the New Hampshire presidential primary to Senator Estes Kefauver of Tennessee. With that defeat, he announced he would not run for reelection in 1952.

K1C2: The Election of 1952

The Republican formula for victory in 1952 was simple. Exploit the Truman administration's obvious weaknesses. Domestically, that did not include the economy, which remained remarkably healthy. Wage and price controls put in place by the administration prevented the sharp inflation that was expected to follow increased wartime spending. But the Republicans could capitalize on the protracted stalemate over Korea. And several of Truman's advisers had been forced to resign for accepting mink coats and deep freezes in return for political favors. The campaign strategy was summed up in the formula K1C2: Korea, corruption, and communism.

The bigger problem for Republicans lay in choosing a candidate. Once General Dwight D. Eisenhower formally joined the Republican party, he became the choice of moderates and the northeastern establishment. Party regulars and the conservative wing were heavily committed to Robert A. Taft, who ran surprisingly well in the party primaries. But Ike's popularity allowed his backers to maneuver their candidate to a first-ballot nomination. To heal the breach with the Taft delegates, the convention chose the staunch anticommunist Senator Richard M. Nixon as Eisenhower's running mate.

With no candidate as popular as Eisenhower, the Democrats drafted Illinois Governor Adlai E. Stevenson. Few candidates could match Stevenson's eloquence, but, like Dewey before him, Stevenson lacked the common touch. Re-

Two strange bedfellows of politics, the moderate Republican presidential candidate Dwight Eisenhower raises the hand of his ardent anticommunist running mate, Richard Nixon.

publican strategists turned his intelligence into a liability by dismissing him and his intellectual supporters as "eggheads." The GOP's campaign against communism and corruption, led by Nixon, left the Democratic candidate on the defensive. Eisenhower, meanwhile, took the high road above the mudslinging and promised voters that if elected, he would go to Korea to seek an end to the war.

Righteous indignation over corruption almost mired the Republicans in a scandal of their own when the New York *Post* revealed that a group of wealthy Californians had provided Richard Nixon with an $18,000 "slush fund" to help cover personal expenses. With his place on the ticket in peril, Nixon made an impassioned television appearance to defend himself as an honest, ordinary American, with car payments, a small life insurance policy, and a mortgage. He could afford to dress his wife only in a sensible "Republican cloth coat," not furs. And yes, his daughter Tricia had received a cocker spaniel puppy named "Checkers," but no matter what his enemies might say, his family was going to keep the dog. The speech was an immediate success, demonstrating clearly the newfound power of television to influence public opinion. More important, Nixon had successfully identified himself with the swelling middle-class center of American society: those who had escaped the Depression and were now determined to secure recent economic advances and savor the taste of prosperity.

The election outcome was never much in doubt. Eisenhower's broad smile and confident manner promised an era of effective leadership, and he received over 55 percent of the vote. The GOP also won a one-vote majority in the Senate and a slim edge in the House. "The great problem of America today," Ike had said during the campaign, "is to take that straight road down the middle." Most Americans who voted for him were comforted to think that was just where they were headed.

If Eisenhower's course pointed to a road down the middle, it is worth noting just how much that sense of "middle" had changed. In 1945, at the end of the war, there were large questions about what kind of peacetime society Americans would return to. The Great Depression had blended almost insensibly into world war. There had been no time to step back and assess the sizable changes that had been wrought. But in a broad sense, the political system was slowly adjusting to the idea that America's economy was inseparably tied to that of the emerging global order. The crash in 1929, with its worldwide effects, had demonstrated the closeness of the links. And the activist policies of the New Deal showed that Americans were willing to give the federal government power to influence American society in major new ways. If anything, the war gave the governments and private businesses greater power to move supplies and shape global policies. So when peace came in 1945, it gradually became clear that the "middle road" did not mean a return to the laissez-faire economics or politics of the 1920s.

Furthermore, the shift from war to peace demonstrated that it was no longer possible to make global war without making a global peace. Under the striking new balance of power in the postwar world, the United States and the Soviet Union stood alone as preeminent "superpowers," swiftly developing the military capability to annihilate each other and the rest of the world. In an environment of competing interests and atomic diplomacy, the suspicions on both sides led to a world where a "limited" war—over Korea, Berlin, Greece, or Iran—could not easily be isolated from larger conflicts. Perhaps the knowledge that there was no retreating from political as well as economic commitment was one reason that the rhetoric of anticommunism became so strident. Life in the shadow of a cold war, too, became part of the middle road Americans walked. And there was no simple way of turning back.

SIGNIFICANT EVENTS

1945	Iran crisis; civil war in Greece
1946	OPA lifts price controls; labor unrest; Kennan's "long telegram"; Stalin and Churchill "cold war" speeches; Republican congressional victories; McMahon Bill creates Atomic Energy Commission; Baruch plan fails at United Nations
1947	Truman Doctrine; Taft–Hartley Act; Marshall announces European recovery plan; Federal Loyalty Oath; HUAC investigates Hollywood; National Security Act creates Defense Department and CIA; Levittown construction begins
1948	Marshall Plan adopted; Berlin blockade; Truman upsets Dewey; Truman recognizes Israel
1949	Soviet A-bomb test; China falls to the Communists; NATO established; Truman orders work on H-bomb
1950	McCarthy's Wheeling, West Virginia, speech; Korean War begins; McCarran Act; NSC-68 adopted; Alger Hiss convicted; Kefauver crime hearings; *McLaurin* and *Sweatt* cases
1951	Rosenbergs accused; Truman fires MacArthur; peace talks in Korea
1952	Fertility rate in the United States reaches new high; Richard Nixon's "Checkers" speech; Eisenhower defeats Stevenson
1957	First black moves into Levittown, Pennsylvania

31

The Suburban Era

If the 1950s had a symbol, it was the automobile: big, boxy, glittering with chrome, sprouting ever more outrageous fins, and careening down the road with the roar of an overpowered V-8 engine. A four-door Plymouth, Ford, or Chevy sedan served both for commuting and for driving the family to church. Rich kids and young-at-heart adults drove sporty convertibles. Harried suburban housewives preferred a station wagon to tote children and groceries. For the upwardly mobile executive or celebrity, a Cadillac, Lincoln, or Imperial was a must. Their huge wheelbases, Torque Flight transmissions, and feather-touch power steering gave them about as much feel for the road as a slab of ice slaloming down the road.

No longer were families scraping together to buy their first car or nursing the old one along until it died. Buyers were trading up, the bigger the better. With the suburbs and new shopping plazas spread so far apart, many families decided they needed two cars in the garage. Kids—mere *teenagers*—were saving enough spare change to buy cars, mostly used. The "hot-rodders" seemed to prefer older coupes, chopped, blocked, and channeled. Their radios would blare out songs like "Mabelline" and "Teen Angel," and guys with greased-back hair courtesy of Vitalis would head off to the drive-in with their girls to watch Steve McQueen in *The Blob*—or even worse, tool up to the overlook at Buena Vista bluff. But what could parents do to stop them? The kids all had jobs, cars, money of their own, and time to kill.

To draw customers to the auto showrooms, manufacturers advertised more than ever before. In an era when the advertising industry was experiencing the biggest boom in its history, 9 out of the top 10 ad campaigns were for cars. (The tenth was for the ubiquitous Coca-Cola.) Chrysler Corporation even hired a psychological consultant from Vienna to lay bare the buyers' automotive ids and egos. When buying a car, Dr. Ernest Dichter reported, a man subconsciously wanted to acquire a mistress. He set his eyes lovingly on a convertible—then, recalling his family responsibilities, settled for a four-door sedan. Chrysler eased the male dilemma by introducing the four-door hardtop, just as convenient, but with the slightly more rakish profile of the convertible.

The "Big Three" auto manufacturers—General Motors, Ford, and Chrysler—raced one another to redesign their annual models, each one boxier and more chrome-laden than the last. Harley Earl, head of the Art and Color Section at General Motors, was inspired by the swept-back silhouette of the Lockheed P-38

In Easter Morning, *Norman Rockwell gently satirized the gap between church membership and attendance. This sheepish suburban father's sanctuary is a "womb" chair designed by one of the most noted architects of the 1950s, Eero Saarinen.*

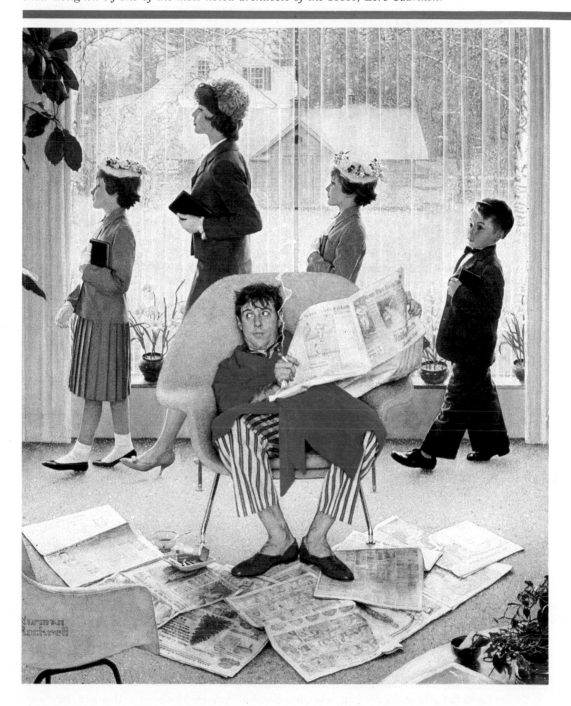

fighter plane to put the first modest tailfins on the 1948 Cadillac. Jet planes in-spired other automakers after 1955 to try ever more outrageous fins. Chrysler's new "Forward Look," created by chief of styling Virgil Exner, embodied the mixture of the big brassy box with futuristic fascination. In the lingo of the Detroit stylists, these designs were "gasaroony," an adjective *Popular Mechanics* maga-zine translated as "terrific, overpowering, weird." By the time the 1959 Cadillac reached showrooms, pedestrians were learning to tread carefully behind the behe-moth creations, lest they be impaled when the car backed up.

Fins, roadside motels, "gaseterias," drive-in burger huts, freeways, interstate highways, shopping centers, and, of course, suburbs were all part of a culture of mobility that was both physical and social in the 1950s. Americans continued their exodus from rural areas to cities and from the cities to the suburbs. As mechaniza-tion transformed cotton farming, blacks left the South in ever larger numbers, heading for industrial centers in the Northeast, Midwest, and West Coast. Mex-ican-Americans concentrated in southwestern cities; Puerto Ricans came largely to New York. And for Americans in the snow belt, the climate of the West and South (at least when civilized by air conditioning) made the Sunbelt irresistible to ever larger numbers.

Social mobility, too, burgeoned as affluence swelled the ranks of middle-class America. Having worried during the Depression era that divisions of class, ethnic-ity, and race might lead to social violence and political disorder, social scientists now spoke about consensus. In a positive light consensus reflected the triumph of the melting pot and an agreement among the wide majority of Americans about fundamental values. They rejected radical ideas at home and opposed the spread of communism abroad. But some social critics worried that too strong a consensus could breed a mindless conformity. In the things they owned, in the places they lived, in their churches and school, and in the values they held, Americans were becoming dangerously homogenized.

The baby boomers who reached adolescence in this era seldom worried about such issues. In the White House President Eisenhower radiated a comforting sense that the affairs of the nation and the world were in capable hands. That left teenagers free to worry about what really mattered: a first date, a first kiss, a first job, a first choice for college, and whether or not to "go all the way" before marriage.

TRANSFORMING WHEELS

The "mass automobility" of the 1950s defined a highly mobile and affluent con-sumer society. Almost every aspect of American life—work, family, and leisure, not to mention sex and personal self-expression—centered on the automobile. Of course, the American love affair with the automobile was hardly new. It had helped define the consumer culture of the 1920s: by the end of that decade nearly 27 million cars were on the road—one for every five Americans. The Depression and the war put a drag on new car sales, but Americans clung to the cars they had, even in hard times. "People give up everything in the world but their car," one observer noted. The postwar boom set autos again in motion. In 1946 Americans purchased 2 million cars; a decade later that figure had jumped to 8 million.

Like a freak of evolution run riot, automotive tailfins metamorphosed from the modest stubs of a 1948 Cadillac (top) into the sweeping wedges of Chrysler's "Forward Look," the batwing curves of a '59 Chevy, and the monstrous protrusions of the 1959 Cadillac (bottom), which also sported bomblike tail lights.

For many, and especially suburbanites, the automobile had become both a status symbol and a necessity. About two out of every three Americans drove a car to work. With about 6 percent of the world's population, Americans owned 50 percent of its automobiles. One out of every six jobs was involved in the manufacture or use of cars. When the automakers flourished, as in 1955, the American economy expanded. During the industry slump of 1958 the economy went into recession. But the automobile affected more than mere prosperity. The transforming power of its wheels changed the way Americans organized their personal lives and the space in which they lived. In the 1950s suburbs grew 40 times faster than cities. By 1960 half of the American people lived in suburbs. Such massive migration affected all aspects of class, religious, ethnic, and race relations. It also altered the economy, as manufacturing and trade followed the population to the suburbs. In the late 1940s almost 75 percent of the Levittowners on Long Island commuted into New York City to work. By the 1960s about 60 percent worked within their home county.

If railroads and mass transit were the vital arteries of urban America, highways carried the lifeblood of suburbia. Nine out of every ten suburban families owned a car and one in five had at least two. Almost all suburban activities depended on the availability of cars, cheap gasoline, and accessible roads. Shopping centers, the predecessors of more elaborate malls, were perhaps the best expression of the new auto-centered life. At the end of World War II the United States had just eight of these retail complexes, their cluster of stores set in a sea of asphalt parking space. By 1960 almost every community had at least one highway strip dotted with drive-in movies, stores, bowling alleys, gas stations, auto dealers, and fast-food joints. Even a few churches and funeral homes provided drive-in facilities to attract people committed to life behind the wheel. By 1960 the nation's approximately 3840 shopping centers covered as much land as all the central business districts.

To ease the burden on congested suburban roads, the Eisenhower administration proposed a 20-year plan for the construction of a massive interstate highway system of some 41,000 miles of freeway. Backed by a commission drawn from the trucking, oil, construction, and automobile industries, Eisenhower argued that not only would the new system ease congestion, but it would also provide easy evacuation of cities in case of nuclear attack. In 1956 Congress passed the Interstate Highway Act, which initiated the largest public works project in history. The federal government picked up 90 percent of the cost through a Highway Trust Fund, financed by special taxes on cars, gas, tires, lubricants, and auto parts.

The Interstate Highway Act had an enormous impact on American life. In all, the country spent some $250 billion on roads and highways in the 25 years after World War II. Average annual driving increased by 400 percent. Travelers had easier access to national parks, historic sites, and vacation areas. Whole new communities sprouted along the beltways around the nation's cities. Yet the new highway system was hardly a panacea. Congestion often worsened as motorists shifted routes to take advantage of the new roads. The massive transfer of dollars from the cities to the suburbs contributed to the eroding quality of urban life: 75 percent of all government transportation dollars (local, state, and federal) went to subsidize travel by car and truck; only 1 percent was earmarked for urban mass transit. Improved highways in turn benefited the largely more affluent suburbanites, who could afford to commute to their jobs. At the same time, many low-paying, unskilled jobs disappeared from the cities, forcing the urban poor into reverse commuting from city to suburb.

As intercity rail service and mass transit deteriorated, cities became less attractive places to live or do business. By the end of the 1950s most cities devoted at least a third of their downtown areas to parking lots and roads to accommodate automobile traffic. Once-thriving shopping districts became virtual ghost towns at night, as commuters returned to their bedroom communities. With fewer well-to-do taxpayers to draw upon, city governments lacked the tax base to finance public services. A vicious cycle ensued that proved most damaging to the urban poor, who had few means of escape.

THE SHAPE OF THE SUBURBS

For those who joined the mass migration to the suburbs, what did they hope to gain and how did they wish to live? First and foremost, the suburban ideal centered on a single-family dwelling owned by those who lived in it. The ideal itself could be traced back to the agrarian dream of being a self-sufficient farmer, carving a homestead from frontier lands. Over the years, the desire for an independent homestead survived the decline of family farming. Like the old agrarian model, suburban living consumed extensive amounts of land. Low-density housing spread over acre after acre of winding tracts, in sharp contrast to densely populated urban apartments. When the booming economy of the 1950s made homeownership possible for many Americans, they leapt at the chance.

Suburban homeownership was popularly associated with the broad middle classes: those workers who held white- or blue-collar jobs and made enough income to afford the housing. Indeed, class distinctions seemed to blur somewhat in the suburbs. "We see eye to eye on most things," commented one Levittown resident, "about raising kids, doing things together with your husband . . . we have practically the same identical background." Unlike many urban neighborhoods, where immigrant parents or grandparents might be living on the same block or even in the same apartment, single-family dwellers often left their relatives and in-laws behind. As a result, ethnic lifestyles were less pronounced in the suburbs. The restrictive immigration policies of the 1920s had also eroded ethnicity by reducing the number of newly arrived foreign-born Americans.

Class distinctions were reduced in other ways. As the GI Bill encouraged colleges and state university systems to expand, college diplomas and professional training became less a badge of the well-to-do. Furthermore, the developing bureaucratic and service economy created new jobs of indeterminate status. Television repair might be similar to blue-collar manufacturing, but what if the repairman also owned his own business? Was teaching or computer programming a higher status job? Class distinctions were more pronounced between suburban communities than within them. The rich tended to cluster in older developments, often centered around country clubs. Working-class suburbs sprouted on the outskirts of large manufacturing centers. Though middle class only on the basis of wages, the residents of blue-collar communities, like most suburbanites, had still escaped the city, owned their own homes, and depended on their cars.

American Civil Religion

If the move to the suburbs gradually stripped many ethnics of their native customs and languages, it seldom forced them to abandon their religious identity. Religion continued to be a distinctive and segregating factor during the 1950s. Catholics, Protestants, and Jews generally married within their own faiths, and in the suburbs they kept their social distance as well. Communities that showed no obvious class distinctions were sometimes deeply divided along religious lines. Catholics attended parochial rather than public schools, formed their own clubs, and gener-

Baptist Billy Graham led the revival of evangelistic denominations and sects. While his message emphasized the traditional fundamentalist themes of sin, redemption, and the Second Coming of Christ, his up-to-date methods took advantage of television, advertising, radio, and paperback books to reach the widest possible audience.

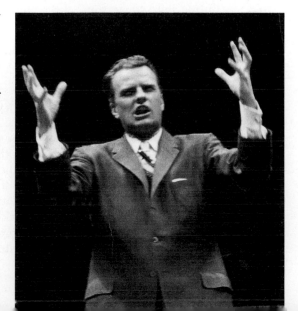

ally did not socialize with their Protestant neighbors. Protestant and Catholic members of the same country club usually did not play golf or tennis in the same foursomes. As for Jews, social historian Richard Polenberg has remarked that whereas a gulf divided many Catholics and Protestants, Jews and Gentiles "seem to have lived on the opposite sides of a religious Grand Canyon." Even superficial signs of friendliness masked underlying mistrust and the persistence of old stereotypes.

Although such religious boundaries remained distinct, the consensus increased that religion was central to American life. Church membership rose to over 50 percent for the first time in the twentieth century, and by 1957 the census bureau reported that 96 percent of the American people cited a specific affiliation when asked the question "What is your religion?" The religious upswing was supported in part by the prevailing cold war mood, since Communists were avowedly atheist. Patriotic and anticommunist themes were quite strong in the preaching of Billy Graham, a Baptist revival preacher who first attracted national attention at a tent meeting in Los Angeles in 1949. Following in the tradition of nineteenth-century revivalists like Charles Finney and Dwight Moody, Graham soon achieved even wider impact by televising his meetings. Though no revivalist, the Roman Catholic Bishop Fulton J. Sheen made the transition from a radio to a television ministry, where he spoke out strongly in favor of traditional values and against communism.

Religion also flourished because it was one crucial way suburbanites maintained a sense of identity and community, even as ethnic identity decreased. For gray-suited "organization men," swallowed up in the stress of corporate competition, religion offered a disciplined calm. So too it offered calm to the suburban homemaker, oppressed by seemingly endless diapers or floors in need of scrubbing. Rabbi Joshua Liebman's *Peace of Mind* became a best seller in 1946; the Reverend Norman Vincent Peale had even greater success with his *Power of Positive Thinking* in 1952. Throughout American culture, the benefits of religion—of *any* religion—were lauded. President Eisenhower made the point quite clear. "Our government makes no sense unless it is founded on a deeply religious faith," he proclaimed, "—and I don't care what it is." Congress, bowing to the popular mood, in 1954 added the phrase "under God" to the pledge of allegiance. And every Friday afternoon children watching "The Howdy Doody Show" were exhorted by "Buffalo Bob" to worship "at the church or synagogue of your choice."

"Homemaking" Women in the Workaday World

The growth of a suburban culture revealed a contradiction in the lives of middle-class women. Never before were their traditional roles as housewives and mothers so central to American society. Yet never before had more women joined the work force outside the home.

For housewives, the single-family dwelling of the suburbs required more labor to keep clean, while the baby boom left mothers with more children to tend with less help from relatives and grandparents, who no longer lived nearby. Increased dependence on automobiles made many a suburban housewife the chauffeur for her family. In the 1920s grocers, milkmen, or knife-sharpeners might deliver their goods or practice their trade from door to door. But by the 1950s delivery services were being replaced by housewives doing "errands."

Yet between 1940 and 1960 the percentage of wives working outside the home doubled from 15 to 30 percent. While the greatest increase occurred among women over 40, whose children were generally grown, by 1960 almost 40 percent of women with children between 6 and 16 held jobs. Some women took jobs simply to help make ends meet, but sheer financial necessity was not the only explanation. Middle-class married women went to work as often as lower class wives, and women with college degrees were the most likely to get a job. Two-income families were able to spend far more on gifts, education, recreation, and household appliances. In addition, women found status and self-fulfillment in their jobs. Wage work was clearly more rewarding to many than unpaid housework. So was the opportunity for social contacts and personal growth.

More women were going to college, too: in 1950 men outnumbered them 2 to 1 on campus, but by 1960 the ratio was only 5 to 3. The increased education did not translate into economic equality, however; the percentage of women holding professional jobs actually dropped between 1950 and 1960. In fact the gap between men's and women's wages was greater than in any other industrial nation. Women professionals earned only 64 percent of what males earned and those in sales earned just 41 percent. Over all, the median wage for women was less than half that for men.

Despite women's wider roles in society, the modern media continued to portray them either as sex objects or as housewives and mothers. A typical article appearing in *Redbook* in 1957 made a heroine of Junior, a "little freckle-faced brunette" who had given up work. As the story closed, Junior nursed her baby at two in the morning, crooning "I'm glad, glad, glad I'm just a housewife." In 1950 Lynn White, the president of Mills College for women, advocated a curriculum that displaced traditional academic subjects with those that were "distinctly feminine." Crafts were more suitable to women than the fine arts, he argued, and home economics had more relevance than a course in post-Kantian philosophy.

The media trivialized women in other ways. Advertisers constantly portrayed them as mindless consumers of household goods. Where the films of the 1930s and 1940s starred strong women like Mae West, Katharine Hepburn, and Barbara Stanwyck, confident in their intelligence, sexuality, and independence, the heroines of the 1950s appeared more vulnerable. Marilyn Monroe's voluptuous sensuality, combined with a little-girl innocence, clearly appealed to male tastes. Similarly, women's fashions portrayed a male vision of femininity. In 1947 Christian Dior introduced his "new look": narrow waistlines emphasizing shapely hips and a full bosom, rarely achieved without constricting foundation garments. The heels on shoes became ever higher and the toes pointier. As historian Lois Banner concluded, "Not since the Victorian era had women's fashions been so confining."

Women's sphere, then, remained limited during the 1950s. But the currents for change were present. Betty Friedan, a college graduate who had given up a career in psychology to raise a family, began to sense that other housewives were similarly frustrated at being merely "a server of food and putter-on of pants and a bedmaker." Her growing disillusionment with such a male-dominated culture led her to catalog its restrictive aspects in *The Feminine Mystique* (1963). By the end of the fifties other women were moving in the same direction.

The "Organization Man" in a Conglomerate World

If the new suburban culture affected middle-class women's lives both at home and at work, the postwar boom of the 1950s shaped the lives of suburban men in new

Daily Lives

PUBLIC SPACE/PRIVATE SPACE

The New Suburbia

Prosperity in the 1950s brought a greater demand for houses that, like automobiles, were larger and more ornamented. By the mid-1950s a builder like William Levitt no longer limited his offerings to the standard 900-square-foot Cape Cod saltbox efficiency house. New development designs, often created by builders rather than architects, haphazardly mixed styles and colors. California single-story ranch houses and one-and-a-half story New England Capes often stood side-by-side in the same developments. "Pink, orange, and turquoise may seem a weird combination," one newspaper commented, but reported that this exterior color scheme won its designer an award and a three-week vacation in Italy.

Despite an eclecticism that sometimes bordered on zaniness, suburban design did evolve from major architectural traditions. The most renowned of all suburban features, the picture window, traced its roots to architect Frank Lloyd Wright. Wright had come of age in the 1890s, at a time when "streetcar suburbs" were expanding around major urban areas. Wright's turn-of-the-century innovations combined open interior space, wide windows for natural lighting, and a horizontal, single-story layout. California architects translated Wright's ideas into the "ranch house," where rooms flowed into each other and indoor spaces opened to the outdoors to take advantage of the mild climate. Houses with fewer walls and defined spaces discouraged formality and even privacy.

Developers across the country seized upon the California "fantasy" style to conjure up for home buyers dreams of informal living along with a touch of glamour. While the reality was usually either a rectangular or L-shaped box, builders followed automobile designers in breaking the boxy profile with longer lines, decorator touches, or different planes defined by shapes, materials, colors, or textures. Developers added picture windows to make small houses seem more spacious, only to discover that they were popular in houses of all sizes and design.

Critics of suburban living suggested that the picture window was a means to ensure conformity. Why, after all, was the window most often placed looking onto the front yard, except to afford homeowners a means to keep an eye on neighbors who were watching them through their own picture windows? In truth, it made sense to have a picture window look onto the street in order to keep an eye on children. More important, it provided about the only vantage point from which people could enjoy their front yards. Few suburbanites sat out front or used the lawn for anything other than ornamental purposes. But since front yards made an important statement about houses and their owners, families decorated and tended them with special care.

By 1955, economics rather than aesthetics forced developers to forsake the basic suburban box. Surveys showed that three-quarters of all would-be buyers wanted a single-story house. But with land prices rising and new zoning codes being enforced, builders could not fit enough floor space onto typical lots. To build a two-story house without seeming to do so, they hit upon the split-level or "raised ranch": something, as one critic wryly noted, that "looked like a ranch-style house that had fallen out of the air and landed on something else." The front door

Daily Lives

This custom-built 1957 house reflected what so many suburban home buyers desired: plenty of glass and an open room structure that encouraged informality.

opened onto a landing halfway between the upper and lower floors, creating an illusion that it was only half the distance from one floor to the next. The basic construction, two simple boxes side-by-side, was cheap to build. By placing half the living space—either the kitchen, dining, and family rooms or the bedrooms—in what would otherwise be a basement, the split level created more habitable living space at little additional cost. Buyers approved, in part because the concept was novel, in larger part because they got more space at an affordable price.

Most of all, homeowners in the 1950s wanted family rooms and "live-in kitchens." One magazine described the family room as "the newest room in the house, but also the oldest," for the concept originated in the middle-class Victorian front parlor. Like it, the 1950s living room acquired more elegant furnishings for use during holidays or special entertaining. That led to the conversion of what often had been a basement "rumpus" room for the kids into a family room. Here, families sought a cozier feel with pine paneling and furniture designed for comfort and dura-

bility, with the television as the focus of the room. The "live-in" kitchen suited the growing families of the late 1950s who needed more space to prepare and eat meals. Earlier kitchens had normally been small and limited largely to food preparation. Meals were eaten in a combined living-dining area. The new larger kitchens were designed, one advertiser claimed, to make "mother a member of the family again," where everyone could gather while mother cooked. The same space would also hold appliances like dishwashers, dual ovens, and televisions, which became common kitchen features.

Clearly, suburban houses were more than

Little boxes on the hillside
Little boxes all the same.

as one folk-singing critic of the 1960s complained. To the people who flocked to suburbia, their homes represented a compromise between fantasy and practicality, fulfilling the American dream, "To own your own home."

ways as well. The 1950s witnessed the first sustained peacetime expansion of the economy since the 1920s. Buoyed by the new prosperity, large corporations moved increasingly toward product diversification and the conglomerate form of mergers. Each was a hedge against conditions that ravaged corporations in the 1930s, when a giant like General Electric, which had concentrated on equipment for generating electric power and light, suddenly found its markets evaporating. General Electric responded by entering markets for appliances, X-ray machines, and elevators, all products that involved application of the fruits of the company's research labs. In the postwar era General Electric diversified even further into nuclear power, jet engines, television, and industrial automation systems.

Diversification was practical for large industrial firms with the manufacturing base and profits to support extensive research and development (R&D). During the 1950s firms in the chemical, electronics, transportation, foods, and petroleum industries led the trend. Most large manufacturers produced in at least five industries, while the largest firms generally operated in twice as many. Large corporations also expanded their overseas operations. They took advantage of weak foreign economies to buy out potential competitors or to establish branches of their domestic operations. Most dynamic in the 1950s were the large integrated oil companies like Mobil and Standard Oil of New Jersey (Exxon), which developed huge oil fields in the Middle East and markets around the free world.

For some giants such as International Telephone and Telegraph (ITT) and for the small but aggressive firms such as Textron, Ling Temco Vought (LTV), and TRW the conglomerate merger served as a way to meet recessions and to seize opportunities for expansion. Unlike the earlier horizontal and vertical mergers, which had been limited to a core industry like automobiles and related manufacturing, conglomerate mergers brought together companies with seemingly unrelated products. Over a 20-year period ITT branched out from its basic communications business into baking, hotels and motels, car rental, home building, and insurance. In this way aggressive entrepreneurs like James Ling of LTV turned tiny local businesses into combinations of as many as 50 formerly independent companies. Between the late 1940s and early 1960s the 200 largest firms increased their share of the value added by manufacturing from around 30 percent to more than 40 percent. But bigger and more diversified did not always mean better or more profitable. Managers who knew how to market toasters did not necessarily know how to run hotels. New layers of managers added to paperwork, complicated decision making, and increased the size of the bureaucracy.

Despite fears that concentration would stifle competition and add to bureaucratic inefficiencies, economists judged concentration and diversification as stabilizing to the economy. In fact, in the critical science-based industries like electronics and chemicals responsible for much of the nation's technological innovation, competition increased. The top six firms in key industries never accounted for more than 45 percent of product value. Economists in banking and research centers like the Brookings Institution produced econometric models, which used statistics to enhance large firms' efficiency in managing inventory and investing revenues.

One key to managing these modern corporate giants was the advent of electronic data processing. In the early 1950s computers were virtually unknown in private industry. But banks and insurance companies saw computers as an answer to their need to manipulate huge quantities of records and statistical data. Manufacturers, especially in the petroleum, chemical, automotive, and electronics industries, began to use computers to monitor their production lines, quality control, and inventory. Americans began to have a sense of the automated workplace: more efficient, quieter, cleaner, and sometimes threateningly impersonal. Many skilled laborers became little more than caretakers of machines. This was a process, of course, that had been well under way since the Civil War. Now large corporations required that middle-level executives submerge their individual goals in the processes and work routines of a large bureaucracy. The corporate structure emphasized the need to work in teams and on committees rather than as individuals pursuing independent ideas.

David Riesman, a sociologist, attracted widespread attention when he outlined the consequences of the new corporate atmosphere in *The Lonely Crowd* (1950). In nineteenth-century America, Riesman argued, Americans had been "inner directed." It was their own consciences that formed their values and drove them to seek success. In contrast, modern workers had developed a personality shaped not so much by inner convictions as by the opinions of their peers. The new "other-directed" society of suburbia preferred security to success. "Go along to get along" was its motto. In a bureaucratized economy, it was important to please others, to conform to the group, and to cooperate. Other-directed people were, Riesman concluded, more superficial or shallow, having no deep convictions of their own.

William Whyte carried Riesman's critique from the workplace to the suburb in *The Organization Man* (1956). Here he found rootless families, shifted from town to town by the whims of impersonal corporations. (IBM, went one standard joke, stood for "I've Been Moved.") The typical "organization man" was sociable but not terribly ambitious. He sought primarily to "keep up with the Joneses" and the number of consumer goods they owned. He seemed all too ready to adopt the tastes and manners of the neighborhood. He lived in a suburban "split-level trap," as one critic put it, one among millions of "haggard" men, "tense and anxious" women, and "the gimme kids," who, like the cartoon character "Dennis the Menace," looked up from the litter under the Christmas tree to ask, "Is that all?"

No doubt such portraits were overdrawn and overly alarmist. (Where, after all, did Riesman's nineteenth-century inner-directed Americans get their values, if not from the society around them?) But they indicated the problems of adjustment faced by those working within large bureaucratic organizations and living in suburbs that were decentralized and self-contained.

THE POLITICS OF CALM

In presiding over these vast changes in American society, President Dwight David Eisenhower projected an aura of paternal calm. Eisenhower had been raised in a large Kansas farm family and his parents, though poor, offered him a warm, caring home steeped in religious faith. In an era of organization men, Eisenhower succeeded by organizing his way to the top of the military pyramid. A graduate of West Point, he was neither a scholar nor an aggressive general like George Patton. Rather, "Ike" had made his way upward by mastering bureaucratic politics. In the placid years between the two world wars, his skills at golf, poker, and bridge often proved as valuable as his military expertise. Yet such genial sociability could not hide his ambition or his ability to judge character shrewdly. It took a gifted organizer to coordinate the D-Day invasion and to hold together the conglomeration of egocentric generals who pushed west to Berlin. After the war Eisenhower presided for a time as president of Columbia University and then as commander of NATO forces in Europe. When the Republicans made the call in 1952, he was ready for a new challenge.

In shaping his administration, Eisenhower called upon his army ways. A good general, he believed, left the details to his staff while concentrating most attention on grand strategy. He also preferred private negotiation to public confrontation and kept such a low political profile that some critics thought he conceived the president to be almost a figurehead, like a constitutional monarch. In reality, he operated more of a "hidden hand" presidency, privately making decisions and setting directions but publicly letting others speak for him (and take the heat). At press conferences, his answers to questions were often garbled or rambling, giving the impression that he didn't always have a firm grasp of his policies. In truth, he was shrewder than his critics believed, sometimes even using his imprecision to bamboozle the press. "Don't worry," he once reassured his press secretary, "if that question comes [up], I'll just confuse them."

Yet for all his ability to organize and negotiate behind the scenes, Eisenhower still remained more aloof than most presidents. He often failed to use his prestige on major issues like civil rights. His chief of staff, Sherman Adams, a New Hampshire businessman and former governor, organized the flow of information so strictly that the president's briefing papers were boiled down to one-page summaries, which could be quickly and easily digested. Ever the organization man, Eisenhower surrounded himself with business executives who were dedicated to the status quo. The *New Republic* described the cabinet as "eight millionaires and a plumber"—the plumber being Secretary of Labor Martin P. Durkin, who soon became uncomfortable hobnobbing with so many thoroughbred Republicans and resigned.* Secretary of Defense Charles Wilson, former president of General Motors, best articulated the probusiness creed of the administration when he told a Senate committee that he had always believed, "What was good for our country was good for General Motors and vice versa."

Modern Republicanism

In office, Eisenhower pursued a course he described as "modern Republicanism." He resisted the demands of conservatives to dismantle New Deal programs and even agreed to increases in Social Security, unemployment insurance, and the minimum wage. He supported a small public housing program and a modest federally supported medical insurance plan for the needy. But he rejected more far-reaching liberal proposals on housing and universal health care through the Social Security system. And his secretary of the treasury, George M. Humphrey, soon became a forceful spokesman for a conservative domestic agenda. Humphrey, the former executive of a profitable conglomerate, cut back federal jobs whenever he could, eliminated construction projects, and resisted any pressure to raise defense spending. He preferred legislation favored by the business community, like the Submerged Lands Act of 1953, a bill that turned rich coastal oil deposits over to the states, which were far more easily influenced by the lobbies of the oil industry.

*When the Department of Health, Education and Welfare was established in 1953, Eisenhower did appoint a woman, Oveta Culp Hobby of Texas, making his cabinet eight millionaires and a millionairess.

To make modern Republicanism successful, Eisenhower had to woo away from the Democrats voters who were joining the newly affluent middle class. Success in that effort hinged on how well the administration could manage the economy. The Democrats of the New Deal had established a tradition of activism: when the economy faltered, deficit spending and tax cuts were used to stimulate it. Eisenhower, in contrast, wanted to reduce federal spending and the government's role in the economy. When a recession struck in 1953–54, the administration was concerned more with balancing the budget and holding inflation in line than with reducing unemployment through government spending. But these policies worked poorly enough (and the voters expressed their resentment in midterm elections) so that when recessions again hit in 1957–1958 and 1960–1961 there was less talk of balancing the budget. Indeed, Eisenhower achieved that goal in only three of eight fiscal years; and in 1959 he faced what was then the largest peacetime deficit in history. The result was that while the economy grew during the Eisenhower years, the pattern of that growth remained uneven, leaving the city and rural poor largely untouched.

Eisenhower followed a similar pragmatic approach in other areas. When major projects called for federal leadership, as with the Highway Act, he supported the policy. In 1954 he signed the St. Lawrence Seaway Act, which joined the United States and Canada in an ambitious engineering project to open the Great Lakes to ocean shipping. Like the highway program, the Seaway was fiscally acceptable because the funding came from user tolls and taxes rather than from general revenues.

In dealing with farmers, Eisenhower was not about to commit political suicide by trying to abolish price supports established during the New Deal. But as more and more government silos filled with farmers' surplus grain, Eisenhower's secretary of agriculture, Ezra Taft Benson, proposed a system of lower support payments designed to discourage farmers from overproducing basic commodities like corn, cotton, and wheat. Benson also established a soil bank program to pay farmers for taking land out of production. Still, agriculture continued to be transformed by the processes of modern technology. Automated harvesters, fertilizers, and new varieties of plants increased farm outputs as prices continued to drop. In an age of continuing centralization, more and more small farms were being replaced by larger agribusinesses.

The Fall of Joseph McCarthy

When Eisenhower hit on the notion of calling himself a modern Republican, he was looking for some way to distance himself from what he called the more "hidebound" members of the GOP. Their continuing anticommunist campaigns were causing him increasing embarrassment. Senator McCarthy's reckless antics, at first directed at Democrats, now had become less discriminating. In 1953 the Wisconsin senator tried to defeat the appointment of Soviet expert Charles E. Bohlen as ambassador to Moscow. Only the parliamentary skill of Senator Robert Taft saved the appointment and grave embarrassment to the administration. By the summer of 1953 the senator was on a rampage. He dispatched two of his staff members, Roy M. Cohn and G. David Schine, to investigate the Voice of America and the State Department's overseas information agency. Behaving more like college pranksters, the two conducted a whirlwind 18-day witch hunt through Western Europe. To the chagrin of the administration, they insisted on purging government library shelves of "subversive" books, including those by John Dewey and Foster Rhea Dulles, a conservative historian and cousin of the secretary of state. Some librarians, fearing for their careers, burned a number of books. That drove President Eisenhower to denounce "book burners," though he soon after reassured McCarthy's rabid supporters that he did not advocate free speech for communists.

Meanwhile, the administration's own behavior contributed to the red hysteria on which McCarthy thrived. The president launched a loyalty campaign, which he claimed resulted in 3000 firings and 5000 resignations of government employees. It was a godsend to McCarthyites: What further proof was needed that subversives were lurking in the federal bureaucracy? In addition, Eisenhower refused pleas to commute the death sentences of Julius and Ethel Rosenberg to life imprisonment. Such a severe sentence was unusual even in cases of espionage (and here the evidence was not conclusive), but the Rosenbergs were still executed on June 13, 1953. A year later the Atomic Energy Commission turned its investigative eyes on physicist J. Robert Oppenheimer. During World War II it was Oppenheimer's administrative and scientific genius that had led to the development of the atomic bomb. Widely respected by his colleagues, he had raised the hackles of many politicians in 1949 when he opposed the construction of a hydrogen bomb. Despite a few left-wing associations from the 1930s (which army officials had known about when Oppenheimer was working on the bomb), no one had ever accused him of passing on national security information. Nonetheless, the Atomic

With the ruthless Roy Cohn (left) and David Schine (right) providing legal counsel, Senator Joseph McCarthy made a minor Senate subcommittee into a major power center and his name synonymous with inquisitional politics.

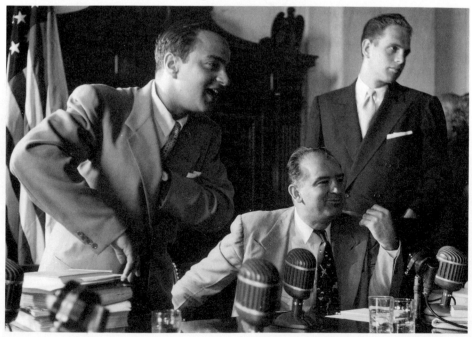

Energy Commission in effect suggested Oppenheimer was a traitor by barring him from sensitive research.

In such a climate—where Democrats remained silent for fear of being called leftists and Eisenhower cautiously refused to "get in the gutter with *that* guy"—McCarthy eventually lost all sense of proportion. In that he was driven on by his overly ambitious and ruthless aide Roy Cohn. When the army denied David Schine a commission, Cohn persuaded McCarthy to investigate communism in the army. The new American Broadcasting Company network, eager to fill its afternoon program slots, decided to televise the hearings. The public had an opportunity to see McCarthy badger witnesses and make a mockery of Senate procedures. When Joseph L. Welch, the outraged lawyer for the army, asked, "Have you no sense of decency, sir?" he laid bare the senator's weak spot, to the applause of the gallery and the satisfaction of the wide television audience. As McCarthy's popularity dwindled and the 1954 elections safely passed, the Senate finally moved to censure him. McCarthy died three years later, destroyed by alcohol and the habit of throwing so many reckless punches.

The Politics of the Middle

Despite his aloof public posture, Eisenhower could not escape partisan politics. Just as Truman had been pricked occasionally by revelations of corrupt aides, key members of Eisenhower's administration were exposed for improperly accepting gifts and peddling influence. Most disturbing to Eisenhower was the resignation in 1958 of Sherman Adams, his most trusted adviser, who had accepted gifts in return for favors. None of these instances involved any hint of corruption on the president's part, and his political stock remained high. But poor economic performance took its toll on the GOP. In the wake of the 1954 recession the Democrats gained a 29-member majority in the House and a one-vote edge in the Senate. Never again would Eisenhower work with a Republican congressional majority. Even when he won a smashing victory over Adlai Stevenson (57 to 42 percent) in the 1956 presidential election, the Democrats' House majority increased to 33. In 1958 recession produced an even greater setback, giving the Democrats a 68-seat majority in the House and 30 seats in the Senate.

Eisenhower's triumph in 1956 had been the one electoral bright spot for the Republicans. A major heart attack in 1955 and abdominal surgery in 1956 had slowed the president, but rather than resulting in questions about his health, led to an outpouring of public sympathy. With the economy strong in 1955–1956 Stevenson never stood a chance. Eisenhower's political strategists also made effective use of television, hiring the advertising firm of Batten, Barton, Durstine, and Osborne to mount a campaign. BBDO pioneered the use of the five-minute trailer, which followed regular programs so that Ike's ads did not disturb the audience.

NATIONALISM IN AN AGE OF SUPERPOWERS

Prosperity at home depended on the maintenance of a stable international system of markets and resources. Before World War II European nations played a central role in that system, particularly in colonial areas of the Middle East, Africa, and Southeast Asia. With the collapse of the European global order, the United States and the Soviet Union had become the dominating superpowers in world affairs. But the war disrupted the old colonial relationships too. In Latin America and the Middle East nationalism often meant freeing states like Venezuela and Iran from burdensome debts and concessions to foreigners. In Asia Vietnamese nationalist forces led by Ho Chi Minh had driven Japanese occupation forces out of Indochina and were continuing their fight against French colonial forces. And within Soviet Eastern Europe, national feeling among nations like Poland and Hungary remained strong.

Given the atmosphere of the cold war, both superpowers tended to see the unrest, revolution, and nationalism in these smaller nations in terms of their bipolar struggle. By fits and starts, both the Soviet Union and the United States waxed hostile then conciliatory toward one another. And both competed for the allegiance of the smaller, newly independent nations across the globe.

To the Brink?

The conduct of foreign policy under Eisenhower was shared by the president with his secretary of state, John Foster Dulles. Eisenhower, of course, was no stranger to world politics, having done his stint of diplomatic maneuvering as a general fighting a global war and as commander of NATO. And Dulles approached his job with a somber enthusiasm; indeed, he had been on a virtual campaign for the position since advising presidential hopeful Thomas Dewey in 1944. Coming from a family of missionaries and diplomats, Dulles had within him a touch of both. He saw the Soviet–American struggle in almost religious terms: a fight of good against evil, in which the differences between the two superpowers were irreconcilable. Admirers praised his global vision of the world; detractors saw him as "the wooliest type of pontificating American." Certainly Dulles did not lack confidence. "With my understanding of the intricate relationship between the peoples of the world," he told Eisenhower, "and your sensitiveness to the political considerations, we will make the most successful team in history."

In the end, the two men's differing temperaments led to a policy that seesawed from confrontation to conciliation. Both men were cautious, but Eisenhower was less consistently aggressive in his attitudes toward the Soviets. Dulles, on the other hand, more often threw up cautionary roadblocks when the Russians suggested compromise. Despite that difference, the two men remained firmly committed to an anticommunist posture. "Freedom is pitted against slavery," Eisenhower declared, "lightness against dark."

The first priority for Eisenhower was to end the Korean War, which had settled into a drawn-out, bone-wearying stalemate. Even before taking office, the president-elect had fulfilled his campaign promise "to go to Korea" and appraise the situation firsthand. Once in office, he and Dulles made ominous noises about resorting to nuclear war against Communist China at the same time that they renewed negotiations with North Korea. On July 27, 1953, the Communists and the United Nations forces signed an armistice ending a "police action" in which 54,000 Americans had died. Korea itself remained divided, almost as it had been in 1950. Communism had been "contained" in Korea, but little more than that.

The administration, however, was determined to turn containment from what they charged had been a defensive strategy under Truman to a more offensive one.

Dulles wanted the United States to aid in liberating the "captive peoples" of Eastern Europe and other Communist nations. That seemed to require a larger military budget, however, at a time when Eisenhower was equally determined to cut back military spending and troop levels in order to keep the budget balanced. The president, who knew how the military services and their allies in defense industries vied for government money, was irked at the "fantastic programs" the Pentagon kept coming up with. "If we demand too much in taxes in order to build planes and ships," he argued, "we will tend to dry up the accumulations of capital that are necessary to provide jobs for the million or more new workers that we must absorb each year."

The solution Eisenhower and Dulles hit on for solving the problem was to rely less on ground forces and more on the threat of massive nuclear retaliation in order to intimidate the Soviets into political accommodations. Dulles proclaimed that Americans could not shrink from the threat of nuclear war. "If you are scared to go to the brink, you are lost," he argued. And as Secretary of Defense Charles Wilson put it, a nuclear strategy was much cheaper—"a bigger bang for the buck." Henceforth American foreign policy would have a "new look," though behind the rhetoric lay an ongoing commitment to containment.

Moving beyond the rhetoric of "brinksmanship" did not prove easy, however. When Dulles announced American intentions to "unleash" Chiang Kai-shek to attack mainland China from his outpost on Taiwan, China's foreign minister Zhou Enlai threatened to liberate Taiwan from the nationalists. At that, Eisenhower ordered the Seventh Fleet into the area to protect rather than unleash Chiang. By

ASIAN TROUBLE SPOTS
After the Geneva accords divided Indochina into North and South Vietnam, Secretary of State John Foster Dulles organized SEATO to resist Communist aggression in Southeast Asia. In addition to the conflict in Vietnam, tensions were fueled by the mutual hostility between mainland Communist China and Chiang Kai-shek's Taiwan, as well as the offshore islands of Quemoy and Matsu.

1955 Dulles had staked the defense of Taiwan on tiny coastal islands, especially Quemoy and Matsu. If the Communists attacked, he bluntly stated, "we'll have to use atomic weapons."

Nuclear weapons also figured in the American response to a crisis in Indochina. Between 1950 and 1954, the United States had given France $1.2 billion in military aid (70 percent of the French military budget) to support the war against Ho Chi Minh. Viewing the countries of Southeast Asia like a row of dominoes, Eisenhower warned that any settlement with the Communists would lead to the loss of the entire region. "You have a row of dominoes set up, you knock over the first one. . . . You could have the beginning of a disintegration that would have the most profound influences."

Worn down by a war they seemed unable to win, the French in 1954 tried to force a final showdown with Ho's forces at Dien Bien Phu. With Vietnamese and Chinese troops holding the surrounding hilltops, the French garrison of 12,000 could not have picked a worse place to do battle. Desperate, the French government pleaded for more American aid, and Admiral Arthur Radford, head of the Joint Chiefs of Staff, volunteered a massive American air raid to relieve the besieged French forces. Radford did not rule out tactical nuclear weapons. But again Eisenhower pulled back. The idea of American involvement in another Asian war aroused opposition from both allies and domestic political leaders like Senate majority leader Lyndon B. Johnson. Without the capacity to win, the French surrendered at Dien Bien Phu in May and convened an international peace conference at Geneva, co-sponsored by the British and Soviet Union. Ho Chi Minh agreed to withdraw his forces north of the 17th parallel in anticipation of elections within two years, confident this would bring him to power in the South as well as the North. But Dulles, having limited the American role to observer at the Geneva peace conference, convinced Eisenhower to support a South Vietnamese government under Ngo Dinh Diem. Diem, Dulles argued, was not bound by the Geneva Accords. The United States then stepped further into the quagmire by sending a military mission to train Diem's army and keep him in power.

The Covert Side of the "New Look"

Dulles and Eisenhower pursued an activist foreign policy in less open ways with the help of John Foster Dulles' brother, Allen Dulles, director of the Central Intelligence Agency (CIA), which had been created in 1947 to coordinate foreign intelligence gathering and conduct covert operations against enemies. In Iran, a nationalist government under Mohammed Mossadeq had in 1951 seized British Petroleum, the British government's single most valuable overseas asset. American oil companies too had developed vast holdings in the region, and government policymakers viewed Iran as a key barrier against Soviet expansion into the Middle East. As relations worsened between Mossadeq and Iran's pro-Western monarch, Shah Mohammad Reza Pahlavi, Dulles feared that Mossadeq would turn to the Soviets. He and Eisenhower approved a covert CIA operation to topple Mossadeq's government. Led by Teddy Roosevelt's grandson, Kermit Roosevelt, "Operation Ajax" recruited a mob to help the Iranian armed forces drive Mossadeq out and return the Shah to his throne in August 1953. The following year a consortium of American oil companies assumed a major role in marketing Iranian oil, and disillusioned nationalists branded the Shah an American puppet.

Seeing how cheaply and quickly American influence had been restored in

Iran, Secretary Dulles looked for similar results in Guatemala. The decision to intervene, however, raised even more vexing ethical questions. Unlike Iran, Guatemala had a duly elected democratic government under Colonel Jacobo Arbenz Guzmán. Arbenz was determined to alleviate the severe poverty in his country by expropriating the idle farmland of rich landowners and giving it to the peasants. Guatemala's richest landowner was the Boston-based United Fruit Company, which had long supported conservative governments, paid few taxes, and shipped its profits back to the United States. Not coincidentally, United Fruit was an old client of Sullivan and Cromwell, a law firm in which both of the Dulles brothers had been partners.

When the Arbenz government seized 400,000 acres from United Fruit, its agents launched a publicity campaign to brand Arbenz a Communist. As the American ambassador to Guatemala later put it, "It seemed to me that the man thought like a communist and talked like a communist, and if not actually one, would do until one came along." When the Soviet Union permitted Czechoslovakia to send Guatemala 1900 tons of small arms, Dulles ordered a CIA-trained band of 1950 Guatemalan and Honduran mercenaries into Guatemala, aided by bombing raids carried out by American P-51 fighter planes. Within a week the army deserted Arbenz, who then fled the country. The leader of the Guatemalan rebels, Carlos Castillo Armas, established a military dictatorship which quickly returned the expropriated lands to United Fruit.

Success in Iran and Guatemala greatly enhanced the reputation of the CIA and created among American policymakers a misplaced faith in covert operations to achieve dramatic results at low cost. But in overthrowing popular governments, the United States gained a dubious reputation in many Third World countries as a foe of national liberation, popular democracy, and social reform. In 1958 the depth of anti-American feeling became obvious when angry crowds in several Latin American countries attacked Vice President Richard Nixon's car, spat at him, and pelted him with eggs and stones.

The Superpowers

Korea, Indochina, Iran, Guatemala—in the eyes of the administration, the crises in all these countries could be traced back to the Soviet dictatorship. Although nationalist movements around the globe were leading nations like India to declare themselves neutral or nonaligned, Dulles continually warned them that they could not sit on the fence: they must choose either the "free world" or the Communist bloc. Throughout the 1950s the secretary of state crisscrossed the globe, setting up mutual defense pacts patterned on NATO, to solidify American security. Yet in all this, it was becoming harder to decide what the motives of the Soviets themselves might be.

Joseph Stalin had died in March 1953, after becoming increasingly isolated, arbitrary, vengeful, and perhaps even paranoiac. For a time the Soviet Union was governed by "collective leadership," but power soon fell to Nikita Khrushchev, a party stalwart with a formidable intellect and peasant origins in the farm country of the Ukraine. In some ways Khrushchev resembled another farm-belt politician, Harry Truman. Both were unsophisticated yet shrewd, earthy in their sense of humor, energetic, irascible, and largely inexperienced in international affairs. Khrushchev kept American diplomats off balance: at times genial and conciliatory, he would suddenly become demanding and boastful.

At home Khrushchev established a relatively moderate regime, gradually shifting the economy toward production of consumer goods. Internationally, the Soviets called for an easing of tensions and reduced forces in Europe, in a bid to wean Western Europeans from dependence on the United States. In Washington the administration was unsure of how to receive the new overtures. The spirit of McCarthyism still reigned, so that compromise with the Soviets involved great political risk. And Secretary Dulles was temperamentally suspicious of all "Godless" Communists. It was actually Winston Churchill who suggested that the Russians might be serious about negotiating. In May 1953 he called on world leaders to hold a summit conference. Dulles and Eisenhower were distinctly cool to the proposition, but further Soviet overtures finally brought the Americans, British, French, and Soviets together in Geneva, Switzerland in 1955.

Little came of the summit other than a cordial "spirit of Geneva," which promised a cooling in the arms race. Neither side had been able to agree about how East and West Germany might be reunified, since both recognized that Germany held the key to Europe's balance of power. Eisenhower did manage a propaganda coup with a policy he called "Open Skies." In a dramatic, unexpected speech, the president announced that the United States would allow the Soviets to photograph American territory from the air and inspect military facilities if the Soviets would grant the same rights to Americans. As the president concluded his remarks to the thunderstruck audience, real lightning suddenly flashed, knocking out the power. The British and French heartily endorsed Open Skies, but Khrushchev condemned it as little more than a "transparent espionage device." Since the Soviets knew the location of American military sites, Open Skies would merely allow the United States to compile more accurate intelligence about the Soviet Union's facilities.

The spirit of Geneva was quickly disturbed by nationalist unrest in 1956. Within the Soviet Union, Khrushchev had undertaken a campaign condemning Stalin's crimes and excesses, and this more liberal attitude encouraged open dissent among Russia's Eastern European allies. Riots erupted in Poland in June, while in Hungary students took to the streets demanding that a coalition government under Imre Nagy replace the Stalinist puppet regime. When the rioting spread, Moscow accepted Nagy and began to remove Soviet tanks from Budapest. But when Nagy announced that Hungary would withdraw from the Warsaw Pact, that was too much. On October 31 tanks rolled into Budapest to crush the uprising. Nagy was imprisoned in Russia and executed in 1957. The American State Department issued formal protests but did nothing to help liberate the "captive nations." For all its tough talk, the "New Look" foreign policy recognized that the Soviets possessed a sphere of influence where the United States would not intervene.

Action would have been difficult because the United States faced a crisis in Egypt. Colonel Gamal Abdel Nasser, a nationalist, had come to power in 1952 and for several years had been attempting to modernize his country and rebuild his army. In 1955 Dulles sought to win Nasser's friendship by offering American aid to build the Aswan Dam, a massive power project on the Nile River. But when Nasser formed an Arab alliance against the young state of Israel and continued to pursue economic ties with the Warsaw bloc, Dulles decided to teach him a lesson. He withdrew the American pledge on Aswan. Nasser angrily upped the ante by seizing the British-owned Universal Suez Canal Company, which ran the waterway through which tankers carried most of Europe's oil.

By 1955 Nikita Khrushchev had emerged as the most powerful Soviet leader. At the Geneva summit (center, front), he was all smiles, claiming, "Things are different now." But like U.S. foreign policy, Khrushchev's waivered between "brinksmanship" and "peaceful coexistence."

Events then began to move quickly. Israel, alarmed at Nasser's Arab alliance, invaded Egypt's Sinai peninsula on October 29, the day Hungary announced it was leaving the Warsaw Pact. Three days later French and British forces seized the canal in an attempt to restore their own interests and prestige. Eisenhower, angered that his allies had not consulted him, for once joined the Soviet Union in supporting a United Nations resolution condemning Britain, France, and Israel and demanding an immediate cease-fire. By December American pressures forced Britain and France to remove their forces. Few events placed so much strain on the Western alliance as the Suez crisis. At the same time Nasser had demonstrated to the industrial powers the potential force of Third World nationalism.

Given the unstable situation, Eisenhower went before Congress in January 1957 and asked for a resolution empowering him to use force in the Middle East against any communist attack. What became known as the Eisenhower Doctrine in effect allowed the president to preempt the war-making authority of Congress in the event of a crisis. Even though the Democrats controlled Congress, fear of Soviet designs on the Middle East persuaded them to give Eisenhower the power he requested. The following year he used it, when Nasser's alliance, known as the United Arab Republic, aided nationalists in ousting a pro-Western government from Iraq. The Christian president of Lebanon, fearing that the unrest would spill into his strife-torn nation, appealed to Eisenhower for aid. Invoking his power under the Eisenhower Doctrine, the president ordered marines into Lebanon. Sunbathers on the beaches of Beirut, Lebanon's capital, were startled on July 15 as 5000 combat-clad marines stormed ashore.

Eventually the United States sent 15,000 troops to Lebanon. No fighting occurred and the American forces turned their peacekeeping role over to the United Nations. Startled by the aggressive American response, Iraq gave assurances that Western oil interests were safe. Nasser, for his part, discovered that Moscow's promise of help amounted to little more than rhetoric. Dulles claimed that the United States had once again turned back the communist drive into the emerging nations, but in reality, nationalism more than communism had been at the root of Middle Eastern turmoil.

Nationalist forces were also in ferment in Latin America, where rapid population growth and maldistribution of wealth and property (2 percent of the people controlled 75 percent of the land) increased social pressures. Repressive dictatorships exercised power and foreign interests—especially American—dominated

Latin American economies, making any conversion to democratic government highly unlikely. Cuba, only 90 miles south of American shores, was typical.

The United States owned many Cuban economic resources, including 80 percent of its utilities, and operated a major naval base at Guantánamo Bay. Cuban dictator Fulgencio Batista had close ties both to the American government and to major crime figures who operated gambling, prostitution, and drug rings in Havana. In 1956 a disgruntled middle-class lawyer, Fidel Castro, sought and quickly gained the support of impoverished peasants in Cuba's mountains to overthrow the corrupt regime. On January 1, 1959, Castro drove Batista from power.

At first many Americans applauded the Cuban revolution, welcoming Castro to the United States in April. But President Eisenhower was distinctly cool to the cigar-smoking Cuban. By summer Castro had filled key positions with Cuban Communists, launched an agricultural reform program, and confiscated American properties. Retaliating, Eisenhower embargoed Cuban sugar and mobilized opposition to Castro in other Latin American countries. Cut off from American markets and aid, Castro turned to the Soviet Union.

Thaws and Freezes

Throughout the series of continuing crises, each superpower found it difficult to interpret the other's motives. The Russians moved to exploit nationalist revolutions where the opportunity offered—more so in Cuba, less in Egypt—and at such times Nikita Khrushchev spoke belligerently of aiding national wars of liberation. "We will bury you," he once admonished the United States, though it was unclear whether this Russian colloquialism meant through peaceful competition or military confrontation. Khrushchev's most outrageous rhetoric came in a speech to the United Nations, where, to make his point, he took off his shoe and pounded it angrily on the table. More seriously, the Soviet premier issued an ultimatum to the Western powers in November 1958 to withdraw their troops from West Berlin within six months, declare it a free city, and negotiate access to it with the East Germans, a government the Western powers had refused to recognize. Eisenhower flatly rejected the ultimatum and Khrushchev backed away from his hardline stance.

By the time John Foster Dulles died of cancer in April 1959, Eisenhower had determined that the last 18 months of his presidency would be devoted to improving Soviet–American relations. In September, at the president's invitation, Khrushchev visited the United States. Though meetings at Camp David produced no significant results, the two leaders agreed to hold another summit meeting in Europe. And Khrushchev concluded his stay with a picturesque tour across America, swapping comments about manure with Iowa farmers, reacting puritanically to movie cancan dancers, and grumping when his visit to the new capitalist marvel, Disneyland, was canceled for security reasons.

Eisenhower's plans for a return visit to the Soviet Union were abruptly canceled on May 17, as the Paris summit conference collapsed. Two weeks earlier the Russians had announced they had shot down a high-altitude U-2 American spy plane. At first Eisenhower claimed that the plane had strayed off course while doing weather research, but Khrushchev sprang his trap: the CIA pilot, Gary Powers, had been captured alive. The president then admitted that he had personally authorized the U-2 overflights for reasons of national security. That epi-

The *Sputnik* launching in 1957 made Americans aware that vast distances no longer protected them from nuclear attack. But even before that discomforting event, Americans had begun devising "fallout shelters" for protection from the aftereffects of a nuclear attack. This one was exhibited in 1955.

sode ended Eisenhower's hopes that his personal diplomacy might create a new framework for Soviet–American relations.

Meanwhile, Congress and the American public had become increasingly worried about Soviet technical achievements. The Russians had developed a hydrogen bomb by 1954. In 1957 they stunned America by launching into outer space the first satellite, dubbed *Sputnik*. And by 1959, when Khrushchev arrived in Washington, the Soviets had crash-landed a much larger payload on the moon. If the Russians could target the moon, they surely could launch nuclear missiles against America, whereas the American space program had been so plagued with delays and mishaps that satellites were being nicknamed "flopniks" and "kaputniks." How had the Soviets managed to catch up with American nuclear technology so quickly? In 1958 Eisenhower joined Congress to pass a National Defense Education Act designed to strengthen graduate education and the teaching of science, mathematics, and foreign languages. At the same time, crash programs proliferated to build basement fallout shelters to protect Americans in case of a nuclear attack.

Democrats charged that the administration had ignored the nation's defense needs. The United States faced an unacceptable "missile gap," they claimed. Disgruntled army officers and defense experts called for a rebuilding of American conventional forces to correct a foreign policy that relied too heavily on nuclear retaliation. Eisenhower knew from American intelligence, but could not admit publicly, that the "missile gap" was not real. While willing to spend more on missile development, he refused to heed his critics' cry for a "crash" defense program at any cost. Eisenhower was not as readily impressed as later presidents by the promises of new weapon systems. He left office with a warning that too much military spending would lead to "an unwarranted influence, whether sought or unsought" by the "military–industrial complex" at the expense of democratic institutions. In looking back over his two terms he could take some comfort from his conduct of foreign policy. A less mature and sophisticated president might have led the United States into more severe conflict or even war. On the other hand, Eisenhower had not been able to place Soviet–American relations in a stable framework.

CIVIL RIGHTS AND THE NEW SOUTH

The history of black Americans and their struggle for equality from the 1940s on is filled with ironies. Just as barriers to legal segregation in the South were tumbling, millions of blacks were leaving for regions where suburbanization imposed new forms of residential discrimination not easily redressed by law. The South they left behind was in the early stages of an economic boom. The cities where they migrated had entered a period of decline that would make them the centers of the nation's worst poverty. Yet, as if to close a circle, the rise of large black voting blocs in major cities created political pressures that forced the nation to dismantle the most blatant legal and institutional barriers to racial equality. For blacks, it might be said that these were the best of times and the worst of times.

The New South's Effect on Blacks

After World War II the southern economy began to grow significantly faster than the national economy. And as it grew, what had for many years been a distinct regional economy was integrated into the larger national and international systems. Where cotton and other agricultural staples had once been king, new centers for manufacturing, the military, petroleum and natural gas, recreation, and finance flourished. None of these newer economic activities depended heavily on the low-wage, unskilled, and non-union labor that had previously been the most distinctive feature of the southern economy.

This remarkable about-face began during the war, with an influx of federal dollars to build and maintain military bases and defense plants. It continued in the postwar period. Congressman Mendel Rivers of South Carolina, for example, was so successful in steering defense projects into his district that critics complained that it might sink under the weight of military installations. As the improved business climate attracted outside capital and skilled labor into the region, wages began to match those elsewhere. And the South attracted new business because it offered a "clean slate." As opposed to more mature economies in the Northeast and Upper Midwest, the region had few unions, little regulation and bureaucracy, and low wages and taxes. Finally, there was the matter of climate, which later became known as the "Sunbelt phenomenon." Especially with improvements in air conditioning, the southern climate and amenities grew more attractive to affluent retirees, skilled professionals, and corporate managers.

Several additional factors more centrally affected the situation of blacks. Before World War II 80 percent of all blacks lived in the South. They constituted a large portion of the low-wage, unskilled labor pool that operated the South's major economic enterprises. The majority worked as sharecroppers and tenant farmers. During the war, about 3 million blacks and whites left farms for the army and urban industrial centers in search of higher wages. After the war that outflow continued.

The departure of so much labor created a crisis in cotton farming, where harvesting remained a labor-intensive task. For the first time cotton farmers had an incentive to mechanize the harvest and International Harvester cooperated by producing a workable machine. In 1950 just 5 percent of the cotton crop was mechanically picked; by 1960 it reached 50 percent. Farmers began to consolidate land into larger holdings. Tenant farmers, sharecroppers, and hired labor of both races, no longer in short supply, left the countryside for the city.

THE MECHANIZATION OF COTTON HARVESTING, 1940–1960

The percentage of cotton harvested by mechanical pickers jumped from only 5 percent in 1950 to 50 percent in 1960 (purple line). As a result, fewer man-hours were needed in the fields (red line), so that after 1949 there was an increasing surplus of labor, spurring black migration out of the cotton belt.

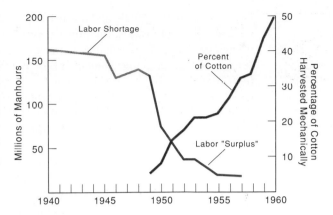

Note: Figure shows unskilled labor for all crops in the Mississippi Delta.

The federal minimum wage also had a profound impact on southern labor. The minimum wage law slowed the growth of low-wage employment everywhere in the country, but nowhere as much as in the South. Low-wage industries like textiles, lumber, paper, furniture, leather, and food processing, which for years had provided the bulk of jobs, became far less important. In addition, steel and other industries with strong national unions and manufacturers with plants around the country set wages by national standards. That brought southern wages close to the national average by the 1960s.

As wages rose and unskilled work disappeared, job opportunities for blacks declined. Outside of cotton farming, the single largest source of jobs for black teenagers was sawmills and lumber factories. As the minimum wage law drove up wages from 1950 to 1960, black teenage employment in lumber dropped 74 percent. New high-wage jobs were reserved for whites. Outside industries arriving in the South made no effort to disturb local employment patterns. So the ultimate irony arose. As per capita income rose and industrialization brought in new jobs, blacks poured out of the region in search of work. They arrived in cities that had little use for their labor or tolerance for racial differences.

The Movement for Civil Rights

In the post–World War II era the NAACP established itself as the great foe of racial segregation. Its chief weapon was the increased national political influence blacks achieved as they migrated in great numbers out of the South. No longer could northern politicians readily ignore the demands black leaders made for greater equality. The Swedish scholar Gunnar Myrdal had amply documented the black case in his landmark work *The American Dilemma* (1944), sponsored by the Carnegie Corporation. Presidents Roosevelt and Truman had taken small but significant steps to address the worst forms of legal and economic discrimination. And across the South black churches and colleges became centers for organized resistance to Jim Crow.

As blacks concentrated their attack on legal forms of discrimination, Thurgood Marshall emerged as the NAACP's leading attorney. Marshall had gone to law school in the 1930s at Howard University in Washington, where the dean, Charles Houston, was in the midst of revamping the school and turning out sharp, dedicated lawyers. Marshall was not only sharp, but he had the common touch. "Before he came along," one observer noted, "the principal black leaders—men like Du Bois and James Weldon Johnson and Charles Houston—didn't talk the language of the people. They were upper-class and upper-middle-class Negroes. Thurgood Marshall was *of* the people. . . . Out in Texas or Oklahoma or down the street here in Washington at the Baptist church, he would make these rousing speeches that would have 'em all jumping out of their seats. . . . 'We ain't gettin' what we should,' was what it came down to, and he made them see that."

During the late 1930s and early 1940s Marshall toured the South (in "a little old beat-up '29 Ford"), typing out legal briefs in the back seat, trying to get teachers to sue for equal pay, and defending blacks accused of murder in a Klan-infested county in Florida. He was friendly with whites, not shy, and blacks who had never even considered the possibility that a member of their race might win a legal battle "would come for miles, some of them on muleback or horseback, to see 'the nigger lawyer' who stood up in white men's courtrooms." For years NAACP lawyers worked hard to organize local chapters, to support members of the community willing to risk their jobs, property, and lives in order to challenge segregation. But they had waged a moderate, pragmatic campaign. They chose not to attack head-on the Supreme Court decision (*Plessy v. Ferguson*, 1896) that permitted "separate but equal" segregated facilities. They simply demonstrated that a black college or school might be separate, but it was hardly equal if it lacked a law school or even indoor plumbing.

But in 1950 the NAACP changed tactics: it would now try to convince the Supreme Court to overturn the separate but equal doctrine itself. Oliver Brown was one of the people who provided a way. Brown was dissatisfied that his daughter Linda had to walk past an all-white school on her way to catch the bus to her segregated black school in Topeka, Kansas. A three-judge federal panel rejected Brown's suit because the schools in Topeka, while segregated, did meet the test of equality. But after two years of arguments the Supreme Court in *Brown v. Board of Education* (1954) overturned the lower court ruling.

Marshall and his colleagues succeeded in part because of a change in the Court itself. The year before, President Eisenhower had appointed Earl Warren, a liberal Republican from California, as Chief Justice. Warren, a forceful advocate, managed to persuade the last of his reluctant judicial colleagues that segregation as defined in *Plessy* rested on an untenable theory of racial supremacy. The Court thus ruled unanimously that separate facilities were inherently unequal. To keep black children segregated solely on the basis of race, it ruled, "generates a feeling of inferiority as to their status in the community that may affect their hearts and minds in a way unlikely ever to be undone."

At the time of the *Brown* decision, 21 states and the District of Columbia operated segregated school systems. All of them had to decide, in some way, how to comply with the new ruling. The Court allowed a certain amount of leeway, handing down a second ruling in 1955 that required that desegregation be carried out "with all deliberate speed." Some border states reluctantly decided to comply, but in the Deep South, many called for diehard defiance. In 1956, a "Southern Manifesto" was issued by 19 United States senators and 81 representatives; it declared their intent to use "all lawful means" to reestablish legalized segregation.

The *Brown* decision did not end segregation, but it combined with political and economic forces to usher in a new era of southern race relations. In December 1955 Rosa Parks, a 43-year-old black civil rights activist, was riding the bus home in Montgomery, Alabama. She was no longer willing to relinquish her seat to a white man, as Alabama Jim Crow laws required. For refusing to do so, she was arrested and fined $10. That incident provoked long-simmering anger in the city's black community. Determined to overturn the law, the leaders organized a boycott of Montgomery buses, whose ridership was predominantly black. The white community, in an effort to halt this unprecedented black challenge, resorted to various forms of legal and physical intimidation. No local agent would insure cars used to carpool black workers. A bomb exploded in the house of the Reverend Martin Luther King, Jr., the key boycott leader. And when that failed to provoke the violence whites could use to justify harsh reprisals, 90 black leaders were arrested for organizing an illegal boycott. Still they held out until November 23, 1956, when the Supreme Court ruled bus segregation was illegal.

The triumph was especially sweet for Martin Luther King, Jr., whose leadership in Montgomery had brought him national fame. Prior to his arrival at the Dexter Street Baptist Church King had little personal contact with the worst forms of white racism. He had grown up in the relatively affluent middle-class black community of Atlanta, Georgia, the son of one of the city's most prominent black ministers. He attended Morehouse College, an academically respected black school in Atlanta, and the Crozer Theological Seminary in Philadelphia before entering the doctoral program in theology at Boston University. He heeded the call to Dexter Street in 1954 with the idea of becoming a theologian after he served his active ministry and finished his dissertation.

Graduate school provided King with the philosophy he would apply as leader of the bus boycott. He built his activism on the Social Gospel of Walter Rauschenbusch and other progressive theological reformers, his vision of modern man's fallen condition on the ideas of theologian Reinhold Niebuhr, and his concept of pacifism and nonviolence on the writings of Henry David Thoreau and Mohandas K. Gandhi, the architect of India's successful drive for independence from Great Britain. The southern black tradition of preaching taught King to speak in the moving "call and response" style, inspiring and energizing his listeners. His powerful sermons and personal magnetism made him the choice of other local black leaders to head the Montgomery Improvement Association (MIA), and to the MIA fell the task of leading the bus boycott.

As the boycott leader it was King's responsibility to rally black support without triggering violence. Since local officials were all too eager for any excuse to use force, King's nonviolent approach was the ideal strategy. King offered his audience two visions. First, he reminded them of the many injustices they had been forced to endure. The boycott, he asserted, was a good way to seek redress. Then he counseled his followers to avoid the actions of their oppressors: "In our protest there will be no cross burnings. No white person will be taken from his home by a hooded Negro mob and brutally murdered." And he evoked the Christian and republican ideals that would become the themes of his civil rights crusade. "If we protest courageously, and yet with dignity and Christian love," he said, "when the future history books are written, somebody will have to say, 'There lived a race of people, of black people, of people who had the moral courage to stand up for their rights. And thereby they injected a new meaning into the history of civilization.'"

Indeed, the blacks of Montgomery did set an example of moral courage that rewrote the pages of American race relations. That made the Supreme Court

Angry white students, opposed to integration, menace black students during a recess at Little Rock's Central High. This was the first civil rights crisis covered by television; for weeks NBC correspondent John Chancellor took a chartered plane daily to Oklahoma City to deliver film footage for the nightly news program.

decision against segregated buses all the more gratifying to King. On December 20, 1956, he took what he described as a "great ride" on the first integrated bus. One white attuned to the decline in municipal services remarked that the boycott had only won blacks "the same lousy service I've been getting every day," but in fact King had won the attention of the national news media as well. He appeared on the cover of conservative *Time* magazine. More important, the probing eye of national news media prevented local whites from greater acts of violence. In Montgomery blacks had developed tactics and leadership that would launch a more aggressive phase of the civil rights movement.

The spotlight moved the following year to Little Rock, Arkansas, a city ironically without a history of racial violence and with a plan for integrating its schools with the most deliberate lack of speed. Nine black students were scheduled to enroll in September 1957 at formerly segregated Central High School. Instead, the school board urged them to stay home when Governor Orval Faubus, generally a moderate on race relations, called out the Arkansas National Guard on the excuse of maintaining order. President Eisenhower tacitly supported Faubus in his defiance of court-ordered integration by remarking "that you cannot change people's hearts merely by laws." The Justice Department won an injunction against Faubus, but as the nine blacks returned on September 23 a mob of 1000 irate and abusive whites greeted them. So great was national attention to the crisis that President Eisenhower was forced to act. To uphold the authority of the federal courts, he sent in 1000 federal troops and took control of the National Guard.

For one year the Guardsmen preserved order until Faubus, in a last-ditch maneuver, closed all the schools. Only in 1959, under the pressure of another federal court ruling, did the Little Rock schools reopen and resume the plan for gradual integration.

Little Rock marked the advent of television news coverage in the civil rights struggle. For weeks, NBC news correspondent John Chancellor appeared on the new "Huntley–Brinkley Report" with film footage of ugly white mobs intimidating neatly dressed and dignified black students. This was only the first in a string of embarrassing racial episodes that television would serve up to national audiences. Moderate southern business leaders recognized they could not attract new industrial development under the shadow of such bad publicity. Often what they advocated to improve the South's image was mere tokenism and an appearance of racial harmony rather than substantive change. Governor James (Big Jim) Folsom of Alabama assured moderates that "we ain't going to force our fine colored folks to go to school with white people."

In the face of such attitudes, Martin Luther King and his followers recognized that the fight had only begun with the skirmishes of Montgomery and Little Rock. Cultural attitudes and customs were not about to give way overnight.

THE CULTURE WARS

The fifties, then, were not a time of consensus on civil rights. Nor, despite the placid surface of the suburban era, were they an era of orthodoxy for either the fine arts or mass entertainment. New York City became an international center for painting and architecture, while mass circulation paperback books revolutionized popular reading habits. American network television became the world's most powerful instrument of mass communication. And rock and roll became the musical idiom of a youth culture spawned by the postwar baby boom. Along with its economic and military power, the United States became a dominant force in world culture.

Cultural ferment provoked widespread commentary, much critical, some even apocalyptic, in warning against moral decadence and spiritual decline. On one level, "highbrow" intellectuals argued that mass culture was vulgarizing and even destroying the great traditions of Western arts. From quite another quarter, the middle class, came the accusation that television, advertising, comic books, movies, and rock music were creating a generation of juvenile delinquents. For both the "highbrow" and "middlebrow" critics, the culture of the 1950s threatened the future of American civilization.

During the 1920s and 1930s many intellectuals had welcomed the idea of mass society. Modern communications, they believed, would break down the barriers of race, class, religion, and nationality. A more homogeneous and harmonious order would emerge. But fascist and communist dictators, with their rabble-rousing mobs and media propaganda, turned these hopes to disillusionment. By the 1950s intellectuals more often argued that the mass media threatened to consume and destroy all valuable culture. In British novelist George Orwell's bleak reading of the future, *1984*, the government's "Ministry of Truth" controlled newspapers, television, film, and radio.

At Columbia University a group of refugees from Nazi Germany, known as the "Frankfurt school," argued that modern media had become the opiate of the masses. The constant repetition of television programs and commercials, Theodor Adorno claimed, tended "to make for automatized reactions and to weaken forces of individual resistance." Dwight Macdonald, another prominent critic, sarcastically attacked the culture of the suburban middle classes, which he called "midcult": books, films, and theater that pretended to be high art but in reality were little more than oversimplified treatments of serious issues. The democratization of American culture, he believed, led to banal conformity and mediocrity. Others, including Leslie Fiedler, stepped in to defend popular tastes. The criticism now leveled against television and popular music echoed criticism of the Elizabethan theater, Fiedler pointed out, as well as the novel, the opera, and film in their early years. Through it all, of course, the vast majority of suburban brows—high, middle, and low—tended to ignore the bombshells critics were lobbing at one another.

Juvenile Delinquency

Many parents and public figures believed that mass media were corrupting America's youth. Dance crazes, outlandish clothing styles, strange jargon, rebelliousness toward parents, and sexual precociousness—all these seemed to be symptoms of more threatening antisocial behavior. America had spawned a generation of rebellious juvenile delinquents. Psychologist Frederic Wertheim told a group of doctors, "You cannot understand present-day juvenile delinquency if you do not take into account the pathogenic and pathoplastic [infectious] influence of comic books." Others laid the blame on films and the lyrics of popular music.

The worry about youth resulted partly from the demographic changes in society. The baby boom children were becoming teenagers in the 1950s. And the general prosperity meant that more of them held after-school jobs, earned more of their own disposable income, and had more leisure time than parents growing up during the Depression and World War II. The center of the new teen culture was the high school. Whether in consolidated rural school districts, new suburban schools, or city systems, the large, comprehensive high schools of the 1950s were often miniature melting pots where middle-class students were exposed to, and often adopted, the style of the lower classes and blacks. Many districts, of course, sustained patterns of social class and racial isolation. All the same, high schools were more likely than neighborhood schools to encourage social integration.

Rock and Roll: Idiom of a Youth Culture

In many ways the argument about juvenile delinquency was an argument about social class and, to a lesser degree, race. When adults complained that "delinquent" teenagers dressed poorly, lacked ambition, were irresponsible and sexually promiscuous, these were the same arguments traditionally used to denigrate other outsiders—immigrants, the poor, and blacks. Nowhere were these racial and class undertones more evident than in the hue and cry which greeted the arrival of rock and roll.

Before 1954 popular music had been divided into three major categories: "pop," country and western, and rhythm and blues. A handful of major record companies with almost exclusively white singers dominated the pop charts. Off on one fringe of the popular field was country and western, often split into cowboy musicians like Roy Rogers and Gene Autry and the hillbilly style associated with

Nashville. The music industry generally treated rhythm and blues as "race music," whose performers and audience were largely black. Nationally, their radio and record market was relatively small. Each of these musical traditions, it is worth noting, grew out of regional cultures. Just as the West and the South saw the gradual breakdown of their colonial economies, so these musical subcultures were being gradually integrated into the national mainstream.

By the mid-1950s the distinctiveness of the three styles began to blur. Singers on the white pop charts recorded a few songs from country and rhythm and blues. The popularity of crossovers such as "Sh-boom," "Tutti-Frutti," and "Earth Angel" indicated that a major shift in taste and market was under way. Lyrics still reflected the pop fields's preoccupation with young love, marriage, and happiness, but the music reflected the rawer and earthier style of rhythm and blues. Country and western singer Bill Haley brought the new blend to the fore in 1954 with "Shake, Rattle, and Roll," the first rock song to reach the top of the pop charts.

And then—calamity! Millions of middle-class roofs nearly blew off with the appearance in 1955 of the rhythmic and raucous Elvis Presley. By background, Elvis was a country boy whose musical style combined elements of gospel, country, and blues. But it was his hip-swinging, pelvis-plunging performances that electrified teenage audiences. To more conservative adults, Presley's long hair, sideburns, and tight jeans seemed menacingly delinquent. His music and sensuous movement appeared to them an expression of hostile rebellion. What they often resented but rarely admitted was that Elvis looked lower class, sounded black, and really could sing.

Two phenomena helped assure the mass popularity of rock and roll. One was the introduction of the 45-rpm record at a price teenage consumers could afford. More important was the development of "top forty" rock radio. Having lost much of their traditional audience to television, radio stations discovered a new market among teenagers. Disc jockeys like Alan Freed developed a frenetic style that reflected the music's excited rhythms.

The Unblinking Eye

No medium played a more central role in the popular culture of the 1950s than television. It had a powerful political impact in the Kefauver hearings, in the 1952 and 1956 elections, and in the Army–McCarthy hearings. No candidate for office could ignore it; no manufacturer could capture the consumer market without it. As a rapidly emerging institution of power and influence, it experienced growing pains and found itself at the center of a debate over its influence in American life.

During the early 1950s advertisers rather than the networks produced most programs. Shows like the "Kraft Television Theater" and "U.S. Steel Hour" were named after the sponsor, not the performers or the content. Without any established history, television at first experimented with ideas drawn from other media such as theater and radio. Eighty percent of all shows were performed live. Original plays, for example, offered a showcase for young writers, directors, and performers such as Sidney Poitier, Paul Newman, and Joanne Woodward. Television news programs like Edward R. Murrow's "See It Now" occasionally probed subjects as sensitive as McCarthyism.

Elvis Presley.

In the mid-1950s television entered a new phase. Controversy surrounding Murrow's probe of McCarthy encouraged the networks to downgrade news and public affairs programs. At the same time they began working out a profitable arrangement with Hollywood film studios. The studios, seeking to regain revenue lost to television, produced telefilm series for the networks, which, in turn, sold time to advertisers. This gave the networks, rather than the sponsors, ultimate control over program content. By 1959 live television was virtually a thing of the past. Westerns, detective shows, and old movies led the ratings. Newscasts, dominated by filmed stories, became an important mechanism for building an audience for prime-time shows.

Critics of television charged that the new shows encouraged violence and juvenile delinquency. Impressionable children, they complained, were regularly exposed to manslaughter and mayhem, followed by appeals for soft drinks and cigarettes, rather than to programs of solid educational value. But those who had the power to regulate television—the president, Congress, the Federal Communications Commission (FCC)—chose not to extend a restraining hand. The only effort to promote "better" programs came in 1952, when the FCC allocated a number of channels, but no funding, to educational television.

Abstract Art and Architecture

Controversy over culture was hardly restricted to the popular arts. The modern paintings and buildings of the postwar era disturbed many Americans dedicated to traditional notions of art and architecture. The avant-garde styles of the 1950s were linked by an international flavor and self-conscious concern for abstraction. Their creators seemed determined to break with the past.

In 1951 the Museum of Modern Art in New York mounted a striking exhibit of American painters whose work baffled many viewers. Artists such as Jackson Pollock, Willem de Kooning, and Mark Rothko specifically rejected the representational style of those like Thomas Hart Benton, popular in the 1930s and 1940s, who celebrated American regional scenes and folkways. Pollock, himself a student of Benton, had become gradually more expressive and abstract, until finally, by dripping and spattering paints rather than brushing them on, he created patterns of action that revealed no controlling influence of the artist's hand. This was abstraction indeed.

For many architects, the decision to build geometric forms sheathed in glass and steel had more to do with economics than aesthetics. Simply put, modern buildings were cheaper to erect. Glass was the material of the decade because it was inexpensive and easy to use. Skilled masons and stonecutters were less available to do the ornate detailing common on public buildings of the prewar era. If modern buildings made any symbolic statement, it was about the faceless bureaucrats housed within the glass and steel boxes that looked like all the other boxes. The best of these, however, earned a well-deserved reputation for innovation and beauty, such as the United Nations complex erected along New York's East River in 1950. Its architects were an international team led by Walter Harrison of New York.

Moving from the East Coast to the West, and from the sublime to the flamboyantly ridiculous, a much more popular style of architecture, dubbed "California Crazy," delighted in producing restaurants in the shape of a hamburger, gas stations that looked like a flying wing, and neon palaces for gamblers in Las Vegas.

Perhaps the ultimate statement of car and home culture came as one architect incorporated the garage into the family room.

Americans in 1960 had reason to be satisfied with the accomplishments of the past decade. Despite periodic recession, income rose dramatically and unemployment remained low. The country had avoided war. The National Aeronautics and Space Administration (NASA) had sent satellites into orbit. A vast highway network linked the nation's urban centers and allowed motorists easier access to both city and countryside. Suburbs had provided millions of families an escape from the crowded center cities.

Yet as the 1950s ended, small cracks appeared in the national consensus. In run-down urban neighborhoods and college towns, motley collections of artists, intellectuals, musicians, and middle-class students had dropped out of mainstream society to form a "beat" subculture. Experimenting openly with drugs, mystical religions, Oriental philosophy, and sex, the "beatniks" self-consciously rejected what they viewed as the excessive materialism and spiritual bankruptcy of America's middle-class culture. A popular president left office warning that an overgrown defense establishment threatened to strangle democratic institutions. The currents of political reform, crushed temporarily by the purges of the McCarthyites, were again on the rise. Antinuclear groups like SANE (Committee for a Sane Nuclear Policy) protested the nuclear arms race. Blacks had shown they were less willing to accept inequality. In the midst of postwar peace and prosperity, the United States began to build a new social and political agenda.

SIGNIFICANT EVENTS

1950	David Riesman's *The Lonely Crowd* published
1951	First major exhibit of abstract expressionism at the Museum of Modern Art
1953	Submerged Lands Act; Rosenbergs executed; Korean armistice; Mossadeq overthrown in Iran
1954	*Brown v. Board of Education;* St. Lawrence Seaway Act; Robert Oppenheimer denied security clearance; Army–McCarthy hearings; McCarthy censured; CIA overthrows Arbenz in Guatemala; Geneva summit
1955	Montgomery bus boycott; Elvis Presley ignites rock and roll
1956	Interstate Highway Act; Eisenhower reelected; Suez crisis; "Southern Manifesto"
1957	*Sputnik* launched; Little Rock crisis; Civil Rights Act; Eisenhower Doctrine
1958	Sherman Adams resigns; Richard Nixon attacked in Latin America; marines sent into Lebanon; Berlin crisis; National Defense Education Act; NASA established
1959	Castro seizes power in Cuba; Khrushchev visits United States; Soviet probe hits moon
1960	Soviet Union captures CIA pilot; Paris summit canceled
1961	Eisenhower farewell address warns of military–industrial complex
1963	Betty Friedan's *The Feminine Mystique* published

32

Liberalism and Beyond

Six-year-old Ruby knew the lessons. Her father and mother had drilled them into her. She was to look straight ahead—not to one side or the other—and especially not at *them*. She was to keep walking. And above all, she was not to look back once she'd passed, because that would encourage them. Ruby knew these things, but it was still hard to keep her eyes straight. The first day of school, and federal marshals were there along with her parents. And hundreds of white people, it seemed, had come from all over New Orleans. The marshals kept them from getting at her, but they came near enough to yell things like, "You little nigger, we'll get you and kill you." Worse things, too, she didn't want to think about. Then she was within the building's quiet halls and alone with her teacher. She was the only person in class: none of the white students had come. As the days went by during that autumn of 1960, the marshals stopped walking with her but the hecklers were still there. And once in a while Ruby couldn't help looking back, trying to see if she recognized the face of one woman in particular.

Ruby's parents were not social activists. They signed their daughter up for the white school because "we thought it was for all the colored to do, and we never thought Ruby would be alone." Her father's white employer fired him and the neighborhood store refused to do business with the family. Letters and phone calls threatened their lives and home. Through it all Ruby seemed remarkably resilient, playing with friends after school and taking things in stride. When she drew pictures, though, some of her feelings came out. White children appeared in large, bold outlines, their features carefully sketched. They had teeth, lips, 10 fingers, and 10 toes. But when she drew herself or other black children, an ear might be missing, or a thumb, or a nose. "When I draw a white girl, I know she'll be okay," she explained once, "but with the colored it's not so okay. So I try to give the colored as even a chance as I can, even if that's not the way it will end up being." Ruby's parents were more disturbed because she was not eating the way she used to. Often she left her school lunch untouched, or refused anything other than packaged food such as potato chips. It was only after a time that the problem was traced to the hecklers. "They tells me I'm going to die, and that it'll be soon. And that one lady tells me every morning I'm getting poisoned soon, when she can fix it." Ruby was convinced that the woman owned the variety store nearby and would carry out her threat by poisoning the family's food.

On August 28, 1963, more than 250,000 demonstrators joined the great civil rights March on Washington. The day belonged to the Reverend Martin Luther King, Jr., who movingly called on blacks and whites to join together in a color-blind society.

Ruby's drawings of a white girl (left) and herself.

Over the course of a year, white students gradually returned to class and life settled into a new routine. By the time Ruby was 10, she had developed a remarkably clear perception of herself. "Maybe because of all the trouble going to school in the beginning I learned more about my people. Maybe I would have anyway; because when you get older you see yourself and the white kids; and you find out the difference. You try to forget it, and say there is none; and if there is you won't say what it be. Then you say it's my own people, and so I can be proud of them instead of ashamed."

If the new ways were hard for Ruby, they were not easy for white southerners either—even those who saw the need for change. One woman, for years a dedicated teacher in Atlanta, vividly recalled a traumatic summer 10 years earlier, when she went north to New York City to take courses in education. There were black students living in the dormitory, an integrated situation she was not used to. One day as she stepped from her shower to dry off, so did a black student from the nearby stall. "When I saw her I didn't know what to do," the woman recalled. "I felt sick all over, and frightened. What I remember—I'll never forget it—is that horrible feeling of being caught in a terrible trap, and not knowing what to do about it. I thought of running out of the room and screaming, or screaming at the woman to get out, or running back into the shower. . . . My sense of propriety was with me, though—miraculously—and I didn't want to hurt the woman. It wasn't *her* that was upsetting me. I knew that, even in that moment of sickness and panic." So she ducked back into the shower until the other woman left.

It took her most of the summer before she felt comfortable eating with blacks at the same table. And when she returned home, she told no one about her experiences. "At that time people would have thought one of two things: I was crazy (for being so upset and ashamed) or a fool who in a summer had become a dangerous 'race mixer.'" She continued to love the South and to speak up for its traditions of dignity, neighborliness, and honor, but she saw the need for change. And so in 1961 she volunteered to teach one of the first integrated high school classes in Atlanta, even though she had her doubts. By the end of two years she concluded that she had never spent a more exciting time teaching. "I've never felt so useful, so constantly useful, not just to the children but to our whole society. American as well as Southern. Those children, all of them, have given me more than I've given them. They've helped me realize that some unpleasant times in my own life were not spent in vain. That's a privilege, to be able to have your life tested and found somewhat consistent, at least over the long haul. I guess I grew up there in New York, and used the strength from it down here later on."

A LIBERAL AGENDA FOR REFORM

The changes that swept America in the 1960s were wrenching to most people. From the schoolrooms and lunch counters of the South to the college campuses of the North, from eastern slums to western migrant labor camps, American society was in ferment. On the face of it, such agitation seemed to be a dramatic reversal of the placid fifties: turbulence and change overturning stability and order.

Yet the new decade grew naturally out of the social conditions that preceded it. Consensus had given society a sense of stability; prosperity bred confidence that nagging problems like poverty might finally be resolved. In the 1960s, wrote one of the era's optimistic liberals, "the world seemed more plastic, more subject to modification by human will"; we believed that "the energy and commitment of multitudes could be linked to compel the enrichment of human life." Such confidence always has the danger of becoming hubris; such hopes too often bring bitter disappointments despite striking successes. So it was with the liberal faith of the 1960s.

The Social Structures of Change

The 1950s sustained an economic expansion unlike any since the 1920s. A general prosperity had enlarged the middle class and given its members money to spend on suburban homes, time-saving appliances, televisions, automobiles. Furthermore, the baby boom created a generation of children who grew up under conditions of relative affluence. They had discretionary income to spend, a greater chance of going to college, and some freedom to think twice about what they might do or become as adults. These were luxuries not available to most young adults during the Depression or World War II.

At the same time, the economic tide of the 1950s did not raise all areas of the nation equally. While suburbs flourished, urban areas decayed. While more whites went to college, more blacks found themselves out of work on southern farms or desperate for jobs in northern ghettos. Mexican-Americans in cities lacked decent housing and jobs. Migrant workers, picking grapes in California or following the harvest north from Texas, felt their employers' sharp hostility with every attempt to unionize and improve their wages. Yet the general prosperity remained for all to see. And the success of the NAACP in wringing a policy of integration from the Supreme Court gave minorities new hopes.

The expansive years of the 1950s, in other words, made it possible for several major reform elements to emerge during the 1960s. The economic boom made minorities aware of the possibilities of economic opportunity. National liberation movements sweeping Africa and other Third World areas gave broader meaning to reforms at home. And the baby-boomers of the middle class came of age at a time when they had enough wealth and leisure to question the prosperity their parents had gained. These social forces, more than politicians or any of society's traditional leaders, were at the root of the decade's change. Time and again, the political system would be challenged to deal with what the 1950s had done—and what had been left undone.

The Election of 1960

The first president to face these currents of reform was John Fitzgerald Kennedy, at 43 the youngest man ever elected to the presidency. On the face of it, Kennedy's 1960 campaign promised to bring the breezes of change to Washington. While Eisenhower played golf, the Russians had launched *Sputnik,* Kennedy complained. While Ike talked about the budget gap, Kennedy pointed to the missile gap and charged that America was losing the cold war. The nation needed to find new challenges and "new frontiers," he proclaimed. The candidate's rhetoric was noble, but the direction in which Kennedy would take the nation was far from clear.

Aside from political issues, there was a social one to be met. Jack Kennedy was a Roman Catholic out of Irish Boston, and no Catholic other than Al Smith in 1928 had run for president as a major party candidate. Conservative Protestants, many concentrated in the heavily Democratic South, were convinced that a Catholic president would never be "free to exercise his own judgment" if the pope ordered otherwise. Despite warnings from his advisers, Kennedy chose to confront the issue head-on. In September he entered the lions' den, addressing an association of hostile ministers in Houston. The speech was the best of his campaign. "I believe in an America where the separation of church and state is absolute," he said, "—where no Catholic prelate would tell the President (should he be Catholic) how to act, and no Protestant minister would tell his parishioners how to vote." House Speaker Sam Rayburn, an old Texas pol, was astonished by Kennedy's bravura performance. "My God! . . . He's eating them blood raw."

Kennedy's opponent, Vice President Richard Nixon, agreed and thus did not make religion a campaign issue. Although Nixon ran on his record as an experienced leader and staunch anticommunist, by October the economy had tailed off into a recession and unemployment was up. Nixon had agreed to a series of debates with Kennedy—the first to be televised nationally. At the time of the first debate he was overtired and his "Lazy Shave" makeup failed to hide his five-o'clock shadow. By contrast, Kennedy seemed relaxed and was able to convince many voters that he had the experience needed to handle the job. Interest in the election ran so high that 64 percent of voters turned out, the largest number in 50 years. Out of 68.3 million ballots cast, Kennedy won by a margin of just 118,000.

In the end religion, ethnicity, and race played decisive roles. One voter was asked if he voted for Kennedy because he was a Catholic. "No, because *I* am," he answered; and in key states Catholic support made a difference. "Hyphenated"

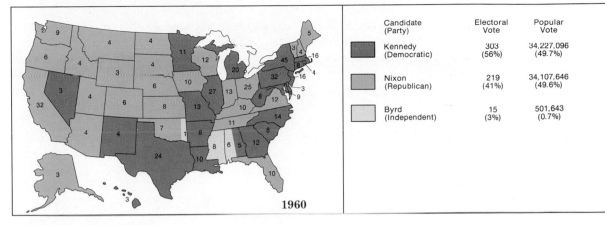

Candidate (Party)	Electoral Vote	Popular Vote
Kennedy (Democratic)	303 (56%)	34,227,096 (49.7%)
Nixon (Republican)	219 (41%)	34,107,646 (49.6%)
Byrd (Independent)	15 (3%)	501,643 (0.7%)

1960

THE ELECTION OF 1960

Americans—Hispanic, Jewish, Irish, Italian, Polish, and German—voted Democratic in record numbers, while much of the black vote which had gone to Eisenhower in 1956 returned to the Democratic fold. Indeed, when Martin Luther King was imprisoned during a civil rights protest in Georgia, Kennedy attracted the support of blacks by telephoning his sympathy to Dr. King's wife. Nixon ran strongest among white Protestant middle Americans. Kennedy became president by a whisker (there was solid evidence of voting fraud in Chicago and Texas), but he was victor nonetheless.

The Hard-Nosed Idealists of Camelot

To many observers, the Kennedy White House seemed to embody the best and brightest of the liberal Democratic promise. The administration was soon dubbed "Camelot," after King Arthur's magical court. In a popular Lerner and Lowe musical of 1960, Camelot had been pictured as a land where skies were fair, men brave, women pretty, and the days full of challenge and excitement. With similar panache, the president invited artists, musicians, and intellectuals to the White House, where his wife Jacqueline proved to be a host with infectious charm. During impromptu touch football games, a rough-and-tumble playfulness shone forth, akin to Arthur's jousting tournaments of old.

Yet Kennedy was by neither birth nor experience a liberal at all. His father, Joseph P. Kennedy, had made a fortune in stock market speculation and Hollywood real estate. Determined to build a family political dynasty, Joe Kennedy sent his boys to prestigious prep schools and then Harvard, to hobnob with the Protestant elite. Jack had followed the appointed regimen, was handsome and intelligent to boot, and possessed an ironic, self-deprecating humor. As a PT boat commander in World War II, he had been decorated for heroism, though he might as easily have been cashiered for carelessness. After the war he was elected to Congress, where he led an undistinguished career, supported Joe McCarthy, and earned a reputation as a lightweight and a playboy. But once Kennedy set his sights on the White House, he was a changed man. He revealed an astonishing capacity for political maneuver and organization. To woo the liberals, he adopted

John F. Kennedy's carefully cultivated image of a "Camelot" administration blended a concern for youth, verve, and life (his son John stands before him) with a determination to appear militarily "tough" against the communists.

their agenda and brought a distinguished group of intellectuals and academics to his campaign staff.

The grand designs of fascism had left many liberals disillusioned with all-encompassing ideologies for change. By the 1960s they had come to favor a pragmatic approach to reforming American society. Economists like John Kenneth Galbraith no longer attacked capitalism, since the strategies of John Maynard Keynes (page 1004) offered a means to make the system work. Rather than embrace a social welfare state, Kennedy liberals preferred to extend benefits piecemeal to solve the nation's lingering social ills. In foreign affairs Kennedy surrounded himself with cold war liberals who were no less dedicated than conservatives to fighting communism.

The Kennedy advisers were convinced that they, more than the likes of John Foster Dulles, had flexible and efficient ways to contain the Soviet Union. McGeorge Bundy, a former intelligence officer and Harvard dean, was both steely and brilliant; he headed the National Security Council. Walt Whitman Rostow, an MIT economist, was known for his theories of how developing nations could prosper and avoid the pitfalls of communism. And as secretary of defense, Robert Strange McNamara came determined to tame the sprawling bureaucracy of the Pentagon. McNamara, a former Harvard Business School professor and president of Ford Motors, specialized in using new quantitative tools like systems analysis to streamline business management. He had been one of the postwar breed of "whiz kids" who moved from the universities into the board rooms of once-staid corporations.

Kennedy liked all these men—witty, brilliant, intellectual—because they seemed not only to have high ideals, but to be at home with power. They were not afraid to use it. If Khrushchev spoke of waging guerrilla "wars of liberation,"

Americans could play that game too. A similar taste was reflected in Kennedy's spare-time reading: the popular James Bond spy novels. Agent 007, with his license to kill, was exactly to the president's taste: sophisticated, a cool womanizer (which Kennedy himself continued to be), and ready to use power and the latest technology to deal with communists or other bizarre enemies. Ironically, Bond demonstrated that there could be plenty of glamour and romance in being "hard-nosed" and pragmatic. That illicit pleasure was the underside, perhaps, of Camelot's high ideals.

NEW FRONTIERS

When Kennedy appointed Dean Rusk secretary of state, he indicated that foreign policy would be conducted from the White House. Rusk was an unassertive diplomat who would preside only over the Department of State, while the president and his national security advisers set broad policy. Kennedy wanted to bring to bear a more flexible range of military and economic options. Above all, he believed that Eisenhower had not realized how much the cold war had shifted from the traditional battlefronts of Europe to the developing nations in Asia, Africa, and Latin America.

Kennedy set the tone for his administration when he announced in the spring of 1961 a new "Alliance for Progress" with the nations of Latin America. The goal of the Alliance was the prevention of future Castro-style revolutions. Kennedy promised to provide $20 billion in foreign aid over 10 years—about four times the aid Latin America had been getting under Truman and Eisenhower. In return, Latin American nations would agree to reform unfair tax policies and begin agricultural land reforms. The administration also set up the Peace Corps, a program that sent idealistic young men and women to Third World nations to provide technical, educational, and public health services. Under the Alliance, a majority of Peace Corps volunteers were assigned to Latin America.

In what seemed the ultimate call to new frontiers, the president established a national commitment to send a man to the moon and bring him back by the end of the decade. But this "star trek" was another phase of the cold war. The Russians had launched their own successful manned space flight in 1959 and Kennedy was eager to beat them in a space race. In May Alan Shepard, Jr., completed a 20-minute suborbital flight. By February 1962 John Glenn had circled the earth three times. Longer flights followed, as Americans discovered in the astronauts heroes for a new age.

But in more down-to-earth ways, high ideals were not easily translated into practical results. Latin American governments were eager to accept aid but much less able or willing to carry out reforms. Few welcomed the intrusive Yankee diplomats who came from north of the border to inspect their programs. Instability remained a key problem, for in the first five years of the Alliance, nine Latin American governments were overthrown by military coups. The Peace Corps, for its part, proved a tremendous public relations success and helped thousands of Third World farmers on a people-to-people basis. But individual Peace Corps workers could do little to change corrupt policies on a national level, and many returned home convinced the Third World needed revolution, not reform.

Kennedy was determined to back economic policies with military measures. As the Alliance for Progress was getting under way, the Pentagon directed jungle warfare schools at Fort Bragg, North Carolina, and in the Canal Zone. These schools trained Latin American police and paramilitary groups to fight guerrilla wars; they also trained American "special forces" like the Green Berets. The administration wanted the capacity to send American forces or their allies into wars of liberation the way the Soviets had.

The prime target for "liberation" was Fidel Castro, whose Communist regime lay only 90 miles south of Florida. Since breaking diplomatic relations in 1960, the Eisenhower administration had authorized the CIA to organize an invasion of Cuba, and Kennedy approved an attack scheduled for April. The CIA assured the president that its 1400-member army of Cuban exiles could inspire their countrymen to overthrow Castro. But the invasion proved to be a mismanaged disaster. The poorly equipped rebel forces landed at the Bay of Pigs in a swamp, with no protective cover for miles. Within two days Castro's army had rounded them up. Taking responsibility for the entire fiasco, Kennedy suffered a bitter humiliation. That did not discourage further covert operations or cold war confrontation. Unrepentent for its first fiasco the CIA secretly hatched plans to embarrass or murder the Cuban leader.* It even tried to enlist the services of organized crime figures eager to renew their profitable operations in Havana.

Kennedy's advisers took a similar approach to the problem of South Vietnam, where a religious war within a civil war was under way. The autocratic government of Prime Minister Ngo Dinh Diem, a Catholic, remained in power, although it was growing more unpopular by the month. South Vietnamese Communists, known as the Vietcong, with support from North Vietnam waged a guerrilla war against Diem. Buddhist elements backed the rebellion. In May 1961, a month after the Bay of Pigs invasion, Kennedy secretly ordered 500 Green Berets and military advisers to Vietnam in hopes of helping Diem defeat the Vietcong. By 1963 the number of "military advisers" had risen to over 16,000 men, who were increasingly being drawn into combat situations. Kennedy publicly defended the aid, supporting Eisenhower's domino theory. "If South Vietnam went, it . . . would give the impression that the wave of the future in Southeast Asia was China and the Communists," he told the press.

By 1963 the situation had badly degenerated. Diem was ruthlessly suppressing Buddhist opposition groups. His corruption and police state tactics created a great deal of bad publicity, and he was not even winning the war. The administration tacitly encouraged a military coup that captured Diem and, to Washington's surprise, shot him in November 1963. Despite Kennedy's policy of pragmatic idealism, the United States found itself mired in a Vietnamese civil war, which it had no clear strategy for winning.

The Missiles of October

Vietnam and Cuba were only two areas in the Third World where the Kennedy administration sought to project its power against Communist forces. But the conflict between the United States and the Soviet Union soon overshadowed developments in Asia, Africa, and Latin America.

*The most notorious of these plans was a special CIA shoe polish, never successfully used, whose ingredients were designed to cause Castro's trademark beard to fall out, thus supposedly embarrassing the revolutionary leader.

June 1961 was the president's first chance to take the measure of Nikita Khrushchev, at a summit meeting held in Vienna. For two long days, Khrushchev was brash and belligerent. Germany must be reunited, he demanded. The Berlin problem must be settled within six months. Kennedy was shocked by the Soviet leader's vehemence and tried to respond in kind, but he left Vienna worried that Khrushchev perceived him as weak and inexperienced. In August his fears were confirmed when the Soviets threw up a heavily guarded wall dividing East from West Berlin, to prevent disillusioned East Germans from escaping to the western sector. But the Soviets did not seal off West Berlin's access to West Germany. Although the president strongly protested the move, the wall became a permanent fixture of Berlin life.

Continuing tensions with the Soviet Union also led the administration to rethink the American approach to nuclear warfare. Under the Dulles doctrine of massive retaliation, almost any incident might trigger a launch of the full arsenal of nuclear missiles. Kennedy and McNamara sought to establish a "flexible response doctrine" that would limit the level of a first nuclear strike and therefore leave room for negotiation. In that case, however, conventional forces in Europe would have to be built up, so that they could better deter aggression. McNamara proposed equipping them with smaller tactical nuclear weapons.

But what if the Soviets were tempted to launch a first-strike attack to knock out American missiles? McNamara's flexible response policy required that enough American missiles survive in order to retaliate. If the Soviets knew the United States could survive a first strike, they would then be less likely to launch a surprise attack. So McNamara began a program to bury missile sites underground and develop submarine-launched missiles. Ironically, American intelligence estimates showed that there was no "missile gap," despite Kennedy's campaign charges. The Soviets had far fewer missiles. Still, the new flexible response policies resulted in a 15 percent increase in the 1961 military budget, compared with only 2 percent increases during the last two Eisenhower years. In this sense, the effort to make American defenses more flexible served only to accelerate the arms race. And critics like George Kennan later concluded that nuclear "flexibility" was a dangerous idea, for there was "no way in which [some] nuclear weapons could be used that would not involve the possibility . . . of escalation into a general nuclear disaster."

The peril of nuclear confrontation became dramatically clear in the Cuban missile crisis of October 1962. In public statements President Kennedy had emphasized repeatedly that the United States would treat any attempt to place offensive weapons in Cuba as an unacceptable threat. Khrushchev had simultaneously promised that the Soviet Union had no such intention. Thus Kennedy was outraged when a CIA U-2 overflight on October 14 confirmed that offensive missile sites were being constructed. "He can't do that to me," the president snapped. For a week, top security advisers met in secret strategy sessions. Hawkish advisers urged Kennedy to order air strikes against the missile sites, but the president worried that such an attack might lead to nuclear war. In the end he decided to impose a naval blockade to intercept "all offensive military equipment under shipment to Cuba." Stunned Americans learned of the crisis on October 22, when the president announced the news on national television.

Tensions mounted as a Soviet submarine approached the line of American ships. On October 25 the navy stopped an oil tanker. Several Soviet ships reversed course. Kennedy was making strenuous efforts to resolve the crisis through diplomatic channels, and on October 26 he received a rambling message from Khrushchev agreeing to remove the missiles in return for an American promise not to invade Cuba. The next day came a more troubling message, insisting the United States must also dismantle its missile bases in Turkey, which bordered on the Soviet Union. Unwilling to strike that deal publicly, Kennedy decided to ignore the second letter and accept the offer in the first. When the Soviets agreed, the faceoff ended on terms that saved either side from overt humiliation.

The Cuban missile crisis was the closest the world had come to full-scale nuclear war, and the confrontation affected both superpowers profoundly. Khru-

---

THE WORLD OF THE SUPERPOWERS
This map shows the extent of the cold war Soviet and American military buildup. The United States established a worldwide network of bases and alliances surrounding Soviet bloc nations, from Japan and South Korea, South Vietnam, Pakistan, and Turkey in Asia to the nations of the NATO alliance in Europe. Soviet efforts to expand its influence in the Third World led to the creation of an outpost in Cuba. Around these strategic perimeters "hotspots" and centers of crisis continued to simmer.

shchev found himself under heavy attack from China and from many of his rivals within the Communist party Politboro, who also chafed at the failure of his economic policies. He was finally removed from power in 1964, but not before the Soviets launched a program to close the real missile gap.

In some ways the crisis sobered Kennedy and his advisers and increased their determination to control the nuclear arms race. "If we cannot end now all our differences, at least we can help make the world safe for diversity," he proclaimed in June 1963. "For . . . we all inhabit this small planet. We all breathe the same air. We all cherish our children's future. And we are all mortal." Following through, the administration negotiated a nuclear test ban with the Soviets, prohibiting all above-ground nuclear tests. A telephone "hotline" was also installed, providing a direct communications link between the White House and the Kremlin for use in times of crisis. At the same time Kennedy's prestige soared for "standing up" to the Soviets. If cold war toughness paid political dividends, then the Kennedy team would look for new contests, confident of their mastery of the subtle uses of power.

The discovery of Soviet offensive missile sites in Cuba, revealed by low-level American reconnaissance flights, led to the first nuclear showdown of the cold war. For several tense days in October 1962, President Kennedy met with his National Security Council to debate alternative responses.

The (Somewhat) New Frontier at Home

President Kennedy had campaigned on a liberal platform, calling for bold initiatives at home as well as abroad. Once in the White House, however, he found himself hemmed in by a Democratic Congress dominated by conservatives. As his vice president Lyndon Johnson quipped, Kennedy had the congressional minnows, but not the whales: the power brokers who controlled committees and determined the course of legislation. As a result, the president's legislative achievements were modest. The Area Redevelopment Act of 1961 provided financial aid to depressed industrial and rural areas while Congress raised the minimum wage to $1.25. But on key issues, including aid to education and medical health insurance, Kennedy made no headway.

He wavered, too, on how to best manage the economy. The president's economic advisers, led by Walter Heller, Paul Samuelson, and John Kenneth Galbraith, were all disciples of Keynes. They favored increased government spending to reduce unemployment, even if that meant a budget deficit. Similarly, they argued that tax cuts could be used to increase consumer spending and so stimulate the economy. Kennedy toyed with both remedies, but conservatives continued to push for a balanced budget—always Eisenhower's goal, and one even Harry Truman endorsed. So Kennedy moved cautiously, relieved at first to discover that the economy was growing quite nicely without a tax cut. Only in 1963 did he send such a proposal to Congress.

Despite his advisers' liberal bent, Kennedy hoped to work amicably with the leaders of big business. He firmly believed that prosperity for large firms spelled growth for the whole nation. Thus the president asked Congress to ease antitrust restrictions and grant investment credits and tax breaks—all actions that perfectly suited corporate interests. But he did believe that the government needed to limit the power of both large corporations and unions to set prices and wages. The alternative was an inflationary spiral, where wage increases would be followed by price increases followed by even higher wage demands.

To prevent that, the Council of Economic Advisors urged that wage increases be given to workers only if their increased productivity allowed prices to remain stable. In April 1962 the United Steel Workers, like most other major unions, agreed to a new contract within the administration's guidelines. The large steel corporations, however, broke their part of the informal bargain, announcing a 3.5 percent rise in steel prices. Feeling betrayed, Kennedy struck back. He called for investigations into price fixing, mounted antitrust proceedings, and shifted Pentagon purchases to smaller steel companies that had not raised prices. Eventually the big companies gave in, but the larger business community remained suspicious of Kennedy's intentions.

The Reforms of the Warren Court

For all of John Kennedy's talk of new frontiers and reform, he remained unwilling— or unable, given the opposition in Congress—to do much more than propose a liberal agenda. Ironically, it was the Supreme Court, traditionally the least activist branch of government, which—under Chief Justice Earl Warren—broke the reform logjam. Until Warren's retirement in 1969, the Court continued to hand down a series of landmark decisions in broad areas of civil liberties and civil rights.

In 1960 the rights of citizens accused of a crime but not yet convicted were often unclear. Those too poor to afford lawyers could be forced to go to trial without representation. The police and the courts often did not inform those accused of crime of their rights guaranteed under the Constitution. In a series of decisions, the Court ruled that the Fourteenth Amendment provided broad guarantees of due process under the law. *Gideon v. Wainwright* (1963), initiated by a Florida prisoner, made it clear that citizens—however poor they might be—were entitled to legal counsel in all cases involving a possible jail sentence. In *Escobedo v. Illinois* (1964) and *Miranda v. Arizona* (1966) the Court declared that individuals detained for a crime must be informed of the charges against them, of their right to remain silent, and of their right to have an attorney present during questioning. Any statement they made might be used against them. Though these decisions applied to all citizens, they were primarily intended to benefit the poor, who were most likely to be in trouble with the law and least likely to understand their rights. As a result, the decisions greatly angered law enforcement agencies and middle-class groups distressed by what they saw as a breakdown of "law and order."

Especially troubling to conservative religious groups was *Engel v. Vitale* (1962), in which the Court ruled that the separation of church and state had been violated in New York State, where the Board of Regents had written a nonsectarian prayer to be recited in school. Even if dissenting children could be excused, the Court ruled, they faced indirect pressure to recite the prayer. *Abington v. Schempp* (1963) extended the ban on school prayer to cover the reading of the Bible and the Lord's Prayer. Reaction against the Court's ruling was so strong that members of Congress introduced nearly 150 proreligious proposals, including one requesting that states require all applicants for a driver's license to state their belief in a supreme being. None were passed.

In a different vein, the Court in *Griswold v. Connecticut* (1964) overturned a nineteenth-century law banning the sale of contraceptives or providing medical advice about their use. And in another step liberalizing the social climate, the Court demonstrated its distaste for book censorship by greatly narrowing the legal definition of obscenity. A book had to be "utterly without redeeming social value" to permit censorship. The combination of decisions reforming criminal rights, prayer, and morality outraged conservatives of almost all social and political backgrounds. The right-wing John Birch Society dotted the landscape with billboards calling for the impeachment of Chief Justice Earl Warren.

The Court's most far-reaching decision was probably one of its least controversial, though politically most sensitive. The explosive growth of cities and suburbs had created enormous problems of legislative apportionment. Rural elements refused to redraw state legislative or congressional district lines to reflect new demographic patterns. In *Baker v. Carr* (1962) and a series of subsequent cases the Court ruled that the states must apportion seats not by "land or trees or pastures," but as closely as possible by the principle of "one person, one vote."

THE CIVIL RIGHTS CRUSADE

Nothing did more to propel the liberalism of the 1960s—and in the end, to push beyond it—than the campaign for civil rights. By the late 1950s a generation of southern blacks, many having moved from farms to cities, was no longer willing to accept second-class citizenship. But how could they overturn the legal bulwarks of segregation in the South as well as the racism evident in everyday life across the nation? As the decade progressed, it became clear that blacks were opting for not one but many strategies. Some tactics were rooted in the doctrines of integration and Christian nonviolence; some focused on winning gains through the courts. More militant blacks sought power over their own lives through direct action or even by separating from white reformers and white society. And from the heat and despair of the ghettos, some blacks spoke with the violence borne of pent-up frustration and rage.

Riding to Freedom

The movement for black civil rights gained momentum not through national movements but through a host of individual decisions by local groups and citizens. When new Orleans schools were desegregated in 1960, young Ruby's parents had not been urged to make a social statement. But once involved, they refused to back down. In Greensboro, North Carolina, that same year, four black students attending North Carolina Agricultural and Technical College happened to read a pamphlet describing the 1955 bus boycott in Montgomery, Alabama. Though all were members of the NAACP Youth Council, they decided to stage an independent sit-in at a segregated lunch counter. "The waitress looked at me as if I were from outer space," recalled one of the protesters. Word of the action spread and within two weeks, 15 sit-ins had taken place across the South. By the end of the year, 50,000 people had demonstrated, 3000 had gone to jail, and black civil rights organizations were actively working to keep the momentum going.

Prior to the 1960s two organizations, the NAACP and the Urban League, had led the civil rights struggle. These groups continued to take legal action to desegregate public facilities, but leadership within the movement had passed by the early 1960s to direct action groups. Since organizing the Montgomery boycott, Martin Luther King and his Southern Christian Leadership Conference (SCLC) had continued to advocate nonviolent protest: "To resist without bitterness; to be cursed and not reply; to be beaten and not hit back." A second key organization, the Congress of Racial Equality (CORE), was more willing than the SCLC to force confrontations with the segregationist system. Another group, the Student Non-Violent Coordinating Committee (SNCC, pronounced "Snick") grew out of the Greensboro sit-in. SNCC represented the more militant, younger generation of black reformers, who, as time went on, became impatient with the slow pace of integration.

In May 1961 CORE director James Farmer led a group of black and white "freedom riders" on a bus trip from Washington to New Orleans. Moving from city to city, they hoped to call attention to segregated facilities—and attention they received. In South Carolina, thugs beat divinity student John Lewis as he tried to enter an all-white waiting room. Freedom riders were also assaulted by mobs in Anniston, Alabama, where one of the buses was burned, and in Birmingham, Alabama.

Like President Roosevelt before him, Kennedy preferred words to action on civil rights. The national attention to freedom riders made his position on the fence uncomfortable. He needed black and liberal votes to win reelection. Yet he also needed the support of southern Democratic committee chairmen to get legislation through Congress. So he hedged on his promise to introduce major civil rights legislation, as he had promised during the campaign. He would, he told black leaders, use executive orders to eliminate discrimination in the government civil service and in businesses filling government contracts. He appointed several blacks to high administrative positions and five, including Thurgood Marshall, to the federal courts. The Justice Department, run by the president's brother Robert Kennedy, beefed up its civil rights enforcement procedures.

When the freedom riders launched their campaign, Kennedy hoped to avoid federal intervention by convincing Alabama officials to protect the demonstrators, so that federal forces would not have to be sent. His hopes were dashed when John Doar, a Justice Department official, relayed what was happening directly to Robert Kennedy from a phone booth outside the bus terminal in Montgomery. "Now the passengers are coming off," Doar reported, as the attorney general listened in shocked silence. "They're standing on a corner of the platform. Oh, there are fists, punching. A bunch of men led by a guy with a bleeding face are beating them. There are no cops. It's terrible. It's terrible. There's not a cop in sight. People are yelling, 'Get 'em, get 'em.' It's awful." Appalled, Robert Kennedy ordered in 400 federal marshals, who barely managed to hold off the mob. Martin Luther King,

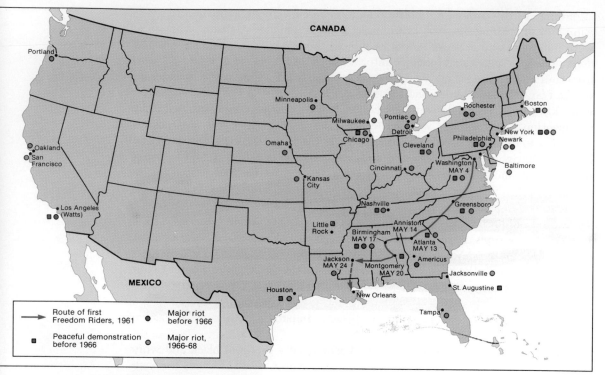

CIVIL RIGHTS: PATTERNS OF PROTEST AND UNREST
The first phase of the civil rights movement was confined largely to the South, where the
Freedom Ride of 1961 dramatized the issue of segregation. Urban unrest beginning in the
summer of 1964 turned the issue of race and politics into a national concern. Severe rioting
followed the murder of Martin Luther King, Jr., in 1968, after which the worst violence
subsided.

who was addressing a church meeting, phoned the attorney general to say that the
situation was becoming desperate. As Kennedy later recalled, "I said that we were
doing the best that we could and that he'd be as dead as Kelsey's nuts if it hadn't
been for the marshals and the efforts that we made."

Liberalism at High Tide

While CORE and the SCLC pulled back temporarily after the confrontation in
Montgomery, the more militant SNCC continued the bus rides from Montgomery
on to Jackson, Mississippi. By summer Robert Kennedy had persuaded SNCC to
shift its efforts from confrontation to voter registration, in hopes that the issue of
voting would prove less controversial. Voting booths, Kennedy noted, were not
like schools, where people would protest, "We don't want our little blond daughter going to school with a Negro." But as SNCC workers arrived in southern towns
the following fall and spring, they encountered legal harassment, jailings, beatings, bombings, and murders. Terrorized workers who called on the administration for protection found it woefully lacking. FBI agents often stood by taking
notes while SNCC workers were assaulted. "Every time I saw FBI men in Albany
[Georgia], they were with the local police force," Dr. King complained. At the
same time, SNCC workers made it clear they intended to stay. Fanning out across

the countryside, they spoke with farmers and poor blacks who had never before been involved in politics.

Confrontation increased, too, when a federal court ordered, over the protests of Governor Ross Barnett, the segregated University of Mississippi to admit James Meredith, a black applicant. In September 1962 Kennedy faced the same crisis that had confronted Eisenhower at Little Rock in 1957. After Governor Barnett personally blocked Meredith's registration, several hundred federal marshals quietly escorted Meredith into a university dormitory. The president announced on national television that the university had been integrated and asked students to follow the law of the land. Instead, a mob moved on campus, shooting out street lights, commandeering a bulldozer, and throwing rocks and bottles. To save the marshals, Kennedy finally sent in federal troops, but not before 2 people were killed and 375 wounded.

In Mississippi, President Kennedy had begun to lose control of the civil rights issue. Black militants urged bolder action than the president was willing to take. The House of Representatives, influenced by television coverage of the violence, introduced a number of civil rights measures. And Martin Luther King led a group to Birmingham, Alabama, to force a showdown against segregation. From a prison cell there, he produced one of the most eloquent documents of the civil rights movement, his "Letter from Birmingham Jail." Addressed to a local minister who had counseled an end to confrontation, King defended the use of civil disobedience. The choice, he warned, was not between obeying the law and nonviolently breaking it to bring about change; it was between his way and streets "flowing with blood," as restive black masses turned toward more militant ideologies.

By May King was again free and leading demonstrations. With arrests depleting his ranks, he organized thousands of children to march. Television cameras were on hand as Birmingham police chief "Bull" Connor, a man with a short fuse, unleashed attack dogs, club-wielding police, and fire hoses powerful enough to

Birmingham, Alabama, firefighters used high-pressure hoses to disperse civil rights demonstrators. The force of the hoses was great enough to tear bark off trees. Pictures like this one aroused widespread sympathy for the civil rights movement.

peel the bark off trees. The scenes enlisted as never before the support of northern liberals for the civil rights cause. But there was a grimmer push for reform in Birmingham. When segregationist bombs went off in black neighborhoods, black mobs retaliated with their own riot, burning a number of shops and businesses owned by whites. In the 10 weeks following the Birmingham demonstration there were over 750 riots in 186 cities and towns, both North and South. King's warning of streets "flowing with blood" seemed no longer far-fetched, and his own nonviolent protest appeared moderate by comparison.

Kennedy sensed that the time had come to take up the civil rights issue. In phrases which, like King's, drew heavily on Christian and republican rhetoric, he asked the nation, "If [an American with dark skin] cannot enjoy the full and free life all of us want, then who among us would be content to have the color of his skin changed and stand in his place? Who among us would then be content with counsels of patience and delay?" The president also threw his weight behind a strong civil rights bill to end segregation and protect black voters. When King announced a massive march on Washington for August 1963, Kennedy at first tried to persuade him that it would undermine support for his bill. "I have never engaged in any direct action movement which did not seem ill-timed," King replied. Faced with the inevitable, Kennedy made the march his own. He convinced the organizers to use the event to publicize and support the administration's bill, much to the disgust of militant CORE and SNCC factions.

On August 28 some 250,000 people gathered at the Lincoln Memorial to demonstrate their support for civil rights and racial harmony. Appropriately, the day belonged to King. In the powerful tones of a southern preacher, he reminded the crowd that the Declaration of Independence was a promise that applied to all people, black and white. "I have a dream," he told them, that one day "all of God's children, black men and white men, Jews and Gentiles, Protestants and Catholics, will be able to join hands and sing in the words of the old Negro spiritual, 'Free at last! Free at last! Thank God Almighty, we are free at last!'" Congress began deliberation of the civil rights bill, which was reported out of the Judiciary Committee on October 23.

The Fire Next Time

Support for civil rights paid Kennedy political dividends. Liberals embraced him as a hero. Though substantial numbers of southern whites and northern ethnics deserted him, appreciative blacks balanced those losses. All the same, the president decided he would make a trip to Texas in an effort to recoup some southern support for his reelection. On November 22, 1963, as his motorcade was making its way along the streets of Dallas, a sniper's rifle fired several times, fatally wounding him. His assassin, Lee Harvey Oswald, was caught hours later. He appeared to be an unstable man who, although having spent several years in the Soviet Union, acted independently and for his own reasons. But Oswald's story was never fully told, because only two days later—in full view of television cameras—he was gunned down by Jack Ruby, a disgruntled nightclub operator. Although an investigative commission headed by Chief Justice Warren concluded that the assassin acted alone, its hasty job prompted critics to suggest that Oswald was part of a larger conspiracy of undetermined origin.

The assassination struck at the heart of the political system. In the face of such violence, could the programs of political liberalism, gradual reform, or nonviolence hold the nation together? A few blacks believed that the Kennedy assassination was a case of a debt being repaid to a system that had tolerated its own racial violence—the "chickens coming home to roost," as black separatist Malcolm X put it. Many younger black leaders were aware that civil rights received the greatest national coverage when white, not black demonstrators were killed. They increasingly questioned how far liberal reform would take them. They wondered too how Kennedy's successor, Lyndon Johnson, a consummate southern politician, would approach the civil rights programs.

The new president, however, saw the need for action. Just as the Catholic issue had tested Kennedy's ability to lead, Johnson knew that without strong leadership on civil rights, "I'd be dead before I could ever begin." On November 23, his first day in office, he promised one civil rights leader after another that he would pass Kennedy's bill. By the following summer a southern filibuster in the Senate had been outmaneuvered and the Civil Rights Act of 1964 was law.

The bill marked one of the great moments in the history of American reform. Embodying all the provisions of the Kennedy bill, it barred discrimination in public accommodations such as lunch counters, bus stations, and hotels; it authorized the attorney general to bring suit to desegregate schools, museums, and other public facilities; it outlawed discrimination in employment by race, color, religion, sex, or national origin; and it gave additional protection to voting rights. Within months, the Supreme Court upheld the controversial public accommodations section, in what Justice Arthur Goldberg described as a "vindication of human dignity."

The Civil Rights Act did not deter some southern registrars from using literacy tests and other technicalities to prevent blacks from voting. Again in 1965 Martin Luther King led a series of demonstrations, culminating in a 54-mile walk

Martin Luther King (left) and his wife Coretta lead the march from Selma to Montgomery in March 1964. Already, however, activists from SNCC and CORE were insisting that tactics more radical than King's were needed.

from Selma to Montgomery, Alabama. President Johnson, who like Kennedy was not eager to offend southern voters, squirmed before federalizing the National Guard to protect the marchers. He then sent Congress even stronger legislation, which was passed in August 1965. The Voting Rights Act suspended literacy tests and other such devices. It also authorized federal officials to supervise elections in districts that had used the tests and in which less than half the population voted in 1964. Never shy about glorifying his own achievements, Johnson with some justice called the act "one of the most monumental laws in the entire history of American freedom." Within a five-year period black registration in the South jumped from 35 to 65 percent. In Mississippi, the scene of so much violence, the number went from 7 to 67 percent.

Black Power at the Ballot Box and on the Street

The civil rights laws, as comprehensive as they were, did not strike at what northern black leaders saw as the most invidious forms of discrimination. These were the de facto systems of segregation not codified in law, but practiced through unwritten custom and long force of habit. In large areas of America, de facto segregation locked blacks out of suburbs, kept them out of decent schools, barred them from exclusive clubs, and denied them all but the most menial jobs. Nor did the Voting Rights Act deal with the sources of urban black poverty, where the median income for blacks was approximately half of what whites earned and where black unemployment was double that of whites and five times as high for black men between the ages of 18 and 25.

In such an atmosphere, militants sharply questioned the liberal goal of integration. Since the 1940s the Black Muslim religious sect, dedicated to complete separation from white society, had attracted as many as 100,000 members, mostly young men. During the early 1960s the sect drew even wider attention through the energetic efforts of Malcolm X, a charismatic leader who spoke the language of the downtrodden from his own experience as a former hustler, gambler, and prison inmate. Malcolm broke with the Black Muslims and was moving toward a more moderate position in 1965, though one that still emphasized black community action, when he was gunned down by rivals. But by 1965–1966, even CORE and SNCC had begun to give up working with white liberals for nonviolent change. They began carrying guns to defend themselves and argued that for blacks to liberate themselves fully, they could not merely accept rights that were "given" to them by whites. They had to claim their rights. In 1966 Stokely Carmichael of SNCC gave the militants a slogan—"Black Power"—and the defiant symbol of a gloved fist raised in the air.

In its moderate form, the black power movement encouraged blacks to recover their cultural roots, their African heritage, and a new sense of identity. African clothes and natural hair styles became popular, while on college campuses black students pressed universities to hire black faculty, institute black studies programs, and provide segregated social and residential space. It was one of the great ironies of the 1960s that just as the civil rights movement broke down the legal barriers to integration, the black nationalist movement pressed for new forms of segregation, though now based on black pride rather than racial inferiority.

Black militants, on the other hand, perceived black power as an element of a broader Marxist ideology that treated violence as a useful revolutionary tool. The most militant among militants was the Black Panther party of Oakland, California. The Panthers, led by Huey P. Newton and Eldridge Cleaver, shocked white sensibilities by calling for the black community to arm themselves. Since California law forbade carrying concealed weapons, Newton and his followers openly brandished their weapons as they patrolled the streets to protect blacks from police harassment. In February 1967 Newton found the showdown he had been looking for, waving his loaded shotgun at one police officer and calling, "O.K., you big fat racist pig, draw your gun!" The police retreated, making Newton a hero in the ghetto.

When Newton was jailed after another gun battle, in which he was shot in the stomach, Eldridge Cleaver assumed leadership of the party and later attracted attention with his searing autobiography, *Soul on Ice*. But even at the height of their power, the Panthers never counted more than 2000 members nationwide. In the end, revolutionary black nationalism faded not because of white repression, but because radicals failed to define a political program that rallied large numbers from the black masses. Most remained committed to the goals defined by the civil rights movement, preferring nonviolence to armed confrontation, integration to segregation.

Beyond any consciously shaped ideology, however, a reservoir of frustration and despair existed in the ghettos. Riots broke out in Harlem and Rochester, New York, in 1964, the Watts area of Los Angeles in 1965, Chicago in 1966, and Newark and Detroit in 1967. Often disturbances were sparked by a seemingly minor incident like an arrest or an argument on the streets. A mob would gather and police cars and white-owned stores would be firebombed or looted. As police and the National Guard were ordered in, the violence escalated. In the riot at Watts, over $200 million in property lay in ruins and 34 people were dead, all of them black. It took nearly 5000 troops to end the bloodiest rioting in Detroit, where 40 died, 2000 were injured, and 5000 were left homeless.

To most whites the violence was unfathomable and inexcusable. Lyndon Johnson echoed the thoughts of many when he argued that "neither old wrongs nor new fears can justify arson and murder." Martin Luther King, still pursuing the tactics of nonviolence, was saddened by the destruction but discovered firsthand some of the anger behind it. Touring Watts only days after the riots, he was approached by a band of young blacks. "We won," they told him proudly. "How can you say you won," King countered, "when thirty-four Negroes are dead, your

A National Guardsman watches as flames consume large areas of the Watts section of Los Angeles during the 1965 riot. Often, a seemingly trivial event set off such scenes of violence, suggesting the depth of explosive rage harbored within the ghettos.

community is destroyed, and whites are using the riot as an excuse for inaction?" The youngsters were unmoved. "We won because we made them pay attention to us."

For Johnson, the explosion of ghetto violence and black militance seemed to mock his efforts to achieve national unity. The Civil Rights and Voting Rights acts were essential parts of the "Great Society" he hoped to build. In that effort he had achieved a legislative record virtually unequaled by any president in the nation's history. What Kennedy had promised, Johnson delivered. But the anger exploding in the nation's cities exposed serious flaws in the theory and practice of liberal reform.

LYNDON JOHNSON AND THE GREAT SOCIETY

Like the state he hailed from, Lyndon Baines Johnson was in all things bigger than life. His gifts were greater, his flaws more glaring. Insecurity was his Achilles heel and the engine that drove him. If Kennedy had been good as president, Johnson would be "the greatest of them all, the whole bunch of them." If FDR won in a landslide in 1936, Johnson would produce an even larger margin in 1964. And to anyone who displeased him, he could be ruthlessly cruel. He was vulgar, too—sometimes astonishingly so. He could summon a foreign dignitary to an audience as he sat, as if enthroned, on his toilet. His scatological language and preoccupation with barnyard sex amused few and offended many. After a 1965 operation, he shocked a national audience by lifting his shirt to expose a jagged scar and corpulent belly. That was not the "plain folks" Americans appreciated. The president was sometimes driven to ask why so few people genuinely liked him; once a courageous diplomat actually answered: "Because, Mr. President, you are not a very likeable man."

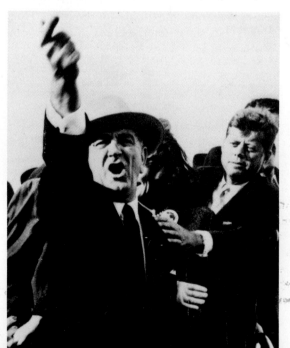

The irrepressible Lyndon Johnson had difficulty playing second fiddle to anyone, even when he was vice president. But his shrewd political instincts and folksy charm, which he knew how to deploy to good effect, often allowed him to outmaneuver his opponents.

Johnson was born in Stonewall, Texas, in the hill country outside Austin, where the dry climate and rough terrain only grudgingly yielded up a living. Schooled in manners by his overbearing mother and in politics by his father and his cronies, Johnson arrived in Washington in 1932 as an ardent New Dealer who loved the political game. When he became majority leader of the Senate in 1954, he cultivated an image as a moderate conservative who knew what strings to pull or levers to jog to get the job done. Johnson knew what made his colleagues run. On an important bill, he latched onto the undecided votes until they succumbed to the famous "Johnson treatment," a combination of arguments, threats, emotional or patriotic appeals, and enticing rewards.

Despite his overbearing nature and insecurity, Johnson possessed certain bedrock strengths. Though he could not help trying to control every person and situation, he was remarkably adept at hammering out compromises among competing interest groups. To those who served him well he could be loyal and generous. As president, he cared sincerely about society's underdogs. His support for civil rights, aid to the poor, education, and the welfare of the elderly came from genuine conviction. He made the betterment of such people the goal of his administration.

The Origins of the Great Society

In the first months after the assassination of John Kennedy, Johnson acted as the conservator of the Kennedy legacy. "Let us continue," he told a grief-stricken nation. Kennedy's assistants would stay on as his assistants; Kennedy's foreign policy would be his foreign policy; Kennedy's domestic agenda would shape his legislative program. Liberals who had dismissed Johnson as an unprincipled power broker begrudgingly came to respect the energy he showed in steering reform through Congress. The Civil Rights Act and tax cut legislation were only two of the most conspicuous pieces of Kennedy business Johnson quickly finished.

Kennedy had come to recognize that prosperity alone would not ease the plight of America's poor. In 1962 Michael Harrington's book *The Other America* brought widespread attention to the mass poverty that persisted in the face of general affluence. Attention focused particularly on the hills of Appalachia, stretching from western Pennsylvania south to Alabama, where in some counties a quarter of the population was trying to survive on a diet of flour and dried-milk paste supplied by federal surplus food programs. Under Kennedy Congress had passed a new food stamp program as well as laws designed to revive the economies of poor areas, replacing urban slums with newer housing and retraining the unemployed. Robert Kennedy also headed a presidential committee to fight juvenile delinquency in urban slums by involving the poor in "community action" programs. Direct participation, they hoped, would help overcome "a sense of resignation and fatalism" that sociologist Oscar Lewis had found while studying the Puerto Rican community of New York City.

It fell to Lyndon Johnson to shape a legislative package that could fight Kennedy's "war on poverty." By August 1964 he had driven through Congress the most sweeping social welfare bill since the New Deal. The Economic Opportunity Act addressed almost every major cause of poverty. It included training programs such as the Job Corps, which brought poor and unemployed recruits to rural or urban camps to receive six-month courses in new job skills. It granted loans to rural families and urban small businesses as well as aid to migrant workers, and it launched a domestic version of the Peace Corps, known as VISTA (Volunteers in Service to America). The price tag for these programs was high. Johnson committed almost $1 billion to Sargent Shriver, a Kennedy brother-in-law, who directed the new Office of Economic Opportunity (OEO). When Michael Harrington complained that even $1 billion could barely scratch the surface, Shriver tartly replied, "Maybe you've spent a billion dollars before, but this is my first time around."

Unfortunately, in his eagerness to move quickly Johnson sponsored a program that presented problems over the long haul. Shriver had to share jurisdiction over OEO programs with the departments of Labor and Health, Education and Welfare. Those bureaucracies had their own well-entrenched constituencies who were reluctant to share power with the politically unorganized poor. To take only one example, the Job Corps was forced to locate many of its retraining centers in remote rural conservation camps, due to the demands of the conservation lobby. Hapless recruits frequently found themselves bused a thousand miles from home. And when OEO workers tried to organize "community action" neighborhood groups, they often found themselves confronting the old-style bosses of city hall, setting up voter registration drives to oust corrupt officials or sponsoring rent strikes to improve conditions in public housing. In Syracuse, New York, the director of city housing reacted typically: "We are experiencing a class struggle in the traditional Karl Marx style in Syracuse, and I do not like it." In such battles for power and bureaucratic turf, federal poverty programs suffered.

The Election of 1964

In 1964, however, these long-term flaws were not yet evident. Johnson's political stock remained high. To an audience at the University of Michigan in May, he announced his ambition to forge a "Great Society," in which poverty and racial injustice no longer existed. The chance to fulfill his dreams seemed open to him, for the Republicans nominated Senator Barry Goldwater of Arizona as their presidential candidate. Few men in politics have been so genuinely well liked as Goldwater. Ruggedly handsome, he was a true son of the West who flew military jets in his spare time and spoke his mind with refreshing candor. But Goldwater's politics were so libertarian, he wished to rein in the federal government much more severely than most Americans believed necessary. Government should not dispense welfare, subsidize farmers, tax incomes on a progressive basis, or aid public education, he argued. At the same time, Goldwater's profound anticommunism led him into an unreserved support for a large defense establishment.

Such extreme views worried even moderate Republicans, and Johnson's election would have seemed a foregone conclusion except for Governor George Wallace of Alabama. Running in several Democratic primaries, Wallace's segregationist campaign won nearly a third or more of the votes in Wisconsin, Indiana, and Maryland—hardly the Deep South. In the end, however, he was persuaded to drop out of the race. In the one-sided contest that followed, Johnson portrayed himself as a responsible moderate, choosing Minnesota's liberal senator Hubert Humphrey to balance the ticket. Goldwater did not help himself by suggesting that the popular Social Security system be made voluntary or that military commanders be given the power to launch tactical nuclear weapons without presidential authority.

The election produced the landslide Johnson craved. Carrying every state except Arizona and four in the Deep South, he received 61 percent of the vote. Democrats gained better than two-to-one majorities in the Senate and House. All the same, the election was probably more a repudiation of Goldwater than a mandate for Johnson. The president was politically shrewd enough to realize that he had to move rapidly to exploit the momentum of his 1964 majority.

The Great Society

In January 1965 Johnson announced a vast legislative program to build the Great Society. In essence he proposed to extend state welfare programs on a scale beyond even Franklin Roosevelt's New Deal. For the poor it meant a doubling of the war on poverty; for the sick and disabled, a program of "Medicare"; for blacks, tougher civil rights enforcement; and for ethnic groups, a reform of restrictive immigration laws. The young would gain from aid to education, and for future generations, environmental legislation would preserve open space and clean up polluted air and water. By the end of 1965 fifty bills had been passed, many of them major pieces of legislation, with more on the agenda for the following year.

Education was a cornerstone of the Johnson program. To compensate the poor for their disadvantaged homes, Johnson as a former teacher wanted a strong educational system. Under the Elementary and Secondary School Act, students in low-income school districts were to receive educational equipment, money for books, and enrichment programs like "Project Headstart" for nursery-age children. But for all its benefits, the bill did not provide money for certain basics, such as badly needed new classrooms or increased teachers' salaries. And although eager schools scrambled to create programs that would tap federal money, they sometimes used the act to fund programs for middle-class as much as poor students. Administrative overhead often cost more than the actual programs. In the end, the Elementary and Secondary School Act gave as many benefits to middle-class educational professionals as to lower income students.

President Johnson also pushed through the Medicare Act, which provided the elderly with mandatory health insurance to cover their hospital costs. Since the days of Harry Truman, Congress had debated whether to provide some kind of health insurance for all Americans. Medicare targeted the elderly, because studies had shown that older people used hospitals three times more than other Ameri-

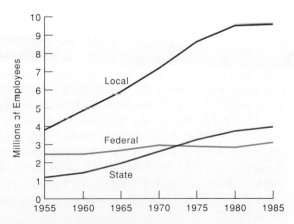

GROWTH OF GOVERNMENT, 1955–1985
Government has been a major growth industry since World War II. But even during the Great Society, government employment was most significant at the state and local levels. It grew more at the federal level during Ronald Reagan's presidency.

Source: U.S. Bureau of the Census.

cans and generally had incomes only half as large. Premiums would be paid into the social security system and financed by it. Citizens could also make voluntary payments that would cover doctors' and surgical fees. Since Medicare made no provision for the poor who were not elderly, Congress also passed a program called Medicaid. Participating states would receive matching grants from the federal government to pay the medical expenses of those on welfare or too poor to afford medical care.

In one sense, Medicare and Medicaid worked. The poor and elderly did receive significantly more help when facing catastrophic illnesses. But as increased numbers of patients used hospital services, Medicare budgets rose. In addition, nothing in the act restricted hospitals or doctors from raising their fees. The cost of the programs soared by over 500 percent in the first 10 years. In the year after Congress approved Medicare, hospitals raised their fees by 14 percent, double the increase of the year before. Doctors began to charge for care they once gave free, raising their fees about 7 percent every year. Those increases wiped out the benefits many of the elderly and poor received, so that actual medical expenses remained constant. What was saved in hospital bills went for more costly drugs, dental work, and doctors' fees not covered under Medicare or Medicaid.

Ten days after signing the Medicare bill, Johnson signed the Omnibus Housing Act, designed to subsidize rents for poor families unable to find adequate public housing. Four days later came the Voting Rights Act. Within two weeks Congress approved creation of a new cabinet-level Department of Housing and Urban Development (HUD) to be headed by Robert Weaver, a former president of the NAACP. And in the tradition of the New Deal, which had patronized the arts under the WPA, Johnson created the National Foundation of the Arts and Humanities. Colleges and their students received support for scholarships and loans, research equipment, and libraries. And on another front, Great Society programs reformed American immigration policy. Although the United States still admitted just 170,000 people each year, the Immigration Act of 1965 abolished the national origins system, which favored northern Europeans over those from other areas of Europe. Racial provisions restricting Asian immigration were eliminated, although limits were still placed on immigration from other parts of the Western Hemisphere.

Nor did Johnson, in his efforts to outdo the New Deal, slight the environment. By the mid-1960s many Americans had become increasingly concerned about the acrid smog from factories and automobiles; lakes and rivers polluted by detergents, pesticides, and industrial wastes; and the disappearance of wildlife. In 1964 Congress had already passed the National Wilderness Preservation System Act to set aside 9.1 million acres of wilderness as "forever wild." Lady Bird Johnson, the president's wife, led a campaign to eliminate the garish billboards and junkyards that marred the views along so many of the nation's roads. And Congress established pollution standards for interstate waterways and a year later provided funds for sewage treatment and water purification. Similar standards were tightened to diminish air pollution. The programs for the environment, like other Great Society measures, often ran afoul of entrenched interests. Mining, cattle-grazing, and lumbering businesses lobbied to continue using portions of public wilderness lands for their own benefit. On the other hand, the new standards did result in a gradual, steady improvement in water and air quality in many areas.

In 1966 Johnson pushed through bills to raise the minimum wage, improve auto safety, aid mass transit, and develop "model cities." But by then he had encountered mounting opposition from legislators worried that they were voting too much power and money to the executive branch. "Doesn't matter what kind of majority you come in with," Johnson had predicted early on. "You've got just one year when they treat you right, and before they start worrying about themselves." Yet as late as 1968 he was able to get major legislation through Congress to ban discrimination in housing (Fair Housing Act), to build public housing, to protect consumers from unfair credit practices (Truth-in-Lending Act), and to protect scenic rivers and expand the national park system.

The unparalleled successes of the Great Society carried a higher price tag than anyone had predicted, and the results were not all unmitigated successes. Statistics suggested that general prosperity, accelerated by the tax cut bill, did more to fight poverty than all the OEO programs. And the inevitable scandals began to surface: Job Corps retrainees burglarizing homes in their off-hours, school equipment purchased that no one knew how to use, and so on. Conservatives and radicals alike objected that the liberal welfare state was intruding into too many areas of people's lives. Ethnic groups like Italian- and Polish-Americans objected to what they considered favoritism accorded blacks and Hispanics under most poverty programs. And the mayors of large cities continued to oppose all community action programs that they did not control themselves.

Most of all, Johnson's consensus collapsed amid the growing controversy over the Vietnam War. By 1966 the war had expanded sharply, and it was no longer clear that the United States could afford to pay for troops and bombs as well as massive social programs. Inflation was one clear result of the president's determination to have both "guns and butter" without higher taxes. Thus the Great Society programs proved to be the high-water mark for the liberal approach to government begun under Franklin Roosevelt. By the mid-1960s civil rights organizations and the poor were not the only groups fighting to reach beyond liberal solutions; dissatisfied members of the middle class—and especially the young—had joined them.

THE COUNTERCULTURE

In the civil rights movement, a young generation of black leaders pushed for more extreme measures. College students had started the sit-in movement at Greensboro, and SNCC continued the freedom rides when CORE felt the situation had become too explosive. As the voting rights drive made headlines in the Deep South, white college students became involved too, getting their first taste of political action. In 1964 some 800 students from Berkeley, Oberlin, and other colleges met to receive training in preparation for the voter registration campaign in the South. Middle-class students who had grown up in peaceful white suburbs found themselves being trained by protest-hardened SNCC coordinators: when beaten by police, assume the fetal position—hands protecting the neck, elbows covering the temples to minimize injuries from nightsticks. It was a sober awakening, and students came back shocked that such things could happen in America.

Activists on the New Left

More than a few students returned home disillusioned with the slow pace of reform, seeing a need to overturn the "establishment"—regardless of whether it

Daily Lives

CLOTHING AND FASHION
The Politics of Dress

Three-piece suits, fur coats, berets, Grateful Dead T-shirts—clothing has always made a statement about the social class and values of the wearer. In the 1950s that statement was conformity. The khaki slacks and brush-cut hair popular with middle-class boys hinted at military regimentation. Rock-and-rollers, lower class kids, and farm boys often wore dungarees and T-shirts, perhaps with a cigarette pack tucked in the rolled-up sleeve. Beatniks advertised their nonconformity by adopting an exotic look: long hair, goatees, turtlenecks, and sandals.

During the 1960s clothing signaled the coming of a political upheaval as nonconformity became the norm. The pattern was closely tied to music, as middle-class teenagers rejected sentimental pop tunes for serious "folk" music or the raucous rhythms of rock and roll. The revolution began in earnest with the coming of the Beatles, four British rockers from working-class Liverpool. John, Paul, George, and Ringo inspired fan hysteria beyond anything seen before. Their "mod"-style British clothes and longish, page-boy hair caused as much commotion as their music. As young Americans embraced the Beatles and all things British, London supplanted Paris and New York as a fashion center.

Suddenly it was the young and working class, not the rich, who set trends in style. At first, women's hemlines rose well above the knees, as the "miniskirt" became the rage, but its popularity was eventually rivaled by the floor-length "maxi." Designer Rudi Gernreich, mostly with his tongue firmly in cheek, introduced the "topless" look with a swimsuit

In men's clothing, flowered prints, bold colors, and zany combinations of style replaced traditionally conservative fashions.

Daily Lives

bottom hung by a thin cord around the neck. Soon anarchy reigned in the world of fashion. Men especially broke with past tradition. Sideburns lengthened and moustaches and beards flourished as they had not since the nineteenth century. Men began to wear jewelry, furs, perfume, and shoulder-length hair. Subdued tweeds and narrow lapels gave way to bell-bottoms, broad floral ties, and wide-collared, sometimes psychedelic shirts.

All these fashions represented a desire to break social constraints in favor of greater sensuality and freedom of expression. Nowhere was that more evident than in the theatrical costuming of the counter-culture. Early in the decade, it was only beatniks and Hell's Angels-style motorcycle gangs who sported long hair and distinctive clothes. Then in the mid-1960s, middle-class students began to let their hair grow and replaced their khakis and pleated skirts with jeans and Army–Navy store military surplus. The original impulse was less rebellion than a distinct youthful identity that blurred social class lines, just as rock and roll did.

"Hippies" added a more colorful twist. They rejected commercial fashion, synthetic fabrics, and cosmetics in favor of a natural look. To express a return to nature, they adopted the Hispanic shawl and serape, the Indian fringed buckskin, beads, and moccasins, and the bright coloring of Oriental and Caribbean cotton fabrics. Much of their clothing and accessories were handcrafted and sold largely through street vendors, medieval style craft fairs, and small shops. Often these same shops, located in college towns and artsy urban neighborhoods, did a lively business selling water pipes, "bongs," rolling papers, roach clips, strobe lights, posters, Indian print bedspreads, and other paraphernalia of the drug culture. Military surplus and the varieties of neo-Indian garb became standard wear at folk and rock music festivals and "be-ins," as well as at political demonstrations.

Fashion had become a function of politics and rebellion. Traditional Americans saw beads, long hair, sandals, drugs, radical politics, and rock and roll as elements of a revolution. To them, hippies and radicals were equally threatening. They struck back by trying to censor and even outlaw the trappings of the counter-culture. Schools expelled boys when their hair was too long and girls when their skirts were too short. It became indecent to desecrate the flag by sewing patches of red, white, and blue on torn blue jeans. Short-haired blue-collar workers harassed long-haired hippies and antiwar protestors. The personal fashions of the youth rebellion came to symbolize a "generation gap" between the young and their elders.

Yet by the early 1970s, even some revolutionaries were having second thoughts. Feminists rejected the more extreme styles as an example of the male-dominated fashion world that treated women as sex objects. Hippie garb, which was impractical in the office, was replaced by knee-length skirts or pants suits. And as the once-shocking innovations became commonplace, even middle-aged men and women donned boots, let their hair grow a bit fuller, and slipped into modified bell-bottoms. Commercial success, not legal repression, had signaled an end to the revolution in fashion. Before long, three-piece suits, khakis, and short hair were back, although the democratic and eclectic spirit of the 1960s persisted. The new informality provided Americans of both sexes with a wider range of choice in fashions.

was liberal or conservative. Tom Hayden, from a working-class family in a suburb of Detroit, went to college at the University of Michigan, then traveled to Berkeley, and soon joined civil rights workers in Mississippi. "At first, you thought, well, the southern system is some kind of historical vestige," he recalled. "Instead, we found out that the structure of power was very tied into the structure of power in the whole U.S. You'd find that Harvard was investing in Mississippi Power and Light, which was a company that economically dominated Mississippi. You'd find that the southern wing of the Democratic Party held all the seniority positions in Congress."

Hayden, along with Al Haber, another student at the University of Michigan, was a driving force in forming the radical Students for a Democratic Society (SDS). Members of SDS had given up on change through the electoral system. They had little sympathy with an "old left" generation of radicals who grew up in the 1930s and were still debating the merits of Marxism. Action was the route that needed to be taken, Hayden argued: through sit-ins, protest marches, and direct confrontation. At a meeting in Port Huron, Michigan, in 1962 the group condemned the modern bureaucratic society exemplified by the "organization man" of the 1950s. The Port Huron Statement called for "participatory democracy," where large organizations run by bureaucrats would be broken down, decentralized, and reformed into face-to-face communities where individual participation mattered.

The bold theories of the Port Huron Statement did not exactly revolutionize America; only 60,000 copies of it were ever sold. The entire nation, however, heard in 1964 about Mario Savio and the Free Speech Movement at Berkeley. To most liberals, Berkeley was the gem of the California state university system. Like so many other universities, it had educated a generation of GIs following World War II. And when the Russians launched *Sputnik,* it had led American universities in setting higher standards. But to people like Tom Hayden and the SDS, Berkeley was a bureaucratic monster, enrolling more than 30,000 students. Like other large universities, it had impersonal lecture halls filled with classes taught by remote professors. Seminars seemed most often to be led by inexperienced graduate students. In the fall of 1964, Berkeley informed students that the one small area where political organizations had been allowed to advertise their causes was now off limits. When university police tried to remove a recruiter for CORE, thousands of angry students surrounded the police car for 32 hours.

Mario Savio, a graduate student in philosophy, soon became the leader of the Free Speech Movement. "In our free-speech fight, we have come up against what may emerge as the greatest problem of our nation—depersonalized, unresponsive bureaucracy," Savio proclaimed. When the university's president, Clark Kerr, threatened to expel him, 6000 students took control of the administration building, stopped classes with a strike, and convinced many faculty members to join them. Kerr backed down, placing no limits to free speech on campus except those that applied to society at large. But the lines between students and administrators had been drawn. Berkeley continued to be a hotbed of political demonstrations throughout the 1960s. And the rebellious spirit spread to other major universities like Michigan, Yale, and Columbia, and then to campuses across the nation.

The Rise of the Counterculture

Political action was only one way the younger generation responded to an impersonal, bureaucratic society. Disaffected rebels also condemned American society

as being too preoccupied with abundance and economic materialism. More alienated students began to grope toward spiritual, nonmaterial goals. "Turn on to the
scene, tune in to what is happening, and drop out of high school, college, grad
school, junior executive," advised Timothy Leary, a Harvard psychology professor
who dropped out himself. Those who heeded Leary's message embraced poverty
as a superior way of life that afforded time to experiment with music, sex, and
drugs. Observers labeled the new movement a "counterculture."

The counterculture of the 1960s had much in common with earlier religious
revival and utopian movements. It admired the quirky individualism of Henry
David Thoreau and, like Thoreau, it turned to Oriental philosophy such as Zen
Buddhism. Like Brook Farm and other nineteenth-century utopian communities,
the new "hippie" communes sought perfection along the fringes of society. Com-
munards built geodesic domes based on the designs of architect Buckminster
Fuller; they "learned how to scrounge materials, tear down abandoned buildings,
use the unusable," as one member of the "Drop City" commune put it. Sexual
freedom became a means to liberate them from the repressive inhibitions that
distorted the lives of their "uptight" parents. Drugs appeared to open the inner
mind to a higher state of consciousness. No longer would people be bound by
conventional relationships and the goals of a liberal, bourgeois society.

The early threads of the sixties counterculture led back to the fifties and the
subculture of the beat generation. The "beats" viewed themselves as being driven
to the margins of society, like the black jazz musicians and underworld "hipsters"
they so admired. "I saw the best minds of my generation destroyed by madness,
starving hysterical naked," wrote Allen Ginsberg in his 1955 poem *Howl*. They
had become "angelheaded hipsters . . . who in poverty and tatters and hollow-
eyed and high sat up smoking in the supernatural darkness of cold-water flats
floating across the tops of cities contemplating jazz." Jack Kerouac tapped the
frenzied energy that lay beneath the beatniks' cool facade in *On the Road* (1957), a
novel based on his travels across the country with his friend Neal Cassady. Kerouac finished the novel in one frenetic three-week binge, feeding a 120-foot roll of
teletype paper through his typewriter and spilling out tales of pot, jazz, crazy sex,
and all-night raps undertaken in a search for "IT"—the ultimate transcendental
moment when mind and experience mesh. Indeed, Neal Cassady ended up driving the bus for a new generation of "hippies" as they sped off in 1964 on another
wild chase across America. The antics of novelist Ken Kesey's "Merry Pranksters"
were recorded in Tom Wolfe's *Electric Kool-Aid Acid Test*.

Unconventional drugs had long been a part of the beat scene of the 1950s, but
their use expanded dramatically during the 1960s. Timothy Leary began experimenting with hallucinogenic mushrooms in Mexico and soon moved on to LSD,
an even more potent drug. It "blew his mind," he announced, and he became so
enthusiastic in making converts that Harvard blew him straight out of its hallowed
doors. By 1966 Leary had joined the psychedelic lecture circuit, going from college to college describing the joys of drug use. Those students who were uncomfortable about taking LSD had the option of smoking marijuana, which by the late
sixties was widely used on many campuses.

The Rock Revolution

While Kerouac, Ginsberg, and others preached sermons of liberation, the hymns
of the movement surfaced in new forms of popular music. In 1958 a group called
the Kingston Trio popularized folk music that appealed more to college than high

school audiences. Compared to the spontaneous and irreverent style of rock and roll, folk music was self-consciously historical and serious. (The Kingston Trio's first hit, "Tom Dooley," was a revival of a nineteenth-century ballad.) As the audience for folk music grew, the lyrics increasingly focused on social or political issues. Joan Baez, with a voice one critic found as pure and clear "as air in autumn," dressed simply, wore no makeup, and rejected the commercialism of popular music. She joined folk singer Bob Dylan in the civil rights march on Washington in 1963, singing "We Shall Overcome" and "Blowin' in the Wind." Such folk singers reflected the activist side of the counterculture as they sought to provoke their audiences to political commitment and social action.

In 1964 a new sound, imported from England, exploded on the American scene. Within a year the Beatles, four musicians from Liverpool, had generated more excitement than any previous phenomenon in popular music. Their concerts and appearances on the Ed Sullivan television show attracted frenzied teen audiences who screamed and swooned as the "mod" crooners sang "I Want to Hold Your Hand." Part of the Beatles' appeal came from their distinctly English style. With hair considered long in the sixties, modish clothes, fresh faces, and irreverent wit, they looked and sounded like nothing young Americans had experienced. Their boyish enthusiasm for life captured the Dionysian spirit of the new counterculture. But the Beatles' enormous commercial success also reflected the creativity of their music. Along with other English groups, like the Rolling Stones, they reconnected American audiences with the rhythm-and-blues roots of rock and roll, which they had drawn upon when creating their own songs.

Until 1965 Bob Dylan was the essential folk artist, writing about nuclear weapons, pollution, and racism. He appeared at concerts with longish frizzy hair, working-class clothes, an unamplified guitar, and a harmonica suspended on a wire support. But then Dylan shocked his fans by donning a black leather jacket and shifting to a "folk-rock" style featuring an electric guitar. His new songs seemed to suggest that the old America was almost beyond redemption. Meanwhile, the Beatles completed a pilgrimage to India to study transcendental meditation and returned to produce *Sergeant Pepper's Lonely Hearts Club Band*, possibly the most influential album of the decade. It blended sound effects with music, alluded to trips taken with "Lucy in the Sky with Diamonds" (LSD), and concluded, "I'd love to turn you on." The new format was innovative, too. No longer were songs limited to the three-minute length of 45-rpm records and popular radio. Out in San Francisco, bands like the Grateful Dead pioneered "acid rock" with long pieces aimed to echo drug-induced states of mind.

The debt of white rock musicians to rhythm and blues led to increased integration in the music world. Prior to the 1960s black rhythm-and-blues bands played primarily to black audiences, in segregated clubs, or over black radio stations. Black artists like Little Richard, Chuck Berry, and Ray Charles wrote numerous hit songs made popular by white performers. With the success of the civil rights movement and a rising black social and political consciousness came "soul" music. Blacks became "soul brothers" and "soul sisters," and for the first time their music was played on major radio stations. One black disc jockey described

Folk singer Bob Dylan became a kind of unofficial spokesperson of the 1960s youth rebellion. His songs expressed the anger, alienation, and despair of both political activists and apolitical cultural dropouts.

soul as "the last to be hired, first to be fired, brown all year round, sit-in-the-back-of-the-bus feeling." Soul was the quality that expressed black pride and separatism: "You've got to live with us or you don't have it." Out of Detroit came the "Motown sound," which combined elements of gospel, blues, and big band jazz. Diana Ross and the Supremes, the Temptations, Stevie Wonder, and other groups under contract to Berry Gordy's Motown Record Company appealed to black and white audiences alike. Yet while soul music promoted black consciousness, it had little to offer by way of social commentary. It evoked the traditional blues themes of unrequited love, workday woes, unhappy marriages, and the troubles between men and women.

The West Coast Scene

For all of its themes of alienation, rebellion, and utopian quest, the counterculture also signaled the increasing importance of the West Coast in American popular culture. In the 1950s the shift of television production from the stages of New York to the film lots of Hollywood helped establish Los Angeles as a communications center. San Francisco became notorious as a center of the beat movement.

Then in 1958 the unthinkable happened. The Brooklyn Dodgers, followed soon after by the New York Giants, two baseball teams that had helped make New York City the national sports capital, fled the East Coast for Los Angeles and San Francisco. When Alaska and Hawaii became states in 1959, the national center of gravity shifted westward. Richard Nixon, a Californian, narrowly missed being elected president in 1960. By 1963 the "surfing sound" of West Coast rock groups like the Beach Boys and Jan and Dean had made Southern California's preoccupation with surfing and cars into a national fad. And Mario Savio and his Free Speech Movement soon attracted the attention of the nation.

Before 1967 Americans were only vaguely aware of another West Coast phenomenon, the "hippies." But in January a loose coalition of drug freaks, Zen cultists, and political activists banded together to hold the first well-publicized "Be-In." Allen Ginsberg was on hand to offer spiritual guidance. The Grateful Dead and Jefferson Airplane, acid rock groups based in San Francisco, provided entertainment. An unknown organization called the Diggers somehow managed to supply free food and drink, while the notorious Hell's Angels motorcycle gang policed the occasion. Drugs of all kinds were plentiful. And a crowd attired in a bizarre mix of Native American, circus, Oriental, army surplus, and other exotic costumes came to enjoy it all. The West Coast had long been a magnet for Americans seeking opportunity, escape, and alternative lifestyles; now the San Francisco Bay Area staked its claim as the spiritual center of the counterculture. The more politically conscious dropouts gravitated toward Berkeley; the apolitical "flower children" moved into Haight–Ashbury, a run-down San Francisco neighborhood of apartments, Victorian houses, and "head shops" selling drug paraphernalia, wall posters, Indian bedspreads, and other coveted accessories.

Haight–Ashbury became a model replicated across the nation. Communes sprang up in the Rocky Mountains; yoga classes appeared in Ohio; Chinese woks were used in Ketchum, Idaho; students enrolled in high schools of ecology in Kennebunk, Maine. Colleges became centers of hip culture, offering alternative courses, eliminating strict requirements, and tolerating the new sexual mores of their students. In the summer of 1969 all the positive forces of the counterculture converged on Bethel, New York, in the Catskill Mountain resort area, to celebrate the promise of peace, love, and freedom. The Woodstock Music Festival attracted 400,000 people to the largest rock concert ever organized. For one long weekend the audience and performers joined to form an ephemeral community based on sex, drugs, and rock and roll.

Even then, the counterculture was dying. Four months after Woodstock, the hippie world reconvened on the West Coast at Altamont, California, to celebrate again, in the last month of the sixties. Over this assemblage presided the Rolling Stones, who delighted in being called "their satanic majesties" and had always cultivated a somewhat hostile, sexually ambiguous image. This time peace and love turned into anger and violence. With Stones leader Mick Jagger singing "Street Fighting Man" and "Sympathy for the Devil," the Hell's Angels police force randomly assaulted members of the audience with chains and broken pool cues. Movie cameras whirred as a group of Angels ran down a black street hood and knifed him to death. Just as Woodstock had symbolized the vitality of the counterculture, Altamont suggested its self-destructive potential.

Violence also intruded on the laid-back urban communities hippies had formed. Organized crime and drug pushers muscled in on the lucrative trade in LSD, amphetamines, and marijuana. Bad drugs and addiction took their toll. Criminals and psychopaths often passed themselves off as hippies. Urban slum dwellers turned hostile to the strange middle-class dropouts who, in ways the poor could not fathom, found poverty ennobling. Free sex often became an excuse for rape, exploitation, and loveless gratification.

Commercial acceptance undermined the counterculture's innocence by integrating its irreverant and rebellious style into mainstream pop culture. Much that had once seemed outrageous in the hippie world was readily absorbed into the marketplace. By 1968, for example, ABC had introduced *The Mod Squad*, a television series featuring three hippie types as undercover police officers. Rock groups became big business enterprises commanding huge fees. Slick concerts with expensive tickets replaced communal dances with psychedelic light shows. Yogurt, granola, and herbal teas appeared on supermarket shelves. Ironically, the world that hippies forged was coopted by the society they had rejected.

By the late 1960s most dreams of human betterment seemed shattered— whether John Kennedy's New Frontier, Lyndon Johnson's Great Society, or the communal society of the hippie counterculture. Recession and inflation brought an end to the easy affluence that made liberal reform programs and alternative lifestyles seem so easily affordable. In 1965 presidential adviser Daniel Patrick Moynihan was still optimistically suggesting that Keynesian management of the economy had created permanent abundance. The challenge, as Moynihan saw it, was to find new problems for reformers to solve. "The immediate *supply* of resources available for social purposes might actually outrun the immediate *demand* of established programs," he speculated in a giddy moment. By the end of the decade that unbridled optimism had turned to gloom, despite the Great Society's successes in altering the political landscape. Poverty and unemployment menaced even middle-class youth who had found havens in communes, colleges, and graduate schools. Racial tensions had divided black militants and the white liberals of the civil rights movement into sometimes hostile camps.

But the Vietnam War more than any other single factor destroyed the promise of Camelot. After 1965 the nation was deeply divided over the American military role in Southeast Asia. Radicals on the left who opposed the war insisted on a new utopian political consciousness that would rid America of a capitalist system that promoted race and class conflict at home and imperialism and military adventurism abroad. Conservatives on the right who supported the war called for a return to more traditional values like law and order. Both the left and the right attacked the liberal center. Their combined opposition helped to undermine the consensus Lyndon Johnson had worked so hard to build.

SIGNIFICANT EVENTS

1958 — Kingston Trio popularizes folk music

1960 — Kennedy–Nixon debates; Greensboro sit-ins; Kennedy elected president

1961 — Alliance for Progress; Peace Corps begun; Alan Shepard, Jr., first American in space; Bay of Pigs invasion; Kennedy steps up U.S. role in Vietnam; Vienna summit; Berlin Wall built; Area Redevelopment Act; CORE freedom rides begin

1962 — John Glenn orbits earth; Michael Harrington's *The Other America* published; Cuban missile crisis; James Meredith desegregates University of Mississippi; *Engel v. Vitale; Baker v. Carr;* SDS Port Huron Statement

1963 — Diem assassinated in Vietnam; nuclear test ban treaty; University of Alabama desegregation crisis; Kennedy introduces Civil Rights Bill; March on Washington; *Gideon v. Wainwright;* Kennedy assassinated

1964 — *Escobedo v. Illinois; Griswold v. Connecticut;* Civil Rights Act passed; SNCC Freedom Summer; Harlem and Rochester race riots; Johnson enacts Kennedy tax cuts; Economic Opportunity Act; VISTA established; Wilderness Preservation System Act; Johnson defeats Goldwater; Berkeley "Free Speech" Movement; Beatles introduce British rock

1965 — Johnson launches the Great Society; King's Selma protest; Voting Rights Act; Watts riots; Malcolm X assassinated; Medicare and Medicaid acts; Elementary and Secondary School Act; Omnibus Housing Act; Immigration Act; escalation in Vietnam

1966 — *Miranda v. Arizona;* Stokely Carmichael of SNCC coins "Black Power" slogan; Model Cities Act; minimum wages raised

1967 — Black Panthers battle Oakland, California, police; first "Be-In"

1968 — Fair Housing Act

1969 — Woodstock Music Festival; Altamont concert

Generations of the Republic

The Baby Boomers (1940–   )

To Americans the end of World War II augured an era of peace, power, and, above all, abundance. The economy was booming, the war had done relatively little damage to the nation's people and natural resources, and U.S. global power was underscored by the monopoly on atomic weapons. For the generation being born at the start of this new era, the contours of abundance shaped their world too.

There was, to begin with, an abundance of postwar children. The baby boom of the mid-twentieth century was especially remarkable given that for two and a half centuries the fertility rate among American women had dropped, as American society changed from a rural-agricultural to an urban-industrial culture. In 1942, however, the rate began a 15-year rise to a high of 122.9 births per thousand in 1957. The baby boom cut across virtually all sectors of American society. Furthermore, the trends also affected other highly industrialized nations.

The sharp rise did not reflect a return to the large-family pattern of earlier centuries, when women married in their early twenties and gave birth, on average, to six or seven children. Baby-boom families were only slightly larger than those of the 1920s and 1930s, jumping from an average of about two children to three. What accounted for the difference was that greater numbers of women were marrying, and at a markedly younger age. Fully one-third of all mothers during the baby-boom years set up housekeeping by the age of 19. Moreover, most chose to stop having children by their early or mid-thirties, unlike most mothers of earlier centuries, who continued to bear children well into their forties.

As young couples moved away from older communities with extended families to single-family suburban tracts, they often found themselves without the advice needed to deal with the challenges of childrearing. They turned eagerly to Dr. Benjamin Spock's *Baby and Child Care* (1946), which eventually sold over 30 million copies, second only to the Bible. Dr. Spock urged parents to follow their instincts, "be flexible and adjust to the baby's needs and happiness." Spock's ideal mother stayed home with her children, while avoiding becoming either over-protective or indifferent to her child's welfare. "Don't be afraid to love him and enjoy him. Every baby needs to be smiled at, talked to, played with, fondled—gently and lovingly—just as much as he needs vitamins and calories."

When the baby boomers went to school, enrollments jumped by over 60 percent. Schools put up new wings and new buildings to accommodate the overflow and struggled to improve curricula to "keep up" with the Russians. During air-raid drills, lines of obedient children were led to basements, or sheltered themselves along interior walls. They were admonished, too, to "duck and cover" if caught at their desks when the first flash of an atomic blast came. Yet the cold war only occasionally intruded on the joys of getting and spending as this generation matured.

Continuing a trend of two centuries, the younger generation took increasingly longer to enter adulthood. The demand for technically skilled labor as well as parents' conviction that children were more likely to succeed with a higher education both served to lengthen the period of adolescence. The average boom child spent 12.9 years in school, with 84 percent finishing high school. Blacks were just as likely as whites to finish high school, but Hispanics lagged behind. As for college education, 44 percent of baby boomers were exposed to at least a year of it, and 25 percent graduated.

Given a prolonged period of adolescence, the 1950s economy of relative abundance was increasingly shaped by teenaged desires, styles and tastes. Adolescents had begun to accumulate money of their own to spend. In 1960 more than 25 percent of all teenaged boys and 14 percent of girls worked at least part time, and less of that money went, as it might have earlier in the century, to support the family. Teenagers controlled some $9.5 billion (out of GNP of $504 billion), which they spent on automobiles, clothes and records, not to mention candy bars, gum, soft drinks, and ice cream.

As a generation of youth came of age in the 1960s, the culture of abundance led many to look beyond the freedom of material well-being to "liberation" in other areas of life. Raised in child-centered, democratic, egalitarian families, college students became less willing to abide by university requirements for military training, chapel services, dress codes, or dormitory closing hours. Similarly, the currents of change touched more conservative courtship rituals. During the 1950s the practice of "going steady" had become common, with college fraternity brothers "pinning" women who would presumably become their wives. The sixties marked a return to more open dating patterns, and for the first time since the 1920s, the rate of premarital intercourse rose significantly. The wider availability of oral contraceptives, beginning in the late 1950s, increased the amount of control young

1920

Birth Year		Age
Before 1846		75 +
1846–50		70–74
1851–55	Males	65–69
1856–60	Females	60–64
1861–65		55–59
1866–70		50–54
1871–75		45–49
1876–80		40–44
1881–85		35–39
1886–90		30–34
1891–95		25–29
1896–1900		20–24
1901–05		15–19
1906–10		10–14
1911–15		5–9
1916–20		0–4

6 5 4 3 2 1 0 1 2 3 4 5 6

adults exerted over their sexual habits.

Liberation, abundance, control over one's future—these were the hallmarks of the new generation. Although only a fringe of the counterculture experimented with open marriage or communal living, liberation for many women meant being able to postpone or subordinate marriage to a full-time career. Often, this was a conscious decision arising out of a new appreciation for women's rights. But even the necessity of working in a blue-collar job fostered independence. One Puerto Rican woman in New York City reacted against the traditional pattern of male dominance in her marriage: "Whether I have a husband or not, I work. So I do what I want,

and if my husband dare to complain, I throw him out." As more women worked, they postponed marriage. In 1980, 20 percent of women between the ages of 25 and 29 were still unmarried—double the percentage a decade earlier and at its highest point since 1890. It was a sharp reversal of the pattern set by the baby boomers' own parents.

With that reversal came an increasing awareness of the limits of a culture of abundance. During the mid-1970s and 1980s, as baby boomers matured, they discovered economic, social, and even biological limits on their independence. As single and even married women increasingly worked full-time outside the home, they increased the competition for jobs. When these pressures were added to the economic problems of the mid-1970s to early 1980s, wages and income levels began to stagnate or even shrink. Families in which wives also worked could make up for much of this loss. But in single-parent families, especially those headed by women, the burden of poverty proved especially heavy. By 1980, one out of seven families was headed by a woman and those families accounted for 40 percent of people below the poverty level.

In addition, women who postponed marriage for the sake of career were, in their mid-thirties, realizing that they would have to begin having children soon or risk the medical complications of an older childbirth. Biological constraints

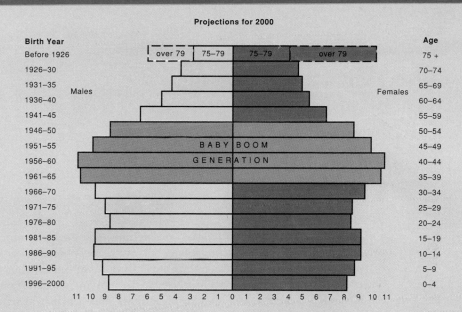

Projections for 2000

Birth Year		Age
Before 1926	over 79 75–79 ‖ 75–79 over 79	75 +
1926–30		70–74
1931–35	Males Females	65–69
1936–40		60–64
1941–45		55–59
1946–50		50–54
1951–55	BABY BOOM	45–49
1956–60	GENERATION	40–44
1961–65		35–39
1966–70		30–34
1971–75		25–29
1976–80		20–24
1981–85		15–19
1986–90		10–14
1991–95		5–9
1996–2000		0–4

11 10 9 8 7 6 5 4 3 2 1 0 1 2 3 4 5 6 7 8 9 10 11

also served to limit social experimentation, as sexually transmitted diseases such as herpes in the 1970s and, more seriously, AIDS in the 1980s made casual sex a riskier proposition.

As baby boomers advanced toward old age, serious long-term issues about the nature of American society were becoming clearer. For most of American history, the shape of the population in any given year resembled a pyramid, as in 1920. The high birth rates provided a broad base at the bottom and mortality rates winnowed the population to a small tip of elderly. But as fertility rates continued their two-century decline and higher living standards made it possible for Americans to live longer, the pyramid was being transformed more nearly into a cylinder. Only the temporary bulge of the baby boom distorted the shape.

With the period of adolescent education lengthening on the one hand and the number of retirees rising on the other hand, the proportion of the population working as productive adults will steadily decrease. At the same time, the burden of supporting both the education of their children and the care of elderly parents seems likely to increase. The generation raised to a sense of abundance, liberation, and control of its own destiny is finding itself experiencing limits that have always been a part of history.

33

The Vietnam Era

ietnam from afar looked almost like an emerald paradise. "I remember getting up on the flight deck and seeing one of the most beautiful visions I've ever seen in my life," recalled Thomas Bird, an army rifleman sent there in 1965: "A beautiful white beach with thick jungle background. The only thing missing was naked women running down the beach, waving and shouting 'Hello, hello, hello.'" Upon landing, Bird and his buddies were each issued a "Nine-Rule" card outlining proper behavior toward the Vietnamese. "Treat the women with respect, we are guests in this country and here to help these people."

But who were they helping and who were they fighting? When American troops sought to engage Vietcong forces, the VC generally disappeared into the jungle beyond the villages and rice fields. John Muir, a Marine rifleman, walked into a typical hamlet with a Korean lieutenant. To Muir the place looked ordinary, but the Korean had been in Vietnam a while. "We have a little old lady and a little old man and two very small children," he pointed out. "According to them, the rest of the family has been spirited away . . . either been drafted into one army or the other. So there's only four of them and they have a pot of rice that's big enough to feed fifty people. And rice, once it's cooked, will not keep. They gotta be feeding the VC." Muir, whose only experience with rice till then had been Minute Rice or Uncle Ben's, watched as the lieutenant set the house on fire. The roof "started cooking off ammunition because all through the thatch they had ammunition stored."

GIs soon learned to walk down jungle trails with a cautious shuffle, looking for a wire or a piece of vine that seemed too straight. "We took more casualties from booby traps than we did from actual combat," recalled David Ross, a medic. "It was very frustrating because how do you fight back against a booby trap? You're just walking along and all of a sudden your buddy doesn't have a leg. Or you don't have a leg." Yet somehow the villagers would walk the same paths and never get hurt. Who was the enemy and who the friend? "It's very easy to slip into a primitive state of mind," noted Marine Douglas Anderson, "particularly if your life is in danger and you can't trust anyone. . . . In one case I saw a young [American soldier], probably eighteen years old, push an old man into his family bunker inside his hootch [hut] and throw a grenade in after him. We'd been hit a lot that week and pressure had been building up. It wasn't anything that happened that day. But I remember this guy distinctly because he had a tattoo of a little red devil

In Vietnam helicopters gave infantry unusual mobility—a critical element in a war with no real front line, since troops could be quickly carried from one battle to another. These soldiers await a pickup amidst rice paddies south of Saigon.

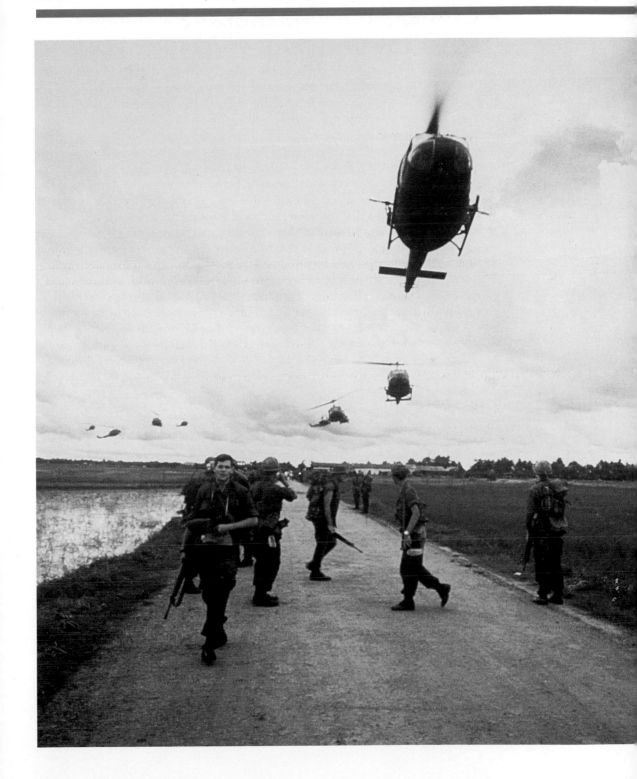

on his left arm and he had his shirt off when he threw the old man into the bunker and threw the grenade in after him."

Who was the friend and who the enemy? The same question was being asked half a globe away, on the campus of Kent State University in May 1970. By then the Vietnam War had dragged on for over five years, had driven President Lyndon Johnson from office and embroiled his successor, Richard Nixon, in a controversy over whether the fighting should be expanded into Cambodia. Kent State, just east of Akron, Ohio, was one of the many campuses that flourished in the 1950s and 1960s to accommodate the children of the baby boom. Normally it was an apolitical community, but opposition to the war had become so intense that 300 students had torn the Constitution from a history text and, in a formal ceremony, buried it, announcing that "President Nixon has murdered it." That evening demonstrators spilled over into the nearby town, smashed shop windows, and returned to campus to burn down an old Army ROTC building. The panicked mayor declared a state of emergency and Governor James Rhodes ordered in 750 of the National Guard. Student dissidents were the "worst type of people we harbor in America," he announced. "We are going to eradicate the problem."

By background and education, the National Guard troops were little different from the students they had come to police. Almost all were white, between 18 and 30, and from Ohio. Most had received only four months of active training before returning to their hometown units. Many treated the Guard much as they would a volunteer fire company. For some it was a second income; for others a weekend off every month with the guys; and for all, a sure way to avoid combat in Vietnam. Still, a political gulf separated most guardsmen from the student protesters. Many soldiers objected to the way antiwar forces criticized the president and the country. The officers, often veterans of World War II or Korea, particularly disap-

Crisis at Kent State: Who was the enemy, who the friend?

proved of students who evaded or openly rejected their military obligations. As his troops arrived at Kent, Guard Commander General Robert Canterbury remarked that "these students are going to have to find out what law and order is all about."

When the demonstrators assembled for a noon rally on the college commons, the Guard ordered them to disperse, although the troops' legal right to break up a peaceful demonstration was debatable. When the protesters did not disband the guardsmen advanced, wearing full battle gear and armed with M-1 rifles, whose high-velocity bullets had a horizontal range of almost two miles. Some students scattered; a few picked up rocks and threw them. The guardsmen then leveled their rifles and fired into the crowd, which included students passing back and forth from classes. Incredulous, a young woman knelt at the side of Jeffrey Miller, a student who lay dead. By the time calm was restored, three other students had been killed and nine more wounded, some caught innocently in the Guard's indiscriminate fire.

News of the killings swept the nation. At Jackson State, a black college in Mississippi, antiwar protesters seized a women's dormitory. On May 14 state police surrounded the building and without evident provocation opened fire, killing two more students and wounding a dozen. In both incidents the demonstrators had been unarmed. Before Kent and Jackson State there were sporadic strikes to protest the U.S. incursion of Cambodia. Afterward, hundreds of schools canceled classes for the week; nearly a third of all colleges had strikes of some sort. The ideals of the United States, it seemed to many, had been betrayed by those forces of law and order who were sworn to protect them.

Who was the friend and who the enemy? Time and again the war in Vietnam propelled conflicts in American society to the center of the political life of the nation. Vietnam did not create the counterculture and the radical student movement, but those elements would never have become so influential if the debate over Vietnam had not moved off college campuses and into the homes of middle Americans, where sons went off to fight and the war came home each night on the evening news. Vietnam did not create the civil rights issue, but it raised questions, as most wars do, of whether Vietnam was a "rich man's war and a poor man's fight," where sons of the upper and middle classes escaped battle by going to college while blacks and other poor draftees became sniper's targets along jungle trails. As no other war had, Vietnam seemed to stand the nation on its head. When American soldiers shot at Vietnamese "hostiles," who could not always be separated from "friendlies," or when National Guardsmen fired on their neighbors across a college green, who were the enemies and who were the friends?

THE ROAD TO VIETNAM

"The enemy must fight his battles far from his home base for a long time," one Vietnamese strategist wrote. "We must further weaken him by drawing him into protracted campaigns. Once his initial dash is broken, it will be easier to destroy him." The enemy in question was not American soldiers or even the French, but the Mongol invaders of A.D. 1284. For several thousand years Vietnam had struggled periodically to fight off foreign invasions. Influenced by Buddhist culture traveling eastward from India, it had also been invaded and ruled periodically by

The Geography of Vietnam

CHINA

NORTH VIETNAM

Lao Cai

Thai Nguyen

BURMA

Dien Bien Phu

Black R.

Red R.

Hanoi

Haiphong

GULF OF TONKIN

Mekong R.

Luang Prabang

PLAIN OF JARS

Thanh Hoa

LAOS

Hainan

Vientiane

Vinh

ANNAMESE

Con Thien

Quang Tri

SOUTH CHINA SEA

THAILAND

Sepone

Khe Sanh

Hue

Da Nang

Yom R.

Ping R.

Mun R.

CORDILLERA

My Lai

Quang Ngai

Po Sak R.

Kong R.

Dak To

Bangkok

Kon Tum

CAMBODIA

Pleiku

Qui Nhon

CENTRAL HIGHLANDS

Tuy Hoa

Tonle Sap

Mekong R.

SOUTH VIETNAM

Pursat

Nha Trang

Da Lat

Phnom Penh

Song Be

GULF OF THAILAND

Chau Doc

PLAIN OF REEDS

Saigon

Ben Tre

Can Tho

MEKONG RIVER DELTA

| 0 | | 100 | | 200 Miles |
| 0 | 100 | | 200 Kilometers | |

| → | Ho Chi Minh Trail |
| ★ | Major battles of Tet offensive |

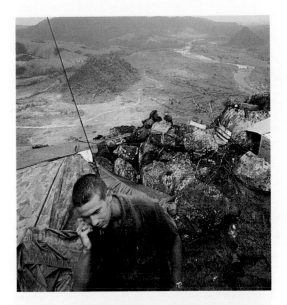

Stretching along a thousand-mile curve along the South China Sea, Vietnam covers an area about 20 percent smaller than California but 20 percent longer. The spine of the peninsula, the Annamese Cordillera, proved a formidable battleground for war. "We were flying parallel to the mountains," Philip Caputo recalled; "the Cordillera spread out before us, and it was the most forbidding thing I had ever seen. An unbroken mass of green stretched westward, one ridgeline and mountain range after another, some more than a mile high and covered with forests that looked solid enough to walk on." Near the border between North and South Vietnam, the terrain was particularly steep. "The Rockpile" (top left) a 1200-foot pyramid near Khe Sanh, commanded a strategic view of five valleys. "Its top had enough flat space for about two medium-sized dinner tables," reported one journalist, "and when weather permitted, helicopters ferried soldiers on and off via a rickety platform inches from a 900-foot drop."

North Vietnam established the Ho Chi Minh Trail through "neutral" Laos (center) in order to supply the Vietcong. In the early stages of the war, supplies were brought in on foot by soldiers carrying knapsacks as well as rice in socks wrapped around their waists. By 1964 the North Vietnamese were building roads and bridges that could handle heavy trucks. Because of the dense rain forest, even low-flying U.S. helicopters found it difficult to locate and bomb the trail.

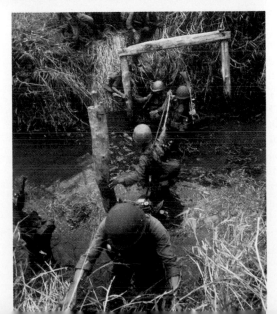

In the flatter terrain of the Mekong River delta to the south, rice paddies and jungle swamps proved equally hazardous (bottom). "On one patrol," recalled an artillery captain, "we had a man who had collected 80 leeches on his body. He died later from exhaustion and loss of blood. Another had a leech crawl through his penis into his bladder. Most of us are wearing prophylactics on patrol to prevent that, because it's painful as hell." In this war, geography, vegetation, and climate often proved as perilous foes as the Vietcong.

Nguyen Ai Quoc, who became Ho Chi Minh, once worked at London's posh Carlton Hotel in the pastry kitchen of the renowned French chef Escoffier. But he was soon swept up in socialist and nationalist politics, appearing at the Versailles Peace Conference (left) to plead for an independent Vietnam. By the time the United States was increasing its involvement in Vietnam, Ho had accumulated a lifetime of anticolonialist and revolutionary activity and become a revered leader of his people.

the Chinese from the north. After 1856 the French entered as a colonial power, bringing with them a strong Catholic tradition.

Ho Chi Minh was one Vietnamese who hoped his country would throw off the French influence as well as the Chinese. In 1912, at the age of 22, Ho gave up the poor life of a schoolteacher and hired out as a messboy on a French ocean liner. Traveling from Asia to Africa to Europe he lived quite literally on the underside of the colonial system: the rich and wealthy vacationing on the upper decks, the darker skinned laborers like Ho serving them below. On a brief visit to America he heard about the campaigns of the Ku Klux Klan. At the end of World War I, when President Wilson came to Versailles calling for self-determination for small nations, Ho bought a formal pin-striped suit at a second-hand store and attended the peace conference, petitioning on behalf of Vietnam. When his plea for independence was ignored, he became a communist, taking the recent Russian Revolution as his model. Visits to Moscow followed, with Ho returning to the Indochina region to organize revolutionary activity.

But it was only after the Japanese were driven out of Vietnam in 1945 that he was able to take advantage of the power vacuum and unite the country under a nationalist government. When France moved to recover control of its old colony, some of Ho's colleagues wanted to approach the Chinese Communists for help. But Ho was first and foremost a nationalist. He saw the age of colonialism dying and worried that Chinese aid might lead to permanent domination. "I prefer to smell French dung for five years rather than Chinese dung for the rest of my life," he concluded, and he allowed the French to return. Negotiations for independence soon broke down, however, so his forces fought eight years of guerrilla war before the French surrendered at Dien Bien Phu in 1954 (page 1136). At a peace conference held in Geneva, Ho agreed to withdraw his forces north of the 17th parallel, limiting his government to North Vietnam in return for the promise of free elections in both the North and the South. When the American-backed government of Ngo Dinh Diem refused to hold elections, South Vietnamese communists—the Vietcong—began their guerrilla war once again. "I think the Americans greatly underestimate the determination of the Vietnamese people," Ho remarked in 1962, as President Kennedy was committing more American advisers to South Vietnam.

Escalation at Tonkin Gulf

For Kennedy, Vietnam had been just one of many communist skirmishes which his activist advisers wanted to fight—in Cuba, in Africa, in Laos (Vietnam's western neighbor). But even 16,000 American "advisers" had been unable to help the unpopular Diem, who was overthrown by the military in November 1963. With renewed attention focused on Vietnam, Kennedy accepted President Eisenhower's "domino theory": if the pro-Western Catholic government fell to the Communists, the other nations of Southeast Asia would collapse like a row of dominos. The United States therefore had to support this government. When Kennedy was assassinated the same month as Diem, the problem of Vietnam was left to Lyndon Johnson.

Johnson's political instincts told him to keep the Vietnam War at arm's length. He felt like a catfish, he remarked, who had "just grabbed a big juicy worm with a right sharp hook in the middle of it." His primary concerns were with domestic issues: passing a tax cut, pushing his war on poverty, and drawing up the Great Society programs. Yet despite his caution, Johnson moved steadily toward deeper American involvement in Vietnam. He shared the cold war assumptions of Kennedy holdovers like National Security Adviser McGeorge Bundy and Defense Secretary Robert McNamara and succumbed to their pressure to apply containment to Vietnam's civil war. Johnson also was sensitive in 1964 to criticism from the Republican presidential candidate Barry Goldwater, who called for an end to appeasement and a "let's-win" policy of total military victory.

Until August 1964 American action had focused on combating the Vietcong within South Vietnam. North Vietnam, for its part, had been infiltrating a modest amount of men and supplies along the Ho Chi Minh Trail, a primitive network of jungle routes threading through Laos and Cambodia into the highlands of South Vietnam. In the summer of 1964 North Vietnam began to modernize the trail, allowing it to handle large trucks in addition to the peasants who carried supplies on their backs or used modified bicycles. At the time American officials were unaware of the change, but they realized all too well that the Vietcong already controlled some 40 percent of South Vietnamese territory. Pressure mounted in Washington to turn matters around. One option was to put more pressure on North Vietnam itself.

So President Johnson sent a number of American ships to the Gulf of Tonkin. Laden with electronic snooping gear, they patrolled the North Vietnamese coast while South Vietnamese ships conducted raids. On August 2, three North Vietnamese patrol boats exchanged fire with the American destroyer *Maddox*—neither side hurting the other—and then the Vietnamese boats fled. An outraged Johnson chided several shamefaced admirals. "You've got a whole fleet and all those airplanes, and you can't even sink three little ol' PT boats?" Two nights later, in inky blackness and a heavy thunderstorm, radar operators on the *C. Turner Joy* reported a torpedo attack. But a follow-up investigation could not be sure whether enemy ships had even been near the scene. "The Gulf is a very funny place," explained one communications officer. "You get inversion layers there that will give you very solid radar contacts . . . that just aren't there. That may have happened to us." The president was not pleased. "For all I know our navy might have been shooting at whales out there," he remarked privately.

Whatever his doubts, the president announced publicly that American ships had been attacked. Calling the incidents "open aggression on the high sea," he ordered retaliatory air raids on North Vietnam. He did not disclose that the Navy and South Vietnamese forces had been conducting secret military operations at the time. Such deception would become standard practice. It abetted Johnson's decision to ask Congress for authority to take "all necessary measures" to "repel any armed attack" on American forces and to "prevent future aggression." Congress jumped at the opportunity, passing what became known as the Gulf of Tonkin resolution by a lopsided vote of 414–0 in the House and 88–2 in the Senate. The action seemed to show Goldwater supporters that Johnson, too, could act firmly, and his popularity rose sharply.

Senator Ernest Gruening of Alaska, who with Wayne Morse of Oregon had been the only lawmakers to object, warned that the Tonkin Gulf Resolution gave the president "a blank check" to declare war, a power which the Constitution specifically reserved to Congress. Johnson insisted—no doubt sincerely at the time—that he had no such intention. But as pressure for an American victory increased, the president exploited the powers the resolution gave him.

Rolling Thunder

No sooner had Johnson taken the oath of office in January 1965 than he received a disturbing memorandum from McGeorge Bundy and Robert McNamara. "Both of us are now pretty well convinced that our present policy can lead only to disastrous defeat," they said. The United States should either increase its attack— "escalate" was the term coined in 1965—or simply withdraw. The idea behind escalation was to increase military pressure to the point at which further resistance cost more than the enemy was willing to risk, either militarily or politically. By taking gradual steps, the United States would demonstrate its resolve to win while leaving the door open to negotiations. But the theory that made so much sense in the planning rooms of the Pentagon did not work well in practice. Each stage of American escalation only hardened the resolve of the Vietcong and North Vietnamese. When a Vietcong mortar attack in February killed seven Marines stationed at Pleiku airbase, Johnson informed the nation that U.S. planes would begin bombing North Vietnam. Privately, McGeorge Bundy admitted that Pleiku was only an excuse to act. "Pleikus are like street cars," he remarked; "there's one every ten minutes."

Restricted air strikes did not satisfy more hawkish leaders like retired Air Force Chief of Staff General Curtis LeMay. "We are swatting flies when we should be going after the whole manure pile," he complained. In March Johnson ordered Operation Rolling Thunder, a systematic bombing campaign aimed at bolstering confidence in South Vietnam and cutting the flow of supplies from the North. At the same time, he declared his willingness to negotiate and consider a vast irrigation project, TVA-style, once North Vietnamese troops had left the South. But

LEVELS OF U.S. TROOPS IN
VIETNAM (AT YEAR-END)

Source : U.S. Department of Defense.

Rolling Thunder achieved none of its goals. An impenetrable jungle canopy made the Ho Chi Minh Trail nearly impossible for American fighter pilots to spot from the air, so that supplies and troops flowed south without interruption. Even when bombs found their targets, North Vietnamese crews quickly filled in craters or spanned rivers with pontoon bridges made of bamboo stalks. Equally discouraging, the ever-changing military governments in South Vietnam carried on ineptly while Ho Chi Minh refused to negotiate unless the bombing stopped and American troops went home.

Once the Americans established bases from which to launch the new air strikes, these too became vulnerable to guerrilla attacks. When General William Westmoreland, the chief of American military operations in Vietnam, requested combat troops to defend the bases, Johnson sent in 3500 Marines, almost without considering the implication of his decision. Until then, only military "advisers" to the South Vietnamese had been sent. Once the crucial decision to commit combat troops had been taken, the urge to send more—to shore up and protect those already there—became strong. Another 40,000 soldiers arrived in May and 50,000 more by July. By then Johnson realized how serious his commitment was, but fearful of a political backlash, he deliberately downplayed the escalation. McNamara ordered the decision carried out in a "low-keyed manner," both to prevent Soviet or Chinese intervention and "to avoid undue concern and excitement in the Congress and in domestic public opinion." By the end of 1965 almost 185,000 American troops had landed—and still the call for more continued. In 1968, at the height of the war, 536,000 American troops were being supported with helicopters, jet aircraft, and other advanced military technologies. This was "escalation" with a vengeance.

SOCIAL CONSEQUENCES OF THE WAR

The greatest social impact of the war, naturally enough, fell first on the baby-boom generation of the 1950s. These young people came of age at a time when, on the one hand, draft calls for the armed services were rising and, on the other, the civil rights movement and the growing counterculture were encouraging students to question the goals of establishment America. The social experiences of both the Americans who fought and those who protested at home eventually forced Americans of all ages to come to grips with Vietnam.

The Soldiers' War

The social structure determining which Americans would be required to fight and which would remain civilian was the draft. The system in place generally favored the middle and upper classes, since college students and graduate students at first received deferments. Thus the Vietnam War increased male enrollment in colleges. As the war escalated the draft was changed, so that some students were called up through a lottery system. Still, those who knew the medical requirements might be able to produce a doctor's affidavit certifying a weak knee, flat feet, or bad eyes—all grounds for flunking the physical. About half of the potential draftees flunked—two to three times the rejection rate of those called up by the NATO allies. Of the 1200 men in Harvard's class of 1970, only 56 served in the military, and only 2 of them in Vietnam. The poorest and least educated were also likely to escape service, because the Armed Forces Qualification Test and the physical often screened them out. Thus the sons of blue-collar America were most likely to accept Uncle Sam's letter of induction, as were the sons of Hispanic and black Americans who, having fewer skills, were more often assigned to combat duty. The draft also made it a relatively young man's war. The average soldier serving in Vietnam was 19, compared with 26 years old for World War II.

Once in Vietnam, life for the ordinary "grunt"—infantry man—was a matter of trying to fight an uncertain enemy. Most soldiers came to Vietnam fairly well trained and with high morale, but the physical and psychological hardships took their toll. In a war of continual small skirmishes, booby traps, and search and destroy missions, it was hard to relax. What was especially frustrating was that success could not be measured in terms of territory gained. An American force would fight its way into a communist-controlled hamlet, clear and burn it, move on—and be ordered back to the same place days or weeks later, because the enemy had moved in again. The main measure of success in such a war soon became the "body count": the number of Vietcong who had been killed. And since most officers wanted to look as good as possible, body counts were inflated as the numbers were passed up the ranks. Furthermore, the strain of not being able to tell who was friendly and who was hostile made it all too easy for GIs to take out their frustrations on innocent civilians.

Other social factors affected morale and the way soldiers fought. Most new recruits were sent to Vietnam as individuals, not as part of units. This was a departure from usual military tradition, and it meant that there was little camaraderie between soldiers—a key requirement for good fighting. Combat veterans felt less sympathy for the raw replacements who joined them and often despised the rear-echelon or "REMF" soldiers who superintended supply depots or received combat pay for being lifeguards at beaches near Da Nang. Paradoxically, the miracles of modern technology also made the war hard to cope with. Because helicopters could whisk GIs from the front lines of a steaming jungle back to Saigon—where they could catch overnight flights to Hawaii or the mainland—the transition from the hell of war to civilian peace could be wrenching. John Kerry, later to become senator from Massachusetts, recalled his homecoming: "There I was, a week out of the jungle, flying from San Francisco to New York. I fell asleep and woke up yelling, probably a nightmare. The other passengers moved away from me—a reaction I noticed more and more in the months ahead. . . . The feeling toward [Vietnam vets] was, 'Stay away—don't contaminate us with whatever you've brought back from Vietnam.'"

Technology and Its Limits

Escalation of the war meant that American forces brought in the most technologically advanced equipment available. The transformation of South Vietnam was astonishing. By 1967 a million tons of supplies was being shipped to Vietnam each month—an average of a hundred pounds a day for every American in the country. Huge cranes, tractors, and barges built warehouses, barracks, and airfields. South Vietnam's airports soon handled more flight traffic than New York, Rome, Tokyo, or any other city in the world. The average soldier carried an automatic rifle that could discharge hundreds of rounds a minute, compared to French forces from the 1950s, whose rifles had clips of 8 or 10 rounds. Ground forces could also count on repeated air strikes to strafe or bomb enemy territory with thousands of shells before they marched in. Troops were provided with infrared sniper scopes and other instruments to help spot nighttime attackers. If technology could have won the war, Americans would have triumphed.

But technology alone could not make the difference, and it raised ethical issues as well. War is always hell, but where friendly and hostile civilian populations were mixed, the chances for deadly error increased. Bombs of napalm (jellied gasoline) and white phosphorus rained liquid fire from the skies, coating everything from village huts to the flesh of fleeing humans. Cluster bombs were designed to explode hundreds of pellets in midair, spraying the enemy with high-velocity shrapnel. To clear jungle canopies and expose Vietcong camps and roads, American planes sprayed more than 100 million pounds of defoliants such as Agent Orange. ("Only You Can Prevent Forests" was the sardonic motto of one unit assigned to the task.) The forests that were destroyed totaled over one-third of South Vietnam's timberlands—an area approximately the size of the state of Rhode Island. The long-term health and ecological effects were severe.

By 1967 the United States was spending more than $2 billion a month on the war. It dropped more bombs on Vietnam than it had during all of World War II. After one air attack on the communist-held provincial capital of Ben Tre, American troops walked into the remains, now mostly ruined buildings and rubble. "We had to destroy the town in order to save it," an officer explained. As the human and material costs of the war increased, that statement stuck in the minds of many observers. How far could the technology of war be taken before it ran headlong into limits? Such questions provoked anguished debate among Americans as the effects of the war came home.

Daily Lives

TIME AND TRAVEL
The Race to the Moon

In campaigning for the presidency in 1960 John F. Kennedy chided the Republicans for a losing effort in the space race with the Soviet Union. While the American program limped along, the Soviets leapt ahead. Only a few months after Kennedy's inauguration, Russian cosmonaut Yuri Gagarin orbited the world in a five-ton spacecraft lifted aloft by rocket engines far more powerful than any the United States possessed. On May 6, 1961, an Atlas rocket did carry Commander Alan Shepard into space, but that was merely a 15-minute suborbital flight of 300 miles. Kennedy feared that in losing the space race, the United States might lose the cold war as well. Nations around the world whose hearts and minds the superpowers struggled to win might conclude that the Soviet Union possessed superior technology and leadership.

Thus Kennedy ordered his science advisers "to shift our efforts in space from low to high gear." To Congress and a national television audience he announced that the United States would do something truly dramatic: land a man on the moon and bring him back alive "before the decade is out." The cost in money and scientific talent would be considerable, but to Kennedy, the investment was sound. "This is not merely a race," he remarked in an allusion to the Soviets' success. "Space is open to us now; and our eagerness to share its meaning is not governed by the efforts of others. We must go into space because whatever mankind must undertake, free men must fully share."

The president's enthusiasm for this enormous undertaking did not win universal acclaim. Former President Eisenhower thought anyone was "nuts" to spend billions for a space spectacular that promised little in the way of scientific discoveries. Nor was it clear that NASA could achieve such a feat in so short a time. Yet Congress, perhaps seeing the space program as a huge pork barrel, voted to fund Kennedy's "great new American enterprise." From then on the space program achieved a string of triumphs. In February 1962 Colonel John Glenn successfully circled the earth three times in "a fireball of a ride"; an unmanned satellite passed Venus later that year; and a Telstar communications satellite began relaying television broadcasts, launching an era of truly global mass communications.

One after another, the space spectaculars continued, much to the public's delight. In March 1965 American astronauts first maneuvered their capsule; in May Edward White took America's first space walk; the following year two vehicles met and docked for the first time. The Gemini program was followed by the Apollo missions, whose Saturn rockets provided the power necessary to launch payloads into lunar orbit. From there, two astronauts planned to pilot a separate module to the moon's surface, while a third remained in the orbiting command module waiting for them and the return trip. Although a fire during ground tests killed three astronauts in 1967, by Christmas eve 1968 a successful Apollo 8 mission was circling the moon. It seemed a "vast, lonely and forbidding sight," one astronaut remarked to hundreds of millions in a live telecast.

On July 20, 1969, the lunar module of Apollo 11 at last touched down on the earth's closest neighbor. Commander Neil Armstrong, moving awkwardly in his bulky spacesuit, worked his way down a ladder to the white, chalky surface. He

Daily Lives

Landing on the moon may have been one small step for a man, but NASA spent $25 billion on the project, over $2 billion for each of the 12 astronauts who took lunar walks.

and left behind devices to measure seismic tremors and solar winds.

Exploration had come a long way in the centuries since the first European mariners pressed westward across the Atlantic. In both cases, exploring parties ventured outward with only the most tenuous links to their home bases. But twentieth-century astronauts were backed by an immense array of instruments, detailed photographic mapping of their proposed landing sites, and hundreds of mission controllers monitoring everything from blood pressure to fuel-tank valves. The economic commitment and the necessary second-by-second coordination could have been provided only by a technologically complex industrial society.

Still, the politics of both eras shaped the course of exploration, whether to the Americas or to the moon. Machines, after all, could have performed most of the moon mission's tasks, at far less risk and expense. Just as Portugal, England, and Spain used explorers to vie for national advantage, so Kennedy seized on the moon missions as a demonstration of American enterprise in the cold war. And NASA bureaucrats cannily recognized that the glamour of a manned space program established the necessary popular support for billion-dollar outlays.

While critics argued that those billions might better have been funneled into research on more earthly problems, Presidents Kennedy, Johnson, and Nixon all responded to the need for symbolic conquests along New Frontiers—and so, apparently, did the public. The creators of television's "Star Trek," a science fiction program originally popular in the 1960s, put its Kennedyesque hero, Captain James T. Kirk, in command of the starship *Enterprise*, "to boldly go where no man has gone before."

was not alone. Besides Edwin Aldrin, who followed him, and Michael Collins, orbiting in the command module, Armstrong brought along a quarter of the world's population, who monitored the moment live on television. "That's one small step for a man, one giant leap for mankind," he proclaimed. By the time the Apollo series concluded its missions in 1972, American astronauts had roamed the lunar surface in roving vehicles, taken geologic samples,

The War Comes Home

College campuses became the center of growing opposition to American involvement in Vietnam. Faculty members held "teach-ins" to explain the issues to concerned students. Scholars familiar with Southeast Asia, like George Kahin at Cornell University and foreign affairs specialist Hans Morgenthau, questioned every major assumption the president used to justify escalation. The United States and South Vietnam had instigated the war, Kahin charged, by violating the Geneva accords of 1954. Moreover, the Vietcong were an indigenous rebel force with legitimate grievances against Saigon's corrupt government. That made the war a civil war among the Vietnamese, not an effort by Soviet or Chinese Communists to conquer Southeast Asia, as Eisenhower, Kennedy, and Johnson had claimed. Finally, dissidents argued that profound differences in Asian and Western culture made it impossible to impose an American solution with troops or diplomacy.

By 1966 national leaders had similarly divided into opposing camps of "hawks" and "doves." The hawks argued that America must win in Vietnam to save Southeast Asia from Communism, to preserve the nation's prestige, and to protect the lives of American soldiers fighting the war. A large majority of the American people supported those views. The doves were nonetheless a prominent minority. They included New Left radicals like Tom Hayden, actress Jane Fonda, and folk singer Joan Baez as well as respected editorialist Walter Lippmann, Senator J. William Fulbright, head of the Foreign Relations Committee, and Dr. Benjamin Spock, the physician whose child-care manuals had raised the generation of baby-boomers sent to fight in Vietnam. Blacks as a group were far less likely than whites to support the war. Some resented the diversion of resources from the cities to the war effort. Even more important, many blacks' heightened sense of racial consciousness led them to identify with the Vietnamese people. Martin Luther King, SNCC, and CORE all opposed the war. Black heavyweight champion Muhammad Ali joined the Black Muslims and the international Islamic movement, refusing to be inducted into the army on religious grounds. And black poet Nikki Giovanni set into vivid phrases her own sense of alienation:

> We kill in Vietnam
> for them
> We kill for UN&NATO&SEATO&US
> And everywhere for all alphabet but BLACK.

By 1967 the antiwar crusade had swept college campuses. Students and faculty turned out in crowds of thousands to express their outrage: "Hey, hey, LBJ, how many kids have you killed today?" Over 300,000 people attended the demonstration organized in April 1967 in New York City. Sixty college protesters organized by SDS leaders from Cornell University burned their draft cards in defiance of federal law. In the fall more violent protests erupted as antiwar radicals stormed a draft induction center in Oakland, California. The next day 55,000 protesters including the novelist Norman Mailer and poet Robert Lowell ringed the Pentagon in Washington. Again, mass arrests followed.

Student protests and demonstrations forced policymakers and citizens to take a sobering look at the justice of the war. But the guerrilla tactics of more radical elements alienated many. It would be hard to exaggerate the shock university communities felt when radicals shut down Columbia University and clashed with

Lyndon Johnson shocked reporters in October 1965 when he publicly exposed his surgical scar from a gallbladder operation. Political caricaturist David Levine caught the underlying tragedy of the Johnson presidency by drawing the scar in the shape of Vietnam.

police for a week in 1968 or the following year when black militant students—bandoleers draped across their shoulders, shotguns at their sides—seized the student union at Cornell. Even more shocking, a graduate student at the University of Wisconsin was killed in his lab when a bomb exploded there. The device had been planted by radicals protesting government-sponsored defense research.

On the other hand, key moderates both within and outside the government became convinced that victory was beyond the resources of the United States. Senator Fulbright, who helped President Johnson push the Tonkin Gulf Resolution through the Senate, held televised hearings that were highly critical of American policy. *Time* and *Life* magazines, run by the hawkish publisher Henry Luce, made a dramatic editorial turnabout in 1967. Even the strongest supporters of the war felt the pressure. Secretary of State Dean Rusk, a hard-liner throughout, was dismayed to hear his relatives back home in Cherokee County, Georgia: "Dean, if you can't tell us when this war is going to end, well then, maybe we just ought to chuck it."

Defense Secretary Robert McNamara became the most dramatic defector from the establishment position. For years the statistically minded secretary had struggled to quantify the success of the war effort. General William Westmoreland duly provided body counts, number of bombs dropped, and pacification reports, all sufficient to convince McNamara that there was indeed a "light at the end of the tunnel." But by 1967 the secretary had become skeptical. If Americans actually were killing 300,000 Vietnamese, enemy forces should be shrinking. Instead, intelligence estimates indicated that North Vietnamese infiltration had risen from 35,000 a year in 1965 to 150,000 by the end of 1967. McNamara had also come to have doubts about the morality of the situation. "The picture of the world's greatest superpower killing or seriously injuring 1,000 non-combatants a week, while trying to pound a tiny, backward nation into submission on an issue whose merits are hotly disputed, is not a pretty one," he advised. Johnson, however, was determined not to be labeled the first American president who lost a war, especially when hawks like Senator John Stennis of Mississippi and General Westmoreland were pressing to escalate further. And so McNamara resigned.

As the war dragged on, it had one other social consequence: inflation. With the president unwilling to negotiate a retreat, the cost of the war soared to over $50 billion a year. Medicare, education, housing, and other Great Society programs raised the domestic budget sharply too. Through it all Johnson refused to raise taxes, and the result was a rise in wages and prices. From 1950 to 1960 the average rate of inflation hovered at about 2 percent a year. From 1965 to 1970, as the war escalated, it jumped to around 4 percent. The rise was not perceived as serious at first, but the seeds were sown for future trouble.

THE UNRAVELING

Almost all the forces dividing America seemed to converge in 1968, when some of the harsh costs of the war became clear. Until January of that year, most Americans had reason to believe that the United States was gaining ground, whatever private doubts had arisen among Lyndon Johnson's advisers and whatever campus protesters might say. Military leaders sent back optimistic figures about mounting enemy casualties. Television relayed home footage of American soldiers on helicopter raids, search and destroy patrols, bombing missions. With the exception of a few correspondents like David Halberstam of the New York *Times* and independent journalists like Bernard Fall, almost no one provided insight into the Vietnamese side of the war. As one network journalist commented, "It's an American war in Asia and that's the only story the American audience is interested in."

Tet Offensive

The Vietcong's Tet offensive in January 1968 changed the American perspective. Tet, the most festive of Vietnamese celebrations, marks the coming of the lunar new year. In previous years it had been observed by an informal cease-fire. But on the night of January 30, 1968, Vietcong guerrillas launched a concerted attack on 36 of the 44 provincial capitals of South Vietnam. Assault targets included Saigon's major airport, the South Vietnamese presidential palace, and Hue, the ancient Vietnamese imperial capital. Perhaps most unnerving to Americans, 19 crack Vietcong commandos blasted a hole in the wall of the American embassy compound in Saigon and stormed in. When they were unable to breach the embassy's heavy main door, they fought in the courtyard until all 19 lay dead. One reporter, stunned by the carnage, compared the courtyard to a "butcher shop."

The Tet offensive had been in the planning for nearly half a year. Deliberately, the North Vietnamese had lured American troops to the hinterlands of South Vietnam to engage in pitched battles at remote outposts like Khe Sanh, Con Thien, Song Be, and Dak To. As American forces were deployed in response, the Vietcong infiltrated major population areas of Saigon and the delta region. Weapons were smuggled in on vegetable carts and a few audacious VC, disguised as South Vietnamese soldiers, even hitched rides on American jeeps and trucks. The attack caught American troops off guard, but they quickly counterattacked, repulsing most of the assaults. Hue, the communists' biggest conquest, took three weeks to retake. Appearing before the American press, General Westmoreland announced that the Vietcong had "very deceitfully" taken advantage of the Vietnamese holiday "to create maximum consternation" and that their "well-laid plans went afoul."

In a narrow military sense, Westmoreland was right. The enemy had been driven back, sustaining perhaps 40,000 deaths compared to 1100 American and 2300 South Vietnamese soldiers' lives lost—a ratio of over 10 to 1 (though 12,500 civilians died). But such military considerations paled beside the message that Americans at home received from Tet. Westmoreland, Johnson, and other officials had repeatedly asserted that the Vietcong were on their last legs. Yet as Ho Chi Minh had cooly informed the French after World War II, "You can kill ten of my men for every one I kill of yours . . . even at those odds, you will lose and I will win." Now the Vietcong had launched a nationwide offense and even penetrated the defenses of the American embassy. Tet created a "credibility gap" between the administration's promises and the harsh reality of the situation. Highly respected CBS news anchor Walter Cronkite drew a gloomy lesson of Tet for his national audience: "To say that we are mired in stalemate seems the only realistic, yet unsatisfactory, conclusion."

The sheer brutality of the war came home, too. Americans were used to combat footage on the nightly news, but few were prepared for an NBC report from Saigon at the height of Tet. It showed South Vietnamese police chief Nguyen Ngoc Loan approaching a recently captured Vietcong suspect, brusquely pulling out his pistol, and shooting him through the head. Two months later, with American troops increasingly edgy about Vietcong attacks, Lieutenant William Calley moved American troops into the hamlet of My Lai, rounded up the villagers, and executed over 200 men, women, and children. The dead of My Lai would have been just more figures in the "body count," except that an army photographer had taken pictures and a helicopter pilot intervened. If returning veterans were to be believed, there had been hundreds of similar incidents, though perhaps few as bloody. On the communist side, vengeance was at times even more severe. Before Hue could be retaken, the Vietcong had shot, clubbed to death, or buried alive perhaps 3000 residents, many of them innocent civilians.

The Tet offensive left Lyndon Johnson sobered and unsure how to react. On the one hand, General Westmoreland was requesting an additional 206,000 troops on top of the half million already in Vietnam. The Joint Chiefs of Staff backed him. But the new secretary of defense, Clark Clifford, became a surprise convert for deescalation. Clifford was a Johnson loyalist through and through, and a stalwart believer in the war. But in sizing up the situation in his new position as defense secretary, he could get no satisfactory answers from his generals. "How long would it take to succeed in Vietnam?" Clifford recalled asking them.

> They didn't know. How many more troops would it take? They couldn't say. Were two hundred thousand the answer? They weren't sure. Might they need more? Yes, they might need more. Could the enemy build up [their own troop strength] in exchange? Probably. So what was the plan to win the war? Well, the only plan was that attrition would wear out the Communists, and they would have had enough. Was there any indication that we've reached that point? No, there wasn't.

Clifford backed up his own judgment by bringing together a panel of "wise men," including such respected pillars of the cold war establishment as Dean Acheson,

Harry Truman's secretary of state; Henry Cabot Lodge, a Republican and former ambassador to South Vietnam; and several distinguished retired generals. The panel told the president that his advisers had led him "down the garden path" on Vietnam. The war could not be won, and he should seek a negotiated settlement.

Meanwhile, the antiwar forces had found a political champion in Senator Eugene McCarthy from Wisconsin. McCarthy was something of a maverick in the Senate—he wrote poetry in his spare time—but he announced that no matter what the odds, he would challenge Johnson by running for the presidency. Idealistic college students, instructed to get haircuts and shaves in order to look "clean for Gene," canvassed New Hampshire voters, lining up support for the first presidential primary. Johnson had not formally entered the 1968 presidential race, but his supporters sponsored a write-in campaign, confident of a decisive win. When the votes were counted, McCarthy had lost by only 300 out of 50,000 votes cast (crossover voting allowed Republicans to vote for him). For the president, so slim a victory was a stunning defeat. It encouraged Robert Kennedy, John Kennedy's younger brother, to announce his own candidacy in opposition to the war.

"I've got to get me a peace proposal," the president told Clifford, and the White House speechwriters went to work. They finally put together an announcement that bombing raids against North Vietnam would be halted, at least partially, in hopes that peace talks could begin. They were still trying to write an ending when Johnson told them, "Don't worry; I may have a little ending of my own." On March 31 he supplied it, announcing: "I have concluded that I should not permit the presidency to become involved in the partisan divisions that are developing in this political year. . . . Accordingly I shall not seek, and I will not accept, the nomination of my party for another term as your president."

The announcement shocked Johnson's advisers and, perhaps even more, those who had opposed him for so long. The Vietnam War had pulled down one of the savviest, most effective politicians of the era. North Vietnam, for its part, responded to the speech by sending delegates to a peace conference in Paris, where negotiations quickly bogged down. And American attention soon focused on the chaotic situation at home, where all the turbulence, discontent, and violence of the 1960s seemed to be coming together.

The Shocks of 1968

On April 4 Martin Luther King, Jr., traveled to Memphis to lead a demonstration in support of striking sanitation workers. He had checked into his motel room and was relaxing on the balcony when James Earl Ray, an escaped convict, fatally shot him with a sniper's rifle. Over the years King had maintained his commitment to nonviolence, despite more militant calls for black power. But the frustration and anger that greeted news of his death could not be contained. Riots broke out that evening in ghetto areas of the nation's capital; by the end of the week, 125 more neighborhoods across the country had seen similar disturbances. Almost before Americans could recover, a disgruntled Arab nationalist, Sirhan Sirhan, assassinated Robert Kennedy on the evening of June 5. Running in opposition to the war, Kennedy had just won a crucial primary victory in California.

The deaths of King and Kennedy raised painful questions about lost possibilities in American politics. In their own ways, both men exemplified the liberal tradition, which reached its high-water mark in the 1960s. King espoused a Christian theology of nonviolence to bring about change without resorting to the lan-

Enthusiastic crowds followed Robert Kennedy on his Democratic primary campaign during the 1968 presidential election. The evening of his victory in California he was assassinated by a Palestinian refugee, Sirhan Sirhan, who later claimed he admired Kennedy.

guage of the gun. He had broadened his campaign in his final years to include the poor of all races. Robert Kennedy had begun his career as a pragmatic politician who, like his brother John, had not hesitated to use power ruthlessly. But Kennedy, like King, had a capacity to change and grow. He had come to reject the war which his brother had supported, and despite his upper-class background he seemed genuinely to sympathize with the poor and minorities. At the same time, he had a good deal of popularity among traditional white ethnics and blue-collar workers. Would the liberal political tradition have had a longer life if these two charismatic figures had survived the turbulence of the sixties?

Violence denied them the chance to answer. And with Eugene McCarthy failing to gain the support of blacks, traditional workers, or party professionals, it became clear that Lyndon Johnson's faithful vice president, Hubert Humphrey, would be the choice of the Democrats when their convention met at Chicago in August. It meant, too, that no major candidate would speak for the growing numbers of Americans disillusioned with the war and searching for ways to bring the currents of reform into the mainstream of politics. The Republicans had already chosen Richard Nixon, a traditional anticommunist (now reborn as the "new," more moderate Nixon), along with little-known conservative governor from Maryland, Spiro Agnew, for vice president. As much as radicals disliked Johnson, they had an even greater distaste for Nixon, "new" or old. And although Hubert Humphrey had begun his career as a progressive and a strong supporter of civil rights, he was now intimately associated with the war and the old-style liberal reforms that could never satisfy radicals.

Chicago, where the Democratic National Convention met, was the fiefdom of

Mayor Richard Daley, long the symbol of machine politics and backroom deals. Daley was determined that the radicals who poured into Chicago would not disrupt "his" convention, just as the radicals were equally determined that they would. For a week the police skirmished with demonstrators: police clubs, riot gear, and tear gas versus the demonstrators' eggs, rocks, and balloons filled with paint and urine. When Daley refused to allow a peaceful march past the convention site, the radicals marched anyway and, with the mayor's blessing, the police turned on the crowd in what a federal commission later labeled a police riot. In one pitched battle, many officers took off their badges and waded into the crowd, nightsticks swinging, chanting, "Kill, kill, kill." Reporters, medics, and other innocent bystanders were injured; at 3:00 a.m. police invaded candidate Eugene McCarthy's hotel headquarters and pulled some of his assistants from their beds. With feelings running so high, President Johnson did not dare to make an appearance at his own party's convention. Theodore White, a veteran journalist covering the assemblage, scribbled his verdict in a notebook as police chased hippies down Michigan Avenue. "The Democrats are finished," he wrote.

Whose Silent Majority?

Radicals were not the only Americans alienated from the political system in 1968. Governor George Wallace of Alabama sensed that the times were ripe for an appeal to disgruntled voters among the "average man on the street, this man in the textile mill, this man in the steel mill, this barber, this beautician, the policeman on the beat." In short, he sought the support of blue-collar workers and the lower middle classes. Wallace had first come to national attention as he stood at the door barring integration of the University of Alabama, and then as a feisty presidential candidate in 1964. For the race in 1968 he formed his own American Independent party and chose as his running mate the hawkish General Curtis LeMay, who spoke belligerently of the United States' ability to bomb North Vietnam "back to the stone age."

Wallace made no effort to mask his appeal to divisiveness. His enemies were the "liberals, intellectuals, and long hairs [who] have run this country for too long." He gleefully taunted the bearded protesters who came to heckle him. "You can come up here and I'll autograph your sandals," he would call, and the pro-Wallace crowd roared its support. Indeed, when security became too tight at a New York City rally, Wallace's managers secretly dispensed a number of tickets to radicals in order to provoke the desired confrontation. On the other hand, Wallace's campaign was not merely an appeal to law and order, militarism, and white backlash; he was too sharp for that. Coming out of a tradition of southern populism, he called for federal job-training programs, stronger unemployment benefits, national health insurance, a higher minimum wage, and a further extension of union rights. Polls in September revealed that many supporters of Robert Kennedy had shifted their allegiance to Wallace. A quarter of all union members backed him, compared with 32 percent for Nixon and 34 percent for Humphrey. Without the tug of party loyalties, many more workers would have defected.

In fact, Wallace had tapped true discontent among the working class. Many blue-collar workers who despised hippies and peace marchers nonetheless wanted the United States out of Vietnam. And they were suspicious, as Wallace was, of the upper-class "establishment" which held power. "We can't understand how all those rich kids—the kids with beards from the suburbs—how they got off when my son had to go over there and maybe get his head shot off," one blue-collar parent complained. Old-style radicals of the 1930s might have tried to channel and organize such discontent, but the leaders of the New Left by and large gave up on traditional workers, preferring to aim their appeal at the newer minorities: students, Hispanics, blacks, and the unorganized poor.

Who, then, would earn the votes of this shifting group of workers, white ethnic groups, and "ordinary" Americans fed up with the war? Martin Luther King and Robert Kennedy had tried to include them in a newer definition of liberal reform. George Wallace appealed to traditional populist themes and underlying racial resentment. And Richard Nixon, too, sought to bring these traditionally Democratic voters, especially disaffected southern Democrats, into the Republican party.

The Republicans, of course, had been reviled by the populists of old as representatives of the Money Power, Monopoly, and the old-line establishment. (Eisenhower's cabinet, after all, had been characterized as "eight millionaires and a plumber.") But Richard Nixon himself had modest roots. His parents owned a general store in Whittier, California, where he had worked to help the family out. His high school grades were good enough to earn him a scholarship to Harvard, but he turned it down in favor of nearby Whittier College, fearing he could not afford the cost of transportation. At Duke Law School he was so pinched for funds he lived in an abandoned toolshed, and his dogged hard work earned him the somewhat dubious nickname of "iron pants." If ever there had been a candidate who had pulled himself up by his bootstraps, Horatio Alger–style, it was Nixon. And he well understood the disdain ordinary laborers felt for "kids with the beards from the suburbs"—hippies who wore flags sewn to the seat of their pants—who seemed always to be insisting, protesting, *demanding*. Nixon believed himself a representative of the "silent majority," as he later described it, not a vocal minority.

He thus set two fundamental requirements for his campaign: to distance himself from President Johnson on Vietnam and to turn Wallace's "average Americans" into a Republican "silent majority." The Vietnam issue was delicate, because Nixon had generally supported the president's desire to end the war and his efforts to work through Soviet leaders to find a solution. He told his aide Richard

THE ELECTION OF 1968

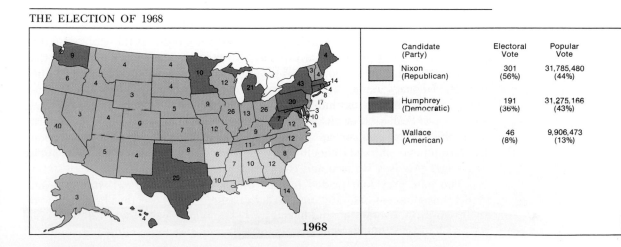

Candidate (Party)	Electoral Vote	Popular Vote
Nixon (Republican)	301 (56%)	31,785,480 (44%)
Humphrey (Democratic)	191 (36%)	31,275,166 (43%)
Wallace (American)	46 (8%)	9,906,473 (13%)

1968

Whalen, "I've come to the conclusion that there's no way to win the war. But we can't say that, of course. In fact, we have to seem to say the opposite." For most of his campaign he hinted that he had a secret plan to end the war but steadfastly refused to disclose it. He pledged only to find an honorable solution.

As for wooing his silent majority, Nixon tried to evoke "the traditional values of middle-class America," as one of his advisers explained: "hard work, individual enterprise, orderly behavior, love of country, moral piety, material progress." He also touched on their fears by promising more police to promote "law and order" while cracking down on "pot," pornography, protest, and permissiveness. He reassured Wallace's populist following that the Republicans would not dismantle the welfare state. At the same time, conservatives took heart in his pledge to unshackle "the greatest engine of progress ever developed in the history of man—American private enterprise."

While Nixon's managers worked to expose their candidate mostly through controlled television appearances, Hubert Humphrey sought to put together a campaign out of the ruins of the Chicago convention. All through September antiwar protesters dogged his trail with "Dump the Hump" posters. Finally the vice president gave a speech distancing his position on Vietnam, however slightly, from that of his unpopular boss. The protests then faded, Humphrey picked up energy, morale, and momentum, and he began appealing to traditional blue-collar Democrats to return to the fold. By November his rallies were enthusiastic and well attended. But the late surge was not enough to turn the tide. Nixon captured 43.4 percent of the popular vote to 42.7 percent for Humphrey and 13.5 percent for Wallace. More important, Nixon's "southern strategy" paid off. He and Wallace carried the entire southern tier of states except Texas. The "Solid South," which had remained in the Democratic camp since the days of Republican carpetbaggers, was solid no longer. And the majority of the American electorate seemed to have turned their back on liberal reform.

THE NIXON ERA

In Richard Nixon, Americans had elected two men to the presidency. On the public side, he appeared as the traditional small-town conservative who cherished individual initiative, Chamber-of-Commerce capitalism, Fourth-of-July patriotism, county-fair culture, and middle-class Victorian mores. At the same time, the private Nixon had worked so hard to make his Horatio Alger story come true that he often became cynical about the symbols of America in which he wrapped himself. His language among intimates was caustic and profane, and he waxed bitter toward those who crossed him. He had never taken naturally to public speaking and was physically rather awkward—a White House aide once found toothmarks on a "child-proof" aspirin cap which the president had been unable to pry open. But Nixon never shirked difficult tasks—indeed, he seemed to search them out as challenges—"crises" to face and conquer.

The new president prided himself on mastering the grand strategies and global consequences of foreign policy. A settlement of the war thus became one of his first priorities upon taking office. He had a congenial ally to work with, National Security Adviser Henry Kissinger. Kissinger at first seemed an unlikely

Nixon protégé. After fleeing Nazi Germany as a young man, he attended Harvard and became a professor there as well as an adviser to Governor Nelson Rockefeller of New York, one of the "eastern liberal" types distrusted by many main-line Republicans. But Kissinger was an intensely ambitious man. He worked for a time for Lyndon Johnson, trying to open negotiations with the North Vietnamese; and when Nixon was running for president, Kissinger secretly supplied the Republicans with information about Johnson's maneuvering. After the election he joined the new administration. Like Nixon, Kissinger strove for a global vision of foreign affairs and the use of grand strategy. Like Nixon, he had a tendency to pursue his ends secretly, circumventing the traditional bureaucracies of government such as the Department of State.

Vietnamization—and Cambodia

Nixon and Kissinger worked closely to devise a new policy for Vietnam. The president wanted to negotiate a settlement that would bring American troops home, but he wanted only "peace with honor," which meant preserving a pro-American South Vietnamese government. The strategy he adopted was "Vietnamization," which involved a carrot and a stick. On its own initiative, the United States began gradually withdrawing troops as a way to advance the peace talks in Paris. The burden of fighting would shift to the South Vietnamese army, equipped now with massive amounts of American supplies. Although to critics this strategy meant little more than "changing the color of the corpses," it helped reduce antiwar protests at home. At the same time the media shifted their focus from the war to the peace talks, thus creating the impression the war was winding down.

Using the stick, President Nixon hoped to drive the North Vietnamese into negotiating peace on American terms. Quite consciously, he traded on his reputation as a cold warrior who would stop at nothing to win. As he explained to his chief of staff Robert Haldeman,

> I call it the Madman Theory, Bob. I want the North Vietnamese to believe that I've reached the point where I might do anything to stop the war. We'll just slip the word to them that, "for God's sake, you know Nixon is obsessed about Communists. We can't restrain him when he's angry—and he has his hand on the nuclear button"—and Ho Chi Minh himself will be in Paris in two days begging for peace.

To underline his point, Nixon launched a series of bombing attacks in the spring of 1969 against North Vietnamese supply depots inside neighboring Cambodia. Johnson had refused to widen the war in this manner, fearing domestic reaction, but Nixon simply kept the raids secret. Over the next 15 months some 100,000 pounds of bombs were dropped in Operation MENU, whose various sorties, in the strange lingo of the Pentagon, were code-named BREAKFAST, LUNCH, SNACK, and DESSERT.

But the North Vietnamese were willing to risk the additional bombing and the threats of the "Madman." Even after Ho Chi Minh died in 1969, his successors continued to reject any offer that did not end with complete American withdrawal and an abandonment of the South Vietnamese military government. And as American bombing raids forced the VC to push deeper into Cambodia, that country became less stable under its neutral government of Prince Sihanouk. Right-wing forces under General Lon Nol overthrew Sihanouk, and a civil war between the communists and the generals ensued.

Once again Nixon decided to turn up the heat. Although his secretaries of defense and state were opposed, he ordered a ground invasion of Cambodia by American troops in order to wipe out North Vietnamese bases there. This, to be sure, was Johnson's old policy of escalation—just the opposite of the withdrawal Nixon had promised. But the Joint Chiefs argued that such an attack would buy time to strengthen the South Vietnamese army, and Nixon decided there would be no point in taking half-measures. He recognized the storm of protest that would arise (the administration was "going to get unshirted hell for doing this," he noted) but decided to "go for all the marbles." On April 30 he announced the "incursion" of American troops into Cambodia, proclaiming that he would not allow "the world's most powerful nation" to act "like a pitiful helpless giant." The wave of protests that followed included the Kent State tragedy as well as another march on Washington by 100,000 protesters. Even Congress was upset enough to repeal the Tonkin Gulf Resolution, a symbolic rejection of Nixon's invasion. After two months American troops left Cambodia, having achieved little.

Morale in a No-Win War

For a time, Vietnamization seemed to be making some headway. More American troops were sent home while the South Vietnamese forces' ability to fight improved modestly. But morale became a serious problem for American GIs. Until the Tet offensive American troops had fought well, however frustrating the conditions of battle. But Tet made it all too clear that the United States was not simply engaged in a "mopping up" operation. The American troops who remained during Vietnamization tended to become more cynical. Obviously the United States was getting out, so why were they still being asked to put their lives on the line? When overly eager officers led their men into battle too often, frustrated GIs became hostile. Fred Hickey, a helicopter pilot, recalled that the men under one arrogant and incompetent lieutenant

> booby-trapped his hooch with a smoke grenade, yellow smoke, which was a warning. But he didn't take any heed. Then they tried another, red smoke, which said the next one was going to be a hand grenade or a white phosphorus grenade. He obviously didn't believe it. The last one was a hand grenade, and he was eliminated and replaced. Grenades leave no fingerprints. Nobody's going to go to jail.

Reports of such "fraggings"—incidents involving fragmentation grenades—rose to over 2000 during the Vietnamization process.

In addition, the same forces that troubled American society were eroding the army's fighting effectiveness. At a time when Timothy Leary was inviting young Americans to "turn on" to marijuana and hallucinogens, the drug culture affected Americans in Vietnam as well. The Pentagon estimated that by 1971 nearly a third of American troops there had experimented with either opium or heroin, easily obtained in Southeast Asia. And just as the civil rights movement sparked increased black consciousness at home, so too abroad. Robert Rawls, a black GI, recalled that his friends "used to make a shoestring that they braided up and tied around their wrist, and everywhere a whole lot of blacks used to go, they'd give a power sign." One white medic noticed that Muhammad Ali's refusal to be drafted had a noticeable effect on the blacks in his unit. They began "to question why they were fighting the Honky's war against other Third World people. I saw very interesting relationships happening between your quick-talking, sharp-witted Northern blacks and your kind of easygoing, laid-back Southern blacks. . . . Many Southern blacks changed their entire point of view by the end of their tour and went home extremely angry."

The problem with morale only underlined the dilemma facing President Nixon. If the troops had become restive, domestic opposition to the war was even greater. By repealing the Gulf of Tonkin Resolution, Congress itself had put the president on notice that he would have to negotiate a settlement soon. Yet the North Vietnamese refused to yield, even after the American assaults in Cambodia.

The Move Toward Détente

As the daily situation reports came in from Vietnam, Nixon attempted to keep the war within a larger global perspective. The United States had a vast—but not limitless—defense arsenal to support the fighting. Committing half a million troops and billions of dollars to Vietnam meant that other resources were stretched. Both Kissinger and Nixon recognized that the United States no longer had the strength to exercise unchallenged dominance across the globe. The Soviets, for one, had undertaken a steady build-up of arms and missiles ever since Khrushchev had backed down at the Cuban missile crisis in 1962. Furthermore, the expanding economies of Japan and Western Europe challenged the dominance in world trade that had benefited the United States following World War II. Continued instability in Southeast Asia, the Middle East, and other Third World areas threatened the strength of the non-Communist bloc. Thus Vietnam had become a bottomless pit consuming valuable military and economic resources.

In what the White House labeled the new "Nixon Doctrine," the United States announced it would no longer expect to fight every battle, win every war, or draw every line to keep the global peace. Instead, Americans would shift some of the military burden for containment to such allies as Japan in the Pacific, the Shah of Iran in the Middle East, Zaire in central Africa, and the apartheid government in South Africa. Over the next six years American foreign military sales jumped from $1.8 billion to $15.2 billion. At the same time, Nixon and Kissinger looked for new ways to contain Soviet power not simply by the traditional threat of arms but through a negotiated easing of tensions. The United States would agree to ease the burdens the cold war placed on the Soviet economy if the Soviets would limit the arms race and put pressure on their Vietnamese allies to negotiate an end to the war. The name of the policy, borrowed from the French, was détente. Kissinger and Nixon also hoped to check Soviet power by playing what they called a "China card." Rather than view Mao Tse-tung as an archenemy, they would open diplomatic relations with the Chinese. By playing on deep-seated Soviet fears of their neighbor, they would force the Soviets to be more conciliatory toward the United States.

The strategy of détente was a remarkable departure from traditional cold war policy, which had long maintained that the Soviets understood force alone and that they were united with China in a monolithic Communist conspiracy. Indeed, although the Soviets had attended a brief summit meeting with Lyndon Johnson in 1967, the new regime of Leonid Brezhnev seemed hardly eager for reform. Nikita Khrushchev had attacked Stalin's excesses, but Brezhnev seemed very

Richard Nixon and Soviet Premier Leonid Brezhnev relax at Brezhnev's dacha on the Black Sea, during a June 1974 summit. For all their differences, the staunch anticommunist and the Soviet bureaucrat were both shrewd, even cynical judges of political power and human nature. Both regarded détente as in their mutual interest.

much in the mold of an old-style Stalinist bureaucrat. In 1968 he had sent Soviet troops into Czechoslovakia to crack down on the more liberal Communist government there. As for the Chinese, beginning in 1966 Mao had led his followers on a "cultural revolution," systematically eradicating all Western influence from China. The Cultural Revolution unleashed a virtual reign of terror at the hands of millions of youthful "Red Guards." Their victims were largely cultural and political figures stigmatized as "capitalist roaders," those who would use capitalist means to promote economic growth. Republicans in particular had regularly denounced the idea of even recognizing Mao's government, although it had been in power for 20 years. Now Richard Nixon, the man who had built a career fighting Communism, was embarked on a policy that broke dramatically with his past.

Characteristically, he and Kissinger moved secretly at first. Quiet talks in Poland between the Chinese and American ambassadors established a bridge, and in 1971 the Chinese indicated they would welcome a vist from an American Ping-Pong team. Since the Chinese were among the world's best Ping-Pong players and the Americans among the worst, bracing athletic competition was clearly not the point. Then in July Henry Kissinger disappeared from public view while visiting Pakistan—nursing a stomachache, according to his aides. A day later he surfaced in Beijing, the Chinese capital, to announce that the president would visit China in early 1972. Nixon's visit lasted nearly a week. He pledged to normalize relations; this included recognizing China's claims on Taiwan as an internal matter, which outraged Chiang Kai-shek, who still controlled the so-called nationalist regime there. Conservative Republicans were irritated, but the president's popularity with the public was high. Only a politician with Nixon's impeccable anticommunist credentials could have managed such an about-face in American foreign policy.

The trip to China was followed by another diplomatic coup, a summit visit to Moscow in May 1972. Brezhnev, troubled by food shortages and a weak consumer economy, was eager to strike a deal for United States grain and technology; for Nixon the Soviet market promised to ease American trade deficits and crop sur-

1218

pluses. The two leaders struck a major wheat deal, but the most important benefit of the meeting was the signing of the first Strategic Arms Limitation Treaty (SALT I). In the agreement, both sides pledged not to develop a new system of antiballistic missiles (ABMs), which would have sparked a costly arms race for both countries. And they agreed to limit the number of intercontinental ballistic missiles (ICBMs) each side would deploy.

Both the China and Moscow visits strengthened Nixon's reputation as a global strategist. But it remained to be seen whether the prestige he gained at lofty summits would help him extricate the United States from Vietnam as well as surmount the domestic divisions the war had raised at home. On those fronts, the president proved less successful.

The New Federalist

As a Republican, Nixon was skeptical of the liberal reliance on federal planning and he looked for ways to decentralize government social policy. "After a third of a century of power flowing from the people and the states to Washington," he argued, "it is time for a New Federalism in which power, funds, and responsibility will flow from Washington to the states and to the people." To accomplish this, he proposed a system of revenue-sharing, where federal money was turned over in block grants to state and local governments. Instead of earmarking the funds for specific purposes, localities could decide which problems needed attention and how best to attack them. Congress passed a revenue-sharing act in 1972, which distributed $30 billion over the following five years.

A similar approach influenced aid to individuals. Liberal programs from Franklin Roosevelt to Lyndon Johnson often provided specific services to individuals: job retraining programs, head-start programs for preschoolers, food supplement programs for nursing mothers. Republicans argued that such a "service strategy" too often assumed that federal bureaucrats best understood what services the poor needed. Nixon favored an "income strategy" instead, which simply gave recipients money and allowed them to spend it as they saw fit. Such grants would encourage individual initiatives, increase personal freedom, and reduce government bureaucracy.

In this spirit Nixon encouraged a renegade liberal academic, Daniel Patrick Moynihan, to develop a program favored by conservatives to reduce the welfare bureaucracy while increasing the incentive for those receiving welfare to find jobs. Moynihan had earlier completed a study which argued that harsh urban conditions and welfare programs had contributed to a serious erosion of the black family. Since the current welfare system favored poor families headed by single females over those with two parents, it sometimes drove fathers away. Moreover, Moynihan was convinced that existing federal programs and civil rights efforts had raised the black standard of living high enough so that further welfare legislation was unnecessary.

He proposed instead a government policy of "benign neglect" and the replacement of the welfare system with a new "Family Assistance Plan." Rather than go through the demeaning welfare process of demonstrating need to unsympathetic bureaucrats, poor families would be guaranteed a minimum annual income of $1600. The emphasis on family would encourage fathers to stay at home. The plan also required recipients to register for employment to satisfy conservative critics who usually envisioned all welfare recipients as able-bodied workers addicted to handouts and too lazy to work. Though Moynihan's proposals died in Congress, they defined the general terms in which poverty and assistance to the poor would be debated in the future.

In the polarized atmosphere of the Vietnam era, Nixon's "new federalism" provoked sharp dissent. Critics feared that if local governments did not have to raise money from local voters, they would have little incentive to spend tax money wisely. In addition, "block grants" would be parceled out to rich and poor districts alike. Why subsidize wealthy suburbs at the expense of underprivileged slums? Furthermore, grants to individuals did not address structural problems in society. A "no-strings-attached" check given to a family whose children needed a good education was of little help if the schools in the area were run-down and inadequate.

In any case, the administration's new federalism was a matter of emphasis, for the new Nixon supported many New Deal–style social programs. In 1970 he signed a bill establishing an Occupational Safety and Health Agency (OSHA) to enforce health and safety standards in the workplace. And although the president was no crusader for the environment, he did support a Clean Air Act to reduce car exhaust emissions as well as a Clean Water Act to make polluters liable for their negligence and to deal with disastrous oil spills. Just as Nixon's pragmatic style allowed him to change course in foreign policy, so too he made accommodations in domestic affairs.

Indeed, the worsening economy stretched his pragmatism even further, for by 1970 the nation had entered its first recession in a decade. Traditionally a recession brought a decrease in demand for goods and a rise in unemployment as workers were laid off. Manufacturers then cut wages and prices in order to preserve profit margins and encourage demand for their goods. But in the recession of 1970, while unemployment rose as expected, wages and prices were also rising in an inflationary spiral. Foreign trade surpluses turned into deficits. Americans were getting the worst of two worlds: a stagnant economy combined with rising prices—or "stagflation." Unfriendly Democrats labeled the phenomenon "Nixonomics," in which "all things that should go up—the stock market, corporate profits, real spendable income, productivity—go down, and all things that should go down—unemployment, prices, interest rates—go up."

But to charge the president with the failings of the economy was hardly fair. Lyndon Johnson had brought on inflation by refusing to raise taxes to pay for the war and Great Society social programs. In addition, wages continued their inflationary rise partly because powerful unions had negotiated automatic cost-of-living increases into their contracts. Similarly, in industries dominated by a few large corporations, like steel and oil, prices did not follow the market forces of a recession. So prices and wages continued to rise as demand and employment fell.

At first Nixon responded by cutting federal spending, hoping that inflation would slow even if unemployment continued to rise. But by December unemployment had risen to 6 percent and so had inflation—the worst level since the Korean War. Interest rates were at their highest point in a century. Mindful that his own "silent majority" were the people most pinched by the slower economy, Nixon decided that unemployment posed a greater threat than inflation. Announcing "I am now a Keynesian," he adopted a deficit budget designed to stimulate the growth of jobs. He announced an even more surprising piece of news in August 1971: to provide short-term relief, wages and prices would be frozen for 90 days. For a Republican to advocate federal wage and price controls was almost as heretical as seeking to establish diplomatic relations with China. Yet Nixon did not hesitate. For another year federal wage and price boards enforced the ground rules for any increases; most controls were lifted in January 1973. Nixon also devalued the dollar in order to reverse the foreign trade deficit. Cheaper dollars raised the price of imports like the popular Volkswagen Beetle and made American exports more competitive in foreign markets.

By the fall of 1972 the economy was again booming. As in foreign policy, Nixon had reversed long-cherished economic policies to achieve practical results.

"SILENT" MAJORITIES AND VOCAL MINORITIES

During the 1968 campaign Richard Nixon had noticed a placard carried by a hopeful voter—"Bring Us Together"—and adopted it as his campaign theme. Yet of necessity political coalitions cannot bring everyone together. Their goal is simply to assemble a majority on election day. Nixon recognized quite well that in the three-way race of 1968, his 43 percent did not add up to a majority. But when Wallace's vote was added, the total came to an impressive 60 percent. Nixon set out to add discontented southerners and blue-collar workers to the traditional GOP base. In doing so, he tried to identify them with the "silent majority," at the same time excluding other vocal minorities who had been actively campaigning for increased civil rights. The black movement had received the most national attention during the mid-1960s, but other minorities also adopted more radical tactics to achieve their ends. Their new, more assertive visibility was crucial to Nixon's attempt to form his own counter-majority.

Hispanic Activism

Outside the southwestern states, southeastern Florida, and New York City few Americans prior to the 1960s and 1970s had much contact with the nation's Hispanic population. The major immigration from Mexico and Puerto Rico began only after World War II and, in the case of Cubans, after the 1959 revolution that brought Castro to power. While historical, cultural, ethnic, and geographic differences among the three major Hispanic groups made it difficult to develop a common political agenda, activist leaders did seek greater Hispanic unity.

The acquisition of Puerto Rico in 1898 gave the United States control over an island population of one million people, whose diverse mixture of classes and races resulted from the intermarriage of African, Indian, and Spanish peoples. Their political status remained uncertain until 1947, when the island acquired a new constitution. Puerto Rico became neither a state nor an independent nation, but a commonwealth. Island people were defined as U.S. citizens subject to the draft, free from federal income taxes, and ineligible for benefits under federal social service programs.

After World War II a weak island economy and the lure of prosperity on the mainland brought over a million Puerto Ricans into New York City. As citizens of the United States, they could move freely to the mainland and back home again. That dual consciousness discouraged many from establishing deep roots stateside. Equally important, the newcomers were startled to discover that, whatever their

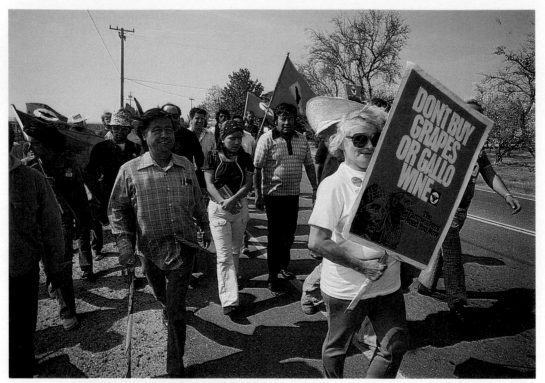

Cesar Chavez mobilized the largely Hispanic migrant workers into the United Farm Workers Union. His demands for recognition of the union by California growers led to a bitter
strike in 1966. A call for boycotts in 1969 against grapes and lettuce gained Chavez and the
union national attention. In July 1970, after five years of conflict, the growers agreed to
recognize the union.

status at home, on the mainland they were subject to racial discrimination and
most often segregated into rundown urban slums. Approximately half of the recent
immigrants lived below the poverty level in 1964, according to the Puerto Rican
Forum, and their unemployment was three times greater than for whites and 50
percent higher than for blacks. When light-skinned migrants escaped those conditions by blending into the middle class as "Latin Americans," the Puerto Rican
community lost some of the leadership it needed to assert its political rights. Still,
a shared island orientation preserved a strong group identity. By the 1960s, the
urban *barrios* gained greater political consciousness as groups like "Aspira"
adopted the strategies of civil rights activists and organizations like the Black and
Puerto Rican Caucus created links with other minority groups.

The Cubans who arrived in the United States after 1959—some 350,000 over
the course of the decade—forged fewer ties with other Hispanics. Most settled
around Miami. An unusually large number came from Cuba's professional, business, and government class, were racially white and politically conservative. Mexican-Americans, on the other hand, constituted the largest segment of the Hispanic population. Until the 1940s most were farmers and farm laborers in Texas,

New Mexico, and California. But during the 1950s, the process of mechanization had affected them, just as it had southern blacks. By 1969 about 85 percent of Mexican-Americans had settled in cities. With urbanization came a slow improvement of the range and quality of jobs they held. A body of skilled workers, middle class professionals, and entrepreneurs emerged.

In 1960, frustrated by years of neglect by major parties, Hispanic political leaders from the region formed the Mexican-American Political Association. MAPA declared its intent to be "proudly Mexican American, *openly* political, and *necessarily* bipartisan." By 1964 four Mexican-Americans had been elected to Congress, but the growing activism across the nation altered traditional Hispanic approaches to politics. Younger Mexican-Americans began to call themselves Chicanos. In 1965 Cesar Chavez gained national attention by his efforts to organize migrant laborers into the United Farm Workers and lead them in *La Huelga*—The Strike—as they struck farm growers and set in motion a national boycott of California lettuce and grapes. Corky Gonzales, a Denver social worker, established *La Crusada Para Justicia* (Crusade for Justice) to support strikes by Chicano high school students, protest police brutality, and oppose the Vietnam War. The more militant Reies Tijerina and his supporters in New Mexico occupied the Kit Carson National Forest to dramatize disputes over old Spanish land titles.

By the late 1960s Mexican-Americans had clearly established an ethnic consciousness and a movement. Like blacks, Chicanos saw themselves as a deculturated people: their heritage rejected, their labor exploited, their opportunity for advancement denied. The new ethnic militancy led to the formation of *La Raza Unida* (The Race United), a third-party movement which sought to gain power in communities where Chicanos were a majority and to extract concessions from the Democrats and Republicans. The more militant "Brown Berets" adopted the paramilitary tactics and radical rhetoric of the Black Panthers.

The Choices of Native Americans

Like blacks and Hispanics, Indians resorted to the strategies of protest and demonstration; yet the unique situation of Native Americans (as many now called themselves) set them apart from other minorities. Despite a largely hostile white culture that had most often worked either to exterminate or assimilate, the traditions and identities of American Indians survived through their tribes, bands, villages, and other kin associations. From a low in population of only 250,000 in 1920, Native Americans grew steadily to around 800,000 by 1970. Leaders of Indian tribal councils, many of them World War II veterans, pressed for expanded civil rights; and in 1948 the Supreme Court required states to grant Indians the right to vote (*Trujillo v. Garley*).

But the growing pressures for civil rights that inspired that decision created another threat to Indian tribal identities. Liberals came to see the reservations not as oases of Indian culture, but as rural ghettos. During the 1950s they joined conservatives eager to repeal the New Deal and western state politicians eyeing tribal resources to adopt a policy of "termination." Under this approach, the Bureau of Indian Affairs would reduce federal services, gradually sell off tribal lands, and push Indians into the "mainstream" of American life. Although most full-blood Indians objected to the policy, some mixed bloods and Indians already assimilated into white society supported the move. The resulting relocation of approximately 35,000 Native Americans accelerated a shift of Indian population from rural areas to cities. The urban population, which had been barely 30,000 in 1940, reached over 300,000 by the 1970s. But the tribal cultures that emphasized communal sharing had not prepared most Indians to deal with regular wage employment, budgeting, the need for personal savings, or an adversary legal system. Less than 10 percent of those relocated in the 1950s found permanent jobs. Unemployment translated into poverty, which in turn led to unusually high levels of disease, alcoholism, and other signs of social disintegration.

The social activism of the 1960s inspired Indian leaders to shape a new political agenda. Tribes in the state of Washington held "fish-ins" to protest restrictions on their fishing rights. In 1968 urban activists in Minneapolis created AIM, the American Indian Movement, and a year later similarly minded Indians living in the San Francisco Bay area formed Indians of All Tribes. Because the Bureau of Indian Affairs refused to address the problems of urban Indians, more militant members of the organization dramatized their dissatisfaction by seizing the abandoned federal prison on Alcatraz Island in San Francisco Bay.

The Alcatraz action inspired a national push for Indian rights, and a determination to join in a pan-Indian movement. Richard Oakes, a Mohawk Indian from New York, declared that the Alcatraz protest was not "a movement to liberate the island, but to liberate ourselves." Then in 1973, AIM organizers Russell Means and Dennis Banks led a dramatic takeover of a trading post at Wounded Knee, on a Sioux reservation in South Dakota. Ever since white cavalry had gunned down more than 200 Sioux in 1890 (page 743), Wounded Knee had symbolized for Indians the betrayal of white promises and the bankruptcy of reservation policy.

At the same time, the Wounded Knee incident demonstrated the problems that Indian activists faced. When federal officers surrounded the trading post, militants discovered that other Indians did not support their tactics, and they were forced to leave. A pan-Indian movement was difficult to achieve when so many tribes were determined to go their own ways, as distinct, self-regulating communities. Less activist tribes often already commanded substantial resources, gained from exploiting oil, timber or mineral rights that went with their lands. Other tribes, like the Penobscot and Passamaquoddy Indians of Maine, turned to the courts to recover land that had been given them in long-ignored treaties. Thus even activists who supported the pan-Indian movement found themselves splintering. During the 1970s over 100 different organizations were formed to unite various tribes pursuing political and legal agendas at the local, state, and federal level.

Social Policies and the Court

The militance of Indian, Hispanic, and black protesters alarmed many of the "silent majority" Nixon hoped to attract to an expanded Republican coalition. The blue-collar and southern Democratic voters he sought to detach distrusted the entire activist counterculture: long-haired demonstrators, drug-users, sexually permissive radicals. In addition, Wallace supporters had been particularly vocal in opposing school desegregation. Nixon capitalized on the themes of law and order in his 1968 campaign and, increasingly, turned his attention to finding an ally in the Supreme Court.

Fifteen years after *Brown v. Board of Education* had ruled that racially separate school systems must be desegregated, many localities still had not complied. Busing was one method of achieving racial balance, but it aroused determined opposition from white neighborhoods, where parents resented their children being bused away from their neighborhood to more distant, formerly all-black schools. For their part, blacks worried about their reception in hostile white neighborhoods, but by and large they supported busing as a means to better education. President Nixon, however, became an outspoken critic of busing and in 1969, when lawyers for Mississippi asked the Supreme Court to delay an integration plan, the Justice Department filed a brief supporting the state. Federal policy had taken a 180-degree turn. The Court rejected that proposal, holding in *United States v. Jefferson County Board of Education* that all state systems, including Mississippi's, had an obligation "to terminate dual systems at once and to operate now and hereafter only unitary schools." Two years later, in *Swann v. Charlotte–Mecklenburg Board of Education* (1971), the Court further ruled that busing, balancing ratios, and redrawing of school district lines were all acceptable ways to achieve integration.

Such decisions indicated that even though Earl Warren had retired as Chief Justice in 1969, the Court was still a force for liberal social policy. Nixon resolved to change that by filling vacancies in the court with more conservative justices. As Earl Warren's replacement as Chief Justice, he nominated Warren Burger, a somewhat lackluster jurist who accepted most of the Court's precedents but had no wish to break new ground. When another vacancy occurred in 1969, Nixon tried twice to appoint conservative southern judges. But both nominees, Clement Haynsworth of South Carolina and G. Harrold Carswell of Florida, had reputations on the federal bench for opposing civil rights and labor unions. Although Haynsworth was an able jurist, he had heard cases in which he had a financial stake. By contrast, Carswell was so undistinguished that one of his defenders, Senator Roman Hruska of Nebraska, was reduced to arguing that the quality of mediocrity deserved "a little representation" on the Court. Congress rejected both.

In the end, Nixon succeeded with Minnesotan Harry Blackmun, a moderate judge of unimpeachable integrity. In 1971 he made two additional appointments: Lewis Powell, a highly regarded Virginia lawyer, and William Rehnquist of Arizona, an extremely conservative attorney who had supported the efforts of the Nixon Justice Department to restrict civil rights and civil liberties. With the successive appointments of Burger, Blackmun, Powell, and Rehnquist, the Court would no longer lead the fight for minority rights. But neither would it reverse the achievements of the Warren Court.

Us versus Them

Shaping the Supreme Court was only one element of Nixon's strategy to fashion a silent majority out of the turmoil of the sixties. He also worked to portray those who opposed him—opponents of the incursion into Cambodia, civil rights activists, liberal Democrats—as standing beyond the bounds of traditional American values. Just as Nixon had tended to equate liberal reformers with communist "pinkos" during the 1950s, now his administration blurred the lines between honest dissent and radical criminals. And in doing so, it reflected a side of the president that tended to see issues in terms of "'us' against 'them,'" as loyal aide

Charles Colson later recalled. Nixon's reaction to Congress when it repealed the Tonkin Gulf Resolution reflected that attitude. There would be no more "screwing around" with Congress, he told his staff. "Don't worry about divisiveness. Having drawn the sword, don't take it out—stick it in hard."

Under Attorney General John Mitchell, the Justice Department launched a systematic campaign against radicals and civil rights activists. The strategy went beyond public denunciations to harassment through legal prosecution. Targets included Vietnam Veterans Against the War, the leaders of demonstrations during the 1968 Democratic convention, socially-conscious members of the Catholic clergy, the Black Panthers, SDS activists, and leaders of the peace movement like Yale chaplain William Sloane Coffin and Dr. Benjamin Spock. Even when Mitchell's department lacked a strong case, it prosecuted anyway, hoping to force dissenters to commit their limited resources to staying out of jail rather than furthering their causes. Meanwhile, in its war against drug users, the administration proposed a bill that would allow police to stage "no-knock" raids and use "preventive detention" to keep suspected criminals in jail without bail. It also lobbied for permission to make greater use of phone taps and other means of electronic surveillance.

In the political arena, Nixon gave Vice President Spiro Agnew the task of traveling the low road, just as Nixon himself had been appointed "point man" during the Eisenhower administration. Aided by speechwriter William Safire, Agnew launched such alliterative assaults as his description of the press and television news commentators as "nattering nabobs of negativism" and "troubadours of trouble" who contributed to the "creeping permissiveness that afflicted America." He reduced antiwar demonstrators to "an effete corps of impudent snobs." Even opponents in the Senate were accused of being "radical liberals." As Agnew's attacks continued, it became clear that his speeches were part of an administration campaign to control or discredit the news media. In the campaign between "us" and "them," the national press corps was clearly seen as "them," a hostile establishment slanting the news. Agnew pointedly reminded the networks that broadcast licenses were subject to public review; to drive the point home, the administration challenged the renewals of two Florida stations owned by the Washington *Post*, a paper critical of the administration.

Triumph

As the election of 1972 approached, Nixon's majority seemed to be falling into place. George Wallace had returned to the Democratic party to run for president, his tone this time a bit more moderate. But at a shopping mall in Maryland a would-be assassin with no evident political motives seriously wounded Wallace and ended his campaign. Some of his support might have gone to Senator Edmund Muskie of Maine, a Democratic moderate who had been a dignified vice-presidential nominee in 1968. But then New Hampshire's largest newspaper, the Manchester *Union-Leader*, printed a letter charging Muskie with disparaging the large French-Canadian population there. When the newspaper's right-wing publisher, William Loeb, added his own slurs about Muskie's wife, the candidate made an impassioned defense, in which tears filled his eyes. And political etiquette damned any man who broke down and cried before the television cameras. Only later was it discovered that the offending letter had been planted by a staff member of the Nixon administration in charge of campaign "dirty tricks."

With Muskie and Wallace effectively out of the race, the antiwar candidacy of Senator George McGovern of South Dakota became unstoppable. Under new party rules, which McGovern had helped write, the delegate selection process was opened to all party members, providing proportional representation for minorities, women, and young people. No longer would party bosses hand-pick the delegates. But with McGovern receiving the nomination, Nixon had his split between "us" and "them" arranged just the way he had hoped. The Democratic platform called for immediate withdrawal from Vietnam, abolition of the draft, amnesty for war resisters, and a minimun guaranteed income for the poor. None of those issues appealed to the traditional New Deal coalition of urban bosses, southerners, labor leaders, and ethnics.

By November the only question was how large Nixon's majority would be. An unsolved burglary at the Watergate complex in Washington, D.C., while vaguely linked to the White House, had not touched the president. He even captured some antiwar sentiment by announcing on election eve that peace in Vietnam was at hand. When the smoke cleared, only liberal Massachusetts and the heavily black District of Columbia gave McGovern a majority. Nixon received almost 61 percent of the popular vote and an impressive 520 out of 538 electoral votes. His biggest gains came among disaffected Democrats in the South and among blue-collar workers. Yet on closer analysis, the smashing victory seemed more a rejection of McGovern than approval of administration policies. In the races for the Senate and governorships the Democrats actually made gains, while losing only 13 House seats. As one pollster concluded, "Richard Nixon's 'new American majority' was the creation of George McGovern."

Victory by a wide margin did not leave the president satisfied. The day after the election, he shocked his White House staff by briefly thanking them for their efforts and then making way for chief of staff H. R. Haldeman, who announced that all cabinet members and senior staff would be required to submit formal letters of resignation so that the president would have the option of "cleaning house." His intentions toward his political opponents were even more ominous "We have not used the power in the first four years, as you know," he remarked to Haldeman during the campaign. "We haven't used the Bureau [FBI] and we haven't used the Justice Department, but things are going to change now. And they *are* going to change and they're going to get it, right?" Haldeman could only agree.

The End of an Era

The president was particularly frustrated because victory still eluded him in Vietnam. Campus protests had subsided after the furor over Cambodia, partly because only 39,000 American troops remained in Vietnam. But the North Vietnamese refused to negotiate any settlement that left the South Vietnamese government of General Nguyen Van Thieu in power. Nixon wanted to subdue his opponents through force, but sending new American reinforcements was out of the question. To step up the pressure he ordered Haiphong harbor mined and blockaded in May 1972, along with a sustained bombing campaign. "The bastards have never been bombed like they're going to be bombed this time," he told one aide. Despite his preelection peace claims, Nixon on December 18 launched an even greater wave of attacks, as American planes dropped more bombs on the North in 12 days than they had during the entire campaign from 1969 to 1971.

Once again, Kissinger returned to Paris, hoping that the combination of threats and conciliation would bring a settlement. Ironically the Americans' ally, General Thieu, threw up the most stumbling blocks, for he was rightly convinced that his regime would not last long once the United States departed. But in January 1973 a treaty was finally arranged, smoothed by Kissinger's promise of aid to the North Vietnamese to help in postwar reconstruction, as well as a secret pledge to Thieu to send troops again if they were needed. By March the last American units were home.

"The enemy must fight his battles . . . [in] protracted campaigns," wrote the Vietnamese strategist in 1284. Ho Chi Minh had taken 8 years to outlast the French and had seen another 15 elapse before he died in 1969 on the way to outlasting the Americans. For all concerned it had been a bloody, wearying conflict. Between 1961 and 1973 the war claimed some 58,000 American lives and left over 300,000 wounded. The cost to Southeast Asia in lives and destruction was almost impossible to calculate. Over a million Vietnamese soldiers and perhaps half a million civilians died. Some 6.5 million South Vietnamese became refugees along with 3 million Cambodians and Laotians.

When the Americans pulled out, they left behind the shell of a mighty military complex. On paper, South Vietnam had the world's fourth largest air force, but probably no more than 10 percent of its planes and helicopters could actually fly. On paper, Nixon achieved the "peace with honor" he had insisted on, but experienced observers predicted that South Vietnam's days were numbered. By any real measure of military success the Vietcong peasant guerrillas and their lightly armed North Vietnamese allies had held off—and in that sense defeated—the world's greatest military power.

For most Americans the lessons of Vietnam were painful. In fundamental ways, the era of optimism rising out of World War II had ended. In those first heady postwar days, the United States had emerged as one of the two preeminent superpowers of the world, embarked on a policy of containment wherever it was needed. Truman had set the policy by becoming a feisty anticommunist; Richard Nixon had begun his political career by attacking Truman for not being tough enough. Yet it was Nixon, in the end, who was pragmatic enough to see that the United States did not have inexhaustible military resources to contain communism everywhere. Sometimes the United States would have to tolerate neutralism and the forces of nationalism. Nixon's policy of détente, based on the rivalry between the Soviet Union and the People's Republic of China, clearly recognized that communism was not monolithic. The enemy too had its divisions and limits.

The scars of Vietnam affected more than just the nation's ability to fight a far-flung guerrilla war. It shattered the liberal optimism of the early sixties: the belief that with enough brilliant intellectuals or enough federal programs, poverty and discontent could be eliminated and the world made safe for democracy. Vietnam was John Kennedy's war as well as Richard Nixon's; and Vietnam brought the reforms of Lyndon Johnson to a halt. Johnson had seen himself as the rightful heir to the liberal Roosevelt, his Great Society a capstone of the New Deal. Like Roosevelt, he had gone to war determined not only to win it, but to triumph over his critics at home, who seemed not to understand his liberal hopes. He died on January 22, 1973, not far from his Texas ranch, one day before the American war in Vietnam ended.

SIGNIFICANT EVENTS

1945 ┼ Ho Chi Minh unifies Vietnam

1947 ┼ Puerto Rico given commonwealth status

1948 ┼ *Trujillo v. Garley*

1954 ┼ French defeat at Dien Bien Phu; Geneva accords

1963 ┼ Diem assassinated; United States has 16,000 "advisers" in Vietnam

1964 ┼ Tonkin Gulf incident; Tonkin Gulf Resolution

1965 ┼ Rolling Thunder begins bombing of North Vietnam; antiwar "teach-ins" on college campuses; Cesar Chavez leads national campaign on behalf of farm workers

1967 ┼ March on the Pentagon; Johnson's advisers oppose war

1968 ┼ U.S. troop levels in Vietnam peak at 536,000; Tet offensive; My Lai massacre; peace talks begin in Paris; Eugene McCarthy challenges Johnson in New Hampshire primary; Johnson withdraws from race; Martin Luther King, Jr., assassinated; Robert Kennedy enters race and is assassinated; riots at Democratic Convention in Chicago; George Wallace candidacy; Nixon wins election

1969 ┼ Secret bombing of Cambodia; Vietnamization leads to reduction of American forces; Nixon Doctrine; Senate defeats Haynsworth and Carswell nominations

1970 ┼ U.S. troops invade Cambodia; killings at Kent State and Jackson State; march on Washington; Clean Air and Water acts; creation of OSHA; recession creates stagflation; repeal of Tonkin Gulf Resolution

1971 ┼ Nixon adopts wage and price controls; *Swann v. Charlotte–Mecklenburg Board of Education;* Pentagon Papers published

1972 ┼ Nixon trip to China; détente with Soviet Union; SALT I; Revenue Sharing Act; Watergate break-in; Nixon reelected; mining of Haiphong Harbor; Christmas bombings of North Vietnam

1973 │ Vietnam peace treaty; AIM supporters occupy Wounded Knee

34

The Age of Limits

In July 1969 newsmen, diplomats, and celebrities from around the world converged on Cape Kennedy to witness the launching of *Apollo 11*, the first manned space flight to the moon. With them came tens of thousands of the curious and a handful of protestors, including a mule-cart procession led by the Reverend Ralph Abernathy, whose Poor People's March hoped to dramatize the problem of poverty. Abernathy, however, was so overwhelmed by the *Saturn 5*'s thunderous ignition and fiery rocket blast that he prayed instead for the safety of the crew. The emotion of the drama caught him up just as it did the millions of Americans who, days later, celebrated when Armstrong and Aldrin walked across a lunar landscape.

President Nixon called the flight of *Apollo 11* the best week's work since the Creation. And undoubtedly the triumph had been epochal. Had not humankind set new outer limits for what it might accomplish? And yet a certain skepticism lingered over what it all meant. One scientist took comfort that after *Apollo* humankind could always go elsewhere, no matter how much a mess was made of the planet earth. That was no small consideration given the increasing problems of smog, water pollution, and toxic wastes. There had been some dramatic warnings. In 1967 an oil tanker, the *Torrey Canyon*, spilled 100,000 tons of oil into the English Channel. Detergents used to clean up the spill left the area clean but without plant and animal life for years after.

Such dangers were of grave concern to city officials in Santa Barbara, California, an outpost of paradise along the Pacific Coast. In the channel stretching between there and Los Angeles, 90 miles to the south, oil companies had drilled some 925 wells in the coastal tidelands. State efforts to impose stringent regulations on federal oil leases offshore had failed, but the Department of Interior repeatedly assured local officials they had "nothing to fear." That changed on January 28, 1969, when Union Oil Company's well A-21 blew a billow of thick crude oil into the channel. Crews quickly capped the hole only to discover that pressure from the well had opened a fissure in the ocean floor, through which natural gas and oil seeped to the surface. "It looked like a massive, inflamed abscess bursting with reddish-brown pus," one dismayed observer commented.

By February 1, an oil slick had covered five miles of Santa Barbara's once-pristine white beaches. Only after 11 days of struggle were oil workers able to seal the leak, which spouted more than 200,000 barrels and left a slick that extended for some 800 miles. Beaches, boats, and wildlife as far south as San Diego were

At the end of a decade in which Americans landed on the moon, a series of down-to-earth crises, like the oil spill that fouled these waters off Santa Barbara, California, underscored the limits of American power and technology both at home and abroad.

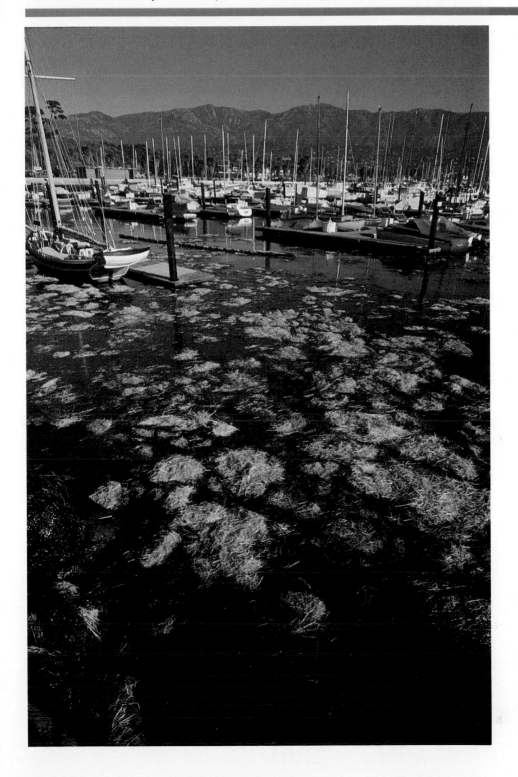

coated with the black, gooey tar. "Cormorants and grebes dived into the the oily swells for fish, most never to surface alive. All along the mucky shoreline, birds lay dead or dying, unable to raise their oil-soaked feathers," one reporter wrote. Despite the heroic efforts of environmentalists, thousands of shore birds died, and detergents claimed the entire population of limpets, abalones, lobsters, sea urchins, mussels, clams, and some fish. One environmentalist warned that "a drastic ecological imbalance" was inevitable.

Few people in Santa Barbara were surprised to learn that Union Oil was operating well below federal and state standards when the well blew. The company was widely known as a polluter and twice in 1967 had been charged with polluting Los Angeles harbor. Two weeks before the Santa Barbara disaster it was accused of dumping 1500 barrels of oil into the Santa Anna River. Outspoken Union Oil President Fred Hartley dismissed the leak as "Mother Earth letting some oil come out." "I'm amazed at the publicity for the loss of a few birds," he told a group of dismayed U.S. Senate conservationists. The Senate responded by passing the Water Quality Improvement Act, which established fines for oil spills.

It was Santa Barbara, not *Apollo 11*, that served as a portent of the coming decade. There would be more Apollo missions, and Vice President Agnew would try briefly to initiate a new race to Mars. But Americans discovered more pressing concerns closer to home: war in the Middle East, the dramatic announcement of the Arab members of the Organization of Petroleum Exporting Countries (OPEC) that they would embargo oil shipments to the West, growing concern over environmental deterioration, the shocking revelations of the Watergate scandals, and the continuing rise of inflation signaled an end to an optimistic faith that American technological know-how could solve any problem or that economic growth was both inevitable and beneficial. No longer could Americans pursue their dreams, whether of conquering space or frontiers closer to home, without calculating the costs. Elliot Richardson, the Nixon administration's secretary of health, education and welfare (HEW), drew the appropriate lesson when he remarked, "We must recognize, as we have with both foreign affairs and natural resources, that resources we thought were boundless . . . are indeed severely limited." The United States had entered an era of limits.

THE LIMITS OF REFORM

Like the space program, the reform movements of the early 1960s had begun with a sense of possibility, of remaking society in a way that preserved both past values and future prospects. But as the decade wore on those movements—for civil rights, against the atomic bomb and the Vietnam War, for a more democratic society, for more meaningful lifestyles—had fragmented into rival, even warring, factions. The nonviolent civil rights movement continued, but so too did radical black nationalism, urban guerrilla violence, and rioting. Out of the radical SDS had come the Weathermen and terrorist Weather Underground. America still seemed a nation in need of reforming, much as it had before, but President Kennedy's call to national sacrifice gave way to narrow preoccupations with self-awareness and personal improvement. According to social observer Tom Wolfe, the self-obsessed "Me Generation" had displaced the crusading New Left.

Amid frustrated hopes, some elements of the reform movement kept alive the idea of restructuring society in substantial ways. Environmentalists, feminists, and consumer advocates utilized many of the same strategies of nonviolent protest and legal maneuver that worked so effectively in the civil rights crusade. But unlike the radicalism of the 1960s, these movements each had long been associated with the American reform tradition. And though they often had radical goals, their leadership most frequently came from the political mainstream and won some major victories, even if they failed ultimately to transform American society.

Environmentalism

The Santa Barbara oil spill was hardly the first warning that Americans were reaching limits to the abuse the environment could take. Searing clouds of acrid smog over Los Angeles had for years hinted at the danger posed by auto emissions in a region where freeways dominated the landscape. Or possibly the first warning came from the recognition that radioactive fallout from nuclear bomb tests in Nevada might well threaten schoolchildren in Troy, New York. Rachel Carson in *Silent Spring* (1962) had so convincingly enumerated the environmental hazards of the pesticide DDT that 40 state legislatures had passed restrictive laws. Certainly, no one with a sense of irony could help but marvel that the Cuyahoga River running through Cleveland, Ohio, had become a major fire hazard. Smog, fallout, dangerous pesticides, hazardous consumer goods, and polluted rivers were all by-products of industrial technology. By the late 1960s Americans started to recognize that a deteriorating environment was the not-so-hidden cost of unbridled economic growth.

The environmental movement that emerged marked a departure from both traditional conservation associated with Teddy Roosevelt, Gifford Pinchot, and Harold Ickes and preservationists like John Muir and the Sierra Club. Conservationists had always stressed the idea of proper *use* of both renewable and nonrenewable resources as a way to ensure the nation's future prosperity. Engineers, lawyers, and economists shaped the conservation agenda. Preservationists shared the Romantics' vision of humankind's spiritual links to nature. They sought largely to save unique wilderness areas like Yellowstone, Yosemite, and the Grand Canyon from development and commercial exploitation.

The new environmental movement incorporated elements of both conservation and preservation into the field of ecology, the biological science that since the early twentieth century has been demonstrating the linkages and dependencies of life processes. Barry Commoner in his book *The Closing Circle* (1971) argued that modern society lived under the illusion it could "improve on nature." In doing so it imposed a terrible price on the environment. American farmers, for example, had shifted from animal manures to artificial fertilizers to increase farm productivity. But the change also raised costs, left soil sterile, and poisoned nearby water sources. After laundry detergents artificially "whitened" clothes, they created foamy scum in lakes and rivers while nourishing deadly algae blooms. Industry profited in the short run, Commoner argued, but in the long run the environment might be bankrupt. Nothing short of a "new social ethic" or transformation of cultural values could produce an ecologically responsible society, warned microbiologist René Dubos.

Increased concern with environmental issues led to greater appreciation of wilderness areas like Yosemite National Park, above. Paradoxically, the influx of new visitors turned once peaceful trails into five-lane thoroughfares, threatening the wilderness with being "loved to death."

By the end of the decade, environmentalists were organizing to implement such an ethic in concrete ways. They brought a lawsuit to block the plan of a consortium of oil companies to build an 800-mile pipeline across Alaska's fragile wilderness. In addition, they successfully lobbied in Congress to defeat a bill authorizing support for the supersonic transport plane, the SST, a plane whose high-altitude flights threatened to deplete the vital ozone layer around the earth. Similarly, a coalition of environmental groups fought a proposed jet airport that threatened south Florida's water supply and the ecology of Florida's Everglades National Park.

The airport battle drew clear lines between the new ethic of environmental restraint and traditional champions of economic growth. Few states have been as receptive to such projects or suffered so much environmental dislocation from development as Florida. Walt Disney, among others, wanted the airport to bring tourists to his huge Disney World project near Orlando; and no one more deeply believed in technology's ability to improve on nature than the king of synthetic culture, Disney himself. At Disneyland in California he had constructed a world that eliminated the accidental or natural in favor of plastic animals, fake forests, and even artificial rocks. Although Disney had a reputation for representing all that was clean and innocent in popular culture, environmentalists defeated the airport project.

"There is a new kind of revolutionary movement under way in this country," declared Senator Henry Jackson of Washington. Even President Nixon, normally a friend of business and real estate interests, responded to the call for more stringent environmental regulation. His administration banned the use of DDT (though not its sale abroad) and supported the National Environmental Policy Act of 1969, which required environmental impact statements for most public projects and made the government responsible for representing the public interest. Nixon also established the Environmental Protection Agency to enforce the law. Echoing Barry Commoner, he announced, "We must learn not how to master nature but how to master ourselves, our institutions, and our technology."

By the spring of 1970 a healthy environment had become such a popular cause that Senator Gaylord Nelson of Wisconsin suggested a national "Earth Day" to celebrate this new consciousness. On April 22, 1970, for at least a few hours pedestrians reclaimed downtown city streets, millions of schoolchildren planted trees and picked up litter, college students demonstrated, and Congress adjourned. The enthusiasm reflected the movement's dual appeal: it combined the rationalism of science with a religious vision of life's organic unity. One California congressman recognized that Americans did not fully appreciate what this celebration could mean: "The Establishment sees this as a great big anti-litter campaign. Wait until they find out what it really means . . . to clean up our earth."

Earth Day was more an end than a beginning. President Nixon, for one, was unwilling to see environmental causes restrict economic development. In his own Earth Day speech he threw the administration's support behind the oil industry's Alaskan pipeline project, which survived a long series of court challenges before construction began in 1973. The president also personally lobbied for the SST. Having helped kill the environmentally destructive Cross-Florida Barge Canal project in 1969, he went to Alabama in 1971 to launch the equally ill-conceived Tombigbee–Tennessee Waterway. "We are not going to allow the environmental issue . . . to destroy the system," he announced in 1972.

Beyond the matter of high principles or pragmatic choices, Nixon's political instincts were shrewd. Conflict between social classes underlay the environmental debate. Many middle-class veterans of the counterculture, civil rights, and anti-war movements had found a new outlet in environmental activism. To workers and the silent majority, facing rising inflation and unemployment, the issue came down to jobs versus the environment. "Out of work? Hungry? Eat an environmentalist," declared one popular bumper sticker. To workers and upwardly mobile middle Americans, environmentalism too often seemed suspiciously like a scenario in which those who already possessed access to the good life wanted to close the door, leaving the less privileged standing on the outside.

Consumerism

In 1965 a thin young man with jet black hair and intense dark eyes shocked the automotive world by publishing *Unsafe at Any Speed*, an exposé that relentlessly criticized the "Big Three" automakers in Detroit for emphasizing style, horsepower, comfort, and sales over any concern with safety, fuel economy, or reliability. The author, Ralph Nader, argued that too many automobiles unnecessarily imperiled their occupants even during minor collisions. Rather than add safety features, the industry lobbied with Washington to block regulation. Nader's particular target was the Chevrolet Corvair, a rear-engined small car which General Motors had produced to compete with the popular German Volkswagen Beetle. Crash reports, as well as internal GM engineering studies, indicated that the

Daily Lives

FOOD AND DRINK

Fast-Food America

If people are what they eat (as well as where and how), American society reveals a good deal about itself through its national eating habits. Three long-term trends in particular became evident during the 1970s: Americans increasingly were eating outside the home; the frequency with which families sat together for the three basic meals of the day declined steadily; and diet itself was altered significantly.

Eating foods prepared by a non–family member was once largely the exclusive privilege of the rich, who had access to servants, restaurants, and clubs; or it was the misfortune of the very poor, who took their meals in prisons, soup kitchens, or other institutional settings. By the 1970s the consumption of prepared foods and meals had become common for most Americans. Fast-food chains, school and office cafeterias, vending machines, and other public facilities served up over 40 percent of the meals Americans ate. Many home meals consisted of packaged foods like TV dinners or frozen entrées that required nothing but temperature change prior to consumption. Whether at home or away, the emphasis at mealtime was increasingly on the speed, convenience, or economy with which food was prepared.

Before the 1960s most American restaurants offered a limited range of foods, featuring meats and potatoes baked, broiled, or fried, vegetables steamed or boiled, eggs over easy, and cakes, pies, and ice cream for dessert. An adventurous eater could discover fine French cooking or ethnic foods in urban areas, but even pizza or sweet-and-sour pork were novelties in suburbia. Affluence in the 1950s and 1960s encouraged Americans to become more cosmopolitan in their eating habits. As people traveled, they experienced the world's cuisine. *Picadinho a Brasileira* and *carbonnades à la Flamande* began to replace beef stew. Immigrants to the United States, especially large numbers of Hispanics and Asians, greatly expanded American tastes. Instead of chop suey and chow mein, diners could choose a variety of regional Chinese styles— Mandarin, Cantonese, or spicy Hunan and Szechwan. Lunch might mean a Kosher delicatessen. Texas and California developed variants of Mexican cooking, as Americans graduated from tacos and Fritos to enchiladas and burritos. California steak houses introduced Americans to salad bars. And many people discovered the differences between northern and southern Italian cooking, as well as the vast array of Asian cuisines from India to Thailand to Korea.

As prepared foods became more popular, meals as social occasions for families became rarer. Common meals required the participants to foresake personal preferences and time schedules to share the same foods, served in the same order, at the same time. But in an age of convenience, fast-food chains, and ethnic takeouts, it became practical for individual family members to eat different foods at the same time or to break the "one-cook-to-one-family" pattern. In the process, eating became desocialized. The two most communal meals, breakfast and dinner, no longer brought families together as they once did. By the end of the 1970s some 75 percent of American families did not have breakfast together, and the average family sat down to dinner less than three times a week for a meal that lasted no more than 20 minutes. As formal meals lost their

Daily Lives

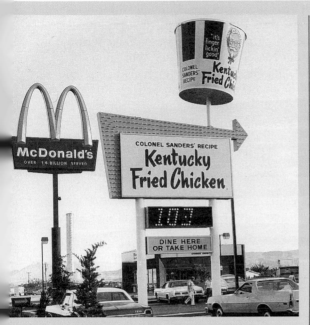

Once limited largely to hamburgers, ice cream, and pancakes, fast food chains now allow Americans to bolt down indifferently synthesized varieties of ethnic and regional foods as well.

importance, snacking became common. Individual family members ingested food in some fashion as often as 20 times a day. More and more often, people combined the consumption of foods with activities other than meals: popcorn and movies, beer and TV sports, coffee and commuting.

As important as where and how people ate were nutritional changes in diet. In earlier societies meals had consisted largely of a core complex carbohydrate (rice, bread, potatoes, or noodles), served up with a fringe complement of meats, vegetables, fruits, and seasoned perhaps with a sauce. The core carbohydrate pro-

vided most nutrition, calories, and satisfaction; the fringe abetted the eating of the core. In modern Western society, including the United States, that pattern reversed over time. By the 1970s the bulk of most Americans' calories had long come from protein foods like meat and eggs, and even more from foods rich in sugars and fats.

As preoccupation with slimness grew, consumption of sugar as a sweetener added to food or eaten in candy declined. But since most Americans ate more and more prepared and precooked foods, the indirect consumption of sugar and sweeteners increased, through desserts, baked goods, soft drinks, and ice cream. Food manufacturers discovered that sugars and dense fats like palm and coconut oil improved flavor, texture, taste, and shelf life. Thus they included sweeteners or fats in places where most people did not expect them: table salt, coatings for fried foods, peanut butter, and "health" foods like granola. By the late 1970s the average American consumed some 130 pounds of sugar and sweeteners per year and about 40 percent of all calories in the form of animal and vegetable fats. The consequence was a steady increase in obesity and diet-related heart diseases and cancers.

An increasing awareness of the relation between diet and disease made the American public, especially the middle and upper classes, more willing to alter eating habits in order to prolong life and health. But with sugars and fats continuing to sell, marketers catered to these preferences. Whether Americans' increasing control over the variety and timing of their meals will eventually lead to long term increases in longevity remains to be seen.

Corvair sometimes tended to roll over in routine turns and quickly lost control when it skidded.

Almost from its beginnings the auto industry had employed carefully orchestrated public relations to shield itself from such criticism. General Motors thus did not take kindly to Nader's revelations. As a defense against this counterculture David, the corporate Goliath decided on a policy of harassment and sent out a private investigator to dig up dirt from Nader's personal life. What they discovered was no hippie disguised in a suit, but an ascetic, penny-pinching example of the American dream. As the son of immigrant parents, he had graduated from Princeton and Harvard Law School. He worked hard, wore his hair short, and never used drugs. And when he discovered GM's intentions, he sued.

GM's embarrassed president James Roche publicly apologized, but by then Nader was a hero and *Unsafe at Any Speed* a best seller. In 1966 Congress passed the National Traffic and Motor Vehicle Safety Act and the Highway Safety Act, which for the first time required safety standards for cars, tires, and roads. Nader used $425,000 from his successful lawsuit against GM to launch his Washington-based Center for the Study of Responsive Law (1969) with a staff of five lawyers and a hundred college volunteers. "Nader's Raiders" as the group soon became known, investigated a wide range of consumer and political issues, including consumer-oriented government agencies, water pollution, Congress, old-age homes, and auto safety.

After 1970 the consumer movement adopted a broad agenda to make business more responsible. It identified unsafe toys, dangerous food additives, and pollutants. It insisted that businesses hire more women and minorities. It brought suit against unethical marketing strategies like "bait-and-switch advertising," against hidden credit costs that plagued the poor, and against defective products, dubbed "lemons." Nader and a host of similar advocates formed powerful lobbying groups and investigating teams; they used legal tools like the "class-action suit," which allowed individuals with common damages from hazardous products or negligence to sue as a group rather than bringing a series of individual suits.

As the consumer movement cast its net more widely, it lost focus. Many of its concerns overlapped with the environmental, civil rights, and women's movements. Like so many leaders from those causes, upper middle-class consumer advocates provoked the skepticism of middle Americans, who worried more about the availability of credit than its fairness. Despite some dramatic victories, consumerism did not shift the location of power in the system. In taking on General Motors once again in the 1970s in Campaign GM, Nader's Raiders had placed their faith in the pressure of public opinion as a way to force corporations to serve the public interest. In response auto executives proved they could appeal to the public as well as Nader's public interest lawyers did. More important, Campaign GM never tapped into the discontent of General Motors workers or forged an alliance with the powerful United Auto Workers Union, which represented them. When public interest lawyers defended the rights of women or minorities or when they attacked specific marketing abuses, they often were more successful. But Nader was never able to establish consumerism as the basis for a mass political reform movement.

Feminism

Undoubtedly the most historically rooted and controversial of the three major "isms" of the 1960s and 1970s was feminism. Organized struggle for women's rights and equality in the United States began before the Civil War. Sustained political efforts had won women the vote in 1920 and shifting economic forces had brought more women into the job market throughout the twentieth century. Yet increasing affluence could not hide the reality that during the post–World War II era, the role of women as housewives and homemakers had been glorified at the expense of two-job families and the aspirations of many women to have careers of their own. In *The Feminine Mystique* (1963) Betty Friedan wrote poignantly about the "problem that has no name," a dispiriting boredom or emptiness in the midst of affluent lives. "Our culture does not permit women to accept or gratify their basic need to grow and fulfill their potentialities as human beings."

The Feminine Mystique acted as an important catalyst to the women's rights movement. The Commission on the Status of Women appointed by President Kennedy proposed the 1963 Equal Pay Act and helped add gender to the forms of discrimination proscribed by the 1964 Civil Rights Act. Women had also assumed an important role in both the civil rights and antiwar movements. But those politically conscious women discovered that like those for whom they struggled, they too were victims of discrimination. During the voter registration drives women were often restricted to behind-the-scenes services such as cooking, doing laundry, and fulfilling others' sexual impulses. Antiwar activists occasionally exploited women's vulnerability as a way to expose the brutality of police and National Guardsmen. As marchers approached hostile forces, up went the cry "Broads on line!" Women who were denied a role in formulating strategy and making decisions were asked to bear much of the violence aimed against protesters.

By 1966 activist women were less willing to see their grievances eclipsed by other political constituencies. Friedan joined a group of 24 women and 2 men who formed the National Organization for Women (NOW). The new feminists sought to force the Johnson administration to take bolder action to eliminate discrimination in such areas as jobs and pay. When feminists argued "sexism" was not qualitatively different from racism, Johnson accepted the argument and in 1967 he included women as well as blacks, Hispanics, and other minorities covered by federal affirmative action programs.

Changes in work, family, education, and sexual mores established a receptive climate for the feminist appeal. After 1957 the birth rate began a rapid decline; affluence and improved methods of contraception, such as the birth control pill, encouraged smaller family size. Women who in the 1950s had children at a young age were free by the 1960s to enter the labor force. By 1970 over 40 percent of all women, an unprecedented number, were employed outside the home. Education also spurred the shift from home to the job market and increased consciousness of women's issues. Higher educational levels allowed women to enter an economy oriented increasingly to white-collar service industries rather than blue-collar manufacturing. Women, especially black women, were more likely than men to be high school graduates.

Between 1960 and 1970 the number of female college students doubled. Former bastions of sexual exclusivity like Yale and Vassar became coeducational. In a social atmosphere that stressed greater freedom for all individuals, college women discovered both the opportunity and pressure for greater experimentation: they contemplated courses in the sciences or careers in law, dated without rules that specified when they had to return to dormitories, and no longer faced a rigid double standard that encouraged men to seek premarital sex that "sweet, marriageable girls" had long been warned to refuse. After college, women could more readily live as singles or in open relationships.

As much as women sought liberation from old restrictions, their new circumstances raised new problems. Men did not readily share traditional family responsibilities with working women; obligations of a job were added to domestic routines. Because they often took part-time jobs or jobs treated as "female" work, women earned far less than men. Many college women continued to view the future "through a wedding band," shunning personal ambition, achievement, and competitiveness as bars to marriage. As a result, they were less likely to choose careers that brought high pay, status, and power. And though greater sexual freedom implied more gender equality, the media continued to promote the image of women as sex objects. To some feminists, the revolution in easy sex and "free" love favored men, since they could more readily escape domestic obligations without loss of sexual companionship.

Such confusing social cross-currents made it difficult for the growing feminist movement to translate its grievances into a coherent political agenda. NOW members could agree in 1967 to a "Bill of Rights" that called for maternity leave for working mothers, federally supported day-care facilities, child-care tax deductions, and equal education and job training. But they divided on two other issues: the passage of an Equal Rights Amendment and a repeal of all state antiabortion laws. Women labor leaders feared that absolute equality would deprive women of necessary protections in the workplace. Socially conservative feminists were offended at the idea that women should have "reproductive freedom." The more radical feminists pushed NOW to adopt both positions.

By the early 1970s the feminists had captured the media's attention. Fifty thousand women participated in NOW's Strike for Equality Parade down New York's Fifth Avenue. Television cameras zeroed in on signs with such slogans as "Don't Cook Dinner—Starve a Rat Today." Some newscasters reported that marchers had burned their bras to protest sexual stereotyping. "Bra burners" became the media's condescending phrase used to deny credibility to militant feminists like Kate Millett, whose *Sexual Politics* (1970) condemned a male-dominated "patriarchal" society.

Political action brought all the major women's organizations together in support of an Equal Rights Amendment (ERA) to the Constitution. A similar effort had gone down to defeat in 1946, but its advocates were more unified by the 1970s. Even the majority of American men were sympathetic to both the ERA and abortion reform. Yet many women feared that the ERA would deprive them of certain protections under the law, while still others saw the amendment as part of a liberation movement they opposed. In 1972 both the House and Senate passed the amendment virtually without opposition. It outlawed all forms of gender discrimination. Within a year 28 of the necessary 38 states had approved the ERA.

Initial success of the ERA drive reflected the growing influence of women in politics. At the 1972 Democratic National Convention the outspoken members of the National Women's Political Caucus captured the party's endorsement for the ERA and helped nominate George McGovern, although the convention would not adopt their platform resolutions supporting gay rights and reproductive freedom. And in 1973 the Supreme Court, even with its conservative Nixon appointees, voted 7–2 in *Roe v. Wade* to strike down 46 state laws restricting a woman's access to abortion. In his opinion for the majority, Justice Harry Blackmun observed that a woman in the nineteenth century had "enjoyed a substantially broader right to terminate a pregnancy than she does in most states today." As legal abortion in the

Feminists recognized the need to strengthen bonds among women in order to provide a new sense of identity not linked to traditional female roles and stereotypes. In this 1970 demonstration they marched to assert their rights, following not only in the footsteps of the New Left but also in the traditions of the women's rights movements of the previous hundred years.

first three months of pregnancy became more readily available, the rate of maternal deaths from illegal operations, especially among minorities, declined.

The early success of the ERA and the feminist triumph with *Roe v. Wade* masked underlying divisions among women's groups in the country. The Supreme Court decision triggered a sharp backlash from many Catholics, Protestant fundamentalists, and socially conservative women. Catholics and fundamentalists alike believed that since human life began with conception, abortion was nothing less than murder under any circumstances. Their outrage inspired a crusade for a "right-to-life" amendment to the Constitution. A similar conservative backlash breathed new life into the "STOP-ERA" crusade of Phyllis Schlafly, an Illinois political organizer who, although a professional herself, believed that women should embrace their traditional role as homemakers subordinate to their husbands. "Every change [that the ERA] requires will deprive women of a right, benefit, or exemption that they now enjoy," Schlafly argued. Many women and men outside the urban professional circle that dominated NOW shared Schlafly's reservations.

In the middle ground stood many women (and a considerable number of men) who wanted the political system to correct the worst inequalities. The forces for moderate reform won several victories, including a ruling forbidding discrimination in colleges receiving federal aid, a court decision ordering the American Telephone and Telegraph Company to open all jobs to women, and the integration of the aggressively masculine military service academies. More far-reaching goals would take longer to achieve. Within a year after Congress passed the ERA, the National Women's Political Caucus conceded that the momentum to pass the amendment had declined. With support waning, Congress in 1979 extended the deadline for ratification from March 22, 1979, to June 30, 1982. Of a necessary 38 state legislatures, 35 had ratified the ERA by 1980, although 5 had rescinded their approval and it was clear that the amendment would fail. Even though determined feminists vowed to continue the fight, they too had discovered the limits of the era.

The Activist Legacy

To say that the organized environmental, consumer, and feminist movements lost ground after the early 1970s is not to say that they failed. Rather, each crusade fell short in its effort to forge a national consensus. There would be no new ecological consciousness, no consumer-directed economy, and no absolute gender equality. Indeed, none of the movements could ever agree just what those ideas would mean in practice.

Instead, the United States was left after the early 1970s with more awareness of ecology, consumer rights, and the blatant and subtle forms of sexism. Advocates of reform had learned to use the media, to lobby politicians, to fight in the courts, and to organize. Old organizations like the National Audobon Society and League of Women Voters had been revitalized. New organizations like NOW and Friends of the Earth had become part of the political infrastructure. Within government the EPA, FTC, and other agencies had a mandate to enforce the court decisions and laws that reformers had won. In that way the advocates of reform achieved a political and social legacy in the tradition of progressivism and the New Deal.

POLITICAL LIMITS: WATERGATE

To Richard Nixon, the triumph of his 1972 reelection must have seemed sweet revenge. In 49 of the 50 states he had defeated George McGovern, the patron saint of liberal environmentalists, consumer advocates, feminists, and the youthful counterculture. Yet while Nixon sought to stem the liberal tide, in the matter of executive power, he continued a trend of concentration and expansion of an "imperial presidency" that had been under way since the early twentieth century. More than any other factor, the cold war with its sense of ongoing crisis had encouraged a steady accumulation of power in the presidency. That expansion involved not only proliferating agencies, both public and secret like the National

Security Agency, but also ever-greater symbolic trappings of political power. Where Franklin Roosevelt had a White House staff of 100, Nixon had over 6000. Emboldened by his victory over McGovern, Nixon determined to use the power of the presidency even more broadly.

The Perils of Power

Part of the president's penchant for wielding power was undoubtedly personal. His lists of enemies and resentments grew ever longer. The impoverished law student who had lived in an abandoned toolshed now reveled in the pomp, the splendor of the presidency, the success and respect it accorded. Where other presidents had seemed content with one or perhaps two vacation retreats, Nixon opted for three. A fleet of 36 planes and helicopters stood ready to ferry members of the White House entourage wherever they might go, while the official yacht *Sequoia* came in for presidential complaint because it was not elegantly enough appointed. Nixon even tried dressing the White House guards in fancy new uniforms, but he was forced to abandon the practice after having them heartily ridiculed as something out of comic opera.

But the matter of power was more than a personal issue. The president and his advisers were particularly eager to act forcefully because they were convinced that the radical reformers of the counterculture menaced American society. As the atmosphere of confrontation during the late sixties encouraged the president to see political debate as a matter of "them" versus "us," members of his staff began compiling an "enemies list"—including everyone from CBS correspondent Daniel Schorr to actress and antiwar activist Jane Fonda. Twenty in particular were targeted for audits by the Internal Revenue Service or similar harassment. In the national debate over Vietnam, Nixon had been particularly irate when in June 1971 the New York *Times* published a secret, often highly critical military study of the war, soon dubbed the Pentagon Papers. Counterattacking, the president authorized his aide John Ehrlichman to organize a team known as "the plumbers," to find and plug security leaks. The government not only prosecuted Daniel Ellsberg, the disillusioned official who had leaked the Pentagon Papers, but the plumbers burglarized the files of Ellsberg's psychiatrist in hopes of finding personally damaging material.

Democrats in Congress had become increasingly concerned about the open assertion of presidential power known as impoundment. When Congress passed a number of social programs Nixon opposed, he simply refused to spend the appropriated money. By 1973 Nixon had used impoundment to make cuts in over a hundred federal programs amounting to some $15 billion. The courts eventually ruled that impoundment was illegal, but meanwhile the president continued his campaign to consolidate power and reshape the more liberal social policies of Congress to his own liking. To that end, he appointed a conservative ideologue to head up Lyndon Johnson's antipoverty agency, the Office of Economic Opportunity, with orders to incapacitate it as much as possible. And Nixon vetoed a host of welfare and environmental bills.

Convinced of the need for firm action in a crisis, suspicious not only of the radical left but also of the liberals in Congress, delighting in personal trappings of power—all these elements made it easier for Richard Nixon to break or bend the rules of power in the service of what he believed was a good cause. In the end, his refusal to acknowledge the limits of power or the ethics of using it brought him down.

Break-In

Nixon's fall began with an apparently minor item that hit the newspapers in June 1972: a petty burglary of Democratic National Committee headquarters, located in Washington's plush Watergate apartment complex. The matter seemed so routine at first that the Washington *Post* assigned the story to a couple of cub reporters, Bob Woodward and Carl Bernstein. But the five burglars proved an unusual lot. They wore business suits, carried walkie-talkies as well as bugging devices and tear-gas guns, and had over $2000 in the form of hundred-dollar bills with sequential serial numbers.

The laconic ivy-league Woodward and the manic, city-smart Bernstein made a true "odd couple." Yet despite their relative inexperience, they sensed the large dimensions of the Watergate affair. One of the burglars, James McCord, had worked for the CIA; another had been captured with an address book whose phone numbers included one belonging to a Howard Hunt at the "W. House." Woodward called the number and discovered that Hunt was indeed a White House consultant. When asked to comment on the story, Nixon's press secretary Ron Ziegler called the break-in "a third rate burglary attempt" and warned that "certain elements may try to stretch this beyond what it is." In August Nixon himself announced that White House Counsel John Dean had conducted a thorough investigation and concluded that "no one on the White House staff . . . was involved in this very bizarre incident. What really hurts in matters of this sort is not the fact that they occur," the president continued. "What really hurts is if you try to cover up."

Matters were not easily settled, however. Woodward and Bernstein traced some of the burglars' money back to the Nixon campaign's Committee to Re-elect the President (popularly known as CREEP). CREEP had "laundered" the money and also established a secret "slush fund" of some $350,000 to be used for projects against the Democrats. The dirty tricks undertaken included forged letters distributed on the letterheads of Democratic candidates, false news leaks, and spying on Democratic campaign workers. But by election time, Woodward and Bernstein had run out of fresh leads. So frustrated was the editor at the Washington *Post*, Benjamin C. Bradlee, that he later confessed that he was "ready to hold both Woodward's and Bernstein's heads in a pail of water until they came up with another story."

In January 1973 the five burglars plus White House aides E. Howard Hunt, Jr., and G. Gordon Liddy went on trial before Judge John J. Sirica. A stern man, "Maximum John" Sirica was not satisfied with the defendants' guilty plea; he wanted to know whether anyone else had directed the burglars and why "these hundred dollar bills were floating around like coupons." Threatened with a stiff jail sentence, James McCord finally cracked. In a letter that Sirica read to the court, McCord admitted that other officials had been involved, that the defendants had been pressured and bribed to plead guilty, and that they had perjured themselves during the trial. In a flight of Orwellian "newspeak," presidential press secretary Ron Ziegler announced on April 17 that all previous administration statements on the Watergate scandal had become "inoperative." With regret, the president announced on April 30 that he had accepted the resignations of his two closest aides,

H.R. Haldeman and John Erlichman. He also fired John W. Dean III, his White House counsel, who had agreed to cooperate with prosecutors.

Over the summer of 1973 televised Senate hearings chaired by Senator Sam Ervin of North Carolina heard testimony from a string of administration officials, each witness taking the trail of the burglary and its cover-up higher and higher into White House circles. It became clear that Attorney General John Mitchell, then the highest ranking law officer of the land, had attended meetings in 1972 where Gordon Liddy outlined preliminary plans for a campaign of dirty tricks, illegal wiretaps, call girl schemes, and burglary of the Democratic National Committee's Watergate office. McCord, Liddy, Hunt, and others had also worked directly for John Erlichman as members of the plumber's unit. When these illegal actions became known, the judge presiding over the Ellsberg Pentagon Papers trial declared a mistrial.

To the Oval Office

Despite these damning revelations most Americans were not quite prepared for the testimony offered by White House counsel John Dean. Young, with a boy scout's face, Dean testified in a quiet monotone that the president had personally been involved in the cover up as recently as April. When McCord threatened to tell all, Dean had met with the president, Haldeman, and Erlichman to discuss raising up to a million dollars in hush money to buy the burglars' silence. Still, Dean was the only witness whose testimony had involved the president. It was his word against Nixon's—until the Senate committee's staff discovered, almost by chance, that the president had been secretly recording all his conversations and phone calls in the Oval Office since 1970. The reliability of Dean's testimony was no longer central, for the tapes could tell all.

Obtaining that evidence proved no easy task. In an effort to restore confidence in the White House, Nixon had appointed Elliot Richardson as attorney general to succeed Richard Kleindienst, who like John Mitchell had fallen under suspicion. Richardson in turn appointed Harvard law professor Archibald Cox as a special prosecutor to investigate the new Watergate disclosures. When Cox subpoenaed the tapes, the president refused to turn them over, citing executive privilege and matters of national security. The courts, however, overruled this position.

As that battle raged and the astonished public wondered if matters could possibly get worse, they did. An investigation unrelated to Watergate found evidence that Vice President Spiro Agnew had systematically solicited graft, not just as governor of Maryland, but while serving in Washington. Agnew loudly denounced the charges while quietly negotiating with prosecutors for permission to plead *nolo contendere* (no contest) to a single charge of federal income tax evasion. In return, he agreed to resign the vice presidency in October. The rambunctious rhetorician of law and order suddenly appeared no better than a petty crook. Under provisions of the Twenty-Fifth Amendment, Nixon appointed popular Michigan congressman Gerald R. Ford to replace Agnew.

Meanwhile, Special Prosecutor Archibald Cox remained unrelenting in his demands to examine the tapes. The president had countered by offering to submit written summaries of conversations rather than the tapes themselves. But trust in the president had by now been so greatly undermined that Cox rejected the offer, especially since the president also demanded that Cox agree to ask for no further

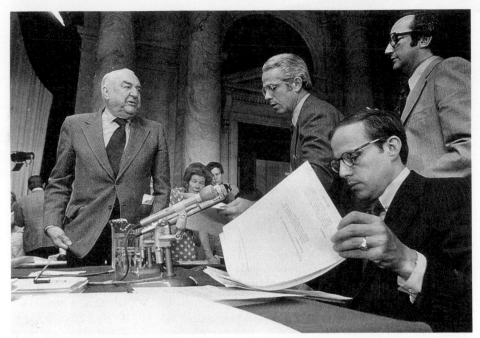

Under the leadership of North Carolina Senator Sam Ervin (left), the Senate Committee investigating the Watergate scandal attracted a large television audience. John Dean (right), the former White House legal counsel, provided the most damning testimony linking President Nixon to the cover-up. But only when the existence of secretly recorded White House tapes became known was there a chance to corroborate his account.

documents. On Saturday night, October 20, Nixon ordered Cox fired. Elliot Richardson and his assistant, William Ruckelshaus, refused and resigned instead; Solicitor General Robert Bork finally fired him. Reaction to the "Saturday Night Massacre" was overwhelming: 150,000 telegrams poured into Washington and by the following Tuesday 84 House members sponsored 16 different bills of impeachment. The beleaguered president agreed to comply with Judge Sirica's order to hand over the tapes. And he appointed Texas lawyer Leon Jaworski as a new special prosecutor.

No sooner had the smoke cleared from the Saturday Night Massacre, however, than White House counsel J. Fred Buzhardt admitted that sections of the subpoenaed tapes were missing, including a crucial 18-minute gap in the conversation in which the president first discussed the Watergate burglary, three days after it occurred. Nixon's loyal secretary Rose Mary Woods tried to take the blame and White House chief of staff Alexander Haig suggested an unaccountable "sinister force" might have caused the blank space, but experts later verified that the gap was the result of intentional erasure.

By April 24, 1974, Jaworski's investigations led him to request additional tapes. Again the president refused; then he grudgingly agreed to supply some 1200 pages of typed transcripts, though not the tapes themselves. Even the transcripts damaged the president's case. The conversations were littered with profanity ("[expletive deleted]," the transcripts read), revealing a vulgar, mean-spirited White House staff. And they suggested a president very much a part of the cover-up process. On March 21, 1973, he had talked with Dean about how to "take care of the jackasses who are in jail." When Dean estimated it might take a million dollars to shut them up, Nixon replied, "We could get that. . . . You could get a million dollars. And you could get it in cash. I know where it could be gotten. I mean it's not easy, but it could be done." And when the matter of perjury came up Nixon suggested a way out: "You can say, 'I don't remember.' You can say, 'I can't recall.'"

Even those devastating revelations did not produce the "smoking gun" the president's defenders demanded as a basis for impeachment. They wanted clear proof that the president had actively participated in the cover-up from its earliest moments. When Jaworski petitioned the Supreme Court to order release of additional tapes to use in the trial of six former Nixon aides, the Court in *United States v. Nixon* on July 24 ruled unanimously in the prosecutor's favor.

The end came quickly. The House Judiciary Committee adopted three articles of impeachment, charging that Nixon had illegally obstructed justice, had abused his constitutional authority in improperly using federal agencies to harass citizens, and had impeded the committee's effort to investigate the cover-up. The tapes produced the smoking gun. Conversations with Haldeman on June 23, 1972, only a few days after the break-in, showed that Nixon knew the burglars were tied to the White House staff, knew that his attorney general had been involved, and knew that Mitchell had acted to limit FBI investigation. Even the president's staunchest supporters deserted him. Knowing that the Senate had the votes to make him the first president convicted in an impeachment trial, Nixon resigned on August 8, 1974. The following day Gerald Ford became president. "The Constitution works," Ford told a relieved nation. "Our long national nightmare is over."

Had the system worked? In one sense, yes. The wheels of justice had turned, even if slowly. For the first time a president had been forced to leave office. Four cabinet officers, John Mitchell, Commerce Secretary Maurice Stans, Agriculture Secretary Earl Butz, and Mitchell's successor Richard Kleindienst were all convicted of crimes. Twenty-five Nixon aides eventually served prison terms ranging from 25 days to over 4 years.

Yet what would have happened if Ben Bradlee had found his pail of water? With the exception of the Washington *Post* and one or two other newspapers, the media had accepted the administration's cover-up at face value. And despite the revelations of widespread political abuses, federal agencies still have it within their power to harass innocent citizens arbitrarily. Later abuses within the executive branch such as the "Irangate" scandals under Ronald Reagan have demonstrated that the imperial powers of the presidency are still largely unchecked. Secret agencies and covert operations remain standard procedure. The Fair Campaign Practices Act adopted in 1974 to eliminate "fat-cat" contributions and to enforce greater financial accountability on campaigns succeeded largely in complicating the efforts of third parties to initiate campaigns. Political action committees (PACs) representing special interest groups became major sources of campaign funding. The system works, as the Founding Fathers understood, only when citizens and public servants respect the limits of government power.

A FORD, NOT A LINCOLN

Gerald Ford inherited a presidential office almost crippled by the Watergate scandals. As the first unelected president, he had no popular mandate. He was little known outside Washington and his home district around Grand Rapids, Michigan. Ford's success as the House minority leader came from personal popularity, political reliability, and plodding determination, qualities that suited a congressman but not an unelected president. Lyndon Johnson once quipped that "Gerry Ford is so dumb he can't walk and chew gum at the same time." Yet Ford had a kind of respect for tradition and inner solidity that came as a relief after the mercurial styles of Johnson and Nixon. He had been a star football player at the University of Michigan and later earned a law degree from Yale. By all instincts a conservative, Ford was determined to continue Nixon's aggressive foreign policy and a domestic program of social and fiscal conservatism.

Kissinger Regnant

As Nixon's star fell, that of his Secretary of State and National Security Advisor Henry Kissinger rapidly rose. Kissinger cultivated reporters who relished his witty quips, intellectual breadth, and willingness to leak stories to the press. He was a ruthless political infighter who rid the White House of his chief rivals. With Nixon desperate for a foreign policy success to offset Watergate in the summer of 1974, he took Kissinger on a trip to Moscow and the Middle East. As the end neared, it was Kissinger who warned military commanders to ignore presidential orders.

Kissinger had struggled to prevent Vietnam and Watergate from eroding the president's power to conduct an independent foreign policy. Congress was too sensitive to public opinion and special interest pressure groups to pursue consistent long-term policies, he warned. But after Vietnam congressional leaders were eager to curtail presidential powers. In 1971 they had repealed the Gulf of Tonkin Resolution (p. 1200), and by 1975 they had passed bills barring American troops from returning to Vietnam or from new involvements in strifetorn Angola without congressional approval. More important, the War Powers Act of 1973 required the president to consult Congress whenever possible before committing troops, to send an explanation for his actions within 2 days, and to withdraw any troops after 60 days unless Congress voted to retain them.

In all his political machinations, Kissinger viewed himself as a realist, a man for whom order and stability were more important than principle. In that way he offended idealists on the political left and right. Quoting the German writer Goethe, Kissinger acknowledged, "If I had to choose between justice and disorder, on the one hand, and injustice and order on the other, I would always choose the latter." He most ruthlessly applied that approach to quell political ferment in Chile.

In 1970 Chile ranked as one of South America's few viable democracies. When a coalition of Socialists, Communists, and radicals succeeeded in electing Salvador Allende Gossens as president, the CIA determined that his victory created a danger to the United States. Kissinger pressed the CIA to bribe the Chilean Congress and to promote a military coup against Allende. When those attempts failed, Kissinger resorted to economic warfare between the United States and the

Allende government. By 1973 a Chilean coalition of disgruntled conservatives, high-paid union workers, and foreign business leaders with CIA backing had joined to drive the Socialists from power. On September 17 the Chilean military attacked the presidential palace and killed Allende. The United States immediately recognized the new government, which over the next decade deteriorated into a brutally repressive dictatorship. Kissinger argued that the United States had the right to destroy this democracy because communists were antidemocratic.

The Decline of American Hegemony

As a political realist, Kissinger understood that the United States no longer had the economic strength to dominate the affairs of the noncommunist bloc of nations. The country faced a process of decolonization that meant loosening its grip in areas like Central America and the Middle East, though it was politically impossible to admit that to the public. Kissinger was particularly vulnerable to hostile Republican conservatives suspicious of his old Rockefeller ties and eager to restore prestige lost during Vietnam.

At home inflation had begun to soar. A short-term economic boom in 1972–1973 following the devaluation of the dollar led to increased prices. American industries with inefficient production, products of poor quality, and high wages struggled against mounting competition from manufacturers in Europe and the Pacific rim (Japan, South Korea, Taiwan, Hong Kong, Singapore, and the Philippines). American-based multinational corporations began to establish their manu-

After having won a Nobel Peace Prize in 1973 for his role in ending the Vietnam War, Henry Kissinger entered the Ford administration as something of a hero. But his efforts to improve relations with the Soviet Union by strengthening détente aroused the ire of the Republican right wing, while liberals accused Kissinger of being too secretive and friendly to dictators.

facturing centers overseas to take advantage of lower costs and cheap labor. The bellwether industry of the American economy, automobiles, steadily lost sales to Japan and Germany. Speaking on behalf of its blue-collar constituency, the AFL–CIO complained that the loss of high-wage manufacturing jobs would create "a nation of hamburger stands, a country stripped of industrial capacity . . . , a nation of citizens busily buying and selling cheeseburgers and root beer floats."

And when it seemed matters could hardly become worse, along came the Yom Kippur War and the OPEC oil boycott. Here was decolonization with a vengeance. On October 6, 1973, Syria and Egypt launched a devastating surprise attack against Israel. The Soviet Union airlifted supplies to the Arabs; the United States countered on October 15 by resupplying its Israeli allies while pressing the two sides to accept a cease-fire. The seven Arab members of OPEC backed Egypt and Syria. They imposed a boycott of oil sales to countries seen as friendly to Israel. Since the 1920s the major multinational oil companies, known after World War II as the Seven Sisters (Exxon, Shell, Gulf, Mobil, British Petroleum, Socal, and Texaco), had dominated world marketing. Never before had the OPEC nations controlled the distribution of their oil, but the boycott from October 1973 until March 1974 devastated the countries of Western Europe and Japan, which imported 80 to 90 percent of their oil from the Middle East. The rise of oil prices from $2 to $8 a barrel set off recessionary pressures that staggered the industrial economies of the world.

Since the United States relied on the Middle East for just 12 percent of its oil consumption (other imports came from Venezuela, Mexico, and Canada), American oil experts were confident that the boycott would end before the United States suffered appreciably. That confidence soon collapsed when it became obvious that Americans were far more dependent on foreign oil than most people had ever appreciated. With just 7 percent of the world's population, the United States consumed about 30 percent of its energy. The nation's postwar prosperity came in large part from the use of cheap energy. Among the technologies that spurred postwar economic growth were high-compression automobile engines, commercial airliners, detergents, artificial fertilizers, synthetic fabrics, plastics, and disposable containers.

In November 1973 President Nixon had announced to the nation, "We are heading toward the most acute shortage of energy since World War II." Americans felt the crunch in every aspect of their lives. As the price of petroleum-based plastics soared, everything from records to raincoats cost more. In some places motorists hoping to buy a few gallons of gas waited for hours in lines miles long. Nixon pledged to "make the United States energy-independent by 1980," but his Watergate woes interfered with efforts to frame a coherent energy policy.

To Kissinger fell the role of shoring up the West's energy fortunes by using American influence to stabilize the politics of the Middle East. If the Arab states saw the United States as a neutral in their conflict with Israel, they would be less likely to resort to future oil blackmail. And in linking the oil boycott to the cold war, Kissinger thought the revival of American prestige would allow him to reduce Soviet influence in the region. Egypt's President Anwar Sadat had recently exposed Soviet vulnerability by expelling 10,000 Russian advisers from his country. From January to April 1974 Kissinger intermittently engaged in "shuttle diplomacy" between Sadat's government in Cairo and the Israeli government of Golda Meir in Jerusalem. By the end of January Kissinger had persuaded Israel to withdraw its troops from the west bank of the Suez Canal; in May he arranged disengagement between Israel and Syria in the Golan Heights.

OIL AND CONFLICT IN THE MIDDLE EAST

What the Balkans had been before World War I the Middle East became after World War II: a vital geopolitical region beset by big-power rivalry and complicated by tribal, ethnic, and religious divisions and political instability. Much of the world's known oil reserves lie along the Persian Gulf. Proximity to the Soviet Union and vital trade routes like the Suez Canal define the region's geographic importance. Revolutions in Iran and Afghanistan, intermittent warfare between Arabs and Jews, the unresolved questions of Israel's borders and a Palestinian homeland, the disintegration of Lebanon, and a long, bloody war between Iran and Iraq have been among the conflicts that have unsettled the region.

That was just one strand in the web Kissinger sought to weave. He also saw the possibility of indirectly asserting American power through a client state. To that end he and Nixon had authorized the sale of the most advanced weapons to the shah of oil-rich Iran. Some 40,000 American military and civilian advisers went to Iran to modernize its military and civilian economies. In regional conflicts the shah, unlike the United States, could threaten pro-Soviet states like Iraq and Syria. In that same spirit Kissinger asserted American power in less strategically vital areas of the Third World, especially in the southwest African nation of Angola. With the departure of Portugal's colonial government, rival factions struggled to gain power. Since the Soviet Union backed the more powerful group, Kissinger ordered the CIA to give covert aid to pro-Western elements.

Kissinger found that despite his almost heroic efforts, he could not stem the erosion of American power. As involvement in Angola stirred memories of Vietnam, Congress prohibited the CIA from spending money for the Angolan civil war. While Kissinger struggled to restore order to the Middle East, the American client government in Vietnam fell. In 1973 President Thieu had broken the cease-fire agreement. By the spring of 1975 the South Vietnamese forces faced certain defeat. President Ford asked Congress for $1 billion in aid to Vietnam, Cambodia, and Laos, but Congress refused to spend more money on a lost cause. The end came almost immediately after. Desperate South Vietnamese civilian and military leaders rushed to escape Communist retribution.

Even in the Western Hemisphere American hegemony eroded. The OPEC boycott heightened the dependence of the United States on Mexico, Venezuela, and Canada for much of its imported energy. While those countries benefited from higher oil prices, oil-dependent economies like Brazil's suffered. As a result, Brazil and other exporters tried to do with coffee and other raw materials what the Arabs had done with oil. Even the normally cooperative Canadians showed an inclination to establish more economic distance. Americans owned or controlled large economic interests in Canada, and much of Canada's popular culture came from the United States. Under Prime Minister Pierre Elliot Trudeau, Canada pursued a more independent foreign policy. It established ties to China and the Soviet Union while limiting the level of foreign investments. And as OPEC tightened its noose, Canada cut back exports to the United States to meet its own energy needs. As much as Kissinger saw Europe, the Middle East, and Asia as the arena for big power initiatives, he could not ignore the growing disaffection between the United States and its hemispheric neighbors.

Détente

Vietnam, Chile, the Yom Kippur War, and Angola indicated that the spirit of détente had not ended Soviet–American rivalry over the Third World. Seeking to ease tensions, Ford met with Soviet leader Leonid Brezhnev in November 1974. Since economic stagnation had dogged the Soviet Union, Brezhnev came to Vladivostok eager for more American trade; Ford and Kissinger wanted a limit on nuclear weapons that preserved the current American advantage. Though many issues could not be resolved, the two sides agreed in principle to a framework for a second SALT treaty.

A similar hope to extend détente brought Ford and Brezhnev together with European leaders at Helsinki, Finland, in August 1975. There they agreed to recognize the political boundaries that had divided Eastern and Western Europe since 1945. For the first time the United States sent an ambassador to East Germany. In return Brezhnev eased restrictions on the rights of Soviet Jews to emigrate. That issue had led numerous senators and congressmen to oppose trade agreements with the Soviet Union.

The erosion of American power, symbolized by Kissinger's overtures to the Soviet Union, led outraged Republican conservatives like 1976 presidential hopeful Ronald Reagan to criticize Ford and Kissinger for trafficking with the Communists. When the administration proposed to return operating control of the Panama Canal to Panama in order to ease tensions in Latin America, the conservatives charged Ford with selling out American interests and weakening the nation's power. In an effort to subdue the critics, Ford in 1976 stripped Kissinger of his post as National Security Advisor.

An Embattled Presidency

Every president has a "honeymoon" during which the press and opposing politicians restrain criticism. Ford's presidential honeymoon was much shorter than most. His first setback came when he appointed former New York governor Nelson A. Rockefeller as vice-president. Liberals had never forgiven Rockefeller for violent police actions in 1971 at Attica Prison which left 33 prisoners and 10 hostages dead. Populist conservatives resented Rockefeller's inherited wealth and viewed him, along with his protégé Henry Kissinger, as the embodiment of the eastern establishment's liberal internationalism.

If the conservatives were angry about Rockefeller, almost everyone was outraged when Ford pardoned Richard Nixon on September 8, 1974. Pardon meant no prosecution, leaving charges unanswered and crimes unpunished. In trying to put Watergate in the past, Ford reopened the wounds. He did the same in refusing charity to the draft resisters from the Vietnam War. He offered them conditional amnesty after review by a government panel. Most of the 350,000 resisters refused the terms, which still held them guilty for an act of conscience. Conservatives and veterans' groups objected to leniency for those they saw as disloyal citizens.

Then Ford inadvertently exposed widespread abuses by the CIA and FBI. Upon taking office, he had incautiously admitted the CIA was involved in the overthrow of Salvador Allende. Soon after, Seymour Hersh of the New York *Times* uncovered illegal CIA domestic espionage operations. A commission headed by Vice President Rockefeller reported that the abuses were more widespread than at first expected. The CIA routinely kept citizens under surveillance, had conducted drug experiments on unwitting subjects, had used Operation CHAOS to infiltrate protest organizations, and had done political dirty work for the White House.

A Senate committee headed by Frank Church of Idaho produced equally disturbing information. The CIA had been involved in numerous assassinations or attempted murders of foreign leaders, including Fidel Castro of Cuba, Patrice Lumumba of the Congo, Rafael Trujillo of the Dominican Republic, and Ngo Dinh Diem of South Vietnam, as well as Allende. The FBI had similarly used illegal means to infiltrate and disrupt domestic dissidents, including an attempt by J. Edgar Hoover to smear Martin Luther King. A chastened President Ford ordered the creation of an Intelligence Oversight Board to monitor the CIA, while the Senate created its own watchdog committee.

Most presidents' fortunes rise and fall with the economy. Ford faced the twin scourges of inflation and recession. As a conservative, he rejected the pressures to impose wage and price controls. Nor did he heed warnings from Democrats to avoid policies that used increased unemployment and lower earnings to fight rising prices. Donning a button with the inscription "WIN" (Whip Inflation Now), he declared inflation the nation's number one problem and opted for a mixture of lower government spending and voluntary restraints. With the economy reeling, the Democrats made major gains during the 1974 election, adding 49 seats in the House and 5 in the Senate as well as 4 governorships.

Election successes masked the deep divisions within the Democratic party in the wake of the 1972 McGovern campaign disaster. No more than the Republicans did the Democrats have a coherent program to restore the economy to health. When Ford went before Congress to give his first State of the Union message in January 1975, the country faced its worst slump since the Great Depression. During the previous quarter the gross national product had fallen over 9 percent, inflation had climbed to almost 14 percent, and unemployment exceeded 7 percent.

At the heart of the economic crisis lay the problem of rising energy costs. By 1976 consumption had returned to 1973 levels, even though domestic oil production had fallen by over 1 million barrels. Imports of Middle Eastern oil priced at almost $14 a barrel were needed to supply the nation's profligate thirst for energy. In 1975 Congress adopted the Energy Policy and Conservation Act, which increased the authority of the Federal Energy Administration to order utilities to burn abundant coal rather than expensive oil. In addition, the act created a strategic petroleum reserve as a hedge against future boycotts and ordered the auto industry to improve energy efficiency (mileage per gallon of fuel). And as a final— but environmentally dangerous—stopgap measure, the government encouraged the rapid development of nuclear power plants.

Rising energy costs struck hardest at the older industrial centers of the Northeast and Upper Midwest, which imported most of their energy. Housing and plants built in the days of cheap energy proved wasteful and inefficient. Nixon's

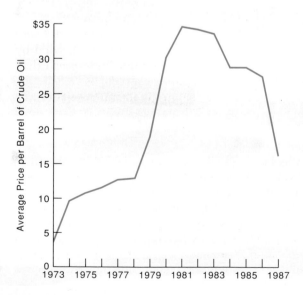

OPEC OIL PRICES, 1973–1987
Prices fell even further than the chart shows after 1980 because the dollar was worth much less than in 1973.

and Ford's fiscal conservatism hurt too. Cutbacks in federal spending fell hardest on major cities with shrinking tax bases, outmoded industries, and heavy social service costs. The crisis for "rust belt" cities came to a head in October 1975 when New York announced it stood on the brink of bankruptcy.

New York's problems stemmed in part from its extensive welfare services, its careless budgetary practices, and its bloated municipal employee unions and in part from the loss of jobs in the private sector. With few ways left to raise taxes or borrow money, Mayor Abraham D. Beame appealed to the federal government for help. When Ford refused, the New York *Daily News'* headline stated, "FORD TO CITY: DROP DEAD." Only after New York had overhauled its finances and won concessions from city workers did Ford authorize loans. His grudging response, which forced much-needed reforms, seemed highly insensitive to the beleaguered people of New York and other strapped municipalities.

The Election of 1976

In the 1976 presidential campaign the greatest debates occurred within rather than between the major parties. Ford's greatest challenge came from former California governor, movie actor, and television pitchman Ronald Reagan. Once a supporter of Franklin Roosevelt, Reagan discovered true conservatism after his marriage to actress Nancy Davis. Although Ford's appearances lost him votes, the polished Reagan won crowds with an aggressive style that radiated amiability. "Under Messrs. Nixon and Ford this nation has become Number Two in military power," he would tell enthusiastic audiences. Reagan had the race deadlocked until the convention, where Ford eked out the nomination while the Reagan forces controlled the party platform, which attacked détente, opposed busing, called for constitutional amendments on balanced budgets, school prayer, and prohibition of abortions, and generally favored reduction of government in Washington wherever possible.

Among Democratic hopefuls James Earl (Jimmy) Carter's anonymity before 1976 proved a strength. His southern accent marked him as a Washington outsider. His image as a "born-again" Christian reassured those Americans searching for renewed faith. And one pledge—"I would not tell a lie"—seemed a welcome antidote to cover-ups and deceptions. Somehow Carter managed to address controversial issues such as abortion or busing without offending large groups on either side. He was "personally opposed to abortion" as a Christian but against a constitutional amendment overturning *Roe v. Wade.* In their platform, rather than their candidate, the Democrats established some distance from the rival GOP. They supported federal health insurance, job programs, and the ERA while opposing an antiabortion amendment and reluctantly accepting busing as a last-ditch tool to achieve integration.

Seldom has an election generated so little interest. "Don't Vote. It Only Encourages Them," one popular bumper sticker proclaimed. No matter who won, American politics in the age of limits would have a conservative flavor. Partisanship proved stronger than ever as most voters (80 percent of Democrats and 90 percent of Republicans) backed their party's candidate. It added up to 50.1 percent for Carter, a popular edge of almost 1.7 million, and a 57-vote lead (297–240) in the Electoral College. Carter's overwhelming margin among blacks (90 percent) carried the South and offset Ford's margin among whites, especially in the western states, which all went Republican. Resounding Democratic majorities in the

Senate (62–38), House (292–143), and governorships (37–12–1) indicated more accurately than the presidential race how much the weak economy had hurt the Republicans.

JIMMY CARTER, RESTORING THE FAITH

"If after the inauguration you find a Cy Vance as secretary of state and Zbigniew Brzezinski as head of national security, then I would say we have failed," Carter's chief aide Hamilton Jordan told reporters during the campaign. The new administration promised to bring fresh faces to Washington. But once elected Carter turned to hiring familiar figures. He appointed establishment lawyer Cyrus Vance as secretary of state and Columbia professor Zbigniew Brzezinski as national security adviser. The New York *Times* warned Carter against such a contradiction because he "lacks the eloquence to hide it." But more than any political shortcoming, the weak economy and small electoral margin denied Carter an opportunity for bold leadership.

The Carter Style

Carter tried to remove some of the trappings from the imperial presidency and infuse a simpler style into the White House. Rather than the usual Inauguration Day ride down Pennsylvania Avenue in the presidential limousine, the president and his wife Rosalynn walked. He shunned the formal morning coat and tails for a business suit. And he cut perquisites and brought into his cabinet many Washington newcomers, whose lack of familiarity with federal administration probably made them unsuitable for high office. Consumer advocate Ralph Nader warned that Carter's "conservatives with high integrity would follow the wrong policies straight instead of crooked."

If Carter had any overriding sense of direction, it remained obscure throughout his administration. He had a tremendous grasp of information but often focused so narrowly on details that he failed to clarify his larger goals. On the one hand, he appointed as ambassador to the United Nations former Georgia congressman and black activist Andrew Young, who hoped to improve American relations with the nonwhite peoples of the Southern Hemisphere. On the other hand, Carter chose as attorney general a Georgian, Griffin Bell, who had belonged to racially and religiously segregated clubs and held generally conservative views on political and social issues. Would the conservative outsider Bell or the liberal Washington veteran Young indicate the course of the new administration?

In foreign policy Carter accepted the realities of decolonization. The United States, he suggested, should exert "leadership without hegemony." Inordinate fear of Communism had led the United States in the past to support any right-wing dictator who happened to oppose Communism. Under Carter, the United States would reassert its moral purpose by giving a higher priority to the preservation of human rights. And in his Inaugural Address, the former nuclear submarine officer established as his ultimate goal "the elimination of all nuclear weapons from this earth." His direction of foreign policy was confused, however, by the rivalry between Zbigniew Brzezinski and Secretary of State Cyrus Vance. Brzezinski profoundly mistrusted the Soviet Union. He had the staunch cold warrior's concern with containing the Communist menace. Vance believed negotiations were both possible and potentially profitable. Stronger economic ties would reduce the risk of superpower conflict. Carter gravitated in both directions.

The president found it most difficult to sustain his good intentions on the domestic front. He set out to make government more efficient, responsive to the people, and ethical. Yet when he first tried to impose these standards by eliminating 19 expensive pork barrel water projects, the leaders of his own party threatened to bury his legislative program. And his efforts to restore faith in government ran afoul of revelations of widespread congressional corruption. Perhaps as many as a hundred congressmen had received bribes from the South Korean government. Others were involved in various kickback schemes and accepted bribes from federal agents posing as Arabs in the "Abscam" investigation. When the dubious financial dealings of his brother Billy and his Georgia friend and budget director Burt Lance came to light, Carter remained loyal to family and friend. But the failure to discipline the two made the president seem hypocritical.

With congressional leaders unwilling and unable to discipline Senate and House members, Carter found it almost impossible to push through a legislative program. And like Gerald Ford, he learned that the wounds of Vietnam were slow to heal. In response to a campaign pledge, he granted amnesty to Vietnam War draft resisters but not to veterans with dishonorable discharges. Conservatives like Barry Goldwater were outraged and many veterans were bitter. As the American Civil Liberties Union pointed out, the veterans with tainted discharges were more likely to be the undereducated poor from minority groups.

The Moral Equivalent of War

In 1977 even the weather seemed to conspire against the Carter administration. One of the most severe winters in modern history created temporary shortages of heating fuels and drove prices up. Heavy snows and fierce cold forced many schools and factories to close. Like Ford, Carter preferred to ask for voluntary restraint rather than enforce mandatory government policies to conserve energy and control fuel costs. To meet the energy crisis the nation had to adopt conservation measures as the "moral equivalent of war," he announced in April 1977.

Carter correctly sensed that conservation was the cheapest and most environmentally desirable way to discourage dependence on foreign oil. But homilies about "helping our neighbors" did not sell the president's program of new taxes aimed to discourage wasteful energy consumption. The American way, as domestic oil producers were quick to argue, was to produce more, not live with less. The oil industry insisted that deregulation of energy prices would stimulate sufficient production to meet the nation's needs. Americans in general were too wedded to large gas-guzzling cars, air conditioners, inefficient electrical appliances, and warm houses to accept limits as long as fuel was available. Although Congress did agree to establish a cabinet-level Department of Energy, it rejected most of Carter's energy taxes and proposals to encourage solar alternatives.

By 1978 the "moral equivalent of war" looked more like its acronym: MEOW. Renewed administration efforts resulted in a weak National Energy Act, which provided tax credits for installation of energy-saving equipment, encouraged utility conversion to coal, and allowed prices to rise for newly discovered natural gas. As a result, the nation was ill-prepared for the dislocation in international oil markets that followed the 1978 revolution against the shah of Iran. Brief shortages allowed OPEC to raise prices 14.5 percent. Carter could only complain that such hikes were unfair while asking Americans to lower thermostats to 65 degrees and, if car trips were essential, observe the new 55 mile per hour speed limit.

As a diversion from the worries of energy shortages, many Americans flocked to see antinuclear activist Jane Fonda in the movie *China Syndrome*, a tale of faulty construction resulting in a meltdown of the core of a nuclear power plant. Then on March 28, 1979, a stuck valve at the Three Mile Island nuclear power plant in Pennsylvania released a cloud of radioactive gas into the atmosphere. It took two weeks before the reactor was shut down. A hundred thousand nearby residents fled their homes. Since the early 1950s public utilities had promoted nuclear power as the answer to future energy needs. Construction of plants raced ahead of technological safeguards and solutions to the problem of nuclear waste disposal. By the time of Three Mile Island, huge construction cost overruns and concerns about safety had inspired a growing antinuclear backlash. Experts now admitted that nuclear plants were no more than a temporary response to the nation's long-term needs.

In the wake of Three Mile Island, President Carter appealed anew for a strong energy program, most of which Congress rejected. By May motorists once

The danger of depending on nuclear power as an alternate source of energy became evident in 1979 when an accident closed this plant at Three Mile Island near Harrisburg, Pennsylvania. The large towers are part of the cooling system in which the accident occurred. Huge construction costs, the unsolved problem of nuclear waste disposal, and safety issues soon soured the public on nuclear energy.

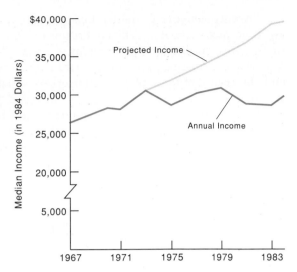

INCOME PROJECTIONS OF TWO-INCOME FAMILIES, 1967–1984

In the age of limits family income stayed relatively even only because more wives entered the work force. Wages for individual workers fell, when calculated in real dollars.

Source: Frank Levy, *Dollars and Dreams: The Changing American Income Distribution* (New York: Norton, 1988), p. 204.

again faced long lines at the gas pumps. OPEC announced plans for a 50 percent price hike. Not until spring 1980 did Congress pass a bill taxing windfall profits (although not significantly), regulating nuclear power more stringently, establishing a Synthetic Fuels Corporation and a solar-energy program, and reviving the Strategic Petroleum Reserve. Carter had promoted sacrifice as a way to "seize control of our common destiny"; Congress preferred halfhearted measures that left America's energy future in OPEC's hands.

A Sick Economy

An economy dependent on inexpensive fuel could hardly absorb rapid OPEC price hikes without serious dislocations. Colleges that had allocated 10 percent of their budgets to energy soon had to pay as much as 50 percent. All costs began a dramatic rise as inflation shot from just below 6 percent in 1976 to almost 14 percent by 1979. Workers' wages could not keep pace. People took home more dollars, but real earnings steadily eroded. Federal policies made matters worse. Government payments to farmers, higher minimum wages, import protection for key industries like steel, and new Social Security taxes added to inflationary pressures. So too did declines in the productivity of American labor, where output for each workhour kept dropping. Outmoded industrial plants, ineffective management practices, burdensome union rules, and inflexible wage contracts with built-in cost-of-living adjustments lowered the competitive standing of American industry in world markets.

As has been true since the early twentieth century, the automobile industry played a determining and symbolic economic role. In 1978 the industry was sick, with the Chrysler Corporation at death's door. The company had for years made serious mistakes in styling and had been unable to design and build small cars in time to respond to shifting consumer demand. Unless the government provided a billion-dollar tax credit, warned Chrysler president Lee Iacocca, the nation's tenth largest business enterprise faced bankruptcy.

"Are we going to guarantee businessmen against their own incompetence?" asked an angry Senator William Proxmire. "No one should hold half a million workers responsible for the decisions of a few officials long since gone," replied Michigan congressman James Blanchard in defense of the Chrysler bailout. In the end the reality of unemployed autoworkers weighed more heavily than the abstractions of free market rhetoric. After wringing wage concessions from Chrysler employees, Congress agreed to guarantee a $1.5 billion loan that did bring Chrysler off the critical list. Still, disgruntled liberals and conservatives appreciated the lyrics of folk singer Tom Paxton as he announced,

> I'm changing my name to Chrysler.
> I'll be waiting in that great receiving line.
> So when they hand a billion grand out,
> I'll be standing with my hand out;
> Mister I'll get by.

The Chrysler loan was little more than a bandage on a badly wounded economy. "Hard choices" were needed to stem inflation, reverse mounting trade deficits, ease rising interest rates, and reduce the federal deficit, the *Wall Street Journal* argued. But Carter called only for voluntary restraints on prices and wages, while seeking to restore the strength of the dollar in international trade. The high interest rates favored by conservatives struck hardest at American consumers addicted to installment and credit-card buying. Before Carter's economic remedies could work, OPEC began another round of oil price hikes that increased energy costs almost 60 percent. Interest rates shot up to almost 20 percent. Mortgage money disappeared. New "housing starts" (the number of homes under construction), second in economic importance only to automobiles, dwindled, while older homes went unsold. With Federal Reserve rates at 15 percent, an anti-inflationary recession in 1980 doomed Carter's political future.

Leadership, Not Hegemony

Presidents battered on the domestic front often see a strong foreign policy as one way to restore power and prestige. Carter achieved a stunning breakthrough in mediating the longstanding hostility between Israel and Egypt, only to fall hostage to OPEC and to Islamic revolutionaries in Iran.

For all the carping from hardboiled liberals and conservatives, Carter's human rights policy did make a difference. At least one Argentinian Nobel Peace Prize winner, Adolfo Pérez Esquivel, claimed he owed his life to it. So did hundreds of others in countries like the Philippines, South Korea, Argentina, and Chile, where dissidents were routinely murdered and tortured. The Carter administration exerted economic pressures to promote more humane policies. Yet when rich minerals, oil, or other national security interests were involved, the administration managed to ignore flagrant abuses. The shah of Iran was so good a customer for American arms and such a major oil exporter that Carter ignored the terror of the shah's secret police, SAVAK, against Iranian political prisoners. Joseph Mobutu, dictator of Zaire in Central Africa, had one of the world's most indefensible records on human rights. His nation also controlled vast mineral resources exploited by European companies, so when rebels from nearby Angola threatened Mobutu, the United States flew in Moroccan and French troops and provided financial aid.

Declining American influence in the Third World underlay a growing debate over Panama. To many Americans the Panama Canal symbolized the American role as a great power. Most Americans believed the United States owned the canal, but in reality it held sovereignty in a ten-mile-wide strip called the Canal Zone and ran the canal under a perpetual lease. Since the 1960s Panamanians had resented and sometimes rioted against American dominance. Pushed by Secretary of State Vance to ease anti-American sentiment in the region, Carter won Senate approval in 1977 of several treaties that returned sovereignty over the canal to Panama by 1999 but maintained the American right to defend and use the waterway. Senator S. I. Hayakawa of California spoke for the defenders of the American imperial tradition when he argued, "It's ours. We stole it fair and square."

Cyrus Vance had pushed the canal treaties as part of a policy of negotiation and conciliation that greatly enhanced American prestige in Central America. From 1979 on, however, it was not Vance but Zbigniew Brzezinski who dominated the administration's foreign policy. Brzezinski was determined to reimpose a cold war framework, even in Latin America. Unrest troubled all the region's struggling nations, especially Nicaragua. The corrupt government of Anastasio Somoza had proven so venal and predatory that it alienated the normally conservative propertied classes. When leading Nicaraguan business figures threw their support behind the rebel Sandinista movement, Carter tried to rally the Organization of American States (OAS) to prevent a rebel victory.

No other nation proved willing to support Somoza and after the rebels assumed power they rejected American aid in favor of a nonaligned status and friendliness toward Cuba. As revolution spread in neighboring El Salvador, the Sandinistas sent supplies. The Carter administration could not make a case for the Salvadoran government, which had systematically murdered its own people as well as four American Catholic churchwomen. Still Carter and his successor Ronald Reagan would assist El Salvador while encouraging the overthrow of the leftist government in Nicaragua.

The United States under Carter was not the only superpower with a flagging economy and problems in the Third World. The Soviet Union struggled with an aging leadership and an economy that produced guns but little butter. Even rising oil prices did not help, although the Russians led the world in oil production. Gains from oil were drained off by inefficient industries, support for impoverished allies in Eastern Europe, Cuba, and Vietnam, and attempts to extend Soviet influence in the Middle East and Africa. Economic weakness made the Soviets receptive to greater cooperation with the United States. In that spirit Carter and Soviet premier Leonid Brezhnev in 1977 issued a joint statement on a Middle East Peace.

Opposition to a Soviet Middle Eastern role was immediate and powerful. Carter quickly learned, as had every politician since Harry Truman, that Soviet bashing made far better domestic politics than did easing of cold war tensions. He quickly rendered his understanding with Brezhnev inoperative. The Soviets then renewed arms shipments to Israel's archenemy, Syria. And in that troubled environment, Zbigniew Brzezinski flew off to Beijing to revive the China card. The United States extended formal recognition to China in 1979. Trade doubled within a single year. The Chinese in return exploited the new relationship to launch a punitive invasion of Vietnam.

For the Russians the China card created a potential Japanese–Chinese–American alliance on their Asian border. In a last attempt to save détente Brezhnev met Carter at a Vienna summit conference in 1979. Their main subject was arms control under SALT II. The treaty did limit nuclear launchers to 2400 and MIRVs (missiles with multiple warheads) to 1320 on each side. But neither side would agree to scrap key weapons systems—the Soviets' 300 huge land-based ICBMs and the new American radar-evading cruise missiles. The cold war lobby led by Paul Nitze, author of NSC-68 (page 1111), killed the treaty even though Brezhnev allowed the emigration of 50,000 Soviet Jews in support of improved Soviet–American relations. Opponents objected to the idea of nuclear weapons' parity as symbolic of declining American power. They never acknowledged that part of the Soviet arsenal was aimed at China, not Western Europe or the United States. Nor did they include in the American arsenal the added potential of British and French nuclear forces.

Stung by hostility to the Vance policy of negotiations and accommodations, Carter turned increasingly to Brzezinski, confrontation, and a military buildup. The president expanded the defense budget, built American bases in the Persian Gulf region, sent aid to anticommunist dictators whatever their record on human rights, and created a Rapid Deployment Force to defend exposed American interests in the Middle East. The Soviet Union responded with similar truculence.

The Middle East: Hope and Hostages

What the unstable Balkans were to Europe in the pre–World War I era the Middle East promised to be for the superpowers in the 1970s and 1980s. Oil and proximity to the Soviet's southern border gave the area its geopolitical importance. Religious, tribal, national, and ethnic rivalries created chronic instability dramatized by the endless bloodletting in Beirut, Lebanon, and the outbreak of war between Israel and its Arab neighbors in 1948, 1956, 1967, and 1973. The United States had strong ties to oil-rich Saudi Arabia, a commitment to the survival of Israel, and a determination to prevent the Soviet Union from extending its influence into the area.

Preservation of the peace was one key to American policy. As a result, Americans were greatly encouraged when President Anwar Sadat of Egypt made an unprecedented trip to Israel to meet with Prime Minister Menachem Begin. To encourage the peace process, Carter invited Begin and Sadat to Camp David in Maryland in September 1978. For 13 days the three men argued, threatened, and cajoled. When it was over, Carter had helped the two reach an agreement ending the 30-year state of war between Israel and Egypt. Israel accommodated Egypt by agreeing to withdraw from the Sinai Peninsula, which it had occupied since 1967; Carter compensated Israel by offering $3 billion in military aid. Begin and Sadat shared a Nobel Peace Prize that might just as fairly have gone to Carter for his critical role in forcing the two to compromise their profound differences.

Camp David established only a momentary hope for Middle Eastern stability. Throughout the 1970s, policymakers had seen the shah of Iran, with his huge American-equipped military forces, as a possible regional policeman. Equally important, a stable Iran blocked Soviet access to the Persian Gulf and its oil. While American intelligence agents scoured the world for signs of potential leftist revolutions, they virtually ignored the possibility of a religious revolution from the

It was at Camp David, in private talks sponsored by President Jimmy Carter (center), that Egyptian President Anwar el-Sadat (left) and Israeli Prime Minister Menachem Begin (right) hammered out a "Framework for Peace in the Middle East" as a first step toward ending decades of war and mistrust. For their efforts Begin and Sadat shared the Nobel Peace Prize of 1978, but the prize justifiably might have gone to Carter.

right in a country as important to the United States as Iran. Thus in the fall of 1978 the dramatic collapse of the Pahlevi dynasty and the rise of Islamic fundamentalists led by the Ayatollah Ruholla Khomeini took the United States almost completely by surprise.

Brzezinski urged Carter to support the shah with troops if necessary; Vance recommended meetings with the revolutionary leaders, distance from the shah, and military restraint. Carter waffled between the two by encouraging the shah to resist with force but holding back any American participation. Indecision created the worst of two worlds. The shah fell in February 1979 and the revolutionaries declared a holy war against the modernizing Western influence the United States had so liberally sowed in Iran. By the fall of 1979 Kissinger, Brzezinski, and other friends of the shah persuaded Carter to admit the dying monarch into the United States for medical treatment. That enraged the Islamic fundamentalists, who saw the shah as a traitor and criminal. They stormed the American embassy in Iran and held 53 Americans hostage.

The hostage crisis seemed to symbolize the inability of the Carter administration to maintain American power and prestige abroad. Concern arose that the Shiite fundamentalists would spread revolutionary instability throughout the region or, worse yet, the Soviets might prey upon a weakened Iran. But the Soviets also worried that religious zeal might spread to restless minorities, especially those within their own borders. With China hostile and Iran in turmoil, Brezhnev on December 27, 1979, ordered Soviet troops into neighboring Afghanistan to subdue anticommunist Muslim guerrillas.

An outraged President Carter condemned the invasion. He withdrew SALT II from the Senate (where it stood no chance of passage), renewed registration for the draft, accelerated the military buildup, embargoed sales of American wheat and technology to the Soviet Union, and forced the United States to withdraw from the 1980 Olympic games in Moscow. And in the tradition of presidents since World War II, he announced the Carter Doctrine, a commitment to intervene unilaterally if the Soviet Union threatened American interests in the Persian Gulf.

The spectacle of "America Held Hostage" shown on nightly newscasts killed Carter's hopes for another term. It did not help that Iran's turmoil led to another round of OPEC price hikes and new inflationary pressures. Nor did it help that Americans eager to confront the Soviet Union were reluctant to sacrifice personally to do so. Agricultural interests, Olympic athletes, the new generation of draft resisters, and feminists all had complaints: Why should the American farmer shoulder the burden of a grain embargo? What do sports have to do with politics? Why should military buildup require draft registration? And shouldn't the draft include women?

Once again Carter faced a test of his leadership. Even more than the 53 Americans in Tehran, Jimmy Carter had been taken hostage by events in the Middle East. His ratings in national polls sank to record lows (77 percent negative). He responded by reviving the cold war rhetoric of the 1950s and accelerating the development of nuclear weapons. But whereas the CIA in 1953 had successfully overthrown an Iranian government, the American military in 1980 proved incapable of organizing a mission to free the hostages (or perhaps to kidnap Khomeini). Eight Marines died in the collision of two helicopters and a plane in Iran's central desert. Cyrus Vance, a lonely voice of moderation, finally resigned.

By 1980 the United States was mired in what Carter himself described as "a crisis of confidence." Visions of Vietnam, Central America, and the Middle East produced a nightmare of waning American power and prestige. Economic dislocations at home revived fears of a depression. And an accompanying spiritual malaise left the American people looking for some way to restore their lost faith. None of these problems had begun with Jimmy Carter. The inflationary cycle and declining American productivity had their roots in the Vietnam era. And ironically, America's lost hegemony reflected long-term success in bringing economic growth to Europe, the Pacific rim, and to a lesser degree Brazil, Mexico, India, and Saudi Arabia.

Thus Carter's failure was more symbolic. He lost the leadership issue to prophets on the political right who campaigned to restore American hegemony by expanding the military and revitalizing the cold war crusade. And in the "me generation" Carter's appeals to sacrifice could not overcome the hawkers of self-help therapy, fundamentalist defenders of the faith, and more traditional commercial vendors of the American dream who promised spiritual renewal in the 1980s.

SIGNIFICANT EVENTS

1962 — Rachel Carson's *Silent Spring* published

1965 — Ralph Nader's *Unsafe at Any Speed* published

1966 — National Traffic and Motor Vehicle Safety Act; NOW established

1969 — Apollo 11 moon mission; Santa Barbara oil spill; National Environmental Policy Act

1970 — First Earth Day; Environmental Protection Agency created; NOW organizes Strike for Equality; CIA assists overthrow of Allende in Chile

1971 — Barry Commoner's *The Closing Circle* published

1972 — Congress passes Equal Rights Amendment; Woodward and Bernstein investigate Watergate burglary

1973 — Watergate burglars convicted; *Roe v. Wade;* Haldeman and Erlichman resign; Ervin Committee hearings; Archibald Cox appointed special prosecutor; Spiro Agnew resigns; Saturday Night Massacre; War Powers Act; OPEC oil boycott triggers U.S. recession

1974 — *United States v. Nixon;* House adopts articles of impeachment; Nixon resigns; Ford becomes president; Fair Campaign Practices Act; Kissinger Arab–Israeli "shuttle" diplomacy; Ford–Brezhnev meeting at Vladivostok; Ford pardons Nixon; Church Committee exposes CIA and FBI abuses

1975 — Thieu government falls in South Vietnam; Helsinki Summit; Energy Policy and Conservation Act; New York City faces bankruptcy

1976 — Carter defeats Ford

1977 — Hyde Amendment limiting abortions; congressional scandals; Department of Energy established; Panama Canal treaties

1978 — Revolution in Iran; Chrysler bailout, Camp David meetings

1979 — Three Mile Island crisis; energy crisis; United States recognizes Peoples' Republic of China; SALT II agreement; Iran hostage crisis; Soviet Union invades Afghanistan

1980 — Inflation and recession hurt economy; Carter adopts sanctions against the Soviet Union; U.S. hostage mission fails

1982 — Ratification of ERA fails

35

A Nation
Still Divisible

In the early 1970s San Diego city officials looked out at a downtown that was growing seedier each year, as stores and shoppers continued their flight to the suburbs. As once-thriving downtown retail centers disintegrated, becoming virtual ghost towns at the close of the business day, the task of revitalizing cities confronted urban planners across the nation. San Diego, with 13 separate malls in suburbs ringing the city's perimeter, was typical. So the city came up with a $3 billion redevelopment plan, calling for a convention center, marina, hotels, and apartment complexes.

The city also intended to beat the suburbs at their own game by erecting Horton Plaza, a mall on a grand scale. By 1985 construction crews had transformed the city center into a shopping complex with the look of an Italian hill town. Stores with stucco facades fronted twisting pedestrian thoroughfares, where Renaissance arches and contrasting-striped stonework lured customers to upscale stores like Banana Republic (which sold safari-style travel clothes), to jewelers, and to sporting goods shops. Jugglers and clowns wandered the streets, while paid guitarists serenaded passersby. Horton Plaza's imitation of Old World architecture in trendy southern California soon followed the zoo and Sea World as San Diego's third-ranked tourist attraction, drawing over 12 million shoppers and tourists in 1986 alone.

Although Horton Plaza was more extravagant than most of its competitors, it was hardly an innovation. The first enclosed mall, Southdale Center, had been completed nearly 20 years earlier in Edina, Minnesota, near Minneapolis. Edina had good reason for enclosure: with chilling winters and 100 days a year of rain, shopping conditions were hardly ideal for outdoor strollers. The mall's planners approached Victor Gruen, an architect who had been seeking ways to reclaim urban downtowns from what he saw as the tyranny of the automobile. Gruen contrasted the pedestrian-dominated streets and fountain-filled squares of European villages with the acres of sterile parking lots surrounding suburban shopping centers. As he noted in his manifesto, *The Tired Heart of Our Cities*, automobiles added pollution and congestion to the urban environment. They decentralized and dehumanized cities with their space-consuming superhighways, inner loops, cloverleafs and exitways, parking lots, gas stations, and auto repair shops. Southdale provided an alternative model: a climate-controlled (68 degrees year-round)

Bringing a touch of Disney World–style magic to urban redevelopment, San Diego succeeded in luring shoppers back to its downtown retail center with Horton Plaza, a replica of an Italian hill town.

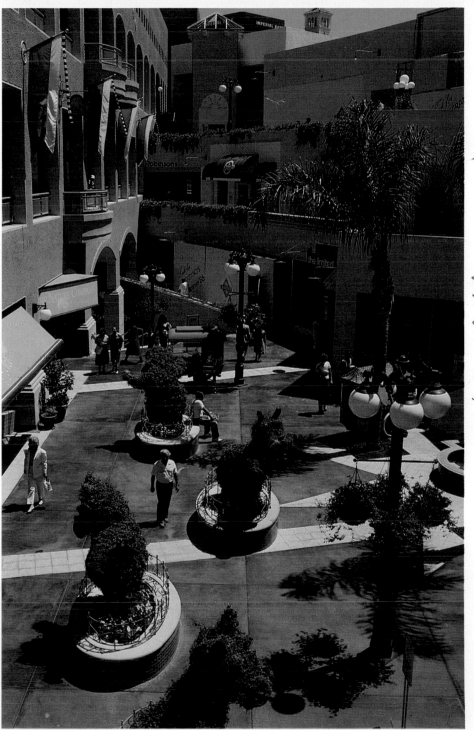

marketplace where shoppers could browse or get a bite to eat at a café without dodging cars or inhaling exhaust fumes.

Retailers elsewhere in the nation were at first reluctant to join the move to malls, fearing that if customers couldn't drive by their stores or park in front, they wouldn't stop and shop. There was no arguing, however, with success: virtually all the new malls turned handsome profits. By 1985, when Horton Plaza opened, Southdale had expanded to a three-level, 144-store complex, spreading over 1.1 million square feet. Nationwide, there were more shopping centers (25,000) than either school districts or hospitals. Some 2800 were enclosed, like Southdale. Furthermore, shopping malls accounted for over 50 percent of all retail sales, excluding the sale of automobile supplies.

Indeed, malls had become money-making machines, crafted to provide the right blend of stores for maximizing a consumer's buying opportunities. The mall manager at Southdale in 1986, Greg Bergan, could call upon sales figures that precisely defined his prime customers as women averaging 40.3 years in age with a household income of $33,750. Their purchases ran most often to clothes; thus 26 separate women's apparel stores took up a fifth of Southdale's floor space. The bottom line in profits was measured in sales per square foot. Jewelry stores led the way, with over $600 per square foot; shoe stores, a popular attraction, averaged over $300. Bergan was continually fine-tuning his retail mix. A Woolworth's store had long occupied a central spot in the mall, but its lease was not renewed. "This was crazy," he explained. "Who was shopping in it? The guy was paying me $3 a square foot." On the other hand a Lens Crafter store, which offered one-hour service on optical prescriptions, seemed a perfect addition. Customers had an hour to kill waiting for their glasses and spent it shopping in other stores. Malls like Southdale had become so profitable that investors with large amounts of capital, like pension funds and insurance companies, sought them out. Southdale was only one of a hundred malls owned by the Equitable Life Assurance Company.

If malls had become rewarding generators of income for investors, to consumers they were the cathedrals of American material culture. Shopping on Sunday seemed to rival churchgoing as the weekly family ritual. Whereas American youth culture had centered on the high school in the 1950s and on college campuses in the 1960s, in the 1970s and 1980s it gravitated toward mall fast-food stores and video amusement arcades. For single men and women malls became a place to find a date. Older people in search of a regimen of moderate exercise discovered that the controlled climate was ideal for "mall walking." For consumers of all stripes, malls were fantasy cities where no one lived but anyone could find a slice of the American dream.

The new cathedrals of consumption serve as an appropriate symbol of a society that in the late 1970s and 1980s turned away from protests and crusades back to the traditions of a consumer culture. Self-improvement replaced social reform as the road to a more perfect society. In the face of declining economic expectations and an age of limits, Americans found it difficult to sustain the commitment to systemic reform or to the liberal philosophies of government intervention. In seeking spiritual fulfillment, they turned in increasing numbers to evangelical religion, with its emphasis on the conversion of "born-again" individuals, private charities, and the virtues of the traditional family. Along less orthodox paths, the "human potential movement" focused on such techniques as yoga, transcendental meditation, and "bioenergetics" to bring inward personal fulfillment.

American politics too had a charismatic leader who celebrated conservative virtues. Against Jimmy Carter's recognition of the inevitability of limits at home and abroad, Ronald Reagan declared it was time for "America to stand tall again." Reagan evoked Puritan John Winthrop's seventeenth-century vision of an American "city on a hill," inspiring the rest of the world. He called for an America liberated from the shackles of the federal government's regulatory jungle, a nation that would resume its position as the number one military power in the world and encourage its citizens to promote the public good through the pursuit of private wealth.

At the same time, Reagan's ideal of limited government failed to address many of the unresolved issues of the 1970s. Indeed, the policies of deregulation, the shift of budget priorities to military spending, and a retreat from social intervention served to increase the gap between the rich and the poor. Environmental decay—whether in the form of acid rain, toxic waste dumps, or nuclear accidents— continued to threaten public health. On many levels the Reagan agenda called for a flight from public responsibility into a fantasy world no more authentic than the Italian hill town nestled in downtown San Diego. At times John Winthrop's austere vision seemed to have become a city on a hill with climate control, where the proprietors of Muzak-filled walkways banished all problems beyond the perimeters of the parking lots. Yet Ronald Reagan tapped the public's deep and abiding feelings of both resentment and hope. He confounded his critics with a capacity to sustain broad support for his image of a born-again America.

THE CONSERVATIVE REBELLION

In 1964 conservative Barry Goldwater had proclaimed his campaign slogan on billboards across America: "In Your Heart You Know He's Right." Beneath one of the billboards an unknown Democratic wag unfurled his own banner: "Yes— Extreme Right." In 1964 most citizens voted with the wag, perceiving Goldwater's platform as too conservative, too extreme, too dangerous for the times.

Two decades later, in the wake of social change at home and a wrenching war abroad, the public mood had changed. During the 1970s economic uncertainties caused by falling real incomes, energy shortages, and rising prices fed a growing resistance to a liberal political or social agenda. Hard-pressed workers resented increased competition from minorities, especially those supported by quotas and government programs. Taxpayers resisted the demands of government, especially at the local and state levels, for increased revenues to support social welfare spending. Rising divorce rates, single-parent households, and declining marriage rates made many Americans fear for the survival of the family. The media, whether television, movies, or popular music, purveyed a culture dominated by explicit sexuality and violence. Sexual permissiveness and the freedom to choose an abortion seemed to many traditional Catholics, orthodox Jews, and evangelical Protestants part of a wholesale assault on decency. Increasingly the political agenda was determined by those who wanted to restore a strong family, traditional religious values, reinvigorated patriotism, and limited government.

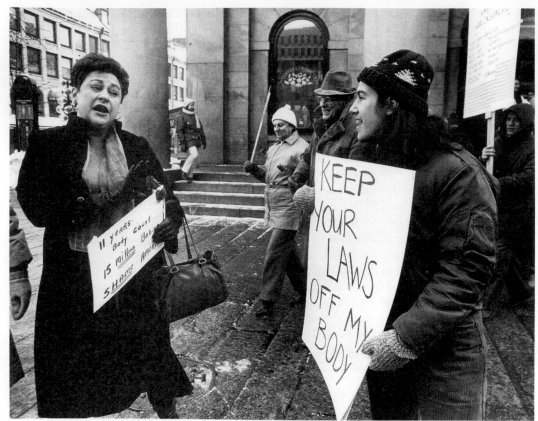

During the late 1970s and the 1980s conservatives increasingly spoke out against abortion and in favor of the right to life for unborn children. Adopting the tactics of protest and civil disobedience once common to radicals in the 1960s, they clash here with pro-choice demonstrators outside Faneuil Hall in Boston.

Born Again

One of the central threads in the conservative rebellion was a call for a renewed revival of religion, and that call came most vocally from white Protestant evangelicals. Fundamentalist Protestants had increasingly separated themselves from the older, more liberal denominations since the 1920s (page 928). In the decades after World War II their membership grew dramatically—between 400 and 700 percent, compared with under 90 percent for the older main-line denominations. By the 1980s they had become a significant third force in Christian America, after Roman Catholics and traditional Protestants. The election of Jimmy Carter, himself a professed born-again Christian, was one reflection of their newfound visibility.

Like most mass movements, evangelical Protestantism was more complex and divided than it appeared to outsiders. Fundamentalists, believing that the Holy Spirit had not spoken to individuals directly since the time of Christ, focused their attention on the literal words and message of the Bible as the key to divine guidance. Pentacostalists, on the other hand, insisted that the Holy Spirit still moved the faithful directly; some believers spoke "in tongues," their bodies and voices contorted by the spirit in them. Thus a fundamentalist like the Reverend Jerry Falwell had strong theological disagreements with a Pentacostalist like the Reverend Pat Robertson. Still, evangelicals found a good deal of common ground in what they saw as the corruptions of American society. They rejected feminism in favor of the patriarchal family, in which men were the breadwinners and spiritual heads and women raised children in the home. They attacked the Supreme Court for decisions which they believed helped open the floodgates of pornography. The demands of homosexuals for "gay rights" particularly offended their belief that the Bible condemned homosexuality as an unqualified sin.

Just as fundamentalists of the 1920s had sought to overturn the trend toward a more secular system of education, the evangelicals of the 1980s sought to refashion it. They pressed states and the federal government to adopt a "school prayer" amendment allowing officially sanctioned prayer in classrooms. They urged the teaching of "Creationism" as an acceptable alternative to Darwinian evolution. When frustrated with public school curricula, they created thousands of "Christian Academies" to insulate their children from the pervasive influence of "secular humanism." Few people charged with being secular humanists knew what the term meant, but to the Christian right it referred generally to the modernist notions that all truths were relative, not absolute, and that ethics were defined by circumstances, not moral verities.

Although evangelicals condemned the modern media as agents of liberalism and secular humanism, they eagerly used the new technology for their own purposes. Cable and satellite broadcasting allowed "televangelists" to reach national audiences. The Reverend Pat Robertson, the son of a Virginia politician, introduced his "700 Club" over the Christian Broadcast Network from Virginia Beach, Virginia. His success inspired a "700 Club" regular, Jim Bakker, to launch a spin-off program called the "Praise the Lord Club"—PTL for short. Within a few years PTL had the largest audience of any daily show in the world. The content was Pentacostal in background: gospel singing, fervent sermons, faith-healing, and speaking in tongues. The format, however, imitated that of sophisticated network "talk shows," including Bakker's Christian monologue, testimonials from celebrity guests, and musical entertainment.

Spiritual leadership easily translated into commercial and political success. Televangelists were determined fund-raisers. By the end of the 1970s, Robertson and Bakker had each received between $25 million and $30 million in contributions. But their coffers were not so full as those of the Reverend Jerry Falwell, spiritual leader of the Thomas Road Baptist Church in Lynchburg, Virginia, and television host of "The Old Time Gospel Hour." It was Falwell who first made the step from religious to political activism. In 1979 he formed the Moral Majority, Inc., an organization to attract campaign contributions and to examine candidates around the country and their views on key issues like school prayer, the Equal Rights Amendment, secular humanism, and abortion. America, Falwell proclaimed, possessed "more God fearing citizens per capita than any other nation on earth," and they needed to make their voices heard politically. Moral Majority soon developed extensive computerized mailing lists to identify donors and target audiences for mass mailings. In the 1980 election it sent out over a billion pieces of mail in an attempt to unseat liberal senators and members of Congress.

American Catholics faced their own decisions about the degree to which religion and politics should mix. In the 1960s conservative Catholics organized opposition to school aid that did not include parochial schools. At the same time liberal

The Reverend Jerry Falwell's Moral Majority attempted to apply religious convictions in the political arena. Falwell actively supported Ronald Reagan's military buildup and political candidates who shared the Moral Majority's social agenda, including opposition to abortion.

Catholics, long commited to social causes, found a vocal leader in Father Robert Drinan, an activist member of Congress from Massachusetts, as well as in the radical priests Philip and Daniel Berrigan, who protested American involvement in the arms race and in Vietnam. Their social activism reflected a more general movement in the church that had arisen out of the church council known as Vatican II (1962–1965). Convened by Pope John XXIII and continued by his successor, Pope Paul VI, the council sought to revitalize the church and to reappraise its role in the modern world. The reforms of Vatican II reduced the amount of Latin in the mass, invited greater lay participation, and encouraged the ecumenical movement for closer ties to other Christians and to Jews.

Catholic conservatives, disturbed by these currents, found support for their views when the charismatic John Paul II assumed the papacy in 1979. The Polish-born John Paul reined in the liberal trends inspired by Vatican II and energetically promoted his views by traveling internationally. His ruling that clergy could not hold political office forced priests like Father Drinan out of politics. He resisted a wider role for women but offered no solution to the crisis American Catholics faced from the sharp decline in young men and women willing to adopt celibate lives as priests and nuns.

Though sometimes wary of one another, conservative Catholics found common cause with Protestant evangelicals. Both groups lobbied for the government to provide federal aid to parochial schools and fundamentalist academies. But it was the issue of abortion that attracted the greatest mutual support. Pope John Paul reaffirmed the church's teaching that all life begins at conception and that abortion amounts to murder of the "unborn." Evangelicals, long suspicious of the power of secular technology and science, attacked abortion as another instance where science had upset the natural moral order of life. Those who believed that women's primary role is motherhood rejected the feminist argument that abortion was "pro-choice" because it allowed women to control their lives.

The Liberal Media

If evangelists like Jerry Falwell and Pat Robertson launched their own shows, and even their own broadcast networks, to champion conservative causes, it was partly because they were convinced that the mass media were staffed and run by an establishment that was liberal in its political orientation and overly permissive in its personal outlook.

The issue was hardly new. In 1928 songwriter Cole Porter teased his audiences with the sly innuendo that "Birds do it, bees do it, even educated fleas do it. . . . Let's fall in love." Indirection was dictated by strict moral standards such as the film industry's Production Code, which forbade graphic violence, offensive language, or any hint of explicit sex or nudity. Even married couples slept in separate beds and had children without ever mentioning the word "pregnant." But by the 1950s a new permissiveness had begun to creep into much of American popular culture. In the case of movies, it reflected in part an effort to recapture some of the mass audience lost to television. Traditional genres like westerns and musicals had lost their appeal, but sex and violence still sold, especially since television was bound by code restrictions. The Supreme Court eased pressures further with a series of landmark decisions on obscenity that limited censorship.

Hollywood did rejuvenate some of its traditional genre subjects without injecting sex or violence. The success of *Planet of the Apes* (1968) launched a series of science fiction film cycles such as *Superman*, *Star Wars*, and *Star Trek*, which recalled much of the innocence of 1930s films. Furthermore, to placate critics, the industry had adopted in 1968 a rating system (G, PG, R, and X) meant to protect moviegoers. This concession could not hide the fact that by the 1970s film had lost any evident moral boundaries or direction. Soft-core pornography with simulated sex and partial nudity gave way to explicit hard-core films like *Deep Throat* and *The Devil in Miss Jones*. *The Texas Chain Saw Massacre* inspired a round of horror and violence films that strove mainly to titillate audiences with mindless murder, dripping gore, and comic mutilation. Even the boundary between horror and patriotism blurred in Sylvester Stallone's *Rambo* series, in which a muscular superpatriot, equipped with enough ammunition to stock several battalions, took on whole nations singlehandedly. Thus the movie industry found itself under attack from two directions. Intellectuals and critics deplored Hollywood's tendency to appeal to the lowest common denominator to attract a mass audience while religious, educational, and community groups were offended by movies that assaulted traditional values.

Television provoked similar condemnation. Parents' organizations charged that young viewers were especially vulnerable to discussions of controversial subject matter, suggestive sexuality and violence, and programs with themes critical of established institutions such as big business, authority, and the family. Women and minorities complained that television portrayed them as stereotypes, when it bothered to portray them at all. Intellectuals despaired that the large majority of Americans spent over five hours a day watching a range of soap operas, quiz shows, rerun movies, series, sports, and news that seldom dealt with any serious issues in a substantial way. Even television's popular "Sixty Minutes," which purported to be the best sort of hard-hitting journalism, combined uneven dashes of muckraking, human interest, and editorializing. The producers routinely reduced hours of interviews to a few selected comments and often gave equal weight to issues of great and minor importance.

Television also attracted criticism because its old standby, the situation comedy (or "sitcom"), became more topical during the 1970s. Traditionally sitcoms had taken lighthearted looks at middle-class family life and avoided controversy. But in 1971 producer Norman Lear introduced the first episode of his new comedy, "All in the Family," with a warning: "The program you are about to see . . . seeks to throw a humorous spotlight on our frailties, prejudices, and concerns." With that advisory, Archie Bunker exploded into prime time. Seething with fears and prejudices, Archie treated his addlepated wife like a doormat, struggled to understand his modestly rebellious daughter, and shouted endless insults at his Polish-American son-in-law. Minority groups, nonconformists, bosses, and liberals all offended his uninformed, blue-collar sensibilities. Out of his mouth came phrases like "Hebes," "Spics," "pansies," "fags," and "Commie crapola" that never before had survived the censors' "bleep." Americans were supposed to laugh at Archie's dumb and outrageous sentiments. "If your Spics and Spades want their rightful share of the American dream, let 'em go out and hustle for it just like I done," Archie shouts at his son-in-law from the shabby security of his living room chair. But large parts of the audience were not laughing. Some minority leaders charged that by making Archie lovable, the show legitimized the very prejudices it seemed to attack.

Benjamin Franklin "Hawkeye" Pierce was every bit as irreverent as Archie Bunker was irascible. Inspired by Robert Altman's movie hit *M*A*S*H* (1970), the television series, launched in 1972, portrayed the lives of army surgeons and nurses during the Korean War. The show's liberal, egalitarian comedy twitted bureaucracy, authority, pretense, bigotry, and snobbery for over 10 years, running 7 years longer than the war itself. During that time the central characters evolved in ways that reflected significant social change in American society. The one major African-American character disappeared during the first season. Hawkeye and his companions began as hard-drinking, womanizing foes of war and army life. Ten years later they still hated the army and war, but Hawkeye had become more vulnerable, respectful to women, and less of a wiseguy. The intensely faithful husband B. J. Hunicutt had replaced the randy "Trapper" John MacIntyre. "Hotlips" Hoolihan was transformed from a military martinet and raving patriot into Margaret Hoolihan, a career woman struggling for respect. Having treated heavy drinking as a mix of college partying and an escape from the horrors of war, the show began to deal with alcoholism.

Critics of television entertainment were most likely to focus their ire on violent cop shows, sexually frank dramatic series, or Saturday morning cartoon mayhem. For children, who were among the heaviest consumers of network programming, television was a virtual wasteland. Even the success of such Public Broadcasting System (PBS) series as "Sesame Street" and "Mister Rogers' Neigh-

Archie Bunker, from "All in the Family", played by Carroll O'Connor.

borhood" could not reduce childhood addiction to commercial television. Advertisements beckoned the undiscriminating young viewer to feast on sugar-laden cereals and candies before dragging their parents off to buy the latest in military toys, space weapons, or leggy Barbie's ever-expanding wardrobe.

Thus television, like the movies, became a battleground over which conservatives and liberals clashed. Norman Lear, Archie Bunker's creator, went on to form a lobbying group, People for the American Way, to push for more diversity in American life and counteract pressure groups like the Moral Majority. The conservatives, looking to take their cause to the political arena, found an amiable actor who had already made a successful transition from movies to politics.

The Election of 1980

Jimmy Carter might be born again, but Ronald Reagan spoke the language of true conservatism. "I think there is a hunger in this land for a spiritual revival, a return to a belief in moral absolutes," he told his followers. Such a commitment to fundamentalist articles of faith was more important than the fact that Reagan actually had no church affiliation and seldom attended services. By contrast, the more religiously active Carter seemed too liberal for the politically conservative Christian right.

The defection of traditionally Democratic evangelical Protestants was just one liability Carter faced. His rapid military buildup and cutbacks in social programs offended liberals, while rampant inflation and a weak economy alienated blue-collar voters. As the Iran hostage crisis dragged on, the president remained preoccupied with it and refrained from vigorous campaigning. By July 1980 only 32 percent of the nation approved of Carter's performance. In Republican primaries, Ronald Reagan easily outdistanced a host of other conservative hopefuls and survived George Bush's charge that his conception of finance amounted to "voodoo economics." As Reagan captured the right and center, Representative John Anderson of Illinois led the frustrated liberal wing into a third party.

THE ELECTION OF 1980

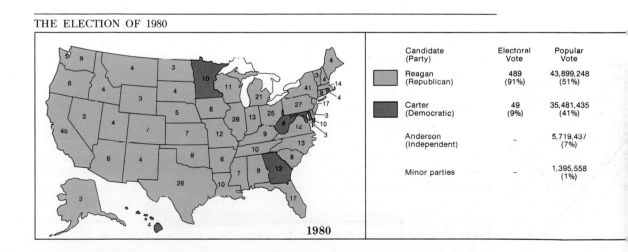

Candidate (Party)	Electoral Vote	Popular Vote
Reagan (Republican)	489 (91%)	43,899,248 (51%)
Carter (Democratic)	49 (9%)	35,481,435 (41%)
Anderson (Independent)	–	5,719,437 (7%)
Minor parties	–	1,395,558 (1%)

1980

Against Reagan's promise to restore America to greatness, Carter tried to sell the less popular notion that the United States needed to sacrifice in order to survive in a world of scarcity. It was an approach Reagan gleefully challenged. In a nationally televised debate he asked the American people, "Are you better off than you were four years ago?" Undecided voters saw in Reagan a candidate with the power to lead. Frustrated by Carter's inability to restore the economy or resolve the hostage crisis, they turned the race into a landslide: 51 percent for Reagan, 41 percent for Carter, 7 percent for Anderson. Equally impressive, the Republicans won their first majority in the Senate since 1954, claiming that the margin of victory was a popular mandate for a conservative agenda.

On that count, however, the verdict was not clear. Certainly the landslide was not of historic proportions: Eisenhower, Lyndon Johnson, and Richard Nixon (in 1972) had all won by larger margins. Only 52 percent of the eligible electorate went to the polls, the lowest total in 32 years. "It's a fed-up vote," argued Carter's political analyst Patrick Caddell. Two-thirds of the voters complained about high taxes, inflation, and unemployment. The more liberal elements, especially the young, blacks, and the poor, stayed away in record numbers, whereas Reagan's majority was greatest among those over 45, white, and earning more than $50,000 per year. Still, Reagan had significantly splintered the New Deal Democratic coalition. He made striking gains among union workers, southern white Protestants, Catholics, and Jews. Whether or not these voters became part of a permanent conservative coalition depended on the new administration's capacity to reduce popular dissatisfaction with government.

PRIME TIME WITH RONALD REAGAN

Jimmy Carter thought simplicity would appeal to Americans fed up with an imperial presidency. Ronald Reagan brought the bright lights of Hollywood to Washington, staging one of the most extravagant inaugurations in the nation's history. White House events took on the air of Hollywood premieres, with celebrities decked out in expensive designer originals. Nancy Reagan became the most fashion-conscious first lady since Jackie Kennedy. The Reagan presidency made the conspicuous display of wealth once again a sign of success and power. During Reagan's first term sales of stretch limousines doubled every year. Poverty rates rose too, as the gulf between rich and poor widened.

The Great Communicator

The message Ronald Reagan brought to Washington was simple and attractive. "It is time to reawaken the industrial giant, to get government back within its means, and to lighten our punitive tax burden," he announced on inauguration day. A strong national defense and a determined effort to revive the cold war crusade against the Soviet Union would reestablish the United States as the number one power in the world. So enthusiastically received was his message that commentators began referring to the president as "the great communicator," whose uncanny ability to use television and radio unsettled his liberal adversaries.

Reagan's skill as a veteran trouper often managed to obscure the contradictions between rhetoric and reality. With his jaunty wave and jutting jaw, he projected physical vitality and the charismatic good looks of John Kennedy. Yet at age 69, he was the oldest president to take office, and none since Calvin Coolidge had slept as soundly or as much. Reagan had begun his political life in the 1930s as an avid New Deal Democrat, but the rise of Stalinism had left him disillusioned, as it had many liberals. By the 1950s Reagan had become an ardent anticommunist who gained a reputation among conservatives as an engaging after-dinner speaker and corporate spokesperson for General Electric. In 1966 he was elected governor of California and served for eight years. As governor he spoke of paring down government programs and balancing budgets, although spending jumped sharply during his term in office. Similarly, he continued to champion family values, although he was divorced and estranged from some of his children.

Similar inconsistencies marked his leadership as president. Outsiders applauded Reagan's "hands-off" management as exactly what the nation needed after Jimmy Carter, the knowledgeable technocrat who immersed himself in details but was unable to inspire or lead. Reagan seemed to set a clear tone and direction, letting his advisers take care of the details. On the other hand, cabinet officials like Secretary of the Treasury Donald Regan were shocked to find the new president remarkably ignorant about important matters of policy and seemingly uninterested in learning more. "The Presidential mind was not cluttered with facts," Regan lamented. Then, too, Reagan appeared uncomfortable with confrontation and disliked reining in members of his administration. To outsiders, that quality appeared to be loyalty; some insiders saw an inability to control his advisers and staff. Nancy Reagan often dictated his schedule (aided by an astrologer), helped select his advisers, and even sometimes determined the major issues the president addressed. Yet the public believed he was firmly in charge and, until the Iran arms scandal in 1986, consistently expressed approval of his handling of the office. His capacity for deflecting responsibility for mistakes from himself to others earned him a reputation as the "Teflon president," since no criticism seemed to stick.

In addition, Reagan was blessed by remarkably good fortune: a number of events beyond his control broke in his favor. The deaths of three aging Soviet leaders, Leonid Brezhnev in 1982, Yuri Andropov in 1984, and Konstantin Chernenko in 1985, compounded that country's persistent economic weakness and reduced Russian influence abroad. Members of the OPEC oil cartel quarreled among themselves, exceeded production quotas, and thus forced oil prices lower, removing one major inflationary pressure. The day Reagan took office, the Iranians released the American hostages, relieving the president of his first major foreign policy crisis. And when a would-be assassin shot the president in the chest on March 30, 1981, the wound was not life threatening. Plans for a conservative Reagan revolution moved ahead.

The Reagan Agenda

Reagan's first task was to restore prestige to a presidential office that Gerald Ford once described as more imperiled than imperial. Here Reagan achieved perhaps his single greatest success. He summoned respect for an executive branch battered by debate over Vietnam, the scandals of Watergate, and the lackluster Ford and Carter administrations. Congress once again looked to the White House to set the legislative agenda. Ironically, Reagan wanted to strengthen the presidency as a way to weaken big government. His budget would become an instrument to reduce bureaucracy and to undermine agencies responsible for what seemed to him excessive meddling in the areas of civil rights, environmental and consumer protection, economic regulation, poverty programs, urban renewal, transportation, the arts, and education. In essence, Reagan wanted to return government to the size and responsibility it had had in the 1950s before the reforms of Kennedy and Johnson. He soon recognized that most programs were so deeply entrenched and their constituencies so attached to them that he could at first only scale back, not destroy them, as his more radical supporters demanded.

At the heart of the Reagan revolution was a commitment to "supply-side" economics, a program with a striking resemblance to the trickle-down economic theories of the Harding–Coolidge era. Supply-side theorists argued that high taxes and government regulation stifled entrepreneurship and economic expansion. If the government wanted employment and the economy to grow, it needed to assure higher profits, reduce the risk of innovation, and guarantee fatter paychecks. More money in private hands would mean more demand for goods. Not coincidentally, the key to this economic revival lay in a politically popular and economically controversial solution, a large tax cut. Such a cut threatened to reduce revenues and increase the deficit, of course—except that supply-side economist Arthur Laffer claimed that the economy would be so stimulated that tax revenues would actually rise, even though the rate was cut.

The second target of Reagan's agenda was the "silent thief," inflation, which had systematically robbed Americans during the Ford–Carter years. Reagan resisted certain traditional cures for inflation: tight money, high interest rates, and wage-and-price controls. He frequently sparred with Federal Reserve Chairman Paul Volker for keeping interest rates high and a tight rein on the money supply. Reagan preferred two approaches unpopular with Democrats, higher unemployment and breaking the power of major unions, which would reduce labor costs.

Lower public spending, a favorite Republican remedy, might have seemed one likely method of reducing inflation. But the third element of Reagan's agenda was a sharp rise in military outlays: a total of $1.5 trillion to be spent over five years. His strategic goal was to provide the United States with the strength to act unilaterally anywhere in the world to beat back any communist threat. This was a remarkably ambitious goal: John Kennedy had wanted the United States prepared to fight two and a half potential wars—one, for example, in Europe, one in Southeast Asia, and a smaller scale skirmish in Central America. Richard Nixon had recognized the rising importance of regional power blocs like Western Europe, with whom the United States might cooperate to guarantee security without bankrupting the economy. Reagan recognized no such limits. The United States would act unilaterally to guarantee its security. And rather than emphasize either nuclear defense or conventional warmaking powers, Defense Secretary Caspar Weinberger lobbied Congress for both.

In opting for such an inclusive approach, the administration seemed undecided about where America's most crucial interests lay if hard choices had to be made. Did the oil-rich Middle East deserve the most attention, or did America's economically and politically unstable neighbor, Latin America? The economically vibrant Pacific rim, or the traditional allies of Europe? All these areas presented important issues to be faced: energy dependence on the Middle East, a mounting Third World debt owed American lenders, the flight of high-wage jobs to low-wage countries, the instability of Eastern Europe. The president tended to view these issues, when he heeded them, through the traditional lenses of the cold warrior. "The Soviet Union underlies all the unrest that is going on. If they weren't engaged in a game of dominoes, there wouldn't be any hot spots in the world," he asserted in 1980. Thus his foreign policy agenda remained staunchly anticommunist.

The Reagan Revolution in Practice

Soon after taking office, the administration found itself with a chance to "hang tough" when PATCO, the union representing air traffic controllers, went on strike. Strikes by civil service employees were technically illegal, but the controllers maintained that a strike was the only way to win better working conditions and ensure greater air safety. Reagan responded in the spirit of Governor Calvin Coolidge breaking the 1919 Boston police strike. Setting aside the merits of the controllers' complaints, he refused to compromise and fired them for violating their contract. The public generally approved what it saw as a blow against big labor's continual appetite for less work at higher wages. Then, too, the air controllers were already receiving solidly middle-class wages for skilled labor, so they hardly appeared to be in the ranks of the downtrodden and impoverished. The administration's hard-line stance, combined with a recession that soon enveloped the nation, allowed major corporations to wrest substantial concessions from unions on wages and work rules. Organized labor witnessed a steady decline in membership and political power.

At the same time, the president's war against government regulation took special aim at rules protecting the environment. Western conservatives had long looked askance at government intervention to preserve wild lands, especially when the policy seemed directed at halting economic development in their areas for the benefit of "nature lovers." Reagan appointed westerner James Watt, an outspoken champion of this "sagebrush rebellion," to head the Interior Department. Watt, in turn, devoted himself to opening federal lands for private development, including lumbering and offshore oil drilling. Similarly, Anne Burford Gorsuch set out to cut back the Environmental Protection Agency's efforts to enforce antipollution regulations. Watt's outrageous statements forced his resignation in 1983 and scandal over mismanagement at the EPA drove Gorsuch out, but the administration continued to oppose most efforts to regulate or protect the environment. Reagan, who once claimed trees were a source of air pollution, refused to accept the conclusion of scientists that the smoke from coal-fired power plants in the Ohio valley was sending destructive acid rain over the lakes and forests of eastern Canada and the United States.

Most important, by the summer of 1981 Reagan had also pushed through Congress his supply-side tax legislation. The Economic Recovery Tax Act (ERTA) provided a 25 percent across-the-board reduction for all taxpayers. The president hailed it, along with recently passed budget cuts, as an antidote to "big government's" addiction to spending and a stimulus to the economy. Opponents called it a bonanza for the rich, pointing out that an "equal" cut of 25 percent for all taxpayers meant a much larger windfall for the wealthy, who paid larger taxes to begin with. Even Budget Director David Stockman admitted that parts of the legislation had been particularly beneficial to special interests. "Do you realize the greed that came to the forefront? The hogs were really feeding," he recalled. "The greed level, the level of opportunism, just got out of control."

The administration's impact on the economy was mixed. By 1982 a recession had pushed unemployment above 10 percent. The Federal Reserve Board's tight money policies and high interest rates deepened the recession. Key industries like automobiles staggered under the pressure of foreign competition and their own inefficiency. But the combination of falling energy costs, the stimulus of federal spending, improved industrial productivity, and easier monetary policy in 1983 brought on an economic expansion that lasted through Reagan's presidency. While many workers earned less per hour, the flow of women into the labor market kept family incomes from falling too much. Recovery also spurred higher corporate profits, but not the increased savings and investment rates that supply-side theorists had predicted. Much of the expansion was financed by borrowing and investment from foreigners, especially the Japanese and British.

Whatever the performance of the economy as a whole, the Reagan tax cut was one of a series of policy changes that brought about a substantial transfer of wealth from the poor and lower middle-class workers to the upper middle classes and the rich. Dedicated to a free market philosophy, the administration barely responded as jobs that paid blue-collar workers relatively high wages flowed to Mexico and Asia, where laborers worked for less. It had no solution either as cheap imported foods cut into the American farmers' share of the domestic market and huge international surpluses created a depression in the agricultural sector. Many once-prosperous farmers found themselves dangerously in debt or their mortgaged farms foreclosed. And Reagan aimed the sharpest edge of his budget axe at programs for the poor. The administration cut most from programs that gave direct benefits to the poor: food stamps, Aid to Families with Dependent Children, Medicaid, school lunches, and housing assistance. The programs least affected were middle-class entitlements like Social Security and Medicare, which affected those over 65 who, as social activist Michael Harrington observed, "are not now, and for a long time have not been, poor."

The shift in wealth distribution caused by the tax cut, rising unemployment, and lost federal benefits hit home for tens of millions of Americans. "For every 25-year-old I read about making $300,000 a year on Wall Street," one economist noted, "there are hundreds of 25-year-olds working as fast-food people or hospital orderlies earning $3.50 an hour." During the 1950s and 1960s family earnings increased some 30 percent each decade. But the 1970s brought a period of decline, which continued into the 1980s.

With a combination of income transfers, agricultural depression, and job flight, the percentage of Americans living below the poverty level rose from 11.7 percent in 1980 to 15 percent by 1982, where it stayed for the rest of the Reagan administration. Reagan's successful war on inflation, which dropped to less than 2 percent by 1986, contributed to a rise in unemployment. Joblessness peaked at over 10 percent (12 million) in 1982 and hovered around 7 percent during the recovery and stock market boom, finally dropping below 6 percent before the 1988 election. (By contrast, the highest rate under Jimmy Carter was 5.9 percent.) Somewhere around 1.5 million people simply gave up trying to find work. Millions of others fled to the booming economies of Texas and the Southwest only to

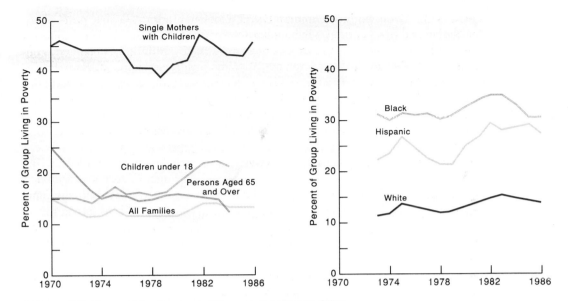

Sources: U.S. Bureau of the Census and Congressional Budget Office.
POVERTY IN AMERICA, 1970–1986
While Social Security and other income supplements to older Americans reduced their rate
of poverty, the circumstances of single mothers with children significantly worsened.

see the bottom fall out as oil prices plunged from over $40 to $13 a barrel and
domestic production slumped. Thus the Reagan recovery was an uneven one,
despite its continued expansion.

The Surge in Military Spending

An equally significant part of the Reagan revolution was the sharp rise in military
spending. Known as "Cap the Knife" for his budget cutting under Richard Nixon,
Defense Secretary Caspar Weinberger surprised many by being more aggressive
than the most hawkish generals in seeking a bigger budget. Outlays rose from
under $200 billion (an average of 4.9 percent of the GNP) under Presidents Ford
and Carter to almost $300 billion (6.2 percent of the GNP) in 1985, when growing
opposition led to some restraint. The largest increases were for strategic nuclear
weapons, especially the B-1 bomber (rejected by Carter as outmoded), aircraft
carrier task forces and Trident missile subs for the navy, the huge land-based MX
intercontinental ballistic missiles, and subsonic cruise missiles. The administration argued that a nuclear buildup would strengthen the position of American
negotiators during arms reductions talks.

This vast buildup inspired three major lines of criticism. First, the rise in
spending accompanied by increasingly tough talk by Reagan defense planners
about the possibility of "winning" a nuclear exchange sparked a revival of antinuclear peace groups across Europe and America. The bishops of the American
Catholic church felt moved to announce their opposition to nuclear war. In *The
Fate of the Earth* (1982), Jonathan Schell speculated on the grisly destruction even
a limited nuclear exchange might cause. Scientists warned that debris in the atmosphere might cause a "nuclear winter" fatal to all life on earth.

Equally vocal were those outraged by the cost and complexity of the Pentagon's armament list. Stories of $600 toilet seats and $7000 coffee pots made headlines, but more serious were the failures of entire multibillion-dollar weapons systems, like the army's Bradley troop carriers and Sergeant York antiaircraft guns. Many weapons were so complicated that they seldom worked and could not be repaired by military personnel. Repeated scandals revealed widespread fraud in defense industry billing and Defense Department procurement.

The public heard little, however, from critics concerned that the military buildup had scant connection to strategic needs. Their primary target was the president's Strategic Defense Initiative (SDI, nicknamed "Star Wars" after the popular futuristic movie series of the era). The goal of SDI was to establish a space-based missile system that would be merely "defensive," knocking enemy missiles out of the sky well before they reached their targets. Almost all reputable scientists argued that the system was technically flawed, yet, beginning in 1983, the administration won billions of dollars each year to pursue development of the idea, hoping as well to wring concessions from the Soviets during arms talks. Critics countered that Reagan's defense buildup amounted to very little bang for trillions of bucks.

The combination of massive defense spending and substantial tax cuts left the federal government awash in red ink. Annual deficits soared to over $200 billion. The vast borrowing required to pay this debt kept interest rates high until recovery set in during 1983–1984. In turn, the high interest rates attracted investors from Europe and Asia, who poured capital into the United States, aggravating the debt crisis in the Third World. But Reagan steadfastly refused any tax increases,

THE FEDERAL BUDGET AND SURPLUS/DEFICIT, 1940–1987 Despite Reagan's campaign pledge to reduce federal spending, the federal deficit soared higher during his presidency than at any other time in the nation's history.

took no steps to curb the rapid growth in foreign oil imports, and ignored mounting foreign trade deficits, as the United States, a creditor nation since World War I, became by 1986 the world's largest debtor.

Whether the large budget deficits were truly a threat to the American economy remained a hotly debated topic. Some economists argued that, just as corporations routinely went into debt and borrowed money to build new factories, it was healthy for the federal government to go into debt to build roads, bridges, schools—the necessary infrastructure of American society. But Reagan largely ignored those expenditures and the general public was convinced cutbacks were needed. Neither the administration nor Congress could agree on where to begin. As a stopgap measure, Congress in 1985 passed the Gramm–Rudman Act, which established a set of steadily declining limits on the federal budget each year, to achieve a balanced budget in 1993. These limits were meant to force Congress and the president to make hard choices; if they did not, automatic across-the-board cuts would go into effect. Not only was the constitutionality of this approach in doubt, but in addition, successive Congresses, as well as presidents Reagan and Bush, accepted unrealistic budget projections that defeated the purpose of the Gramm–Rudman Act.

The Election of 1984

No matter how loudly Reagan's critics complained, the president remained popular with the American people. Even among African-Americans and other minorities he received generally favorable ratings, despite his hostility to affirmative action and social welfare programs. Massive foreign borrowing and deficit spending fueled an economic expansion that assured the president, though not the Republican party, electoral success. The only real questions in 1984 were which

In the 1984 presidential campaign, Jesse Jackson called for a "Rainbow coalition" of citizens of all colors who had been hurt by the Reagan revolution. But his positions seemed too liberal for most Americans at the time.

LOS ANGELES CITY COLLEGE

Democrat would lose to Reagan and by how much. A challenge by Jesse Jackson and his "Rainbow Coalition" raised the prospect of an African-American candidate. But the honor went to the former Carter vice president, Walter Mondale of Minnesota, a moderate who embraced traditional New Deal liberalism.

The Democrats perceived one small ray of hope in what pollsters had identified as a gender gap. Reagan's standing among women was lower than with men, even though he had appointed Sandra Day O'Connor the first female justice of the Supreme Court and Elizabeth Hanford Dole secretary of transportation. Most of his appointments went, however, to white Protestant males who met the conservative test of ideological purity on issues like abortion, tax cuts, military spending, and anticommunist crusades in the Third World. To exploit the gender gap, Mondale chose Representative Geraldine Ferraro of New York as his running mate. In doing so, he paid his debt to the National Organization for Women for its support and fulfilled his campaign pledge to work for greater opportunity for all Americans.

But the continuing economic recovery, along with the president's affable charm, brought to Reagan even greater numbers of traditional New Deal Democrats, especially southern evangelicals and blue-collar workers. Baby-boom voters also favored Reagan by wide margins. He even won a majority of the women's vote (57 percent) as well as a crushing majority (59 percent) of the popular vote and victory in 49 states. Women suffered an additional political setback as 9 women candidates for the Senate and all but 2 women out of the 41 running for Congress went down to defeat. At least in 1984, the gender gap did not translate into an identifiable women's vote.

SECOND-TERM BLUES

Second terms have been hard on many popular presidents, especially those re-elected by wide margins. For George Washington it was factionalism that marred his second term; for Thomas Jefferson, the embargo; for Franklin Roosevelt, the Court-packing plan; for Lyndon Johnson, the Vietnam War; and for Richard Nixon, Watergate. So too Ronald Reagan suffered a precipitous drop in his political fortunes as scandals racked his administration.

A good deal of the problem could be traced to the president's hands-off approach to governing. In March 1987, at the administration's low point, former senator Howard Baker of Tennessee was brought in as chief-of-staff to reorganize the White House. One of Baker's aides was shocked to discover how far matters had slipped:

> There was no pattern of analysis, no coming together. Individual cabinet members were just doing what they wanted to do—the ones that were smart had realized that the White House really didn't matter. . . . [Aides] felt free to sign [the president's] initials on documents without noting that they were acting for him. When I asked a group of them, who among them thought they had authority to sign in the president's name, there was a long, uncomfortable silence. Then one answered, "Well—everybody, and nobody."

Yet Reagan again confounded his critics with his political resilience. The Iran–Contra scandal, the worst of his problems, passed without precipitating an impeachment, as Watergate had. The president presided over an economic expansion that became the longest in peacetime history without a recession, and he concluded with the Soviet Union an Intermediate Nuclear Force Treaty (INF) that promised to eliminate a whole class of missiles from Europe. He left office with his personal popularity still high.

Triumph Before the Storm

Indeed, the second term began well enough, with inflation under control, the economy continuing to expand, and the stock market reaching new highs. The president could claim partial credit for a major reform in the tax system, though its passage owed just as much to the persistence of Senator Bill Bradley of New Jersey and Representative Richard Gephardt of Missouri. The bill, passed in August 1986, was designed to be "revenue neutral"—that is, the changes would not raise or lower the total amount of taxes collected. But it removed many of the old inequities and loopholes that had often allowed the people with the highest incomes to pay the lowest taxes. Tax avoidance had become something of a national obsession, influencing when and what people bought in order to gain tax deductions. Under the new law individuals were far less likely to base a spending decision on tax consequences rather than on whether it made economic sense on its own merits.

Furthermore, vacancies in the Supreme Court allowed the president to shift its ideological balance further to the right. When Chief Justice Warren Burger resigned in 1986, Reagan elevated Justice William Rehnquist to that position, filling Rehnquist's vacancy with distinguished conservative jurist Antonin Scalia. But the limits of the president's influence became clear when the Senate rejected Robert Bork, a more combative conservative. Bork's long history of polemical articles and speeches challenging long-established Court policies on privacy and civil rights made many Republicans hesitate. Even so, a moderately conservative judge from California, Anthony Kennedy, won easy approval in 1988.

As of July 1986, the president's popularity seemed unassailable as he stood in the glare of Fourth-of-July patriotic fireworks, lighting the torch of a newly refurbished Statue of Liberty. "The 75-year-old man is hitting home runs," rhapsodized *Time* magazine. In reality, he was about to enter the most wrenching years of his presidency. The crisis was sparked by two longstanding traits of the administration: Reagan's indifference to the details of his office and his determination to pursue a more aggressive anticommunist foreign policy abroad.

Standing Tall

In his public life Ronald Reagan had stood firm in defense of the principles of liberty and freedom. Most often, his administration focused attention on human rights abuses in communist nations, turning a blind eye toward the excesses of right-wing dictatorships. This ideological approach, as one analyst pointed out, tended to give Reagan policymakers an "absolute certainty of their own rightness." Since they were operating with "pure hearts," they found it all too easy to justify working with "dirty hands." In some cases, noble ends were used to justify dubious tactics.

Three areas of the world commanded the administration's attention. First, Reagan was determined to counter a Soviet arms buildup and adventurism with American arms and interventionism. In Central America, the shadow of Fidel Castro's communist regime loomed, the Sandinistas of Nicaragua had established a leftist government, and instability threatened to spread revolution. Finally, the Reaganites sought to stabilize the Middle East, where Soviet troops were bogged down in Afghanistan, a bloody war dragged on between Iran and Iraq, the governments of Syria and Libya supported international terrorists, chaos engulfed Lebanon, and tensions between Israel and its neighbors simmered.

The administration's first test came in 1982, after Israel invaded war-torn Lebanon to drive out the guerrilla forces of the Palestine Liberation Organization (PLO). Once Israeli troops reached Beirut, Syrian-armed Muslim groups struck back. A bloody stalemate resulted. Secretary of State George Shultz proposed that the Israelis be replaced by a European–American peacekeeping force. Although Defense Secretary Weinberger objected that troops might be drawn into an indefensible situation with an uncertain mission, Reagan agreed with Shultz and sent American marines to support the embattled Christian minority government. Soon the peacekeeping forces became the target of rival Muslim factions. Terrorists backed by the Khomeini regime in Iran succeeded in bombing the American Embassy and, six months later in October 1983, blew up a U.S. Marine barracks, killing 239. At Weinberger's urging, the president reconsidered his position and ordered American troops withdrawn. In Lebanon, Reagan found it difficult to project American force.

Grenada, a Caribbean island with a medical school attended by a number of American students, proved more susceptible to forceful intervention. With civil war threatening to bring a Marxist government to power there, the president sent in an invasion force that not only airlifted the American students to safety, but crushed the forces of the unpopular leftist rebels. Although troop actions were not particularly well coordinated (one desperate officer was forced to open a communications link with his air cover by making a collect call to Washington over a local pay phone), the American public generally approved the show of force. The military, the president seemed to be saying, would no longer be shackled by the agony of Vietnam.

Still, a constructive response to the Middle East with its wars, political upheavals, and terrorists eluded the Reagan administration. In 1985 Iranian-backed terrorists took additional hostages in Lebanon, a number of them American. Terrorists also struck airlines. In the most dramatic incident they hijacked a TWA flight between Athens and Rome in June 1985. In such situations, Reagan's public response was always uncompromising: "Let terrorists beware: when the rules of international behavior are violated, our policy will be one of swift and effective retribution." But against whom should the United States seek revenge? There was little intelligence about the many political and terrorist factions. Only in the case of the hijacked cruise ship *Achille Lauro* did the United States strike back effectively. When Egyptian authorities allowed the captured terrorists to quietly board a plane for Tunisia, American F-14 Tomcat fighters forced the plane to land in Italy.

In its war on terrorists, the Reagan government increasingly focused on Libya and its eccentric, vocally anti-American leader Colonel Muammar Qadhafi. Intelligence sources indicated that Qadhafi's supporters were behind at least some of the terrorist attacks on American tourists and servicemen. In the Gulf of Sidra, Libyan gunboats periodically played cat-and-mouse with an American naval task force, while American jets retaliated with attacks on radar installations. Then a terrorist bombing killed a U.S. serviceman in West Berlin. Reagan ordered 30 air force and navy bombers to attack selected targets, including Qadhafi's headquarters. The show of force impressed the American public, although European leaders, with the exception of Prime Minister Margaret Thatcher of Great Britain, opposed the raids. Later intelligence reports indicated that the majority of terrorist attacks were supported not by Libya, but by Syria—a nation much less isolated from the international community, and one the administration seemed more wary of challenging openly.

Clean Hearts and Dirty Hands in Central America

In South and Central America the gap between American ideals and American power proved even larger. The greatest long-term crisis involved the mounting debts that undermined the economic and political stability of the region. So large were the sums involved that paying the interest alone strained the debtor nations' economies. American banks, which had loaned billions of dollars, were themselves threatened if the nations decided to default. By 1988 the debt crisis across the entire Third World had expanded to $1.2 trillion. As interest rates rose, hard-pressed debtor nations were forced to spend valuable resources servicing interest on their debt rather than promoting industry, building needed roads and hospitals, or offering public services. Since the problem seemed intractable, the administration did little to look for ways to ease the crisis.

Communism, not economics, preoccupied Reagan. In El Salvador, leftist rebels increasingly gained ground in their attempt to overthrow the reigning dictatorship. In response, private right-wing "death squads" exacted their own retribution, murdering anyone suspected of opposition, including a few Americans in the area. Thus moderate forces were caught in the crossfire, with approximately 40,000 civilians killed in the period between 1979 and 1984. The combination of American pressure and foreign aid finally led to the election of a moderate conservative government for El Salvador under José Napoleón Duarte. A slowdown in the guerrilla war and civilian murders followed, but there was little improvement in conditions for El Salvador's impoverished peasants.

In neighboring Nicaragua the circumstances were reversed. Since 1979 the left-wing Sandinista government had gravitated steadily toward Cuba and had repressed the country's internal political opposition. For all that, most neutral observers conceded that a majority of Nicaraguans supported Sandinista efforts to introduce land, educational, and health reforms. Reagan had campaigned in 1980 for a harder line against Nicaragua, however, and cut off American aid during his first year in office. At the same time, he extended help to the rebel "Contra" forces trying to overthrow the Sandinistas. When critics accused Reagan of fomenting another Vietnam in Central America, he called the Contras "freedom fighters," comparing them to the Founding Fathers. While the Contras did include disaffected Sandinistas and moderate democrats, a good many of their leaders were refugees from the Somoza dictatorship, whose repressive policies had helped make the Sandinistas so welcome to Nicaraguans.

Congress at first refused to support the Contras with anything more than limited supplies for "humanitarian" purposes. Most Central American governments were similarly loathe to intervene; indeed, four of Nicaragua's regional neighbors, known as the Contadora group—Venezuela, Mexico, Panama, and Colombia—sought to negotiate a solution and avoid an expanded war. But Reagan was determined to overthrow the Sandinistas. The CIA helped the Contras to mine the harbor at Managua, damaging seven foreign ships and violating international law in the process. Even conservative senators like Barry Goldwater were outraged, and Congress adopted (and the president signed) an amendment sponsored by Representative Edward Boland of Massachusetts explicitly forbidding the CIA or "any other agency or entity involved in intelligence activities" from spending money to support the Contras "directly or indirectly." Despite administration pressures, Congress remained leery of providing more military aid.

The Iran–Contra Connection

Thus by mid-1985 Reagan policymakers felt two major frustrations. For one, Congress had limited their support of the Contras in Central America; and second, Iranian-backed terrorists continued to hold hostages in Lebanon. In the summer of 1985, soon after the anguishing TWA hijacking, a course of events was set in motion that eventually linked these two issues.

The president made it increasingly clear he wanted to find a way to free the remaining hostages in Lebanon. Robert McFarlane, his stoic national security adviser, suggested the administration try to open a channel to moderate factions in the Iranian government. A former Israeli intelligence officer had hinted that such moderates did exist and hoped to improve relations with Western nations, especially since Iran was embroiled in a protracted war with Iraq. If the United States sold Iran a few weapons, the grateful Iranians might use their influence in Lebanon to free the hostages.

There were major problems with this scenario. No one knew whether any influential moderates existed in Iran. The only available contact was a glib-tongued, arms-dealing Iranian named Manucher Ghorbanifar. Even if an agreement exchanging arms for hostages could be made, it violated the president's often-repeated vow never to negotiate or pay ransom to terrorists. "This is almost too absurd to comment on," Secretary Weinberger replied, upon hearing of the idea to supply Iran with arms. "It's like asking Qadhafi to Washington for a cozy chat." Still, the president apparently approved the initiative—or at least McFarlane believed he had. In August 500 missiles were shipped to Iran from Israel, while the United States replaced the missiles in Israel's arsenal.

Over the following year, three more secret arms shipments were made to Iran, once using Israel as a go-between and twice more directly. The man who seemed to pull so much of the negotiations together was a junior officer under McFarlane in the National Security Council, Lieutenant Colonel Oliver North. North, a decorated Vietnam veteran with a flair for the dramatic, had already orchestrated the bold midair interception of the *Achille Lauro* terrorists. He was a "can-do" sort, impatient with bureaucrats and bureaucratic procedures. In the most astonishing initiative to Iran he and McFarlane flew to the capital, Teheran, in May 1986, using false Irish passports, carrying gift-wrapped .357-caliber pistols, a chocolate layer cake, and poison pills, in case the mission went awry. Despite four separate arms shipments, only one hostage was released.

Secretaries Weinberger and Shultz had strongly opposed the idea of exchang-

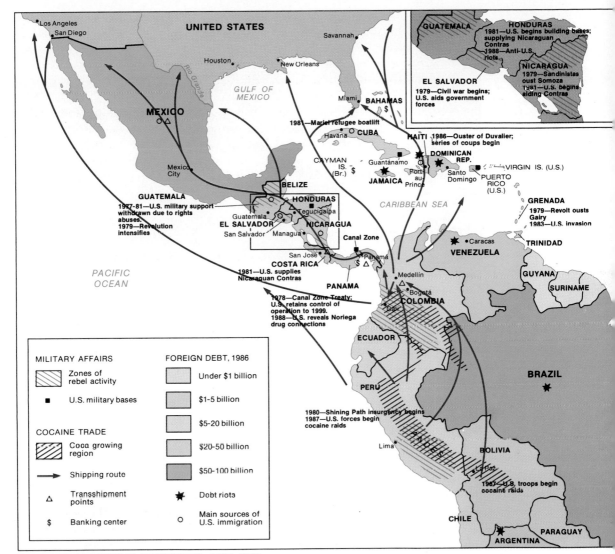

CENTRAL AMERICAN CONFLICTS, 1974–1988
President Reagan's attempts to overthrow the Sandinista government in Nicaragua and to contain communism focused American attention on Latin America. So too did the staggering debts Latin countries owed to banks in America and elsewhere. Equally distorting to the hemisphere's social and economic fabric was the sharp rise in the drug trade organized by criminal syndicates. Most notorious was the Medellin cartel, which operated from a remote region in Colombia, shipping drugs through havens in Panama and the Bahamas into the United States while depositing its enormous profits in banks in Miami and offshore banking centers like the Cayman Islands.

ing arms for hostages. What was perhaps most astonishing is that they were largely uninformed of the initiatives, precisely because their opposition was well known. McFarlane's successor as national security adviser, Admiral John Poindexter, had the president sign a secret intelligence "finding" that allowed him, North, and others to pursue their mission without informing anyone in Congress or even four

Oliver North successfully took the offensive in his testimony before the congressional committee investigating the Iran–Contra scandals. Here he delivers a pro-Contra lecture to his interrogators.

of the eight members of Poindexter's own National Security Council, including the secretaries of defense and state. With the president so inattentive to the details of foreign policy, McFarlane, Poindexter, and North derived an immense amount of power to act on their own.

North and McFarlane had already been acting without the knowledge of Congress to supply the Contras with arms in Central America. To do so, they devised ways to circumvent the Boland Amendment and its prohibitions against military aid. McFarlane made clear to Saudi Arabia and several other friendly allies that the Contras were desperately in need of funds. Between the summers of 1984 and 1985, the Saudis deposited at least $30 million in Swiss bank accounts set up to launder the money. North then recruited to the cause Richard Secord, a former major general who had been forced to retire from the air force under suspicion of having sold arms at a profit to Libya. Secord set up a delivery system, buying weapons with the laundered money, making a tidy profit, and delivering them to Central America. In addition, North illegally helped private conservative fund-raisers within the United States raise money for what he nobly referred to as Project Democracy. Secord, his sights set a trifle lower, merely referred to it as "the Enterprise."

The two strands of North's secret missions came together in January 1986, in a meeting with Ghorbanifar to work out the third arms sale to Iran. It occurred to North that the excess profits from the sale of U.S. missiles could be deposited in a Swiss account and then siphoned off to benefit the Contras. Ghorbanifar thought the idea a capital one: "I think this is now, Ollie, the best chance, because . . . we never get such good money out of this," he laughed, as he was recorded on a tape North himself made. "We do everything. We do hostages free of charge; we do all terrorists free of charge; Central America free of charge." By secretly selling government property at a profit, funds were made available for a rogue covert operation, without having the funds appropriated by Congress through the usual constitutional process.

Cover Blown

Through the fall of 1986, both operations had remained hidden from view, but that changed abruptly as the congressional elections drew near. A hostage, David Jacobsen, was released in return for a fifth shipment of TOW missiles. But the news that McFarlane and North had visited Teheran in May was leaked to a Lebanese newspaper, *Al Shiraa,* which gleefully published it. As corroborating evidence appeared, the administration was swamped by incredulous reporters, trying to determine how its policy of secret arms sales could be squared with its vocal antiterrorist campaign. Within the administration, both Weinberger and Shultz were outraged that the negotiations had been kept from them (although critics claimed they had too easily turned a blind eye, once they had seen that their advice was being rejected). Then, during the investigation of the Iranian affair, the link between the arms sales and the Contras was discovered. Attorney General Edwin Meese undertook an investigation to piece together the complete story, but he was so leisurely in pursuing the matter that North and his secretary were able to spend the bulk of one weekend shredding crucial documents. Enough of a paper trail remained, however—along with crucial computer files that had not been erased—that the dimensions of Project Democracy became clear.

As the controversy unfolded, the president defended the arms sales to Iran as negotiations unrelated to the release of hostages. He accepted Poindexter's resignation and dismissed Oliver North, though referring to him as a national hero. He seemed singularly uninterested in discovering what his subordinates had been doing, ostensibly in his name, but because of the public outcry agreed to appoint an investigative commission of three, led by former senator John Tower of Texas. The following week, on December 4, the House and Senate launched their own nine-month joint investigation into the Iran–Contra affair. And Attorney General Meese reluctantly appointed Lawrence Walsh as an independent prosecutor to investigate possible illegalities.

The press immediately began referring to the scandal as "Irangate," making the obvious comparison to Richard Nixon's Watergate scandal. But the two episodes had different dynamics and different outcomes. Watergate led eventually to the Oval Office, implicating the president in a cover-up from the very beginning. But the Iran–Contra congressional hearings, held during the summer of 1987, left the role of the president unexplained. "I assumed that the president was aware of what I was doing and had, through my superiors, approved it," North told Congress. But his superior, Admiral Poindexter, claimed he had deliberately kept Reagan in ignorance, "so that I could insulate him from the decision. . . . On this whole issue, you know, the buck stops here, with me." Since the committee had no desire to proceed with impeachment, the hearings came to a sputtering end, although the independent prosecutor did win convictions against North in 1989 and Poindexter in 1990.

So Irangate was not Watergate; perhaps it was worse. Harry Truman coined the phrase "The buck stops here," meaning that the president bore final responsibility for the actions of his subordinates. Iran–Contra revealed a presidency in which an unelected segment within the government took upon itself the power to intercept the buck's upward movement and launch a series of illegal diversions of government money to finance an unapproved war. "Dirty hands" worked diligently for the ideals of "clean hearts."

From Cold War to *Glasnost*

Still, the president's Teflon coating held. By the end of his term, Reagan's popularity returned, in part because of substantial progress achieved in Soviet–American relations. The 1980s had been difficult for the Soviet Union, with its stagnant economy, unstable leadership, and the loss of influence in Africa and the Middle East. The war in Afghanistan had become a Russian Vietnam. When Soviet jets in 1983 shot down a South Korean airliner that had penetrated its air space, killing all 269 passengers (including a member of Congress from Georgia), the world community condemned the brutality. Reagan, aware of the strains in the Soviet economy, at first accelerated the arms race to place additional pressure on the Russians to negotiate. In 1983 the United States deployed both intermediate-range Pershing II and cruise missiles in Europe, placing Moscow within a 10-minute missile flight from the launch site. Despite the pressure, the beleaguered Soviets walked out of the negotiations.

By 1985 the choice of Mikhail Gorbachev as premier created new possibilities in Soviet–American relations. Unlike his aged predecessors, Gorbachev was young, saw the need for reform within the Soviet Union, and rivaled Reagan as a shaper of world opinion. The fundamental restructuring, or *perestroika*, conceived by Gorbachev entailed improving relations with the United States, reduc-

---

Soviet Premier Gorbachev (right) used his summits with Ronald Reagan to reduce Soviet–American tensions, although the spirit of *glasnost* did not ease the skirmishes between his wife Raisa and Nancy Reagan, who waged a quiet war over fashion and ideology. Gorbachev came to rival Reagan as a "great communicator," with many Americans applauding his efforts to reform Soviet society and to slow the arms race.

ing military commitments, and adopting a policy of openness (*glasnost*) about problems in the Soviet Union. The Reagan administration soon found itself on the defensive over arms limitations. Gorbachev unilaterally ended all nuclear tests; Reagan refused to make a similar move, since American tests were needed to develop his controversial Strategic Defense Initiative. To many foreign observers it seemed Reagan was determined to extend the arms race into space. In June 1986, he announced that the United States would unilaterally exceed the limits of SALT II, an agreement which, though never ratified, had been since 1979 the only fragile restraint on the arms race.

In October, when the two leaders held their second summit in Reykjavík, Iceland, Gorbachev dangled the possibility of abolishing all nuclear weapons. Reagan seemed receptive to the idea, apparently unaware that if both sides eliminated all nuclear weapons, Soviet conventional forces would far outnumber NATO troops in Europe. In the end, the president refused to sacrifice his Star Wars for an all-or-nothing Soviet proposal. Many of his advisers were stunned that he had been so ill-prepared to negotiate. Although the Reykjavík summit proved a giddy exercise in hasty diplomacy, negotiations continued. In December 1987 Reagan traveled to Moscow, where he signed an agreement to eliminate an entire class of missiles. These intermediate-range nuclear forces (INFs) were land-based missiles, with ranges of 600 to 3400 miles. Both sides agreed to allow on-site inspections of missile bases and facilities where missiles were destroyed. Only two significant groups objected. Western European leaders feared a weakening of their defenses, and the right wing of Reagan's own party refused to believe that the Soviets could be trusted. They were not convinced, as Reagan was, that Gorbachev needed to shift resources from military buildup to domestic economic reforms. On May 27, 1988, the Senate approved the treaty by a 93–5 margin, marking a major step back from the brink of nuclear confrontation.

THE REAGAN LEGACY AND AN UNFINISHED SOCIAL AGENDA

As the election of 1988 approached, Ronald Reagan, against all odds, appeared to have made a comeback. What remained less clear was the long-term consequences of his years in office. The aura of prosperity, like the president's own aura of amiability, seemed at times to mask deeper problems requiring serious attention if the republic was to prosper and grow.

The Uncertain Legacy

The Reagan era most certainly proved that conservatives remained alive and well in America. For many years, the intellectual high ground of political thought had been held by liberal think tanks like the Brookings Institution. By the 1980s, conservative centers like the Hoover Institute and the American Enterprise Institute were energetically providing the Reagan administration with personnel and advice. Few Democrats seemed willing to call themselves liberals, and such traditional constituencies as labor unions were increasingly condemned as unhealthy interest groups.

Daily Lives

POLITICAL CULTURE
Life in the Underclass

During the 1880s Jacob Riis "discovered" a class of people largely invisible to the "better half" of society. Drawing on his investigative reporting for the New York *Tribune*, he described them as "individuals who have lost connection with home life, or never had any, or whose homes had ceased to be sufficiently separated, decent, and desireable to afford what are regarded as ordinary wholesome influences of home and family." A century later investigators for the Chicago *Tribune* discovered that there still existed in American cities "a lost society dwelling in enclaves of despair and chaos that infect and threaten the communities at large." This world, comprising as many as 5 million Americans, was also invisible, except when its behavior became so violent or criminal that newspapers and television news could not ignore it.

The trials of this underclass, numbing when seen as aggregate statistics, were searing when the *Tribune* reporters described individual lives, like that of Dorothy Sands. In 1957 Dorothy, her mother, Ora Streeter, and the rest of her family lived in a one-room shack in rural Mississippi. The family made a bare living picking cotton. But Dorothy's stepfather drank heavily and beat her mother in his intoxication, until finally Ora decided to escape the South, her job, and her abusive husband to take six small children to Chicago, where her mother lived. For young Dorothy, "It was something like going to a new world."

Life in Chicago imposed disappointments and cruelties of its own. Streeter's husband tracked the family down. After a brief reconciliation, the drinking and the

Early teen pregnancies trapped many poverty-stricken families in a recurring cycle of poverty.

beatings began anew. The couple separated and Streeter moved her children to a poorer neighborhood, where rents were lower. When arthritis prevented her from working she signed up for public assistance. Dorothy, the oldest child, assumed responsibility for the household, caring for the other children. With what little time she had for herself, she reached the ninth grade at school. But when she was 15 her dream of a nursing career ended when she discovered she was pregnant. In 1965, after her mother died, Dorothy began a relationship with Carra Little, a man who promised he could not get her pregnant.

Daily Lives

Within a year, Dorothy had her second child. She asked the doctors to sterilize her, but they refused. And the children kept arriving—four more of them. "When you are young, you don't really think about the future," Dorothy recalled. "You say, 'if I have another baby, then I have another child.'"

Though Little and Dorothy never married, he shared some of the household burdens and had regular work. But he also drank heavily, had affairs with other women, and beat her. And in 1976 he died of a heart attack. The household soon disintegrated. Dorothy did not even notice until seven months had passed that her oldest daughter, Barbara, like her mother and grandmother before her, was pregnant at age 15. By 1985 Dorothy was suffering from chronic depression and had considered suicide. At age 37 she was a grandmother living in a three-room apartment with five of her six children, her daughter LaWanda's new boyfriend, two grandchildren ages 7 and 2, and two teenaged girls who had run away from home. In 20 years the family had never been off welfare and no one in the household had held a regular job. Only one of her children attended school for more than brief periods.

With public assistance money Dorothy could afford only to house her family in a dilapidated three-story building on Chicago's West Side, where they were the sole tenants in eight apartments. Each evening people from the neighborhood pried open the front door to do "crack" or drink 100 percent grain alcohol. Sometime in 1985 the family stopped bathing because every time they turned on the water, plaster fell into the tub. The building manager reneged on his promise to make repairs. So the children just stood over the sink and washed their clothes by hand. An electrical wire attached to a bare bulb doubled as a clothesline.

This apartment, without heat or gas for cooking, rented for $275, which Dorothy paid out of her welfare allotment of $868 a month, comprising support payments and food stamps. Only she had a room of her own, which she kept neat and cleaned. To protect her few personal items from her family or intruders, she kept them padlocked in a closet. The girls slept on canvas cots in one room, while the boys took turns between cots and a mattress on the living room floor. Meals were irregular affairs, since money was scarce and no one liked to cook. For two weeks each month the family splurged on eggs for breakfast and Spam for dinner. More often they got by on hot dogs, rice, and beans.

Of this neighborhood's 61,500 people, over half received some form of welfare. People lucky enough to find work quickly moved away. The social agencies that existed to help people in trouble had largely stopped trying, leaving what one government official described as "a caste of people almost totally dependent on the state, with little hope of breaking free." The combination of Reagan administration cuts in welfare, inept and overburdened public agencies, depressed urban economies, as well as crime, drug addiction, and other social pathologies had left a permanent urban underclass. As citizens too depressed, apathetic, distracted, or ignorant of electoral procedures to vote, these people remained a largely voiceless part of the body politic.

For the rest of the American people, more fortunate in their circumstances, a question persisted: How could the problems of the largely invisible underclass be solved before the violence and desperation of the streets threatened the identity of American democracy itself?

There seemed limits, however, to the conservative rebellion. Although Ronald Reagan championed the agenda of conservative religious leaders, he did little to act on the issues they raised, including school prayer, amendments to the Constitution requiring a balanced budget and outlawing abortion, and forceful antidrug legislation. Moreover, the taint of self-interest and scandal hampered the administration's effectiveness. Key Reagan advisers Lyn Nofziger and Michael Deaver were both indicted and later convicted for profiting illegally from their connections with the president and his administration. Attorney General Edwin Meese was never indicted but was so often criticized for misusing his office to help friends in private business that the Justice Department's own committee on ethics issued a critical report after his resignation. In all, over 100 members of the Reagan administration had either resigned or been forced out of office by criticism of their ethical or legal conduct.

The Democratic Congress might have provided the counterweight of visible, effective leadership, but for the most part, Congress seemed unwilling to grapple with serious issues. The tax reform legislation of 1986 was an exception; so, in 1988, was a compromise between conservatives and liberals for overhauling the welfare system. That bill incorporated liberal demands for increases in child-care payments, Medicaid, and welfare with conservative requirements for recipients either to work or to enroll in job training and educational programs. In other areas, however, Congress remained skittish. Virtually all members condemned the record-high deficits of the Reagan years, but with the president so adamantly opposed to new taxes, they appointed a bipartisan commission to issue recommendations, which turned out to be useless. As the rising tide of drug traffic placed increasing pressure on the urban social fabric, Congress passed a hastily drawn bill to strengthen law enforcement and treatment programs during the election year—but failed to fund the programs adequately.

Unsolved Problems

The seeming inability of both the executive and legislative branches to act vigorously was even more alarming because of deeper structural problems in the economy and society. Ironically, one crisis stemmed from the Reagan administration's inability to put into practice its "free enterprise" philosophy of reining in government bureaucracy. The bureaucracy most in need of reining in was the military's. Investigations of Pentagon procurement procedures showed that millions of dollars were being misspent when contracts were not let out for competitive bidding, as they would have under free-market conditions. On the other hand, the lack of oversight at the military's nuclear power plants showed that the bureaucracy suffered equally from too little regulation. By the end of the Reagan years, 17 sites had been closed down due to safety hazards involved in processing nuclear wastes. Because these sites were military installations, they were exempt from—and had often ignored—some of the most elementary regulations in place for civilian nuclear power plants. The prolonged inattention meant that the cost of repair might reach $200 billion. Similar problems plagued the space program, as the explosion of the space shuttle *Challenger* demonstrated in January 1986. Flaws in other military rocket designs left the American space program temporarily crippled.

In the area of public health, the spread of AIDS (acquired immune deficiency syndrome) posed a challenge that caught the administration particularly unprepared. The disease at first struck especially hard at the male homosexual community, at a time when both lesbians and gays were becoming more vocal in asserting their rights as citizens. Since the 1970s increasing numbers of people had begun to "come out of the closet" by making their sexual orientation known publicly and fighting for "gay rights" and an end to legal discrimination. Although a number of outspoken conservatives were themselves gay, most evangelical Christians, conservative Catholics, and other traditional groups continued to condemn homosexual acts as immoral. Intravenous drug users also were hard-hit by AIDS. Public health officials warned that the enormous expense of treating AIDS patients threatened the health care system, but the Reagan administration moved with extreme caution in providing research funds or care for those afflicted. Much of the burden fell on states like New York and California, where a high percentage of the gay and drug-addicted population lived.

The health of the nation's financial system seemed equally shaky, despite the continuing prosperity. After a surging bull market broke repreated records, on October 19, 1987, the Dow Jones industrial averages dropped over 500 points. On paper, that meant a loss of almost 20 percent in the value of stocks in a single day, forcing investors to recall the catastrophic crash of 1929. A presidential commission found evidence that the severe loss came from unregulated market practices like buying and selling on the basis of computer programs, not from weakness in the economy. Yet neither Congress nor the administration acted on the commission's recommendations. At the same time, savings and loans banks around the country were failing at the highest rate since the Great Depression. The Reagan administration had significantly cut back its regulation of savings and loan industry investments. Under the new, more liberal rules, many savings banks jumped into highly speculative deals or even engaged in outright fraud. Since depositors' money was backed by the Federal Savings and Loan Insurance Corporation (FSLIC), the government was faced with paying back depositors if these thrift institutions failed. The administration ignored the problem, as experts warned that a bailout might cost as much as $250 billion.

While the administration's economic policy had helped create 14.5 million jobs through 1988, the jobs were spread unevenly through the economic sector. Over 2 million of them were in finance, insurance, real estate, and law, all services used by the wealthy, not the poor. In the highly paid "Wall Street" jobs—those involving financial services—over 70 percent went to white males, only 2 percent to African-Americans. New employment for women was concentrated in the areas of health, education, social services, and government, where approximately 3 million jobs opened, most dependent on government support. New jobs for the poor (over 3 million) were largely restricted to minimum wage or poverty-level employment in hotels, fast-food restaurants, and retail stores. Here, in unskilled, often part-time, and usually dead-end jobs, almost 2 million blacks and Hispanics found work. Finally, there were almost 2.5 million new jobs for people (mostly male) who handled or moved things. Jobs for "light truck drivers," for example, increased five times as fast as any other employment.

For the wealthiest 20 percent of Americans, the 1980s had been the best of times. Demand for doctors, lawyers, engineers, and MBAs soared. What counterculture hippies were to the 1960s, high-salaried yuppies (young, upwardly mobile professionals) were to the 1980s. While the middle 60 percent of the population saw their earnings fall slightly, earnings dropped 8 percent for the poorest 20 percent and rose 9 percent for the top 20 percent. Over one-third of all tax savings ($3.6 billion) went to those 162,000 American families earning over $200,000, compared to $2.9 billion to the 31.7 million families with incomes under $15,000 a year.

A Question of Civil Rights

By the 1980s the African-American community had seemingly split in two. A significant minority had successfully lived the American dream. Almost three times more African-Americans were elected to public office in the 1970s and 1980s than in the 1960s. Tom Bradley in Los Angeles, Andrew Young in Atlanta, Harold Washington in Chicago, and Wilson Goode in Philadelphia had become mayors of some of the nation's largest cities. Blacks made substantial strides in the professions, management, sports, and entertainment. The earnings of households headed by blacks rose faster than those for whites in the 1970s, although they remained 20 percent lower.

But the surge of African-Americans into middle-class occupations tended to disguise the persistence of poverty tied to race, along with age and sex. In the 1970s and 1980s, while many of the elderly escaped poverty with the aid of Social Security payments, more young families were counted among the nation's poor. Those families were increasingly headed by single women. Over 40 percent of all black families (versus 12 percent for whites) were headed by women, and the number was growing. Here was the hard core of poverty. And for blacks as well as whites the divorce rate continued to rise. To make matters worse, the largest numbers of black families were concentrated in urban areas hard hit by the recessionary economy. Black unemployment, particularly severe among teenagers and young adults, was twice the national average.

The issue of racial prejudice, one of the oldest problems in American history, provided new cause for concern in the 1980s. During the 1970s, judicially active courts had forced officials in many large cities to take affirmative action to counter the long-term effects of segregation. That trend was challenged when the Supreme Court decided *Bakke v. Regents of the University of California* (1978). Allan Bakke, a white man, had been rejected by the medical school at the University of California at Davis, even though he had higher grades than most of the minority applicants admitted under a quota system. In a divided, ambiguous ruling, the Court ruled 5–4 that fixed quotas were illegal and that Bakke was to be admitted. On the other hand, Justice Powell's concurring opinion acknowledged that race could be a factor in admissions programs in order to secure a more diversified student body. Similar cases (decided in closely split decisions) left many observers unsure of the Court's direction, except that in general it was taking a more stringent attitude toward quota systems and affirmative action.

In the realm of everyday life, African-Americans received all too many signs that prejudice continued to operate in American society. Howard Beach, a white area of New York City, attracted national attention in 1987 when a gang of white youths beat several blacks who had strayed into the neighborhood, chasing one onto a highway where he was run over and killed. Racial incidents increased on college campuses, including the universities of Michigan and Massachusetts and the ivy league campus of Dartmouth. Equally disturbing, a black agent working for the Federal Bureau of Investigation, the nation's highest law enforcement agency, accused white co-workers of harassing him with death threats. The combination of persisting race discrimination and an economy that perpetuated a despairing underclass posed problems that could not be ignored.

The New Immigration

During the 1980s, according to provisional figures, about 6 million immigrants entered the country legally—more than in any decade in American history except

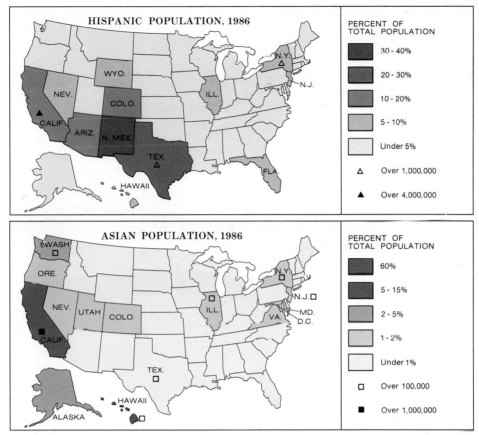

HISPANIC AND ASIAN POPULATIONS

Hispanics and Asians have been the two fastest-growing population groups in the United States over the past several decades. Demographers predict that Hispanics will soon displace African-Americans as the nation's single largest minority group. Both Asians and Hispanics have been especially drawn to the climate and job opportunities in California.

1901–1910. Adding another 300,000 to 500,000 illegal immigrants each year, the total was even greater than the 8.8 million arriving in the first decade of the century.

Latin American immigrants accounted for approximately 35 to 40 percent of the influx each year, as they had since the 1960s. The greatest number settled in sunbelt states of Florida, Texas, and California, as well as Illinois and New York. However, the increased visibility of Hispanics did not readily translate into economic gains. In an economy increasingly divided between highly skilled jobs in the service sectors and low-paying unskilled jobs, Hispanics lagged behind anglos and blacks in education. Often, the lack of adequate English-language skills discouraged academic success. As housing costs soared during the late 1970s, only 43 percent of Hispanics owned their homes, compared to 63 percent of all Americans.

Larger families with less money translated into crowded conditions. Like immigrant families at the turn of the century, the more established Hispanic families provided housing for newer immigrants, who were often single. The new-comers hoped to save enough money from their weekly paycheck to send it to relatives in Mexico or Central America.

At the same time, some of the new immigration patterns reversed established ones. Traditionally, the majority of immigrants arriving in America have taken the lowest paying jobs, gradually assimilating into society and working their way up. Census figures from the mid-1980s indicated, however, that newcomers often did better than natives. Thus foreign-born black and Hispanic people appeared more likely to have jobs than native-born ones. Riots in Miami during 1989 revealed growing tension between newly arrived Haitians and African-Americans. Heavy immigration also disturbed relations between Hispanics and Central Americans.

By the 1980s Asians had surpassed Hispanics in numbers of legal immigrants. By eliminating the national origins quota system, the Immigration Act of 1965 opened the door on a first-come, first-qualified basis, making possible the influx of people from China and Taiwan, Korea, Japan, the Philippines, Vietnam, Cambodia, Laos, Thailand, and India. As of 1990 about 6.5 million Asian-Americans lived in the United States. Like earlier immigrants from Europe, those from the Pacific rim came in waves. Some, like the Vietnamese "boat people" of the late 1970s, were driven from their homes by economic or political turmoil; others were drawn to reunite families or realize greater opportunities in the Western Hemisphere. Professional and educated Asian Indians emigrated in search of better jobs in the United States. Doctors and nurses constituted a large percentage of the early Korean immigrants. But letters home to relatives and other nationals soon attracted a more diverse population, which concentrated in small businesses. By the mid-1980s Indians owned over 50 percent of the non–chain motels in the United States, and Koreans often replaced Jews and Italians as owners of small inner-city delicatessens and produce stores.

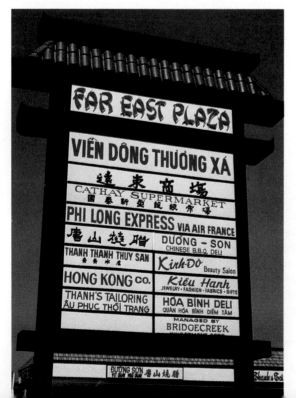

A wave of Asian immigrants has changed the style of America's cities much as European immigrants did a century before. This shopping plaza in Westminster, California, includes both a Chinese supermarket and "B.B.Q. Deli" as well as various Vietnamese enterprises. The overseas package and mail service indicates continued links to Asia.

The presence of other Asian-Americans and an international atmosphere drew many Asian-Americans to New York City, but climate made Hawaii and California particularly popular destinations. In 1977 alone some 40,000 Filipinos, many eager to escape from the corrupt regime of dictator Ferdinand Marcos, migrated to Honolulu. Of the 400,000 Korean-Americans in 1980 some 100,000 lived around Los Angeles. So, too, the half million Japanese-Americans settled primarily in California and Hawaii. By contrast, the federal government attempted to disperse the large influx of Vietnamese (as well as Cambodians and Laotians) who fled after the American withdrawal from Southeast Asia.

Many of the new immigrants achieved success while facing subtle forms of discrimination. With the exception of the Vietnamese, whose average income had been lowered by the presence of newly arrived boat people, the census bureau's 1980 figures of average yearly income showed many Asians leading not only other immigrant groups, but full-time American wage earners:

Asian Indian	$18,707
Japanese	16,829
Chinese	15,753
White	15,572
Korean	14,224
Filipino	13,690
Hispanic	11,650
Vietnamese	11,641
African-American	11,327

The high rate of success resulted partly from previous business and educational experience, as well as a powerful work ethic. One survey indicated that while the average American student spent 19.6 hours a week on academic work, the average Japanese-American spent 32.6 hours and Chinese-Americans, 40.4.

Racial tensions, made worse by job losses and the U.S. trade deficit with Asian countries, soon gave way to scattered acts of violence. In the ports of Texas and Louisiana the Ku Klux Klan joined with angry shrimp fishermen to mount a campaign of harassment and terror against newly arrived Vietnamese shrimpers. During a 1982 recession, some Detroit blue-collar workers vented their fear of Japanese auto imports by beating a Chinese-American to death. Many inner-city Korean merchants faced vandalism from local street gangs. The increasing numbers of both Asians and Hispanics also raised fears that they would not assimilate into American society. To spur acculturation conservatives called for the elimination of bilingual education. In 1981 the outspoken Max Rafferty, a nativist California educator, told Hispanics, "Immigrating was *your* idea. So the burden of learning the new language falls upon you—or should." In 1986 California voters reinforced the message. They passed a state referendum ending bilingual education. Other states such as Florida followed suit.

Congress also attacked the problem of increasing illegal immigration along the nation's southern border. After debating the issue for several years, in 1987 it passed a compromise version of the Simpson–Mazzoli Bill, which for the first time punished employers for hiring illegal aliens. To ease the plight of those aliens illegally in the country, the new law allowed those resident since January 1982 to become citizens. The Immigration and Naturalization Service used stricter guidelines for determining which immigrants would be granted political asylum, although critics complained that the anticommunist Reagan administration was much more generous in admitting Nicaraguans fleeing the Sandinistas than it was El Salvadoreans fleeing the American-backed government.

The new wave of immigration created serious local stresses. In the long view, though, it did not constitute a pressing crisis. Despite the "flood" of new arrivals, incoming immigrants made up only 0.3 percent of the population every year—about half the percentage that had entered, on average, over the past two centuries. In 1985, the total foreign-born population in the United States was 7 percent, compared with 11 percent for France, 16 percent for Canada, and 20 percent for Australia. In general, the traditional forces favoring assimilation seemed still at work.

The Election of 1988

All of these underlying problems—the role of the military bureaucracy, the savings and loan crisis, the need for racial tolerance, and the place of new immigrants—were fit topics for discussion in the election of 1988. Yet both candidates avoided them. The race to succeed Ronald Reagan in the White House proved a drawn-out affair that failed, above all, to define a new political agenda. Among seven major Democratic candidates only Jesse Jackson showed a real ability to excite the voters, both positively and negatively. He called for a national crusade to ease the plight of the poor. But as an African-American with a record of distinctly liberal ideas, Jackson could not capture the center of the Democratic party. That was the target of Massachusetts governor Michael Dukakis. Little-known outside New England, Dukakis ran a cautious but effective primary campaign

George Bush accepts the 1988 Republican nomination for president. Despite his controversial selection of Senator J. Danforth Quayle (looking on) as his vice-presidential running mate, Bush defeated the Democratic nominee, Michael Dukakis.

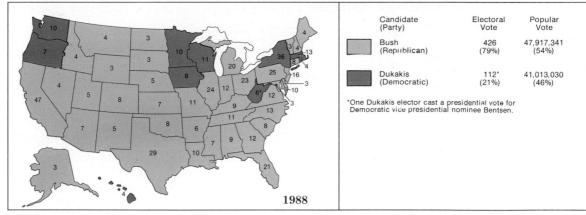

Candidate (Party)	Electoral Vote	Popular Vote
Bush (Republican)	426 (79%)	47,917,341 (54%)
Dukakis (Democratic)	112* (21%)	41,013,030 (46%)

*One Dukakis elector cast a presidential vote for Democratic vice presidential nominee Bentsen.

1988

THE ELECTION OF 1988

based on a record of administrative competence and a call to revive the economic fortunes of the poor and middle classes.

As the heir apparent to Ronald Reagan, George Bush appealed most to Republican party professionals and the affluent middle class that had benefited from Reagonomics. Bush had some evident weaknesses. He had been involved in the disastrous decision to trade arms for hostages. Women voters showed a preference for Dukakis and his support for free choice on the abortion issue. Many blue-collar workers hurt by the loss of high-wage jobs seemed ready to return to the Democratic fold. To emphasize his own stature, Bush selected one of the least qualified candidates in American political history, conservative Senator J. Danforth Quayle of Indiana, as his running mate.

More than Dukakis, Bush evaded major campaign issues and draped himself in the flag. Like Reagan, he emphasized the Republican themes of strong national defense and anti-Soviet policies. In addition, Americans seemed reluctant to change the political course so long as the economy kept growing. In a campaign that ultimately focused on media images rather than issues, Bush won by a comfortable margin (54 to 46 percent) while achieving an Electoral College advantage of 426 to 112. The people had spoken, though not very loudly.

George Washington had begun his first term in office exactly 200 years earlier, presiding over a fragile republic whose future seemed uncertain at best. Yet that republic survived, flourished, and developed a remarkably democratic system for adjudicating the rival needs and claims of its diverse citizenry. To George Bush fell the responsibility of articulating an agenda for a nation of nations that remained divided, as always, along lines of class, gender, race, religion, section, generation, and ideology.

SIGNIFICANT EVENTS

1978 — *Bakke v. Regents of the University of California*

1979 — Moral Majority established; Sandinistas overthrow Somoza in Nicaragua

1980 — Reagan defeats Carter

1980s — Asians pass Hispanics in numbers of legal immigrants

1981 — Reagan shot; military buildup; Reagan breaks PATCO strike; recession sets in; Economic Recovery Tax Act; United States begins aiding Nicaraguan Contras

1982 — Jonathan Schell's *Fate of the Earth* published; attack on U.S. Marine barracks in Lebanon

1983 — Reagan proposes SDI; invasion of Grenada; Soviets shoot down South Korean airliner; Pershing missiles deployed in Europe

1984 — Boland Amendment passed; Geraldine Ferraro nominated for vice president; Reagan defeats Mondale

1985 — Gramm–Rudman Act; U.S. bombing raid on Libya; increase in hostages taken by terrorists; United States begins secret arms-for-hostages negotiations with Iran

1986 — *Challenger* shuttle disaster; Oliver North begins diverting Iran arms sales profits to Contras; California restricts bilingual education; Tax Reform Act; American jets attack Libya; Reykjavík summit; Immigration Reform Act; Iran–Contra scandal breaks

1987 — Iran–Contra hearings; United States and Soviet Union agree on INF treaty; stock market plunge

1988 — Congress passes drug and welfare reform bills; Bush defeats Dukakis

1989 — Miami riots; Oliver North convicted

APPENDIX

THE DECLARATION OF INDEPENDENCE

In Congress, July 4, 1776,

THE UNANIMOUS DECLARATION OF THE
THIRTEEN UNITED STATES OF AMERICA

When, in the course of human events, it becomes necessary for one people to dissolve the political bands which have connected them with another, and to assume, among the powers of the earth, the separate and equal station to which the laws of nature and of nature's God entitle them, a decent respect to the opinions of mankind requires that they should declare the causes which impel them to the separation.

We hold these truths to be self-evident, that all men are created equal; that they are endowed by their Creator with certain unalienable rights; that among these, are life, liberty, and the pursuit of happiness. That, to secure these rights, governments are instituted among men, deriving their just powers from the consent of the governed; that, whenever any form of government becomes destructive of these ends, it is the right of the people to alter or to abolish it, and to institute a new government, laying its foundation on such principles, and organizing its powers in such form, as to them shall seem most likely to effect their safety and happiness. Prudence, indeed, will dictate that governments long established, should not be changed for light and transient causes; and, accordingly, all experience hath shown, that mankind are more disposed to suffer, while evils are sufferable, than to right themselves by abolishing the forms to which they are accustomed. But, when a long train of abuses and usurpations, pursuing invariably the same object, evinces a design to reduce them under absolute despotism, it is their right, it is their duty, to throw off such government and to provide new guards for their future security. Such has been the patient sufferance of these colonies, and such is now the necessity which constrains them to alter their former systems of government. The history of the present King of Great Britain is a history of repeated injuries and usurpations, all having, in direct object, the establishment of an absolute tyranny over these States. To prove this, let facts be submitted to a candid world:

He has refused his assent to laws the most wholesome and necessary for the public good.

He has forbidden his governors to pass laws of immediate and pressing importance, unless suspended in their operation till his assent should be obtained; and, when so suspended, he has utterly neglected to attend to them.

He has refused to pass other laws for the accommodation of large districts of people, unless those people would relinquish the right of representation in the legislature; a right inestimable to them, and formidable to tyrants only.

He has called together legislative bodies at places unusual, uncomfortable, and distant from the depository of their public records, for the sole purpose of fatiguing them into compliance with his measures.

He has dissolved representative houses repeatedly for opposing, with manly firmness, his invasions on the rights of the people.

He has refused, for a long time after such dissolutions, to cause others to be elected; whereby the legislative powers, incapable of annihilation, have returned to the people at large for their exercise; the state remaining, in the meantime, exposed to all the danger of invasion from without, and convulsions within.

He has endeavored to prevent the population of these States; for that purpose, obstructing the laws for naturalization of foreigners, refusing to pass others to encourage their migration hither, and raising the conditions of new appropriations of lands.

He had obstructed the administration of justice, by refusing his assent to laws for establishing judiciary powers.

He has made judges dependent on his will alone, for the tenure of their offices, and the amount and payment of their salaries.

He has erected a multitude of new offices, and sent hither swarms of officers to harass our people, and eat out their substance.

He has kept among us, in time of peace, standing armies, without the consent of our legislatures.

He has affected to render the military independent of, and superior to, the civil power.

He has combined, with others, to subject us to a jurisdiction foreign to our Constitution, and unacknowledged by our laws; giving his assent to their acts of pretended legislation:

For quartering large bodies of armed troops among us:

For protecting them by a mock trial, from punishment, for any murders which they should commit on the inhabitants of these States:

For cutting off our trade with all parts of the world:

For imposing taxes on us without our consent:

For depriving us, in many cases, of the benefit of trial by jury:

For transporting us beyond seas to be tried for pretended offences:

For abolishing the free system of English laws in a neighboring province, establishing therein an arbitrary government, and enlarging its boundaries, so as to render it at once an example and fit instrument for introducing the same absolute rule into these colonies:

For taking away our charters, abolishing our most valuable laws, and altering, fundamentally, the powers of our governments:

For suspending our own legislatures, and declaring themselves invested with power to legislate for us in all cases whatsoever.

He had abdicated government here, by declaring us out of his protection, and waging war against us.

He has plundered our seas, ravaged our coasts, burnt our towns, and destroyed the lives of our people.

He is, at this time, transporting large armies of foreign mercenaries to complete the works of death, desolation, and tyranny, already begun, with circumstances of cruelty and perfidy scarcely paralleled in the most barbarous ages, and totally unworthy the head of a civilized nation.

He has constrained our fellow citizens, taken captive on the high seas, to bear arms against their country, to become the executioners of their friends, and brethren, or to fall themselves by their hands.

He has excited domestic insurrections amongst us, and has endeavored to bring on the inhabitants of our frontiers, the merciless Indian savages, whose known rule of warfare is an undistinguished destruction of all ages, sexes, and conditions.

In every stage of these oppressions, we have petitioned for redress, in the most humble terms; our repeated petitions have been answered only by repeated injury. A prince, whose character is thus marked by every act which may define a tyrant, is unfit to be the ruler of a free people.

Nor have we been wanting in attention to our British brethren. We have warned them, from time to time, of attempts made by their legislature to extend an unwarrantable jurisdiction over us. We have reminded them of the circumstances of our emigration and settlement here. We have appealed to their native justice and magnanimity, and we have conjured them, by the ties of our common kindred, to disavow these usurpations, which would inevitably interrupt our connections and correspondence. They, too, have been deaf to the voice of justice and consanguinity. We must, therefore, acquiesce in the necessity which denounces our separation, and hold them as we hold the rest of mankind, enemies in war, in peace, friends.

We, therefore, the representatives of the United States of America, in general Congress assembled, appealing to the Supreme Judge of the world for the rectitude of our intentions, do, in the name, and by the authority of the good people of these colonies, solemnly publish and declare, that these united colonies are, and of right ought to be, free and independent states: that they are absolved from all allegiance to the British Crown, and that all political connection between them and the state of Great Britain is, and ought to be, totally dissolved; and that, as free and independent states, they have full power to levy war, conclude peace, contract alliances, establish commerce, and to do all other acts and things which independent states may of right do. And, for the support of this declaration, with a firm reliance on the protection of Divine Providence, we mutually pledge to each other our lives, our fortunes, and our sacred honor.

The foregoing Declaration was, by order of Congress, engrossed, and signed by the following members:

JOHN HANCOCK

New Hampshire
Josiah Bartlett
William Whipple
Matthew Thornton

New York
William Floyd
Philip Livingston
Francis Lewis
Lewis Morris

Delaware
Caesar Rodney
George Reed
Thomas M'Kean

North Carolina
William Hooper
Joseph Hewes
John Penn

Massachusetts Bay
Samuel Adams
John Adams
Robert Treat Paine
Elbridge Gerry

New Jersey
Richard Stockton
John Witherspoon
Francis Hopkinson
John Hart
Abraham Clark

Maryland
Samuel Chase
William Paca
Thomas Stone
Charles Carroll,
    of Carrollton

South Carolina
Edward Rutledge
Thomas Heyward, Jr.
Thomas Lynch, Jr.
Arthur Middleton

Rhode Island
Stephen Hopkins
William Ellery

Connecticut
Roger Sherman
Samuel Huntington
William Williams
Oliver Wolcott

Pennsylvania
Robert Morris
Benjamin Rush
Benjamin Franklin
John Morton
George Clymer
James Smith
George Taylor
James Wilson
George Ross

Virginia
George Wythe
Richard Henry Lee
Thomas Jefferson
Benjamin Harrison
Thomas Nelson, Jr.
Francis Lightfoot Lee
Carter Braxton

Georgia
Button Gwinnett
Lyman Hall
George Walton

Resolved, That copies of the Declaration be sent to the several assemblies, conventions, and committees, or councils of safety, and to the several commanding officers of the continental troops; that it be proclaimed in each of the United States, at the head of the army.

THE CONSTITUTION OF THE UNITED STATES OF AMERICA[1]

We the People of the United States, in Order to form a more perfect Union, establish Justice, insure domestic Tranquility, provide for the common defence, promote the general Welfare, and secure the Blessings of Liberty to ourselves and our Posterity, do ordain and establish this CONSTITUTION for the United States of America.

ARTICLE 1

Section 1. All legislative Powers herein granted shall be vested in a Congress of the United States, which shall consist of a Senate and House of Representatives.

Section 2. The House of Representatives shall be composed of Members chosen every second Year by the People of the several States, and the Electors in each State shall have the Qualifications requisite for Electors of the most numerous Branch of the State Legislature.

No Person shall be a Representative who shall not have attained to the Age of twenty-five Years, and been seven Years a Citizen of the United States, and who shall not, when elected, be an Inhabitant of that State in which he shall be chosen.

[Representatives and direct Taxes[2] shall be apportioned among the several States which may be included within this Union, according to their respective Numbers, which shall be determined by adding to the whole Number of free Persons, including those bound to Service for a Term of Years, and excluding Indians not taxed, three fifths of all other Persons.][3] The actual Enumeration shall be made within three Years after the first Meeting of the Congress of the United States, and within every subsequent Term of ten Years, in such Manner as they shall by Law direct. The Number of Representatives shall not exceed one for every thirty Thousand, but each State shall have at Least one Repre-

sentative; and until such enumeration shall be made, the State of New Hampshire shall be entitled to chuse three, Massachusetts eight, Rhode-Island and Providence Plantations one, Connecticut five, New York six, New Jersey four, Pennsylvania eight, Delaware one, Maryland six, Virginia ten, North Carolina five, South Carolina five, and Georgia three.

When vacancies happen in the Representation from any State, the Executive Authority thereof shall issue Writs of Election to fill such Vacancies.

The House of Representatives shall chuse their Speaker and other Officers; and shall have the sole Power of Impeachment.

Section 3. The Senate of the United States shall be composed of two Senators from each State, chosen by the Legislature thereof, for six Years; and each Senator shall have one Vote.

Immediately after they shall be assembled in Consequence of the first Election, they shall be divided as equally as may be into three Classes. The Seats of the Senators of the first Class shall be vacated at the Expiration of the second Year, of the second Class at the Expiration of the fourth Year, and of the third Class at the Expiration of the sixth Year, so that one-third may be chosen every second Year; and if Vacancies happen by Resignation, or otherwise, during the Recess of the Legislature of any State, the Executive thereof may make temporary Appointments until the next Meeting of the Legislature, which shall then fill such Vacancies.

No Person shall be a Senator who shall not have attained to the Age of thirty Years, and been nine Years a Citizen of the United States, and who shall not, when elected, be an Inhabitant of that State for which he shall be chosen.

The Vice President of the United States shall be President of the Senate, but shall have no vote, unless they be equally divided.

The Senate shall chuse their other Officers, and also a President pro tempore, in the absence of the Vice President, or when he shall exercise the Office of President of the United States.

The Senate shall have the sole Power to try all Impeachments. When sitting for that pur-

---

[1]This version follows the original Constitution in capitalization and spelling. It is adapted from the text published by the United States Department of the Interior, Office of Education.

[2]Altered by the Sixteenth Amendment.

[3]Negated by the Fourteenth Amendment.

pose they shall be on Oath or Affirmation. When the President of the United States is tried, the Chief Justice shall preside: And no person shall be convicted without the Concurrence of two thirds of the Members present.

Judgment in Cases of Impeachment shall not extend further than to removal from Office, and disqualification to hold and enjoy any Office of honor, Trust, or Profit under the United States: but the Party convicted shall nevertheless be liable and subject to Indictment, Trial, Judgment, and Punishment, according to Law.

Section 4. The Times, Places and Manner of holding Elections for Senators and Representatives, shall be prescribed in each State by the Legislature thereof; but the Congress may at any time by Law make or alter such Regulations, except as to the Places of Chusing Senators.

The Congress shall assemble at least once in every Year, and such Meeting shall be on the first Monday in December, unless they shall by Law appoint a different Day.

Section 5. Each House shall be the Judge of the Elections, Returns and Qualifications of its own Members, and a Majority of each shall constitute a Quorum to do Business; but a smaller number may adjourn from day to day, and may be authorized to compel the Attendance of absent Members, in such Manner, and under such Penalties, as each House may provide.

Each House may determine the Rules of its Proceedings, punish its Members for disorderly Behaviour, and, with the Concurrence of two thirds, expel a Member.

Each House shall keep a Journal of its Proceedings, and from time to time publish the same, excepting such Parts as may in their Judgment require Secrecy; and the Yeas and Nays of the Members of either House on any question shall, at the Desire of one fifth of those Present, be entered on the Journal.

Neither House, during the Session of Congress, shall, without the Consent of the other, adjourn for more than three days, nor to any other Place than that in which the two Houses shall be sitting.

Section 6. The Senators and Representatives shall receive a Compensation for their Services, to be ascertained by Law, and paid out of the Treasury of the United States. They shall in all Cases, except Treason, Felony, and Breach of the Peace, be privileged from Arrest during their Attendance at the Session of their respective Houses, and in going to and returning from the same; and for any Speech or Debate in either House, they shall not be questioned in any other Place.

No Senator or Representative shall, during the Time for which he was elected, be appointed to any civil Office under the Authority of the United States, which shall have been created, or the Emoluments whereof shall have been increased, during such time; and no Person holding any Office under the United States shall be a Member of either House during his continuance in Office.

Section 7. All Bills for raising Revenue shall originate in the House of Representatives; but the Senate may propose or concur with Amendments as on other bills.

Every Bill which shall have passed the House of Representatives and the Senate, shall, before it become a Law, be presented to the President of the United States; If he approve he shall sign it, but if not he shall return it, with his Objections, to that House in which it shall have originated, who shall enter the Objections at large on their Journal, and proceed to reconsider it. If after such Reconsideration two thirds of that House shall agree to pass the bill, it shall be sent, together with the objections, to the other House, by which it shall likewise be reconsidered, and if approved by two thirds of that House, it shall become a Law. But in all such Cases the Votes of both Houses shall be determined by Yeas and Nays, and the Names of the Persons voting for and against the Bill shall be entered on the Journal of each House respectively. If any Bill shall not be returned by the President within ten Days (Sundays excepted) after it shall have been presented to him, the Same shall be a Law, in like Manner as if he had signed it, unless the Congress by their Adjournment prevent its Return, in which Case it shall not be a Law.

Every Order, Resolution, or Vote to which the Concurrence of the Senate and House of Representatives may be necessary (except on a question of Adjournment) shall be presented to the President of the United States; and before the Same shall take Effect, shall be approved by him, or being disapproved by him, shall be repassed by two thirds of the Senate and House of Representatives, according to the Rules and Limitations prescribed in the Case of a Bill.

Section 8. The Congress shall have Power To lay and collect Taxes, Duties, Imposts and Excises, to pay the Debts and provide for the common Defence and general Welfare of the United States; but all Duties, Imposts and Excises shall be uniform throughout the United States;

To borrow money on the credit of the United States;

To regulate Commerce with foreign Nations, and among the several States, and with the Indian Tribes;

To establish an uniform rule of Naturalization, and uniform Laws on the subject of Bankruptcies throughout the United States;

To coin Money, regulate the Value thereof, and of foreign Coin, and fix the Standard of Weights and Measures;

To provide for the Punishment of counterfeiting the Securities and current Coin of the United States;

To establish Post Offices and post Roads;

To promote the Progress of Science and useful Arts, by securing for limited Times to Authors and Inventors the exclusive Right to their respective Writings and Discoveries;

To constitute Tribunals inferior to the Supreme Court;

To define and punish Piracies and Felonies committed on the high Seas, and Offenses against the Law of Nations;

To declare War, grant Letters of Marque and Reprisal, and make Rules concerning Captures on Land and Water;

To raise and support Armies, but no Appropriation of Money to that Use shall be for a longer Term than two Years;

To provide and maintain a Navy;

To make Rules for the Government and Regulation of the land and naval forces;

To provide for calling forth the Militia to execute the Laws of the Union, suppress Insurrections and repel Invasions;

To provide for organizing, arming, and disciplining the Militia, and for governing such Part of them as may be employed in the Service of the United States, reserving to the States respectively, the Appointment of the Officers, and the Authority of training the Militia according to the discipline prescribed by Congress;

To exercise exclusive Legislation in all Cases whatsoever, over such District (not exceeding ten Miles square) as may, by Cession of particular States, and the acceptance of Congress, become the Seat of the Government of the United States, and to exercise like Authority over all Places purchased by the Consent of the Legislature of the State in which the Same shall be, for the Erection of Forts, Magazines, Arsenals, Dock-yards, and other needful Buildings;—And

To make all Laws which shall be necessary and proper for carrying into Execution the foregoing Powers, and all other Powers vested by this Constitution in the Government of the United States, or in any Department or Officer thereof.

Section 9. The Migration or Importation of such Persons as any of the States now existing shall think proper to admit, shall not be prohibited by the Congress prior to the Year one thousand eight hundred and eight, but a tax or duty may be imposed on such Importation, not exceeding ten dollars for each Person.

The privilege of the Writ of Habeas Corpus shall not be suspended, unless when in Cases of Rebellion or Invasion the public Safety may require it.

No bill of Attainder or ex post facto Law shall be passed.

No capitation, or other direct, Tax shall be laid unless in Proportion to the Census or Enumeration herein before directed to be taken.

No Tax or Duty shall be laid on Articles exported from any State.

No Preference shall be given by any Regulation of Commerce or Revenue to the Ports of one State over those of another: nor shall Vessels bound to, or from, one State, be obliged to enter, clear, or pay Duties in another.

No Money shall be drawn from the Treasury, but in Consequence of Appropriations made by Law; and a regular Statement and Account of the Receipts and Expenditures of all public Money shall be published from time to time.

No Title of Nobility shall be granted by the United States: And no Person holding any Office of Profit or Trust under them, shall, without the Consent of the Congress, accept of any present, Emolument, Office, or Title, of any kind whatever, from any King, Prince, or foreign State.

Section 10. No State shall enter into any Treaty, Alliance, or Confederation; grant Letters of Marque and Reprisal; coin Money; emit Bills of Credit; make any Thing but gold and silver Coin a Tender in Payment of Debts; pass any Bill of Attainder, ex post facto Law, or Law impairing the Obligation of Contracts, or grant any Title of Nobility.

No State shall, without the Consent of the Congress, lay any Imposts or Duties on Imports or Exports, except what may be absolutely necessary for executing its inspection Laws; and the net Produce of all Duties and Imposts, laid by any State on Imports or Exports, shall be for the use of the Treasury of the United States; and all such Laws shall be subject to the Revision and Control of the Congress.

No state shall, without the Consent of Congress, lay any duty of Tonnage, keep Troops, or Ships of War in time of Peace, enter into any Agreement or Compact with another State, or with a foreign Power, or engage in War, unless actually invaded, or in such imminent Danger as will not admit of delay.

ARTICLE II

Section 1. The executive Power shall be vested in a President of the United States of America. He shall hold his Office during the Term of four years, and, together with the Vice President, chosen for the same Term, be elected, as follows:

Each State shall appoint, in such Manner as the Legislature thereof may direct, a Number of Electors, equal to the whole Number of Senators and Representatives to which the State may be entitled in the Congress: but no Senator or Representative, or Person holding an Office of Trust or Profit under the United States, shall be appointed an Elector.

[The Electors shall meet in their respective States, and vote by Ballot for two persons, of whom one at least shall not be an Inhabitant of the same State with themselves. And they shall make a List of all the Persons voted for, and of the Number of Votes for each; which List they shall sign and certify, and transmit sealed to the Seat of the Government of the United States, directed to the President of the Senate. The President of the Senate shall, in the Presence of the Senate and House of Representatives, open all the Certificates, and the Votes shall then be counted. The Person having the greatest Number of Votes shall be the President, if such Number be a Majority of the whole Number of Electors appointed; and if there be more than one who have such Majority, and have an equal Number of Votes, then the House of Representatives shall immediately chuse by Ballot one of them for President; and if no Person have a Majority, then from the five highest on the List the said House shall in like Manner chuse the President. But in chusing the President, the Votes shall be taken by States, the Representation from each State having one Vote; a quorum for this Purpose shall consist of a Member or Members from two-thirds of the States, and a Majority of all the States shall be necessary to a Choice. In every Case, after the Choice of the President, the Person having the greatest Number of Votes of the Electors shall be the Vice President. But if there should remain two or more who have equal votes, the Senate shall chuse from them by Ballot the Vice President.]⁴

The Congress may determine the Time of chusing the Electors, and the Day on which they shall give their Votes; which Day shall be the same throughout the United States.

No person except a natural-born Citizen, or a Citizen of the United States, at the time of the Adoption of this Constitution, shall be eligible to the Office of President; neither shall any Person be eligible to that Office who shall not have attained to the Age of thirty-five years, and been fourteen Years a Resident within the United States.

In Case of the Removal of the President from Office, or of his Death, Resignation, or Inability to discharge the Powers and Duties of the said Office, the same shall devolve on the Vice President, and the Congress may by Law provide for the Case of Removal, Death, Resignation, or Inability, both of the President and Vice President, declaring what Officer shall then act as President, and such Officer shall act accordingly, until the disability be removed, or a President shall be elected.

The President shall, at stated Times, receive for his Services a Compensation, which shall neither be increased nor diminished during the Period for which he shall have been elected, and he shall not receive within that Period any other Emolument from the United States, or any of them.

Before he enter on the execution of his Office, he shall take the following Oath or Affirma-

---

⁴Revised by the Twelfth Amendment.

tion:—"I do solemnly swear (or affirm) that I will faithfully execute the Office of President of the United States, and will, to the best of my Ability, preserve, protect, and defend the Constitution of the United States."

Section 2. The President shall be Commander in Chief of the Army and Navy of the United States, and of the Militia of the several States, when called into the actual Service of the United States; he may require the Opinion, in writing, of the principal Officer in each of the executive Departments, upon any subject relating to the Duties of their respective Offices, and he shall have Power to Grant Reprieves and Pardons for Offenses against the United States, except in Cases of Impeachment.

He shall have Power, by and with the Advice and Consent of the Senate, to make Treaties, provided two-thirds of the Senators present concur; and he shall nominate, and by and with the Advice and Consent of the Senate, shall appoint Ambassadors, other public Ministers and Consuls, Judges of the supreme Court, and all other Officers of the United States, whose Appointments are not herein otherwise provided for, and which shall be established by Law: but the Congress may by Law vest the Appointment of such inferior Officers, as they think proper, in the President alone, in the Courts of Law, or in the Heads of Departments.

The President shall have Power to fill up all Vacancies that may happen during the Recess of the Senate, by granting Commissions which shall expire at the End of their next Session.

Section 3. He shall from time to time give to the Congress Information of the State of the Union, and recommend to their Consideration such Measures as he shall judge necessary and expedient; he may, on extraordinary occasions, convene both Houses, or either of them, and in Case of Disagreement between them, with respect to the Time of Adjournment, he may adjourn them to such Time as he shall think proper; he shall receive Ambassadors and other public Ministers; he shall take care that the Laws be faithfully executed, and shall Commission all the Officers of the United States.

Section 4. The President, Vice President and all civil Officers of the United States, shall be removed from Office on Impeachment for, and Conviction of, Treason, Bribery, or other high Crimes and Misdemeanors.

ARTICLE III

Section 1. The judicial Power of the United States, shall be vested in one supreme Court, and in such inferior Courts as the Congress may from time to time ordain and establish. The Judges, both of the supreme and inferior Courts, shall hold their Offices during good Behaviour, and shall, at stated Times, receive for their Services, a Compensation, which shall not be diminished during their Continuance in Office.

Section 2. The judicial Power shall extend to all Cases, in Law and Equity, arising under this Constitution, the Laws of the United States, and Treaties made, or which shall be made, under their Authority;—to all Cases affecting ambassadors, other public ministers and consuls;—to all cases of admiralty and maritime Jurisdiction;—to Controversies to which the United States shall be a Party;—to Controversies between two or more States;—between a State and Citizens of another State;[5]—between Citizens of different States—between Citizens of the same State claiming Lands under Grants of different States, and between a State, or the Citizens thereof, and foreign States, Citizens, or Subjects.

In all Cases affecting Ambassadors, other public Ministers and Consuls, and those in which a State shall be Party, the supreme Court shall have original Jurisdiction. In all the other Cases before mentioned, the supreme Court shall have appellate Jurisdiction, both as to Law and Fact, with such Exceptions, and under such Regulations as the Congress shall make.

The trial of all Crimes, except in Cases of Impeachment, shall be by Jury; and such Trial shall be held in the State where the said Crimes shall have been committed; but when not committed within any State, the Trial shall be at such Place or Places as the Congress may by Law have directed.

Section 3. Treason against the United States, shall consist only in levying War against them,

[5]Qualified by the Eleventh Amendment.

or in adhering to their Enemies, giving them Aid and Comfort. No Person shall be convicted of Treason unless on the Testimony of two Witnesses to the same overt Act, or on Confession in open Court.

The Congress shall have power to declare the Punishment of Treason, but no Attainder of Treason shall work Corruption of Blood, or Forfeiture except during the Life of the Person attainted.

ARTICLE IV

Section 1. Full Faith and Credit shall be given in each State to the public Acts, Records, and judicial Proceedings of every other State. And the Congress may by general Laws prescribe the Manner in which such Acts, Records and Proceedings shall be proved, and the Effect thereof.

Section 2. The Citizens of each State shall be entitled to all Privileges and Immunities of Citizens in the several States.

A Person charged in any State with Treason, Felony, or other Crime, who shall flee from Justice, and be found in another State, shall on demand of the executive Authority of the State from which he fled, be delivered up, to be removed to the State having Jurisdiction of the crime.

No Person held to Service or Labour in one State, under the Laws thereof, escaping into another, shall, in Consequence of any Law or Regulation therein, be discharged from such Service or Labour, but shall be delivered up on Claim of the Party to whom such Service or Labour may be due.

Section 3. New States may be admitted by the Congress into this Union; but no new State shall be formed or erected within the Jurisdiction of any other State; nor any State be formed by the Junction of two or more States, or parts of States, without the Consent of the Legislatures of the States concerned as well as of the Congress.

The Congress shall have Power to dispose of and make all needful Rules and Regulations respecting the Territory or other Property belonging to the United States; and nothing in this Constitution shall be so construed as to Prejudice any Claims of the United States, or of any particular State.

Section 4. The United States shall guarantee to every State in this Union a Republican Form of Government, and shall protect each of them against Invasion; and on Application of the Legislature, or of the Executive (when the Legislature cannot be convened) against domestic Violence.

ARTICLE V

The Congress, whenever two-thirds of both Houses shall deem it necessary, shall propose Amendments to this Constitution, or, on the Application of the Legislatures of two-thirds of the several States, shall call a Convention for proposing Amendments, which, in either Case, shall be valid to all Intents and Purposes, as part of this Constitution, when ratified by the Legislatures of three-fourths of the several States, or by Conventions in three-fourths thereof, as the one or the other Mode of Ratification may be proposed by the Congress; Provided that no Amendment which may be made prior to the Year One thousand eight hundred and eight shall in any Manner affect the first and fourth Clauses in the Ninth Section of the first Article; and that no State, without its Consent, shall be deprived of its equal Suffrage in the Senate.

ARTICLE VI

All Debts contracted and Engagements entered into, before the Adoption of this Constitution, shall be as valid against the United States under this Constitution, as under the Confederation.

This Constitution, and the Laws of the United States which shall be made in Pursuance thereof; and all Treaties made, or which shall be made, under the Authority of the United States, shall be the supreme Law of the Land; and the Judges in every State shall be bound thereby, any Thing in the Constitution or Laws of any State to the Contrary notwithstanding.

The Senators and Representatives before mentioned, and the Members of the several State Legislatures, and all executive and judicial Officers, both of the United States and of the several States, shall be bound by Oath or Affirmation to support this Constitution; but no religious Tests shall ever be required as a qualification to any Office or public Trust under the United States.

ARTICLE VII

The Ratification of the Conventions of nine States shall be sufficient for the Establishment of this Constitution between the States so ratifying the same.

Done in Convention by the Unanimous Consent of the States present the Seventeenth Day of September in the Year of our Lord one thousand seven hundred and Eighty seven, and of the Independence of the United States of America the Twelfth. In Witness whereof We have hereunto subscribed our Names.[6]

GEORGE WASHINGTON

PRESIDENT AND DEPUTY FROM VIRGINIA

New Hampshire
John Langdon
Nicholas Gilman

Massachusetts
Nathaniel Gorham
Rufus King

Connecticut
William Samuel
   Johnson
Roger Sherman

New York
Alexander Hamilton

New Jersey
William Livingston
David Brearley
William Paterson
Jonathan Dayton

Pennsylvania
Benjamin Franklin
Thomas Mifflin
Robert Morris
George Clymer
Thomas FitzSimons
Jared Ingersoll
James Wilson
Gouverneur Morris

Delaware
George Read
Gunning Bedford, Jr.
John Dickinson
Richard Bassett
Jacob Broom

Maryland
James McHenry
Daniel of
   St. Thomas Jenifer
Daniel Carroll

Virginia
John Blair
James Madison, Jr.

North Carolina
William Blount
Richard Dobbs
   Spaight
Hugh Williamson

South Carolina
John Rutledge
Charles Cotesworth
   Pinckney
Charles Pinckney
Pierce Butler

Georgia
William Few
Abraham Baldwin

Articles in Addition to, and Amendment of, the Constitution of the United States of America, Proposed by Congress, and Ratified by the Legislatures of the Several States, Pursuant to the Fifth Article of the Original Constitution[7]

[AMENDMENT I]

Congress shall make no law respecting an establishment of religion, or prohibiting the free exercise thereof; or abridging the freedom of speech, or of the press; or the right of the people peaceably to assemble, and to petition the Government for a redress of grievances.

[AMENDMENT II]

A well regulated Militia, being necessary to the security of a free State, the right of the people to keep and bear Arms shall not be infringed.

[AMENDMENT III]

No Soldier shall, in time of peace, be quartered in any house, without the consent of the Owner, nor in time of war, but in a manner to be prescribed by law.

[AMENDMENT IV]

The right of the people to be secure in their persons, houses, papers, and effects, against unreasonable searches and seizures, shall not be violated, and no Warrants shall issue, but

[6]These are the full names of the signers, which in some cases are not the signatures on the document.

[7]This heading appears only in the joint resolution submitting the first ten amendments, known as the Bill of Rights.

upon probable cause, supported by Oath or affirmation, and particularly describing the place to be searched, and the persons or things to be seized.

[AMENDMENT V]

No person shall be held to answer for a capital or otherwise infamous crime, unless on a presentment or indictment of a Grand Jury, except in cases arising in the land or naval forces, or in the Militia, when in actual service in time of War or public danger; nor shall any person be subject for the same offence to be twice put in jeopardy of life or limb; nor shall be compelled in any criminal case to be a witness against himself, nor be deprived of life, liberty, or property, without due process of law; nor shall private property be taken for public use, without just compensation.

[AMENDMENT VI]

In all criminal prosecutions, the accused shall enjoy the right to a speedy and public trial, by an impartial jury of the State and district wherein the crime shall have been committed, which district shall have been previously ascertained by law, and to be informed of the nature and cause of the accusation; to be confronted with the witnesses against him; to have compulsory process for obtaining witnesses in his favour, and to have the Assistance of Counsel for his defence.

[AMENDMENT VII]

In suits at common law, where the value in controversy shall exceed twenty dollars, the right of trial by jury shall be preserved, and no fact tried by a jury, shall be otherwise reexamined in any Court of the United States, than according to the rules of the common law.

[AMENDMENT VIII]

Excessive bail shall not be required, nor excessive fines imposed, nor cruel and unusual punishments inflicted.

[AMENDMENT IX]

The enumeration of the Constitution, of certain rights, shall not be construed to deny or disparage others retained by the people.

[AMENDMENT X]

The powers not delegated to the United States by the Constitution, nor prohibited by it to the States, are reserved to the States respectively, or to the people.
   [Amendments I–X, in force 1791.]

[AMENDMENT XI][8]

The Judicial power of the United States shall not be construed to extend to any suit in law or equity, commenced or prosecuted against one of the United States by Citizens of another State, or by Citizens or Subjects of any Foreign State.

[AMENDMENT XII][9]

The Electors shall meet in their respective States and vote by ballot for President and Vice-President, one of whom, at least, shall not be an inhabitant of the same State with themselves; they shall name in their ballots the person voted for as President, and in distinct ballots the person voted for as Vice-President, and they shall make distinct lists of all persons voted for as President, and of all persons voted for as Vice-President, and of the number of votes for each, which lists they shall sign and certify, and transmit sealed to the seal of the government of the United States, directed to the President of the Senate;—The President of the Senate shall, in the presence of the Senate and House of Representatives, open all the certificates and the votes shall then be counted;—The person having the greatest number of votes for President, shall be the President, if such number be a majority of the whole number of Electors appointed; and if no person have such majority, then from the persons having the highest numbers not exceeding three on the list of those

---

[8]Adopted in 1798.
[9]Adopted in 1804.

voted for as President, the House of Representatives shall choose immediately, by ballot, the President. But in choosing the President, the votes shall be taken by states, the representation from each state having one vote; a quorum for this purpose shall consist of a member or members from two-thirds of the states, and a majority of all the states shall be necessary to a choice. And if the House of Representatives shall not choose a President whenever the right of choice shall devolve upon them, before the fourth day of March next following, then the Vice-President shall act as President, as in the case of the death or other constitutional disability of the President.—The person having the greatest number of votes as Vice-President, shall be the Vice-President, if such number be a majority of the whole number of Electors appointed, and if no person have a majority, then from the two highest numbers on the list, the Senate shall choose the Vice-President; a quorum for the purpose shall consist of two-thirds of the whole number of Senators, and a majority of the whole number shall be necessary to a choice. But no person constitutionally ineligible to the office of President shall be eligible to that of Vice-President of the United States.

[AMENDMENT XIII][10]

Section 1. Neither slavery nor involuntary servitude, except as a punishment for crime whereof the party shall have been duly convicted, shall exist within the United States, or any place subject to their jurisdiction.

Section 2. Congress shall have power to enforce this article by appropriate legislation.

[AMENDMENT XIV][11]

Section 1. All persons born or naturalized in the United States, and subject to the jurisdiction thereof, are citizens of the United States and of the State wherein they reside. No State shall abridge the privileges or immunities of citizens of the United States; nor shall any State deprive any person of life, liberty, or property, without due process of law, nor deny to any

[10]Adopted in 1865.
[11]Adopted in 1868.

person within its jurisdiction the equal protection of the laws.

Section 2. Representatives shall be apportioned among the several States according to their respective numbers, counting the whole number of persons in each State, excluding Indians not taxed. But when the right to vote at any election for the choice of electors for President and Vice-President of the United States, Representatives in Congress, the Executive and Judicial officers of a State, or the members of the Legislature thereof, is denied to any of the male inhabitants of such State, being twenty-one years of age, and citizens of the United States, or in any way abridged, except for participation in rebellion, or other crime, the basis of representation therein shall be reduced in the proportion which the number of such male citizens shall bear to the whole number of male citizens twenty-one years of age in such State.

Section 3. No person shall be a Senator or Representative in Congress, or elector of President and Vice-President, or hold any office, civil or military, under the United States, or under and State, who, having previously taken an oath, as a member of Congress, or as an officer of the United States, or as a member of any State legislature, or as an executive or judicial officer of any State, to support the Constitution of the United States, shall have engaged in insurrection or rebellion against the same, or given aid or comfort to the enemies thereof. But Congress may by a vote of two-thirds of each House, remove such disability.

Section 4. The validity of the public debt of the United States, authorized by law, including debts incurred for payment of pensions and bounties for services in suppressing insurrection or rebellion, shall not be questioned. But neither the United States nor any State shall assume or pay any debts or obligation incurred in aid of insurrection or rebellion against the United States, or any claim for the loss or emancipation of any slave; but all such debts, obligations, and claims shall be held illegal and void.

Section 5. The Congress shall have the power to enforce, by appropriate legislation, the provisions of this article.

[AMENDMENT XV][12]

Section 1. The right of citizens of the United States to vote shall not be denied or abridged by the United States or by any State on account of race, color, or previous condition of servitude—

Section 2. The Congress shall have power to enforce this article by appropriate legislation.

[AMENDMENT XVI][13]

The Congress shall have power to lay and collect taxes on incomes, from whatever source derived, without apportionment among the several States, and without regard to any census or enumeration.

[AMENDMENT XVII][14]

The Senate of the United States shall be composed of two Senators from each State, elected by the people thereof, for six years; and each Senator shall have one vote. The electors in each State shall have the qualifications requisite for electors of the most numerous branch of the State legislatures.

When vacancies happen in the representation of any State in the Senate, the executive authority of such State shall issue writs of election to fill such vacancies: *Provided,* That the legislature of any State may empower the executive thereof to make temporary appointments until the people fill the vacancies by election as the legislature may direct.

This amendment shall not be so construed as to affect the election or term of any Senator chosen before it becomes valid as part of the Constitution.

[AMENDMENT XVIII][15]

Section 1. After one year from the ratification of this article the manufacture, sale, or transportation of intoxicating liquors within, the importation thereof into, or the exportation

[12]Adopted in 1870.

[13]Adopted in 1913.

[14]Adopted in 1913.

[15]Adopted in 1918.

thereof from the United States and all territory subject to the jurisdiction thereof for beverage purposes is hereby prohibited.

Section 2. The Congress and the several States shall have concurrent power to enforce this article by appropriate legislation.

Section 3. This article shall be inoperative unless it shall have been ratified as an amendment to the Constitution by the legislatures of the several States, as provided in the Constitution, within seven years from the date of the submission hereof to the States by the Congress.

[AMENDMENT XIX][16]

The right of citizens of the United States to vote shall not be denied or abridged by the United States or by any State on account of sex.

Congress shall have power to enforce this article by appropriate legislation.

[AMENDMENT XX][17]

Section 1. The terms of the President and Vice-President shall end at noon on the 20th day of January, and the terms of Senators and Representatives at noon on the 3d day of January, of the years in which such terms would have ended if this article had not been ratified; and the terms of their successors shall then begin.

Section 2. The Congress shall assemble at least once in every year, and such meeting shall begin at noon on the 3d day of January, unless they shall by law appoint a different day.

Section 3. If, at the time fixed for the beginning of the term of the President, the President elect shall have died, the Vice-President elect shall become President. If a President shall not have been chosen before the time fixed for the beginning of his term or if the President elect shall have failed to quality, then the Vice-President elect shall act as President until a President shall have qualified; and the Congress may by law provide for the case wherein neither a President elect nor a Vice-President elect shall

[16]Adopted in 1920.

[17]Adopted in 1933.

have qualified, declaring who shall then act as President, or the manner in which one who is to act shall be selected, and such person shall act accordingly until a President or Vice-President shall have qualified.

Section 4. The Congress may by law provide for the case of the death of any of the persons from whom the House of Representatives may choose a President whenever the right of choice shall have devolved upon them, and for the case of the death of any of the persons from whom the Senate may choose a Vice-President whenever the right of choice shall have devolved upon them.

Section 5. Sections 1 and 2 shall take effect on the 15th day of October following the ratification of this article.

Section 6. This article shall be inoperative unless it shall have been ratified as an amendment to the Constitution by the legislatures of three-fourths of the several States within seven years from the date of its submission.

[AMENDMENT XXI][18]

Section 1. The eighteenth article of amendment to the Constitution of the United States is hereby repealed.

Section 2. The transportation or importation into any State, Territory, or possession of the United States for delivery or use therein of intoxicating liquors, in violation of the laws thereof, is hereby prohibited.

Section 3. This article shall be inoperative unless it shall have been ratified as an amendment to the Constitution by conventions in the several States, as provided in the Constitution, within seven years from the date of the submission hereof to the States by the Congress.

[AMENDMENT XXII][19]

No person shall be elected to the office of the President more than twice, and no person who has held the office of President, or acted as President, for more than two years of a term to

[18]Adopted in 1933.

[19]Adopted in 1961.

which some other person was elected President shall be elected to the office of the President more than once.

But this Article shall not apply to any person holding the office of President when this Article was proposed by the Congress, and shall not prevent any person who may be holding the office of President, or acting as President, during the term within which this Article becomes operative from holding the office of President or acting as President during the remainder of such term.

This article shall be inoperative unless it shall have been ratified as an amendment to the Constitution by the legislatures of three-fourths of the several states within seven years from the date of its submission to the states by the Congress.

[AMENDMENT XXIII][20]

Section 1. The District constituting the seat of Government of the United States shall appoint in such manner as the Congress may direct:

A number of electors of President and Vice-President equal to the whole number of Senators and Representatives in Congress to which the District would be entitled if it were a State, but in no event more than the least populous State; they shall be in addition to those appointed by the States, but they shall be considered, for the purpose of the election of President and Vice-President, to be electors appointed by a State; and they shall meet in the District and perform such duties as provided by the twelfth article of amendment.

Section 2. The Congress shall have power to enforce this article by appropriate legislation.

[AMENDMENT XXIV][21]

Section 1. The right of citizens of the United States to vote in any primary or other election for President or Vice-President, for electors for President or Vice-President, or for Senator or Representative in Congress, shall not be denied or abridged by the United States or any state by reason of failure to pay any poll tax or other tax.

[20]Adopted in 1961.

[21]Adopted in 1964.

Section 2. The Congress shall have the power to enforce this article by appropriate legislation.

[AMENDMENT XXV][22]

Section 1. In case of the removal of the President from office or of his death or resignation, the Vice-President shall become President.

Section 2. Whenever there is a vacancy in the office of the Vice President, the President shall nominate a Vice President who shall take office upon confirmation by a majority vote of both Houses of Congress.

Section 3. Whenever the President transmits to the President Pro Tempore of the Senate and the Speaker of the House of Representatives his written declaration that he is unable to discharge the powers and duties of his office, and until he transmits to them a written declaration to the contrary, such powers and duties shall be discharged by the Vice-President as Acting President.

Section 4. Whenever the Vice-President and a majority of either the principal officers of the executive departments or of such other body as Congress may by law provide, transmit to the President Pro Tempore of the Senate and the Speaker of the House of Representatives their written declaration that the President is unable to discharge the powers and duties of his office, the Vice President shall immediately assume the powers and duties of the office as Acting President.

Thereafter, when the President transmits to the President Pro Tempore of the Senate and the Speaker of the House of Representatives his written declaration that no inability exists, he shall resume the powers and duties of his office unless the Vice President and a majority of either the principal officers of the executive departments or of such other body as Congress may by law provide, transmit within four days to the President Pro Tempore of the Senate and the Speaker of the House of Representatives their written declaration that the President is unable to discharge the powers and duties of his office. Thereupon Congress shall decide the issue, assembling within forty-eight hours for that purpose if not in session. If the Congress, within twenty-one days after receipt of the latter written declaration, or, if Congress is not in session, within twenty-one days after Congress is required to assemble, determines by two-thirds vote of both Houses that the President is unable to discharge the powers and duties of his office, the Vice President shall continue to discharge the same as Acting President; otherwise, the President shall resume the powers and duties of his office.

[AMENDMENT XXVI][23]

Section 1. The right of citizens of the United States, who are eighteen years of age or older, to vote shall not be denied or abridged by the United States or by any State on account of age.

Section 2. The Congress shall have power to enforce this article by appropriate legislation.

---

[22]Adopted in 1967.

[23]Adopted in 1971.

PRESIDENTIAL ELECTIONS

Year	Candidates	Parties	Popular Vote	% of Popular Vote	Electoral Vote	% Voter Partici- pation
1789	**George Washington**				69	
	John Adams				34	
	Other candidates				35	
1792	**George Washington**				132	
	John Adams				77	
	George Clinton				50	
	Other candidates				5	
1796	**John Adams**	Federalist			71	
	Thomas Jefferson	Dem.-Rep.			68	
	Thomas Pinckney	Federalist			59	
	Aaron Burr	Dem.-Rep.			30	
	Other candidates				48	
1800	**Thomas Jefferson**	Dem.-Rep.			73	
	Aaron Burr	Dem.-Rep.			73	
	John Adams	Federalist			65	
	Charles C. Pinckney	Federalist			64	
	John Jay	Federalist			1	
1804	**Thomas Jefferson**	Dem.-Rep.			162	
	Charles C. Pinckney	Federalist			14	
1808	**James Madison**	Dem.-Rep.			122	
	Charles C. Pinckney	Federalist			47	
	George Clinton	Dem.-Rep.			6	
1812	**James Madison**	Dem.-Rep.			128	
	DeWitt Clinton	Federalist			89	
1816	**James Monroe**	Dem.-Rep.			183	
	Rufus King	Federalist			34	
1820	**James Monroe**	Dem.-Rep.			231	
	John Quincy Adams	Indep.-Rep.			1	
1824	**John Quincy Adams**	Dem.-Rep.	108,740	31	84	26.9
	Andrew Jackson	Dem.-Rep.	153,544	43	99	
	Henry Clay	Dem.-Rep.	47,136	13	37	
	William H. Crawford	Dem.-Rep.	46,618	13	41	
1828	**Andrew Jackson**	Democratic	647,286	56.0	178	57.6
	John Quincy Adams	National Republican	508,064	44.0	83	
1832	**Andrew Jackson**	Democratic	688,242	54.5	219	55.4
	Henry Clay	National Republican	473,462	37.5	49	
	William Wirt	Anti-Masonic ⎫	101,051	8.0	7	
	John Floyd	Democratic ⎭			11	
1836	**Martin Van Buren**	Democratic	765,483	50.9	170	57.8
	William H. Harrison	Whig ⎫			73	
	Hugh L. White	Whig ⎪	739,795	49.1	26	
	Daniel Webster	Whig ⎬			14	
	W. P. Mangum	Whig ⎭			11	

Year	Candidates	Parties	Popular Vote	% of Popular Vote	Electoral Vote	% Voter Partici- pation
1840	**William H. Harrison**	Whig	1,275,016	53	234	80.2
	Martin Van Buren	Democratic	1,129,102	47	60	
1844	**James K. Polk**	Democratic	1,338,464	49.6	170	78.9
	Henry Clay	Whig	1,300,097	48.1	105	
	James G. Birney	Liberty	62,300	2.3		
1848	**Zachary Taylor**	Whig	1,360,967	47.4	163	72.7
	Lewis Cass	Democratic	1,222,342	42.5	127	
	Martin Van Buren	Free Soil	291,263	10.1		
1852	**Franklin Pierce**	Democratic	1,601,117	50.9	254	69.6
	Winfield Scott	Whig	1,385,453	44.1	42	
	John P. Hale	Free Soil	155,825	5.0		
1856	**James Buchanan**	Democratic	1,832,955	45.3	174	78.9
	John C. Fremont	Republican	1,339,932	33.1	114	
	Millard Fillmore	American	871,731	21.6	8	
1860	**Abraham Lincoln**	Republican	1,866,452	39.8	180	81.2
	Stephen A. Douglas	Democratic	1,375,157	29.5	12	
	John C. Breckinridge	Democratic	847,953	18.1	72	
	John Bell	Constitutional Union	590,631	12.6	39	
1864	**Abraham Lincoln**	Republican	2,206,938	55.0	212	73.8
	George B. McClellan	Democratic	1,803,787	45.0	21	
1868	**Ulysses S. Grant**	Republican	3,013,421	52.7	214	78.1
	Horatio Seymour	Democratic	2,706,829	47.3	80	
1872	**Ulysses S. Grant**	Republican	3,596,745	55.6	286	71.3
	Horace Greeley	Democratic	2,843,446	43.9	66	
1876	**Rutherford B. Hayes**	Republican	4,036,298	48.0	185	81.8
	Samuel J. Tilden	Democratic	4,300,590	51.0	184	
1880	**James A. Garfield**	Republican	4,453,295	48.5	214	79.4
	Winfield S. Hancock	Democratic	4,414,082	48.1	155	
	James B. Weaver	Greenback-Labor	308,578	3.4		
1884	**Grover Cleveland**	Democratic	4,879,507	48.5	219	77.5
	James G. Blaine	Republican	4,850,293	48.2	182	
	Benjamin F. Butler	Greenback-Labor	175,370	1.8		
	John P. St. John	Prohibition	150,369	1.5		
1888	**Benjamin Harrison**	Republican	5,477,129	47.9	233	79.3
	Grover Cleveland	Democratic	5,537,857	48.6	168	
	Clinton B. Fisk	Prohibition	249,506	2.2		
	Anson J. Streeter	Union Labor	146,935	1.3		
1892	**Grover Cleveland**	Democratic	5,555,426	46.1	277	74.7
	Benjamin Harrison	Republican	5,182,690	43.0	145	
	James B. Weaver	People's	1,029,846	8.5	22	
	John Bidwell	Prohibition	264,133	2.2		
1896	**William McKinley**	Republican	7,104,779	52.0	271	79.3
	William J. Bryan	Democratic	6,502,925	48.0	176	
1900	**William McKinley**	Republican	7,218,491	51.7	292	73.2
	William J. Bryan	Democratic; Populist	6,356,734	45.5	155	
	John C. Wooley	Prohibition	208,914	1.5		
1904	**Theodore Roosevelt**	Republican	7,628,461	57.4	336	65.2
	Alton B. Parker	Democratic	5,084,223	37.6	140	
	Eugene V. Debs	Socialist	402,283	3.0		
	Silas C. Swallow	Prohibition	258,536	1.9		

Year	Candidates	Parties	Popular Vote	% of Popular Vote	Electoral Vote	% Voter Participation
1908	**William H. Taft**	Republican	7,675,320	51.6	321	65.4
	William J. Bryan	Democratic	6,412,294	43.1	162	
	Eugene V. Debs	Socialist	420,793	2.8		
	Eugene W. Chafin	Prohibition	253,840	1.7		
1912	**Woodrow Wilson**	Democratic	6,293,454	42.0	435	58.8
	Theodore Roosevelt	Progressive	4,119,538	28.0	88	
	William H. Taft	Republican	3,484,980	24.0	8	
	Eugene V. Debs	Socialist	900,672	6.0		
	Eugene W. Chafin	Prohibition	206,275	1.4		
1916	**Woodrow Wilson**	Democratic	9,129,606	49.4	277	61.6
	Charles E. Hughes	Republican	8,538,221	46.2	254	
	A. L. Benson	Socialist	585,113	3.2		
	J. Frank Hanly	Prohibition	220,506	1.2		
1920	**Warren G. Harding**	Republican	16,143,407	60.4	404	49.2
	James M. Cox	Democratic	9,130,328	34.2	127	
	Eugene V. Debs	Socialist	919,799	3.4		
	P. P. Christensen	Farmer-Labor	265,411	1.0		
1924	**Calvin Coolidge**	Republican	15,718,211	54.0	382	48.9
	John W. Davis	Democratic	8,385,283	28.8	136	
	Robert M. La Follette	Progressive	4,831,289	16.6	13	
1928	**Herbert C. Hoover**	Republican	21,391,381	58.2	444	56.9
	Alfred E. Smith	Democratic	15,016,443	40.9	87	
1932	**Franklin D. Roosevelt**	Democratic	22,821,857	57.4	472	56.9
	Herbert C. Hoover	Republican	15,761,841	39.7	59	
	Norman Thomas	Socialist	881,951	2.2		
1936	**Franklin D. Roosevelt**	Democratic	27,751,597	60.8	523	61.0
	Alfred M. Landon	Republican	16,679,583	36.5	8	
	William Lemke	Union	882,479	1.9		
1940	**Franklin D. Roosevelt**	Democratic	27,307,819	54.8	449	62.5
	Wendell L. Wilkie	Republican	22,321,018	44.8	82	
1944	**Franklin D. Roosevelt**	Democratic	25,606,585	53.5	432	55.9
	Thomas E. Dewey	Republican	22,014,745	46.0	99	
1948	**Harry S Truman**	Democratic	24,105,812	50.0	303	53.0
	Thomas E. Dewey	Republican	21,970,065	46.0	189	
	J. Strom Thurmond	States' Rights	1,169,021	2	39	
	Henry A. Wallace	Progressive	1,157,172	2		
1952	**Dwight D. Eisenhower**	Republican	33,936,234	55.1	442	63.3
	Adlai E. Stevenson	Democratic	27,314,992	44.4	89	
1956	**Dwight D. Eisenhower**	Republican	35,590,472	57.6	457	60.6
	Adlai E. Stevenson	Democratic	26,022,752	42.1	73	
1960	**John F. Kennedy**	Democratic	34,227,096	49.7	303	62.8
	Richard M. Nixon	Republican	34,107,646	49.6	219	
	Harry F. Byrd	Independent	501,643		15	
1964	**Lyndon B. Johnson**	Democratic	43,129,566	61.1	486	61.7
	Barry M. Goldwater	Republican	27,178,188	38.5	52	
1968	**Richard M. Nixon**	Republican	31,785,480	44.0	301	60.6
	Hubert H. Humphrey	Democratic	31,275,166	42.7	191	
	George C. Wallace	American Independent	9,906,473	13.5	46	
1972	**Richard M. Nixon**	Republican	47,169,911	60.7	520	55.2
	George S. McGovern	Democratic	29,170,383	37.5	17	
	John G. Schmitz	American	1,099,482	1.4		

Year	Candidates	Parties	Popular Vote	% of Popular Vote	Electoral Vote	% Voter Partici- pation
1976	**Jimmy Carter**	Democratic	40,830,763	50.1	297	53.5
	Gerald R. Ford	Republican	39,147,793	48.0	240	
1980	**Ronald Reagan**	Republican	43,899,248	51.0	489	52.6
	Jimmy Carter	Democratic	35,481,432	41.0	49	
	John B. Anderson	Independent	5,719,437	7.0	0	
	Ed Clark	Libertarian	920,859	1.0	0	
1984	**Ronald Reagan**	Republican	54,451,521	58.8	525	53.3
	Walter Mondale	Democratic	37,565,334	40.5	13	
1988	**George H. Bush**	Republican	47,917,341	54.0	426	48.6*
	Michael Dukakis	Democratic	41,013,030	46.0	112	

*Estimate

PRESIDENTIAL ADMINISTRATIONS

The Washington Administration (1789–1797)

Vice President	John Adams	1789–1797
Secretary of State	Thomas Jefferson	1789–1793
	Edmund Randolph	1794–1795
	Timothy Pickering	1795–1797
Secretary of Treasury	Alexander Hamilton	1789–1795
	Oliver Wolcott	1795–1797
Secretary of War	Henry Knox	1789–1794
	Timothy Pickering	1795–1796
	James McHenry	1796–1797
Attorney General	Edmund Randolph	1789–1793
	William Bradford	1794–1795
	Charles Lee	1795–1797
Postmaster General	Samuel Osgood	1789–1791
	Timothy Pickering	1791–1794
	Joseph Habersham	1795–1797

The John Adams Administration (1797–1801)

Vice President	Thomas Jefferson	1797–1801
Secretary of State	Timothy Pickering	1797–1800
	John Marshall	1800–1801
Secretary of Treasury	Oliver Wolcott	1797–1800
	Samuel Dexter	1800–1801
Secretary of War	James McHenry	1797–1800
	Samuel Dexter	1800–1801
Attorney General	Charles Lee	1797–1801
Postmaster General	Joseph Habersham	1797–1801
Secretary of Navy	Benjamin Stoddert	1798–1801

The Jefferson Administration (1801–1809)

Vice President	Aaron Burr	1801–1805
	George Clinton	1805–1809
Secretary of State	James Madison	1801–1809
Secretary of Treasury	Samuel Dexter	1801
	Albert Gallatin	1801–1809
Secretary of War	Henry Dearborn	1801–1809
Attorney General	Levi Lincoln	1801–1805
	Robert Smith	1805
	John Breckinridge	1805–1806
	Caesar Rodney	1807–1809
Postmaster General	Joseph Habersham	1801
	Gideon Granger	1801–1809
Secretary of Navy	Robert Smith	1801–1809

The Madison Administration (1809–1817)

Vice President	George Clinton	1809–1813
	Elbridge Gerry	1813–1817
Secretary of State	Robert Smith	1809–1811
	James Monroe	1811–1817
Secretary of Treasury	Albert Gallatin	1809–1813
	George Campbell	1814
	Alexander Dallas	1814–1816
	William Crawford	1816–1817
Secretary of War	William Eustis	1809–1812
	John Armstrong	1813–1814
	James Monroe	1814–1815
	William Crawford	1815–1817
Attorney General	Caesar Rodney	1809–1811
	William Pinkney	1811–1814
	Richard Rush	1814–1817
Postmaster General	Gideon Granger	1809–1814
	Return Meigs	1814–1817
Secretary of Navy	Paul Hamilton	1809–1813
	William Jones	1813–1814
	Benjamin Crowninshield	1814–1817

The Monroe Administration (1817–1825)

Vice President	Daniel Tompkins	1817–1825
Secretary of State	John Quincy Adams	1817–1825
Secretary of Treasury	William Crawford	1817–1825
Secretary of War	George Graham	1817
	John C. Calhoun	1817–1825
Attorney General	Richard Rush	1817
	William Wirt	1817–1825
Postmaster General	Return Meigs	1817–1823
	John McLean	1823–1825
Secretary of Navy	Benjamin Crowninshield	1817–1818
	Smith Thompson	1818–1823
	Samuel Southard	1823–1825

The John Quincy Adams Administration (1825–1829)

Vice President	John C. Calhoun	1825–1829
Secretary of State	Henry Clay	1825–1829
Secretary of Treasury	Richard Rush	1825–1829
Secretary of War	James Barbour	1825–1828
	Peter Porter	1828–1829

Attorney General	William Wirt	1825–1829
Postmaster General	John McLean	1825–1829
Secretary of Navy	Samuel Southard	1825–1829

The Jackson Administration (1829–1837)

Vice President	John C. Calhoun	1829–1833
	Martin Van Buren	1833–1837
Secretary of State	Martin Van Buren	1829–1831
	Edward Livingston	1831–1833
	Louis McLane	1833–1834
	John Forsyth	1834–1837
Secretary of Treasury	Samuel Ingham	1829–1831
	Louis McLane	1831–1833
	William Duane	1833
	Roger B. Taney	1833–1834
	Levi Woodbury	1834–1837
Secretary of War	John H. Eaton	1829–1831
	Lewis Cass	1831–1837
	Benjamin Butler	1837
Attorney General	John M. Berrien	1829–1831
	Roger B. Taney	1831–1833
	Benjamin Butler	1833–1837
Postmaster General	William Barry	1829–1835
	Amos Kendall	1835–1837
Secretary of Navy	John Branch	1829–1831
	Levi Woodbury	1831–1834
	Mahlon Dickerson	1834–1837

The Van Buren Administration (1837–1841)

Vice President	Richard M. Johnson	1837–1841
Secretary of State	John Forsyth	1837–1841
Secretary of Treasury	Levi Woodbury	1837–1841
Secretary of War	Joel Poinsett	1837–1841
Attorney General	Benjamin Butler	1837–1838
	Felix Grundy	1838–1840
	Henry D. Gilpin	1840–1841
Postmaster General	Amos Kendall	1837–1840
	John M. Niles	1840–1841
Secretary of Navy	Mahlon Dickerson	1837–1838
	James Paulding	1838–1841

The William Harrison Administration (1841)

Vice President	John Tyler	1841
Secretary of State	Daniel Webster	1841
Secretary of Treasury	Thomas Ewing	1841

Secretary of War	John Bell	1841
Attorney General	John J. Crittenden	1841
Postmaster General	Francis Granger	1841
Secretary of Navy	George Badger	1841

The Tyler Administration (1841–1845)

Vice President	None	
Secretary of State	Daniel Webster	1841–1843
	Hugh S. Legaré	1843
Secretary of State	Abel P. Upshur	1843–1844
	John C. Calhoun	1844–1845
Secretary of Treasury	Thomas Ewing	1841
	Walter Forward	1841–1843
	John C. Spencer	1843–1844
	George Bibb	1844–1845
Secretary of War	John Bell	1841
	John C. Spencer	1841–1843
	James M. Porter	1843–1844
	William Wilkins	1844–1845
Attorney General	John J. Crittenden	1841
	Hugh S. Legaré	1841–1843
	John Nelson	1843–1845
Postmaster General	Francis Granger	1841
	Charles Wickliffe	1841
Secretary of Navy	George Badger	1841
	Abel P. Upshur	1841
	David Henshaw	1843–1844
	Thomas Gilmer	1844
	John Y. Mason	1844–1845

The Polk Administration (1845–1849)

Vice President	George M. Dallas	1845–1849
Secretary of State	James Buchanan	1845–1849
Secretary of Treasury	Robert J. Walker	1845–1849
Secretary of War	William L. Marcy	1845–1849
Attorney General	John Y. Mason	1845–1846
	Nathan Clifford	1846–1848
	Isaac Toucey	1848–1849
Postmaster General	Cave Johnson	1845–1849
Secretary of Navy	George Bancroft	1845–1846
	John Y. Mason	1846–1849

The Taylor Administration (1849–1850)

Vice President	Millard Fillmore	1849–1850
Secretary of State	John M. Clayton	1849–1850

The Taylor Administration (1849–1850)
(continued)

Secretary of Treasury	William Meredith	1849–1850
Secretary of War	George Crawford	1849–1850
Attorney General	Reverdy Johnson	1849–1850
Postmaster General	Jacob Collamer	1849–1850
Secretary of Navy	William Preston	1849–1850
Secretary of Interior	Thomas Ewing	1849–1850

The Fillmore Administration (1850–1853)

Vice President	None	
Secretary of State	Daniel Webster	1850–1852
	Edward Everett	1852–1853
Secretary of Treasury	Thomas Corwin	1850–1853
Secretary of War	Charles Conrad	1850–1853
Attorney General	John J. Crittenden	1850–1853
Postmaster General	Nathan Hall	1850–1852
	Sam D. Hubbard	1852–1853
Secretary of Navy	William A. Graham	1850–1852
	John P. Kennedy	1852–1853
Secretary of Interior	Thomas McKennan	1850
	Alexander Stuart	1850–1853

The Pierce Administration (1853–1857)

Vice President	William R. King	1853–1857
Secretary of State	William L. Marcy	1853–1857
Secretary of Treasury	James Guthrie	1853–1857
Secretary of War	Jefferson Davis	1853–1857
Attorney General	Caleb Cushing	1853–1857
Postmaster General	James Campbell	1853–1857
Secretary of Navy	James C. Dobbin	1853–1857
Secretary of Interior	Robert McClelland	1853–1857

The Buchanan Administration (1857–1861)

Vice President	John C. Breckinridge	1857–1861
Secretary of State	Lewis Cass	1857–1860
	Jeremiah S. Black	1860–1861
Secretary of Treasury	Howell Cobb	1857–1860
	Philip Thomas	1860–1861
	John A. Dix	1861
Secretary of War	John B. Floyd	1857–1861
	Joseph Holt	1861
Attorney General	Jeremiah S. Black	1857–1860
	Edwin M. Stanton	1860–1861
Postmaster General	Aaron V. Brown	1857–1859
	Joseph Holt	1859–1861
	Horatio King	1861
Secretary of Navy	Isaac Toucey	1857–1861
Secretary of Interior	Jacob Thompson	1857–1861

The Lincoln Administration (1861–1865)

Vice President	Hannibal Hamlin	1861–1865
	Andrew Johnson	1865
Secretary of State	William H. Seward	1861–1865
Secretary of Treasury	Samuel P. Chase	1861–1864
	William P. Fessenden	1864–1865
	Hugh McCulloch	1865
Secretary of War	Simon Cameron	1861–1862
	Edwin M. Stanton	1862–1865
Attorney General	Edward Bates	1861–1864
	James Speed	1864–1865
Postmaster General	Horatio King	1861
	Montgomery Blair	1861–1864
	William Dennison	1864–1865
Secretary of Navy	Gideon Welles	1861–1865
Secretary of Interior	Caleb B. Smith	1861–1863
	John P. Usher	1863–1865

The Andrew Johnson Administration (1865–1869)

Vice President	None	
Secretary of State	William H. Seward	1865–1869
Secretary of Treasury	Hugh McCulloch	1865–1869
Secretary of War	Edwin M. Stanton	1865–1867
	Ulysses S. Grant	1867–1868
	Lorenzo Thomas	1868
	John M. Schofield	1868–1869

Attorney General	James Speed	1865–1866
	Henry Stanbery	1866–1868
	William M. Evarts	1868–1869
Postmaster General	William Dennison	1865–1866
	Alexander Randall	1866–1869
Secretary of Navy	Gideon Welles	1865–1869
Secretary of Interior	John P. Usher	1865
	James Harlan	1865–1866
	Orville H. Browning	1866–1869

The Grant Administration (1869–1877)

Vice President	Schuyler Colfax	1869–1873
	Henry Wilson	1873–1877
Secretary of State	Elihu B. Washburne	1869
	Hamilton Fish	1869–1877
Secretary of Treasury	George S. Boutwell	1869–1873
	William Richardson	1873–1874
	Benjamin Bristow	1874–1876
	Lot M. Morrill	1876–1877
Secretary of War	John A. Rawlins	1869
	William T. Sherman	1869
	William W. Belknap	1869–1876
	Alphonso Taft	1876
	James D. Cameron	1876–1877
Attorney General	Ebenezer Hoar	1869–1870
	Amos T. Ackerman	1870–1871
	G. H. Williams	1871–1875
	Edwards Pierrepont	1875–1876
	Alphonso Taft	1876–1877
Postmaster General	John A. J. Creswell	1869–1874
	James W. Marshall	1874
	Marshall Jewell	1874–1876
	James N. Tyner	1876–1877
Secretary of Navy	Adolph E. Borie	1869
	George M. Robeson	1869–1877
Secretary of Interior	Jacob D. Cox	1869–1870
	Columbus Delano	1870–1875
	Zachariah Chandler	1875–1877

The Hayes Administration (1877–1881)

Vice President	William A. Wheeler	1877–1881
Secretary of State	William M. Evarts	1877–1881
Secretary of Treasury	John Sherman	1877–1881
Secretary of War	George W. McCrary	1877–1879
	Alex Ramsey	1879–1881
Attorney General	Charles Devens	1877–1881
Postmaster General	David M. Key	1877–1880
	Horace Maynard	1880–1881
Secretary of Navy	Richard W. Thompson	1877–1880
	Nathan Goff, Jr.	1881
Secretary of Interior	Carl Schurz	1877–1881

The Garfield Administration (1881)

Vice President	Chester A. Arthur	1881
Secretary of State	James G. Blaine	1881
Secretary of Treasury	William Windom	1881
Secretary of War	Robert T. Lincoln	1881
Attorney General	Wayne MacVeagh	1881
Postmaster General	Thomas L. James	1881
Secretary of Navy	William H. Hunt	1881
Secretary of Interior	Samuel J. Kirkwood	1881

The Arthur Administration (1881–1885)

Vice President	None	
Secretary of State	F. T. Frelinghuysen	1881–1885
Secretary of Treasury	Charles J. Folger	1881–1884
	Walter Q. Gresham	1884
	Hugh McCulloch	1884–1885
Secretary of War	Robert T. Lincoln	1881–1885
Attorney General	Benjamin H. Brewster	1881–1885
Postmaster General	Timothy O. Howe	1881–1883
	Walter Q. Gresham	1883–1884
	Frank Hatton	1884–1885
Secretary of Navy	William H. Hunt	1881–1882
	William E. Chandler	1882–1885
Secretary of Interior	Samuel J. Kirkwood	1881–1882
	Henry M. Teller	1882–1885

The Cleveland Administration (1885–1889)

Vice President	Thomas A. Hendricks	1885–1889
Secretary of State	Thomas F. Bayard	1885–1889
Secretary of Treasury	Daniel Manning	1885–1887
	Charles S. Fairchild	1887–1889
Secretary of War	William C. Endicott	1885–1889
Attorney General	Augustus H. Garland	1885–1889
Postmaster General	William F. Vilas	1885–1888
	Don M. Dickinson	1888–1889
Secretary of Navy	William C. Whitney	1885–1889
Secretary of Interior	Lucius Q. C. Lamar	1885–1888
	William F. Vilas	1888–1889
Secretary of Agriculture	Norman J. Colman	1889

The Benjamin Harrison Administration (1889–1893)

Vice President	Levi P. Morton	1889–1893
Secretary of State	James G. Blaine	1889–1892
	John W. Foster	1892–1893
Secretary of Treasury	William Windom	1889–1891
	Charles Foster	1891–1893
Secretary of War	Redfield Proctor	1889–1891
	Stephen B. Elkins	1891–1893
Attorney General	William H. H. Miller	1889–1891
Postmaster General	John Wanamaker	1889–1893
Secretary of Navy	Benjamin F. Tracy	1889–1893
Secretary of Interior	John W. Noble	1889–1893
Secretary of Agriculture	Jeremiah M. Rusk	1889–1893

The Cleveland Administration (1893–1897)

Vice President	Adlai E. Stevenson	1893–1897
Secretary of State	Walter Q. Gresham	1893–1895
	Richard Olney	1895–1897
Secretary of Treasury	John G. Carlisle	1893–1897
Secretary of War	Daniel S. Lamont	1893–1897
Attorney General	Richard Olney	1893–1895
	James Harmon	1895–1897
Postmaster General	Wilson S. Bissell	1893–1895
	William L. Wilson	1895–1897
Secretary of Navy	Hilary A. Herbert	1893–1897
Secretary of Interior	Hoke Smith	1893–1896
	David R. Francis	1896–1897
Secretary of Agriculture	Julius S. Morton	1893–1897

The McKinley Administration (1897–1901)

Vice President	Garret A. Hobart	1897–1901
Secretary of State	Theodore Roosevelt	1901
	John Sherman	1897–1898
	William R. Day	1898
	John Hay	1898–1901
Secretary of Treasury	Lyman J. Gage	1897–1901
Secretary of War	Russell A. Alger	1897–1899
	Elihu Root	1899–1901
Attorney General	Joseph McKenna	1897–1898
	John W. Griggs	1898–1901
	Philander C. Knox	1901
Postmaster General	James A. Gary	1897–1898
	Charles E. Smith	1898–1901
Secretary of Navy	John D. Long	1897–1901
Secretary of Interior	Cornelius N. Bliss	1897–1899
	Ethan A. Hitchcock	1899–1901
Secretary of Agriculture	James Wilson	1897–1901

The Theodore Roosevelt Administration (1901–1909)

Vice President	Charles Fairbanks	1905–1909
Secretary of State	John Hay	1901–1905
	Elihu Root	1905–1909
	Robert Bacon	1909
Secretary of Treasury	Lyman J. Gage	1901–1902
	Leslie M. Shaw	1902–1907
	George B. Cortelyou	1907–1909
Secretary of War	Elihu Root	1901–1904
	William H. Taft	1904–1908
	Luke E. Wright	1908–1909
Attorney General	Philander C. Knox	1901–1904
	William H. Moody	1904–1906
	Charles J. Bonaparte	1906–1909
Postmaster General	Charles E. Smith	1901–1902
	Henry C. Payne	1902–1904
	Robert J. Wynne	1904–1905

	George B. Cortelyou	1905–1907
	George von L. Meyer	1907–1909
Secretary of Navy	John D. Long	1901–1902
	William H. Moody	1902–1904
	Paul Morton	1904–1905
	Charles J. Bonaparte	1905–1906
	Victor H. Metcalf	1906–1908
	Truman H. Newberry	1908–1909
Secretary of Interior	Ethan A. Hitchcock	1901–1907
	James R. Garfield	1907–1909
Secretary of Agriculture	James Wilson	1901–1909
Secretary of Labor and Commerce	George B. Cortelyou	1903–1904
	Victor H. Metcalf	1904–1906
	Oscar S. Straus	1906–1909
	Charles Nagel	1909

The Taft Administration (1909–1913)

Vice President	James S. Sherman	1909–1913
Secretary of State	Philander C. Knox	1909–1913
Secretary of Treasury	Franklin MacVeagh	1909–1913
Secretary of War	Jacob M. Dickinson	1909–1911
	Henry L. Stimson	1911–1913
Attorney General	George W. Wickersham	1909–1913
Postmaster General	Frank H. Hitchcock	1909–1913
Secretary of Navy	George von L. Meyer	1909–1913
Secretary of Interior	Richard A. Ballinger	1909–1911
	Walter L. Fisher	1911–1913
Secretary of Agriculture	James Wilson	1909–1913
Secretary of Labor and Commerce	Charles Nagel	1909–1913

The Wilson Administration (1913–1921)

Vice President	Thomas R. Marshall	1913–1921
Secretary of State	William J. Bryan	1913–1915
	Robert Lansing	1915–1920
	Bainbridge Colby	1920–1921
Secretary of Treasury	William G. McAdoo	1913–1918
	Carter Glass	1918–1920
	David F. Houston	1920–1921
Secretary of War	Lindley M. Garrison	1913–1916
	Newton D. Baker	1916–1921
Attorney General	James C. McReyolds	1913–1914
	Thomas W. Gregory	1914–1919
	A. Mitchell Palmer	1919–1921
Postmaster General	Albert S. Burleson	1913–1921
Secretary of Navy	Josephus Daniels	1913–1921
Secretary of Interior	Franklin K. Lane	1913–1920
	John B. Payne	1920–1921
Secretary of Agriculture	David F. Houston	1913–1920
	Edwin T. Meredith	1920–1921
Secretary of Commerce	William C. Redfield	1913–1919
	Joshua W. Alexander	1919–1921
Secretary of Labor	William B. Wilson	1913–1921

The Harding Administration (1921–1923)

Vice President	Calvin Coolidge	1921–1923
Secretary of State	Charles E. Hughes	1921–1923
Secretary of Treasury	Andrew Mellon	1921–1923
Secretary of War	John W. Weeks	1921–1923
Attorney General	Harry M. Daugherty	1921–1923
Postmaster General	Will H. Hays	1921–1922
	Hubert Work	1922–1923
	Harry S. New	1923
Secretary of Navy	Edwin Denby	1921–1923
Secretary of Interior	Albert B. Fall	1921–1923
	Hubert Work	1923
Secretary of Agriculture	Henry C. Wallace	1921–1923
Secretary of Commerce	Herbert C. Hoover	1921–1923
Secretary of Labor	James J. Davis	1921–1923

The Coolidge Administration (1923–1929)

Vice President	Charles G. Dawes	1925–1929
Secretary of State	Charles E. Hughes	1923–1925
	Frank B. Kellogg	1925–1929
Secretary of Treasury	Andrew Mellon	1923–1929
Secretary of War	John W. Weeks	1923–1925
	Dwight F. Davis	1925–1929
Attorney General	Henry M. Daugherty	1923–1924
	Harlan F. Stone	1924–1925
	John G. Sargent	1925–1929
Postmaster General	Harry S. New	1923–1929
Secretary of Navy	Edwin Derby	1923–1924
	Curtis D. Wilbur	1924–1929
Secretary of Interior	Hubert Work	1923–1928
	Roy O. West	1928–1929
Secretary of Agriculture	Henry C. Wallace	1923–1924
	Howard M. Gore	1924–1925
	William M. Jardine	1925–1929
Secretary of Commerce	Herbert C. Hoover	1923–1928
	William F. Whiting	1928–1929
Secretary of Labor	James J. Davis	1923–1929

The Hoover Administration (1929–1933)

Vice President	Charles Curtis	1929–1933
Secretary of State	Henry L. Stimson	1929–1933
Secretary of Treasury	Andrew Mellon	1929–1932
	Ogden L. Mills	1932–1933
Secretary of War	James W. Good	1929
	Patrick J. Hurley	1929–1933
Attorney General	William D. Mitchell	1929–1933
Postmaster General	Walter F. Brown	1929–1933
Secretary of Navy	Charles F. Adams	1929–1933
Secretary of Interior	Ray L. Wilbur	1929–1933
Secretary of Agriculture	Arthur M. Hyde	1929–1933
Secretary of Commerce	Robert P. Lamont	1929–1932
	Roy D. Chapin	1932–1933
Secretary of Labor	James J. Davis	1929–1930
	William N. Doak	1930–1933

The Franklin D. Roosevelt Administration (1933–1945)

Vice President	John Nance Garner	1933–1941
	Henry A. Wallace	1941–1945
	Harry S. Truman	1945
Secretary of State	Cordell Hull	1933–1944
	Edward R. Stettinius, Jr.	1944–1945
Secretary of Treasury	William H. Woodin	1933–1934
	Henry Morgenthau, Jr.	1934–1945
Secretary of War	George H. Dern	1933–1936
	Henry A. Woodring	1936–1940
	Henry L. Stimson	1940–1945
Attorney General	Homer S. Cummings	1933–1939
	Frank Murphy	1939–1940
	Robert H. Jackson	1940–1941
Attorney General	Francis Biddle	1941–1945
Postmaster General	James A. Farley	1933–1940
	Frank C. Walker	1940–1945
Secretary of Navy	Claude A. Swanson	1933–1940
	Charles Edison	1940
	Frank Knox	1940–1944
	James V. Forrestal	1944–1945
Secretary of Interior	Harold L. Ickes	1933–1945
Secretary of Agriculture	Henry A. Wallace	1933–1940
	Claude R. Wickard	1940–1945
Secretary of Commerce	Daniel C. Roper	1933–1939
	Harry L. Hopkins	1939–1940
	Jesse Jones	1940–1945
	Henry A. Wallace	1945
Secretary of Labor	Frances Perkins	1933–1945

The Truman Administration (1945–1953)

Vice President	Alben W. Barkley	1949–1953
Secretary of State	Edward R. Stettinius, Jr.	1945
	James F. Byrnes	1945–1947
	George C. Marshall	1947–1949
	Dean G. Acheson	1949–1953
Secretary of Treasury	Fred M. Vinson	1945–1946
	John W. Snyder	1946–1953
Secretary of War	Robert P. Patterson	1945–1947
	Kenneth C. Royall	1947

Attorney General	Tom C. Clark	1945–1949
	J. Howard McGrath	1949–1952
	James P. McGranery	1952–1953
Postmaster General	Frank C. Walker	1945
	Robert E. Hannegan	1945–1947
	Jesse M. Donaldson	1947–1953
Secretary of Navy	James V. Forrestal	1945–1947
Secretary of Interior	Harold L. Ickes	1945–1946
	Julius A. Krug	1946–1949
	Oscar L. Chapman	1949–1953
Secretary of Agriculture	Clinton P. Anderson	1945–1948
	Charles F. Brannan	1948–1953
Secretary of Commerce	Henry A. Wallace	1945–1946
	W. Averell Harriman	1946–1948
	Charles W. Sawyer	1948–1953
Secretary of Labor	Lewis B. Schwellenbach	1945–1948
	Maurice J. Tobin	1948–1953
Secretary of Defense	James V. Forrestal	1947–1949
	Louis A. Johnson	1949–1950
	George C. Marshall	1950–1951
	Robert A. Lovett	1951–1953

The Eisenhower Administration (1953–1961)

Vice President	Richard M. Nixon	1953–1961
Secretary of State	John Foster Dulles	1953–1959
	Christian A. Herter	1959–1961
Secretary of Treasury	George M. Humphrey	1953–1957
	Robert B. Anderson	1957–1961
Attorney General	Herbert Brownell, Jr.	1953–1958
	William P. Rogers	1958–1961
Postmaster General	Arthur E. Summerfield	1953–1961
Secretary of Interior	Douglas McKay	1953–1956
	Fred A. Seaton	1956–1961
Secretary of Agriculture	Ezra T. Benson	1953–1961
Secretary of Commerce	Sinclair Weeks	1953–1958
	Lewis L. Strauss	1958–1959
	Frederick H. Mueller	1959–1961

Secretary of Labor	Martin P. Durkin	1953
	James P. Mitchell	1953–1961
Secretary of Defense	Charles E. Wilson	1953–1957
	Neil H. McElroy	1957–1959
	Thomas S. Gates Jr.	1959–1961
Secretary of Health, Education, and Welfare	Oveta Culp Hobby	1953–1955
	Marion B. Folsom	1955–1958
	Arthur S. Flemming	1958–1961

The Kennedy Administration (1961–1963)

Vice President	Lyndon B. Johnson	1961–1963
Secretary of State	Dean Rusk	1961–1963
Secretary of Treasury	C. Douglas Dillon	1961–1963
Attorney General	Robert F. Kennedy	1961–1963
Postmaster General	J. Edward Day	1961–1963
	John A. Gronouski	1963
Secretary of Interior	Stewart L. Udall	1961–1963
Secretary of Agriculture	Orville L. Freeman	1961–1963
Secretary of Commerce	Luther H. Hodges	1961–1963
Secretary of Labor	Arthur J. Goldberg	1961–1962
	W. Willard Wirtz	1962–1963
Secretary of Defense	Robert S. McNamara	1961–1963
Secretary of Health, Education, and Welfare	Abraham A. Ribicoff	1961–1962
	Anthony J. Celebrezze	1962–1963

The Lyndon Johnson Administration (1963–1969)

Vice President	Hubert H. Humphrey	1965–1969
Secretary of State	Dean Rusk	1963–1969
Secretary of Treasury	C. Douglas Dillon	1963–1965
	Henry H. Fowler	1965–1969
Attorney General	Robert F. Kennedy	1963–1964
	Nicholas Katzenbach	1965–1966
	Ramsey Clark	1967–1969
Postmaster General	John A. Gronouski	1963–1965
	Lawrence F. O'Brien	1965–1968
	Marvin Watson	1968–1969

The Lyndon Johnson Administration (1963–1969)

Secretary of Interior	Stewart L. Udall	1963–1969
Secretary of Agriculture	Orville L. Freeman	1963–1969
Secretary of Commerce	Luther H. Hodges	1963–1064
	John T. Connor	1964–1967
	Alexander B. Trowbridge	1967–1968
	Cyrus R. Smith	1968–1969
Secretary of Labor	W. Willard Wirtz	1963–1969
Secretary of Defense	Robert F. McNamara	1963–1968
	Clark Clifford	1968–1969
Secretary of Health, Education, and Welfare	Anthony J. Celebrezze	1963–1965
	John W. Gardner	1965–1968
	Wilbur J. Cohen	1968–1969
Secretary of Housing and Urban Development	Robert C. Weaver	1966–1969
	Robert C. Wood	1969
Secretary of Transportation	Alan S. Boyd	1967–1969

The Nixon Administration (1969–1974)

Vice President	Spiro T. Agnew	1969–1973
	Gerald R. Ford	1973–1974
Secretary of State	William P. Rogers	1969–1973
	Henry A. Kissinger	1973–1974
Secretary of Treasury	David M. Kennedy	1969–1970
	John B. Connally	1971–1972
	George P. Shultz	1972–1974
	William E. Simon	1974
Attorney General	John N. Mitchell	1969–1972
	Richard G. Kleindienst	1972–1973
	Elliot L. Richardson	1973
	William B. Saxbe	1973–1974
Postmaster General	Winton M. Blount	1969–1971
Secretary of Interior	Walter J. Hickel	1969–1970
	Rogers Morton	1971–1974
Secretary of Agriculture	Clifford M. Hardin	1969–1971
	Earl L. Butz	1971–1974
Secretary of Commerce	Maurice H. Stans	1969–1972
	Peter G. Peterson	1972–1973
	Frederick B. Dent	1973–1974

Secretary of Labor	George P. Shultz	1969–1970
	James D. Hodgson	1970–1973
	Peter J. Brennan	1973–1974
Secretary of Defense	Melvin R. Laird	1969–1973
	Elliot L. Richardson	1973
	James R. Schlesinger	1973–1974
Secretary of Health, Education, and Welfare	Robert H. Finch	1969–1970
	Elliot L. Richardson	1970–1973
	Caspar W. Weinberger	1973–1974
Secretary of Housing and Urban Development	George Romney	1969–1973
	James T. Lynn	1973–1974
Secretary of Transportation	John A. Volpe	1969–1973
	Claude S. Brinegar	1973–1974

The Ford Administration (1974–1977)

Vice President	Nelson A. Rockefeller	1974–1977
Secretary of State	Henry A. Kissinger	1974–1977
Secretary of Treasury	William E. Simon	1974–1977
Attorney General	William Saxbe	1974–1975
	Edward Levi	1975–1977
Secretary of Interior	Rogers Morton	1974–1975
	Stanley K. Hathaway	1975
	Thomas Kleppe	1975–1977
Secretary of Agriculture	Earl L. Butz	194–1976
	John A. Knebel	1976–1977
Secretary of Commerce	Frederick B. Dent	1974–1975
	Rogers Morton	1975–1976
	Elliot L. Richardson	1976–1977
Secretary of Labor	Peter J. Brennan	1974–1975
	John T. Dunlop	1975–1976
	W. J. Usery	1976–1977
Secretary of Defense	James R. Schlesinger	1974–1975
	Donald Rumsfeld	1975–1977
Secretary of Health, Education, and Welfare	Caspar Weinberger	1974–1975
	Forrest D. Mathews	1975–1977
Secretary of Housing and Urban Development	James T. Lynn	1974–1975
	Carla A. Hills	1975–1977
Secretary of Transportation	Claude Brinegar	1974–1975
	William T. Coleman	1975–1977

The Carter Administration (1977–1981)

Vice President	Walter F. Mondale	1977–1981
Secretary of State	Cyrus R. Vance	1977–1980
	Edmund Muskie	1980–1981
Secretary of Treasury	W. Michael Blumenthal	1977–1979
	G. William Miller	1979–1981
Attorney General	Griffin Bell	1977–1979
	Benjamin R. Civiletti	1979–1981
Secretary of Interior	Cecil D. Andrus	1977–1981
Secretary of Agriculture	Robert Bergland	1977–1981
Secretary of Commerce	Juanita M. Kreps	1977–1979
	Philip M. Klutznick	1979–1981
Secretary of Labor	F. Ray Marshall	1977–1981
Secretary of Defense	Harold Brown	1977–1981
Secretary of Health, Education, and Welfare	Joseph A. Califano	1977–1979
	Patricia R. Harris	1979
Secretary of Health and Human Services	Patricia R. Harris	1979–1981
Secretary of Education	Shirley M. Hufstedler	1979–1981
Secretary of Housing and Urban Development	Patricia R. Harris	1977–1979
	Moon Landrieu	1979–1981
Secretary of Transportation	Brock Adams	1977–1979
	Neil E. Goldschmidt	1979–1981
Secretary of Energy	James R. Schlesinger	1977–1979
	Charles W. Duncan	1979–1981

The Reagan Administration (1981–1989)

Vice President	George Bush	1981–1989
Secretary of State	Alexander M. Haig	1981–1982
	George P. Shultz	1982–1989
Secretary of Treasury	Donald Regan	1981–1985
	James A. Baker, III	1985–1988
	Nicholas Brady	1988–1989
Attorney General	William F. Smith	1981–1985
	Edwin A. Meese, III	1985–1988
	Richard Thornburgh	1988–1989
Secretary of Interior	James Watt	1981–1983
	William P. Clark, Jr.	1983–1985
	Donald P. Hodel	1985–1989
Secretary of Agriculture	John Block	1981–1986
	Richard E. Lyng	1986–1989
Secretary of Commerce	Malcolm Baldridge	1981–1987
	C. William Verity, Jr.	1987–1989
Secretary of Labor	Raymond Donovan	1981–1985
	William E. Brock	1985–1987
	Ann D. McLaughlin	1987–1989
Secretary of Defense	Caspar Weinberger	1981–1987
	Frank Carlucci	1987–1989
Secretary of Health and Human Services	Richard Schweiker	1981–1983
	Margaret Heckler	1983–1985
	Otis R. Bowen	1985–1989
Secretary of Education	Terrel H. Bell	1981–1985
	William J. Bennett	1985–1988
	Laura F. Cavazos	1988–1989
Secretary of Housing and Urban Development	Samuel Pierce	1981–1989
Secretary of Transportation	Drew Lewis	1981–1983
	Elizabeth Dole	1983–1987
	James H. Burnley	1987–1989
Secretary of Energy	James Edwards	1981–1982
	Donald P. Hodel	1982–1985
	John S. Herrington	1985–

The Bush Administration (1989–   )

Vice President	J. Danforth Quayle	1989–
Secretary of State	James A. Baker III	1989–
Secretary of Treasury	Nicholas Brady	1989–
Attorney General	Richard Thornburgh	1989–
Secretary of Interior	Manuel Lujan	1989–
Secretary of Agriculture	Clayton Yeutter	1989–
Secretary of Commerce	Robert Mosbacher	1989–
Secretary of Labor	Elizabeth Dole	1989–
Secretary of Defense	Richard Cheney	1989–

The Bush Administration (1989–) (continued)		
Secretary of Health and Human Services	Louis W. Sullivan	1989–
Secretary of Housing and Urban Development	Jack Kemp	1989–

Secretary of Transportation	Samuel K. Skinner	1989–
Secretary of Energy	James Watkins	1989–
Secretary of Veterans Affairs	Edwin Derwinski	1989–

JUSTICES OF THE SUPREME COURT

	Term of Service	Years of Service	Life Span		Term of Service	Years of Service	Life Span
John Jay	1789–1795	5	1745–1829	John M. Harlan	1877–1911	34	1833–1911
John Rutledge	1789–1791	1	1739–1800	William B. Woods	1880–1887	7	1824–1887
William Cushing	1789–1810	20	1732–1810	Stanley Matthews	1881–1889	7	1824–1889
James Wilson	1789–1798	8	1742–1798	Horace Gray	1882–1902	20	1828–1902
John Blair	1789–1796	6	1732–1800	Samuel Blatchford	1882–1893	11	1820–1893
Robert H. Harrison	1789–1790	—	1745–1790	Lucius Q. C. Lamar	1888–1893	5	1825–1893
James Iredell	1790–1799	9	1751–1799	*Melville W. Fuller*	1888–1910	21	1833–1910
Thomas Johnson	1791–1793	1	1732–1819	David J. Brewer	1890–1910	20	1837–1910
William Paterson	1793–1806	13	1745–1806	Henry B. Brown	1890–1906	16	1836–1913
*John Rutledge**	1795	—	1739–1800	George Shiras, Jr.	1892–1903	10	1832–1924
Samuel Chase	1796–1811	15	1741–1811	Howell E. Jackson	1893–1895	2	1832–1895
Oliver Ellsworth	1796–1800	4	1745–1807	Edward D. White	1894–1910	16	1845–1921
Bushrod Washington	1798–1829	31	1762–1829	Rufus W. Peckham	1895–1909	14	1838–1909
Alfred Moore	1799–1804	4	1755–1810	Joseph McKenna	1898–1925	26	1843–1926
John Marshall	1801–1835	34	1755–1835	Oliver W. Holmes	1902–1932	30	1841–1935
William Johnson	1804–1834	30	1771–1834	William R. Day	1903–1922	19	1849–1923
H. Brockholst Livingston	1806–1823	16	1757–1823	William H. Moody	1906–1910	3	1853–1917
Thomas Todd	1807–1826	18	1765–1826	Horace H. Lurton	1910–1914	4	1844–1914
Joseph Story	1811–1845	33	1779–1845	Charles E. Hughes	1910–1916	5	1862–1948
Gabriel Duval	1811–1835	24	1752–1844	Willis Van Devanter	1911–1937	26	1859–1941
Smith Thompson	1823–1843	20	1768–1843	Joseph R. Lamar	1911–1916	5	1857–1916
Robert Trimble	1826–1828	2	1777–1828	*Edward D. White*	1910–1921	11	1845–1921
John McLean	1829–1861	32	1785–1861	Mahlon Pitney	1912–1922	10	1858–1924
Henry Baldwin	1830–1844	14	1780–1844	James C. McReynolds	1914–1941	26	1862–1946
James M. Wayne	1835–1867	32	1790–1867	Louis D. Brandeis	1916–1939	22	1856–1941
Roger B. Taney	1836–1864	28	1777–1864	John H. Clarke	1916–1922	6	1857–1945
Philip P. Barbour	1836–1841	4	1783–1841	William H. Taft	1921–1930	8	1857–1930
John Catron	1837–1865	28	1786–1865	George Sutherland	1922–1938	15	1862–1942
John McKinley	1837–1852	15	1780–1852	Pierce Butler	1922–1939	16	1866–1939
Peter V. Daniel	1841–1860	19	1784–1860	Edward T. Sanford	1923–1930	7	1865–1930
Samuel Nelson	1845–1872	27	1792–1873	Harlan F. Stone	1925–1941	16	1872–1946
Levi Woodbury	1845–1851	5	1789–1851	*Charles E. Hughes*	1930–1941	11	1862–1948
Robert C. Grier	1846–1870	23	1794–1870	Owen J. Roberts	1930–1945	15	1875–1955
Benjamin R. Curtis	1851–1857	6	1809–1874	Benjamin N. Cardozo	1932–1938	6	1870–1938
John A. Campbell	1853–1861	8	1811–1889	Hugo L. Black	1937–1971	34	1886–1971
Nathan Clifford	1858–1881	23	1803–1881	Stanley F. Reed	1938–1957	19	1884–1980
Noah H. Swayne	1862–1881	18	1804–1884	Felix Frankfurter	1939–1962	23	1882–1965
Samuel F. Miller	1862–1890	28	1816–1890	William O. Douglas	1939–1975	36	1898–1980
David Davis	1862–1877	14	1815–1886	Frank Murphy	1940–1949	9	1890–1949
Stephen J. Field	1863–1897	34	1816–1899	*Harlan F. Stone*	1941–1946	5	1872–1946
Salmon P. Chase	1864–1873	8	1808–1873	James F. Byrnes	1941–1942	1	1879–1972
William Strong	1870–1880	10	1808–1895	Robert H. Jackson	1941–1954	13	1892–1954
Joseph P. Bradley	1870–1892	22	1813–1892	Wiley B. Rutledge	1943–1949	6	1894–1949
Ward Hunt	1873–1882	9	1810–1886	Harold H. Burton	1945–1958	13	1888–1964
Morrison R. Waite	1874–1888	14	1816–1888	*Fred M. Vinson*	1946–1953	7	1890–1953
				Tom C. Clark	1949–1967	18	1899–1977

	Term of Service	Years of Service	Life Span		Term of Service	Years of Service	Life Span
Sherman Minton	1949–1956	7	1890–1965	Abe Fortas	1965–1969	4	1910–
Earl Warren	1953–1969	16	1891–1974	Thurgood Marshall	1967–	—	1908–
John Marshall Harlan	1955–1971	16	1899–1971	*Warren C. Burger*	1969–	—	1907–
William J. Brennan, Jr.	1956–	—	1906–	Harry A. Blackmun	1970–	—	1908–
Charles E. Whittaker	1957–1962	5	1901–1973	Lewis F. Powell, Jr.	1971–	—	1907–
Potter Stewart	1958–1981	23	1915–	William H. Rehnquist	1971–	—	1924–
Byron R. White	1962–	—	1917–	John P. Stevens, III	1975–	—	1920–
Arthur J. Goldberg	1962–1965	3	1908–	Sandra Day O'Connor	1981–	—	1930–
				William H. Rehnquist	1986–	—	1924–
				Antonin Scalia	1986–	—	1936–
				Anthony M. Kennedy	1987–	—	1936–

*Appointed and served one term, but not confirmed by the Senate.

Note: Chief justices are in italics.

A SOCIAL PROFILE OF THE AMERICAN REPUBLIC

POPULATION

Year	Population	Percent Increase	Population Per Square Mile	Percent Urban/ Rural	Percent Male/ Female	Percent White/ Nonwhite	Persons Per Household	Median Age
1790	3,929,214		4.5	5.1/94.9	NA/NA	80.7/19.3	5.79	NA
1800	5,308,483	35.1	6.1	6.1/93.9	NA/NA	81.1/18.9	NA	NA
1810	7,239,881	36.4	4.3	7.3/92.7	NA/NA	81.0/19.0	NA	NA
1820	9,638,453	33.1	5.5	7.2/92.8	50.8/49.2	81.6/18.4	NA	16.7
1830	12,866,020	33.5	7.4	8.8/91.2	50.8/18.1	81.9/18.1	NA	17.2
1840	17,069,453	32.7	9.8	10.8/89.2	50.9/49.1	83.2/16.8	NA	17.8
1850	23,191,876	35.9	7.9	15.3/84.7	51.0/49.0	84.3/15.7	5.55	18.9
1860	31,443,321	35.6	10.6	19.8/80.2	51.2/48.8	85.6/14.4	5.28	19.4
1870	39,818,449	26.6	13.4	25.7/74.3	50.6/49.4	86.2/13.8	5.09	20.2
1880	50,155,783	26.0	16.9	28.2/71.8	50.9/49.1	86.5/13.5	5.04	20.9
1890	62,947,714	25.5	21.2	35.1/64.9	51.2/48.8	87.5/12.5	4.93	22.0
1900	75,994,575	20.7	25.6	39.6/60.4	51.1/48.9	87.9/12.1	4.76	22.9
1910	91,972,266	21.0	31.0	45.6/54.4	51.5/48.5	88.9/11.1	4.54	24.1
1920	105,710,620	14.9	35.6	51.2/48.8	51.0/49.0	89.7/10.3	4.34	25.3
1930	122,775,046	16.1	41.2	56.1/43.9	50.6/49.4	89.8/10.2	4.11	26.4
1940	131,669,275	7.2	44.2	56.5/43.5	50.2/49.8	89.8/10.2	3.67	29.0
1950	150,697,361	14.5	50.7	64.0/36.0	49.7/50.3	89.5/10.5	3.37	30.2
1960	179,323,175	18.5	50.6	69.9/30.1	49.3/50.7	88.6/11.4	3.33	29.5
1970	203,302,031	13.4	57.4	73.5/26.5	48.7/51.3	87.6/12.4	3.14	28.0
1980	226,545,805	11.4	64.0	73.7/26.3	48.6/51.4	86.0/14.0	2.76	30.0
1990*	250,410,000	9.9	70.8	NA	48.8/51.2	84.1/15.9	NA	32.1**
2000*	268,266,000	7.1	75.8	NA	48.9/51.1	82.6/17.4	NA	NA

NA = Not available.
* Projections.
**1987 figure.

VITAL STATISTICS (rates per thousand)

Year	Births	Year	Births	Deaths*	Marriage*	Divorces*
1800	55.0	1900	32.3	17.2	NA	NA
1810	54.3	1910	30.1	14.7	NA	NA
1820	55.2	1920	27.7	13.0	12.0	1.6
1830	51.4	1930	21.3	11.3	9.2	1.6
1840	51.8	1940	19.4	10.8	12.1	2.0
1850	43.3	1950	24.1	9.6	11.1	2.6
1860	44.3	1960	23.7	9.5	8.5	2.2
1870	38.3	1970	18.4	9.5	10.6	3.5
1880	39.8	1980	15.9	8.8	10.6	5.2
1890	31.5	1987	15.7	8.7	9.9	4.8

NA = Not available.
*Data not available before 1900.

LIFE EXPECTANCY (in years)

Year	Total Population	White Females	Nonwhite Females	White Males	Nonwhite Males
1900	47.3	48.7	33.5	46.6	32.5
1910	50.1	52.0	37.5	48.6	33.8
1920	54.1	55.6	45.2	54.4	45.5
1930	59.7	63.5	49.2	59.7	47.3
1940	62.9	66.6	54.9	62.1	51.5
1950	68.2	72.2	62.9	66.5	59.1
1960	69.7	74.1	66.3	67.4	61.1
1970	70.9	75.6	69.4	68.0	61.3
1980	73.7	78.1	73.6	70.7	65.3
1987	74.9	78.3	75.4	71.5	67.6

THE CHANGING AGE STRUCTURE

For more explanation of these population pyramids, see pages 714–15 and 1190–91.

REGIONAL ORIGIN OF IMMIGRANTS (percent)

Years	Total Number of Immigrants	Total Europe	North and West	East and Central	South and Other	Western Hemisphere	Asia
			Europe				
1821–1830	143,389	69.2	67.1	—	2.1	8.4	—
1831–1840	599,125	82.8	81.8	—	1.0	5.5	—
1841–1850	1,713,251	93.8	92.9	0.1	0.3	3.6	—
1851–1860	2,598,214	94.4	93.6	0.1	0.8	2.9	1.6
1861–1870	2,314,824	89.2	87.8	0.5	0.9	7.2	2.8
1871–1880	2,812,191	80.8	73.6	4.5	2.7	14.4	4.4
1881–1890	5,246,613	90.3	72.0	11.9	6.3	8.1	1.3
1891–1900	3,687,546	96.5	44.5	32.8	19.1	1.1	1.9
1901–1910	8,795,386	92.5	21.7	44.5	6.3	4.1	2.8
1911–1920	5,735,811	76.3	17.4	33.4	25.5	19.9	3.4
1921–1930	4,107,209	60.3	31.7	14.4	14.3	36.9	2.4
1931–1940	528,431	65.9	38.8	11.0	16.1	30.3	2.8
1941–1950	1,035,039	60.1	47.5	4.6	7.9	34.3	3.1
1951–1960	2,515,479	52.8	17.7	24.3	10,8	39.6	6.0
1961–1970	3,321,677	33.8	11.7	9.4	12.9	51.7	12.9
1971–1980	4,384,000	18.3	4.3	5.6	8.4	44.0	37.3

Dash indicates less than 0.1 percent.

RECENT TRENDS IN IMMIGRATION (in thousands)

	1961–1970	1971–1980	Percent 1961–1970	Percent 1971–1980	1985	1987
All countries	3,321.7	4,493.3	100.0	100.0	570.0	601.5
Europe	1,123.5	800.4	33.8	17.8	69.5	68.0
Austria	20.6	9.5	0.6	0.2	1.9	2.4
Hungary	5.4	6.6	0.2	0.1	0.6	—
Belgium	9.2	5.3	0.3	0.1	0.8	0.9
Czechoslovakia	3.3	6.0	0.1	0.1	0.7	0.7
Denmark	9.2	4.4	0.3	0.1	0.5	0.5
Finland	4.2	2.9	0.1	0.1	0.2	0.3
France	45.2	25.1	1.4	0.6	3.5	3.8
Germany	190.8	74.4	5.7	1.7	10.2	9.9
Great Britain	214.5	137.4	6.5	3.1	15.6	15.9
Greece	86.0	92.4	2.6	2.1	3.5	4.1
Ireland	33.0	11.5	1.0	0.3	1.3	3.0
Italy	214.1	129.4	6.4	7.9	6.4	4.7
Netherlands	30.6	10.5	.9	0.2	1.2	1.3
Norway	15.5	3.9	.5	0.1	0.4	0.4
Poland	53.5	37.2	1.6	0.8	7.4	5.8
Portugal	76.1	101.7	2.3	2.3	3.8	4.0
Spain	44.7	39.1	1.3	0.9	2.3	2.1
Sweden	17.1	6.5	.5	0.1	1.2	1.2
Switzerland	18.5	8.2	.6	0.2	1.0	0.1
U.S.S.R.	2.5	39.0	.1	0.9	1.5	1.1
Yugoslavia	20.4	30.5	.6	0.7	1.5	1.8
Other Europe	9.1	18.9	.2	0.2	4.0	4.0
Asia	427.6	1,588.2	12.9	35.2	255.2	248.3
China	34.8	124.3	1.0	2.8	33.1	18.6
Hong Kong	75.0	113.5	2.3	2.5	10.8	8.8
India	27.2	164.1	0.8	3.7	24.5	26.4

RECENT TRENDS IN IMMIGRATION (continued)

	1961–1970	1971–1980	Percent 1961–1970	Percent 1971–1980	1985	1987
Iran	10.3	45.1	0.3	1.0	12.3	10.3
Israel	29.6	37.7	0.9	0.8	4.3	4.8
Japan	40.0	49.8	1.2	1.1	4.6	4.7
Jordan	11.7	27.5	0.4	0.6	2.7	2.8
Korea	34.5	267.6	1.0	6.0	34.8	35.4
Lebanon	15.2	41.3	0.5	0.9	2.5	3.0
Philippines	98.4	355.0	3.0	7.9	53.1	58.3
Turkey	10.1	13.4	0.3	0.3	1.7	2.1
Vietnam	4.3	172.8	1.1	3.8	20.4	13.1
Other Asia	36.5	176.1	1.1	3.8	50.4	60.0
America	1,716.4	1,982.5	51.7	44.3	225.5	265.0
Argentina	49.7	29.9	1.5	0.7	1.9	2.2
Brazil	29.3	17.8	0.9	0.4	2.6	2.7
Canada	413.3	169.9	12.4	3.8	16.4	16.7
Colombia	72.0	77.3	2.2	1.7	11.8	11.5
Cuba	208.5	264.9	6.3	5.9	17.1	27.4
Dominican Rep.	93.3	148.1	2.8	3.3	23.9	24.9
Ecuador	36.8	50.1	1.1	1.1	4.6	4.7
El Salvador	15.0	34.4	0.5	0.8	10.1	10.6
Guatemala	15.9	25.9	0.5	0.6	4.4	5.8
Haiti	34.5	56.3	1.0	1.3	9.9	14.8
Honduras	15.7	17.4	0.5	0.4	3.7	72.5
Mexico	453.9	640.3	13.7	14.3	61.3	2.8
Panamá	19.4	23.5	0.6	0.5	3.2	5.8
Peru	19.1	29.2	0.6	0.6	4.1	5.8
West Indies	133.9	271.8	4.0	6.1	28.5	48.3
Other America	106.1	125.7	3.1	2.8	22.0	9.7

Figures may not add to total due to rounding.

AMERICAN WORKERS AND FARMERS

Year	Total Number of Workers (thousands)	Percent of Workers Male/Female	Percent of Female Workers Married	Percent of Workers in Female Population	Percent of Workers in Labor Unions	Farm Population (thousands)	Farm Population as Percent of Total Population
1870	12,506	85/15	NA	NA	NA	NA	NA
1880	17,392	85/15	NA	NA	NA	21,973	43.8
1890	23,318	83/17	13.9	18.9	NA	24,771	42.3
1900	29,073	82/18	15.4	20.6	3	29,875	41.9
1910	38,167	79/21	24.7	25.4	6	32,077	34.9
1920	41,614	79/21	23.0	23.7	12	31,974	30.1
1930	48,830	78/22	28.9	24.8	7	30,529	24.9
1940	53,011	76/24	36.4	27.4	27	30,547	23.2
1950	59,643	72/28	52.1	31.4	25	23,048	15.3
1960	69,877	68/32	59.9	37.7	26	15,635	8.7
1970	82,049	63/37	63.4	43.4	25	9,712	4.8
1980	108,544	58/42	59.7	51.5	23	6,051	2.7
1987	119,865	55/45	59.1	55.4	19	4,986	2.0

THE ECONOMY AND FEDERAL SPENDING

Year	Gross National Product (GNP) (in billions)	Foreign Trade (in millions)			Federal Budget (in billions)	Federal Surplus/Deficit (in billions)	Federal Debt (in billions)
		Exports	Imports	Balance of Trade			
1790	NA	$ 20	$ 23	$ −3	$ 0.004	$ +0.00015	$ 0.076
1800	NA	71	91	−20	0.011	+0.0006	0.083
1810	NA	67	85	−18	0.008	+0.0012	0.053
1820	NA	70	74	−4	0.018	−0.0004	0.091
1830	NA	74	71	+3	0.015	+0.100	0.049
1840	NA	132	107	+25	0.024	−0.005	0.004
1850	NA	152	178	−26	0.040	+0.004	0.064
1860	NA	400	362	−38	0.063	−0.01	0.065
1870	$ 7.4	451	462	−11	0.310	+0.10	2.4
1880	11.2	853	761	+92	0.268	+0.07	2.1
1890	13.1	910	823	+87	0.318	+0.09	1.2
1900	18.7	1,499	930	+569	0.521	+0.05	1.2
1910	35.3	1,919	1,646	+273	0.694	−0.02	1.1
1920	91.5	8,664	5,784	+2,880	6.357	+0.3	24.3
1930	90.7	4,013	3,500	+513	3.320	+0.7	16.3
1940	100.0	4,030	7,433	−3,403	9.6	−2.7	43.0
1950	286.5	10,816	9,125	+1,691	43.1	−2.2	257.4
1960	506.5	19,600	15,046	+4,556	92.2	+0.3	286.3
1970	992.7	42,700	40,189	+2,511	195.6	−2.8	371.0
1980	2,631.7	220,783	244,871	+24,088	590.9	−73.8	907.7
1987	4,526.7	252,866	424,082	−171,216	1,015.6	−173.2	2,350.3

80°N

GREENLAND
(KALALLIT-NUNAAT)
(Den.)

ALASKA
(U.S.)

60°N

CANADA

NORTH
AMERICA

40°N

UNITED STATES

ATLANTIC
OCEAN

BERMUDA
(Br.)

HAWAII
(U.S.)

MEXICO

BAHAMAS

CUBA

DOMINICAN
REP. 18

CAPE
VERDE

20°N

HAITI
BELIZE
PUERTO 27
RICO (U.S.)
29
26
25
23

GUATEMALA
EL SALVADOR
HONDURAS 20
NICARAGUA
COSTA RICA
21
24
22
19
28

PACIFIC
OCEAN

VENEZUELA
GUYANA
SURINAME
FR. GUIANA

PANAMA
COLOMBIA

ECUADOR

0° Equator

SOUTH
AMERICA

WESTERN
SAMOA

PERU

BRAZIL

AMERICAN
SAMOA

FRENCH
POLYNESIA

BOLIVIA

20°S

TONGA

PARAGUAY

URUGUAY

CHILE

ARGENTINA

40°S

FALKLAND
IS. (Br.)

60°S

80°S

160°W 140°W 120°W 100°W 80°W 60°W

0   1000   2000 Miles

0   1000   2000 Kilometers

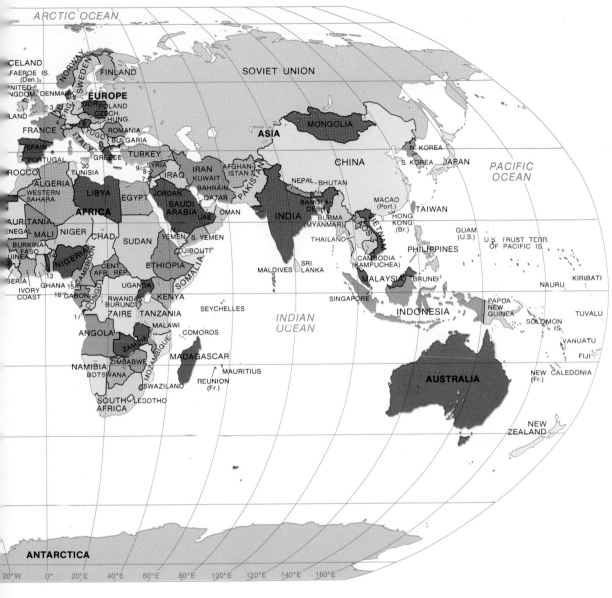

ARCTIC OCEAN

ICELAND
FAEROE IS.
(Den.)
UNITED
KINGDOM
IRELAND
FRANCE
SPAIN
PORTUGAL
MOROCCO
ALGERIA
WESTERN
SAHARA
MAURITANIA
SENEGAL
MALI
GUINEA
LIBERIA
IVORY
COAST
GHANA
GABON
ANGOLA
NAMIBIA
BOTSWANA
SOUTH
AFRICA

NORWAY
SWEDEN
FINLAND
DENMARK
EUROPE
GDR
FRG
POLAND
CZECH.
HUNG.
ROMANIA
YUGO
ITALY
BULGARIA
GREECE
TUNISIA
TURKEY
SYRIA
IRAQ
JORDAN
EGYPT
LIBYA
SAUDI
ARABIA
UAE
OMAN
NIGER
CHAD
SUDAN
N.
YEMEN
S. YEMEN
DJIBOUTI
NIGERIA
CAMEROON
CENT.
AFR. REP.
CONGO
ZAIRE
RWANDA
BURUNDI
UGANDA
KENYA
TANZANIA
MALAWI
ZAMBIA
ZIMBABWE
SWAZILAND
LESOTHO
BURKINA
FASO

AFRICA

SOVIET UNION

MONGOLIA

ASIA

CHINA

N. KOREA
S. KOREA
JAPAN

IRAN
AFGHAN-
ISTAN
KUWAIT
BAHRAIN
QATAR
PAKISTAN
NEPAL
BHUTAN
INDIA
BANGLA-
DESH
BURMA
(MYANMAR)
THAILAND
LAOS
VIETNAM
CAMBODIA
(KAMPUCHEA)
MACAO
(Port.)
HONG
KONG
(Br.)
TAIWAN

PACIFIC
OCEAN

GUAM
(U.S.)
U.S. TRUST TERR.
OF PACIFIC IS.

PHILIPPINES

KIRIBATI
NAURU

MALDIVES
SRI
LANKA

MALAYSIA
BRUNEI

SINGAPORE

INDONESIA

SEYCHELLES

INDIAN
OCEAN

COMOROS
MADAGASCAR
MOZAMBIQUE
MAURITIUS
REUNION
(Fr.)

PAPUA
NEW
GUINEA
SOLOMON
IS.
TUVALU
VANUATU
FIJI
NEW CALEDONIA
(Fr.)

AUSTRALIA

NEW
ZEALAND

ANTARCTICA

20°W   0°   20°E   40°E   60°E   80°E   100°E   120°E   140°E   160°E

1. SWITZERLAND
2. NETHERLANDS
3. BELGIUM
4. LUXEMBOURG
5. ALBANIA
6. AUSTRIA
7. ISRAEL
8. LEBANON
9. CYPRUS
10. GAMBIA
11. GUINEA-BISSAU
12. SIERRA LEONE
13. TOGO
14. BENIN
15. EQUATORIAL GUINEA

16. SÃO TOMÉ AND PRÍNCIPE
17. CABINDA (Angola)
18. VIRGIN IS. (U.S./Br.)
19. BARBADOS
20. NETHERLANDS ANTILLES
21. GRENADA
22. ST. VINCENT
23. ST. LUCIA
24. DOMINICA
25. FRENCH ANTILLES
26. ANTIGUA AND BARBUDA
27. ST. KITTS AND NEVIS
28. TRINIDAD AND TOBAGO
29. JAMAICA
30. MALTA

BIBLIOGRAPHY

CHAPTER 17

General Histories
Eric Foner, *Reconstruction: America's Unfinished Revolution, 1863–1877* (1988); James McPherson, *Ordeal by Fire: The Civil War and Reconstruction* (1982); James G. Randall and David Donald, *The Civil War and Reconstruction*, 2d ed. (1961); Kenneth M. Stampp, *The Era of Reconstruction, 1865–1877* (1965).

Biographies
Fawn M. Brodie, *Thaddeus Stevens: Scourge of the South* (1959); David Donald, *Charles Sumner and the Rights of Man* (1970); William S. McFeely, *Yankee Stepfather: General O. O. Howard and the Freedmen* (1968), and *Grant: A Biography* (1981).

National Politics
Richard H. Abbott, *The Republican Party and the South, 1855–1877: The First Southern Strategy* (1986); Herman Belz, *Emancipation and Equal Rights: Politics and Constitutionalism in the Civil War Era* (1978); Michael Les Benedict, *A Compromise of Principle: Congressional Republicans and Reconstruction* (1974), and *The Impeachment and Trial of Andrew Johnson* (1973); W. R. Brock, *An American Crisis: Congress and Reconstruction, 1865–1867* (1963); John Cox and LaWanda Cox, *Politics, Principles, and Prejudice, 1865–1866* (1963); Eric L. McKitrick, *Andrew Johnson and Reconstruction* (1966); James M. McPherson, *The Struggle for Equality: Abolitionists and the Negro in the Civil War and Reconstruction* (1964); John G. Sproat, *"The Best Men": Liberal Reformers in the Gilded Age* (1968); Hans L. Trefousse, *The Radical Republicans: Lincoln's Vanguard for Racial Justice* (1969).

Reconstruction and the Constitution
William Gillette, *The Right to Vote: Politics and the Passage of the Fifteenth Amendment* (1965); Harold M. Hyman, *A More Perfect Union: The Impact of the Civil War and Reconstruction on the Constitution* (1973); Joseph James, *The Framing of the Fourteenth Amendment* (1956); Stanley I. Kutler, *Judicial Power and Reconstruction Politics* (1968).

The Black Experience in Reconstruction
Herbert G. Gutman, *The Black Family in Slavery and Freedom, 1750–1925* (1976); Janet Sharp Hermann, *The Pursuit of a Dream* (1981); Thomas Holt, *Black Over White: Negro Political Leadership in South Carolina* (1977); Leon Litwack, *Been in the Storm So Long: The Aftermath of Slavery* (1979); Howard Rabinowitz, ed., *Southern Black Leaders in Reconstruction* (1982); Willie Lee Rose, *Rehearsal for Reconstruction: The Port Royal Experiment* (1964); Vernon L. Wharton, *The Negro in Mississippi, 1865–1890* (1947); Joel Williamson, *After Slavery: The Negro in South Carolina During Reconstruction* (1966).

Reconstruction in the South
Dan T. Carter, *When the War Was Over: The Failure of Self-Reconstruction in the South, 1865–1867* (1985); Richard N. Current, *Those Terrible Carpetbaggers: A Reinterpretation* (1988); William C. Harris, *Day of the Carpetbagger: Republican Reconstruction in Mississippi* (1979); Elizabeth Studley Nathans, *Losing the Peace: Georgia Republicans and Reconstruction, 1865–1871* (1968); Michael Perman, *Reunion Without Compromise: The South and Reconstruction, 1865–1868* (1973), and *The Road to Redemption: Southern Politics, 1869–1880* (1984); George C. Rable, *But There Was No Peace: The Role of Violence in the Politics of Reconstruction* (1984); James Sefton, *The United States Army and Reconstruction, 1865–1877* (1967); Allen Trelease, *White Terror: The Ku Klux Klan Conspiracy and Southern Reconstruction* (1967); Ted Tunnell, *Crucible of Reconstruction: War, Radicalism, and Race in Louisiana, 1862–1877* (1974); Sarah Woolfolk Wiggins, *The Scalawag in Alabama Politics, 1865–1881* (1977).

Social and Economic Reconstruction
George R. Bentley, *A History of the Freedmen's Bureau* (1955); Eric Foner, *Nothing But Freedom: Emancipation and Its Legacy* (1983); Steven Hahn, *The Roots of Southern Populism: Yeoman Farmers and the Transformation of the Georgia Upcountry, 1850–1890* (1983); Jacqueline Jones, *Soldiers of Light and Love: Northern Teachers and Georgia Blacks, 1865–1873* (1980); Donald Nieman, *To Set the Law in Motion: The Freedmen's Bureau and the Legal Rights of Blacks, 1865–1868* (1979); Lawrence N. Powell, *New Masters: Northern Planters During the Civil War and Reconstruction* (1984); Roger L. Ransom and Richard Sutch, *One Kind of Freedom: The Economic*

Consequences of Emancipation (1977); James Roark, *Masters Without Slaves: Southern Planters in the Civil War and Reconstruction* (1977); Mark W. Summers, *Railroads, Reconstruction, and the Gospel of Prosperity* (1984).

The End of Reconstruction
Paul Buck, *The Road to Reunion, 1865–1900* (1937); William Gillette, *Retreat from Reconstruction, 1869–1879* (1980); Keith Ian Polakoff, *The Politics of Inertia: The Election of 1876 and the End of Reconstruction* (1973); C. Vann Woodward, *Reunion and Reaction: The Compromise of 1877 and the End of Reconstruction* (1951).

CHAPTER 18

General Studies
Daniel Boorstin, *The Americans: The Democratic Experience* (1973); John A. Garraty, *The New Commonwealth* (1968); Ray Ginger, *The Age of Excess* (1963); Samuel P. Hays, *The Response to Industrialism, 1885–1914* (1957); Edward C. Kirkland, *Industry Comes of Age: Business, Labor and Public Policy, 1860–1897* (1961); Robert Wiebe, *The Search for Order, 1877–1920* (1968).

The Economy
Frederick Lewis Allen, *The Great Pierpont Morgan* (1949); W. Elliott Brownlee, *Dynamics of Ascent: A History of the American Economy*, rev. ed. (1979); Stuart Brunchey, *Growth of the Modern American Economy* (1975); Milton Friedman and Anna Schwartz, *Monetary History of the United States, 1867–1960* (1963); Robert L. Heilbroner, *The Economic Transformation of America* (1977); Robert Higgs, *The Transformation of the American Economy, 1865–1914* (1971); Susan Previant Lee and Peter Passell, *A New Economic View of American History* (1979).

The Railroads
Alfred D. Chandler, Jr., *The Railroads: The Nation's First Big Business* (1965); Robert Fogel, *Railroads and American Economic Growth* (1964); Julius Grodinsky, *Jay Gould* (1957); Gabriel Kolko, *Railroads and Regulation, 1877–1916* (1965); Albro Martin, *James J. Hill and the Opening of the Northwest* (1976); George H. Miller, *Railroads and the Granger Laws* (1971); John F. Stover, *American Railroads* (1970).

The Rise of Big Business
Alfred Chandler, *Pierre S. DuPont and the Making of the Modern Corporation* (1971); Alfred Chandler, *Strategy and Structure: Chapters in the History of American Industrial Enterprise* (1962), and *The Visible Hand: The Managerial Revolution in American Business* (1977); Thomas Cochrane, *Business in American Life* (1972); Harold C. Livesay, *Andrew Carnegie and the Rise of Big Business* (1975); Alan Nevins, *Study in Power: John D. Rockefeller*, 2 vols. (1953); Glenn Porter, *The Rise of Big Business* (1973); Alan Trachtenberg, *The Incorporation of America* (1982); Joseph Wall, *Andrew Carnegie* (1970).

Invention and Industry
Robert Bruce, *Alexander Graham Bell and the Conquest of Solitude* (1973); Robert Conot, *A Streak of Luck* (1979); John F. Kasson, *Civilizing the Machine* (1976); Harold Passer, *The Electrical Manufacturers, 1875–1900* (1953); Nathan Rosenberg, *Technology and American Economic Growth* (1972); Peter Temin, *Iron and Steel in Nineteenth Century America* (1964); Frederick A. White, *American Industrial Research Laboratories* (1961).

Capitalism and Its Critics
Robert Bannister, *Social Darwinism: Science and Myth in Anglo-American Social Thought* (1979); Sidney Fine, *Laissez Faire and the General Welfare State: A Study of Conflict in American Thought, 1865–1900* (1956); Louis Galambos, *The Public Image of Big Business in America, 1880–1940: A Quantitative Study of Social Change* (1975); Richard Hofstader, *Social Darwinism in American Thought* (rev. ed., 1955); Edward C. Kirkland, *Dream and Thought in the Business Community, 1860–1900* (1956); T. Jackson Lears, *No Place of Grace: Antimodernism and the Transformation of American Culture, 1880–1920* (1981); John Thomas, *Alternative America: Henry George, Edward Bellamy, and the Adversary Tradition* (1983).

The Culture of Work
John Bodnar, *Immigration and Industrialization: Ethnicity in an American Mill Town* (1977); Michael Frisch and Daniel Walkowitz, eds., *Working-Class America: Essays on Labor, Community, and American Society* (1983); James R. Green, *World of the Worker: Labor in Twentieth Century America* (1980); Herbert Gutman, *Work, Culture, and Society in Industrializing America* (1976); Tamara Hareven, *Family, Time, and Industrial Time: The Relationship Between the Family and Work in a New England Industrial Community* (1982); Susan Kennedy, *If All We Did Was To Weep At Home: A History of White Working Class Women in America* (1979); Alice Kessler-Harris, *Out of Work: A History of Wage-Earning Women in the United States* (1982); Walter Licht, *Working for the Railroad: The Organization of Work in the Nineteenth Century* (1983); David Montgomery, *Workers' Control in America: Studies in the History of Work, Technology, and Labor Struggles* (1979); Daniel Nelson, *Managers and Workers: Origins of the New Factory System* (1975); Daniel T. Rodgers, *The Work Ethic in Industrial America, 1850–1920* (1978); Stephan Thernstrom, *The Other Bostonians: Poverty and Progress in the American Metropolis, 1880–1970* (1973).

The Labor Movement
Mari Jo Buhle, *Women and American Socialism, 1870–1920* (1981); Melvyn Dubofsky, *Industrialism and the American Worker, 1865–1920* (1975); Melvyn Dubofsky, *We Shall Be All: A History of the Industrial Workers of the World* (1969); Leon Fink, *Workingmen's Discovery: The Knights of Labor and American Politics* (1983); Philip Foner, *Women and the American Labor Movement*, 2 vols. (1979); William H. Harris, *The Harder We Run: Black Workers Since the Civil War* (1982); Stuart Kaufman, *Samuel Gompers and the Origins of the American Federation of Labor* (1973); Gwendolyn Mink, *Old Labor and New Immigrants in American Political Development: Union, Party, and State, 1875–1920* (1986); Nick Salvatore, *Eugene V. Debs: Citizen and Socialist* (1982); David Shannon, *The Socialist Party* (1955); Lloyd

Ulman, *The Rise of the National Trade Union: The Development and Significance of Its Structure, Governing Institutions, and Economic Policies* (1955).

CHAPTER 19

General Studies
Howard P. Chudacoff, *The Evolution of American Urban Society* (rev. ed., 1981); Charles Glabb and A. Theodore Brown, *A History of Urban America* (rev. ed., 1976); Blake McKelvey, *The Urbanization of America, 1860–1915* (1963); Allan Pred, *Spatial Dynamics of U.S. Urban Growth, 1800–1914* (1971); John Stilgoe, *Borderland: Origins of the American Suburb, 1820–1939* (1988); Stephan Thernstrom and Richard Sennett, eds., *19th Century Cities: Essays in the New Urban History* (1969); Sam Bass Warner, Jr., *Streetcar Suburbs* (1962), and *The Urban Wilderness* (1972).

Immigration and Immigrants
Josef Barton, *Peasants and Strangers: Italians, Rumanians, and Slovaks in an American City* (1975); Jack Chen, *The Chinese of America* (1980); Leonard Dinnerstein, Roger Nichols, and David Reimers, *Natives and Strangers* (1979); John Duff, *The Irish in the United States* (1971); Mario Garcia, *Desert Immigrants: The Mexicans of El Paso, 1880–1920* (1981); Yuji Ichioka, *The Issei: The World of the First Generation Japanese Americans, 1885–1924* (1988); Edward Kantowicz, *Polish-American Politics in Chicago* (1975); Thomas Kessner, *The Golden Door: Italian and Jewish Immigrant Mobility in New York City, 1880–1915* (1977); Alan M. Kraut, *The Huddled Masses: The Immigrant in American Society, 1880–1921* (1982); Joseph Lopreato, *Italian Americans* (1970); James Stuart Olsen, *The Ethnic Dimension in American History*, vol. II (1979); Moses Richin, *The Promised City: New York's Jews* (1962); Jacob Riis, *How the Other Half Lives* (1890); Philip Taylor, *The Distant Magnet: European Emigration to the U.S.A.* (1971); Virginia Yans-McLaughlin, *Family and Community: Italian Immigrants in Buffalo, 1880–1930* (1977); Olivier Zunz, *The Changing Face of Inequality: Urbanization, Industrial Development, and Immigrants in Detroit, 1880–1920* (1982).

Nativism and Race
Louis Harlan, *Booker T. Washington: The Making of a Black Leader, 1856–1901* (1972), and *Booker T. Washington: The Wizard of Tuskegee, 1901–1915* (1953); John Higham, *Strangers in the Land: Patterns of American Nativism, 1880–1925* (1955), and *Send These to Me* (1975); Kenneth Kusmer, *A Ghetto Takes Shape* (1976); Gilbert Osofsky, *Harlem: The Making of a Ghetto* (1966); Allan H. Spear, *Black Chicago* (1967); Donald Spivey, *Schooling for the New Slavery: Black Industrial Education, 1868–1915* (1978).

Politics and Poverty
John Allswang, *Bosses, Machines, and Urban Voters* (1977); Robert H. Bremmer, *From the Depths: The Discovery of Poverty in the United States* (1956); Lyle Dorsett, *The Pendergast Machine* (1968); Steven Eric, *Rainbow's End: Irish-Americans and the Dilemmas of Urban Machine Politics, 1840–1985* (1988); Leo Hershkowitz, *Tweed's New York: Another Look* (1977); Zane Miller, *Boss Cox's Cincinnati* (1968); James T. Patterson, *America's Struggle Against Poverty* (1981); Thomas Philpott, *The Slum and the Ghetto* (1978); William L. Riordan, *Plunkitt of Tammany Hall* (1963); Lloyd Wendt and Herman Kogan, *Bosses in Lusty Chicago* (2d. ed., 1971).

Reform
Jane Addams, *Twenty Years at Hull-House* (1910); Ruth Bordin, *Woman and Temperance: The Quest for Power and Liberty, 1860–1900* (1981); Allen Davis, *Spearheads for Reform: The Social Settlements and the Progressive Movement, 1890–1914* (1967), and *American Heroine: The Life and Legend of Jane Addams* (1973); Marvin Lazerson, *Origins of the Urban School* (1971); Eric Monkonnen, *Police in Urban America, 1860–1920* (1981); David Pivar, *Purity Crusade: Sexual Morality and Social Control, 1868–1900* (1973); Barbara Rosencrantz, *Public Health and the State* (1972); Martin Schiesl, *The Politics of Efficiency: Municipal Administration and Reform in America* (1977); David Tyack, *The One Best System: A History of American Urban Education* (1974); Morris Vogel, *The Invention of the Modern Hospital: Boston, 1870–1930* (1980); James C. Whorton, *Crusaders for Fitness: The History of American Health Reformers* (1982).

Urban Life, Work, and Culture
Cindy Aron, *Ladies and Gentlemen of the Civil Service: Middle Class Workers in Victorian America* (1987); Gunther Barth, *City People: The Rise of Modern City Culture in 19th Century America* (1980); Allan Brandt, *No Magic Bullet: A Social History of Venereal Disease in the United States Since 1880* (rev. ed., 1985); Robert Cross, *The Church and the City* (1967); Ronald Davies, *A History of Music in American Life, Volume II: The Gilded Years, 1865–1920* (1980); Tamara K. Hareven and Randolph Langenbach, *Amoskeag: Life and Work in an American Factory* (1978); Neil Harris, *Humbug: The Art of P. T. Barnum* (1973); Lawrence Kasson, *Amusing the Million: Coney Island at the Turn of the Century* (1978); Richard Lingeman, *Theodore Dreiser: At the Gates of the City, 1871–1907* (1986); John Lucas and Ronald Smith, *Saga of American Sport* (1978); Henry F. May, *Protestant Churches and Urban America* (1949); Katherine Morello, *The Invisible Bar: The Woman Lawyer in America, 1638 to the Present* (1986); Joseph Musselman, *Music in the Cultured Generation: A Social History of Music in America, 1870–1900* (1971); Russel Nye, *The Unembarrassed Muse: The Popular Arts in America* (1970); Roy Rosenzweig, *Eight Hours for What We Will: Workers & Leisure in An Industrial City, 1870–1920* (1983); Robert H. Walker, *Life in the Age of Enterprise, 1865–1900* (1967).

Women and Family
Harvey Green, *The Light of the Home: An Intimate View of the Lives of Women in Victorian America* (1983); John S. Haller and Robin M. Haller, *The Physician and Sexuality in Victorian America* (1986); N. Ray Hiner and Joseph Hawes, eds., *Growing Up in America: Children in Historical Perspective* (1985); David Katzman, *Seven Days a Week: Women and Domestic Service in Industrializing America* (1978); Judith Leavitt, *Brought to Bed: Childbearing in America, 1750–1950* (1988); Elaine May, *Great Expectations: Marriage and Divorce in Post-Victorian America* (1980); Steven Mintz, *A Prison of Expectations: The Family in Victorian Culture* (1983);

Steven Mintz and Susan Kellogg, *Domestic Revolutions: A Social History of American Family Life* (1988); Ellen Rothman, *Hands and Hearts: A History of Courtship in America* (1984); Carroll Smith-Rosenberg, *Disorderly Conduct: Visions of Gender in Victorian America* (1986); Susan Strasser, *Never Done: A History of American Housework* (1983).

CHAPTER 20

The New South: History, Politics, and Culture

Orville Vernon Burton, *In My Father's House* (1985); W. J. Cash, *The Mind of the South* (1941); Thomas D. Clark and Albert Kirwan, *The South Since Appomattox* (1967); Thomas L. Connelly, *God and General Longstreet: The Lost Cause and the Southern Mind* (1982); John M. Cooper, *Walter Hines Page: The Southerner as American, 1855–1918* (1977); Carl N. Degler, *The Other South: Southern Dissenters in the Nineteenth Century* (1974); Vincent P. DeSantis, *Republicans Face the Southern Question: The New Departure Years, 1877–1897* (1959); Robert Durden, *The Self-Inflicted Wound: Southern Politics in the Nineteenth Century* (1985); John S. Ezell, *The South Since 1865* (1975); Paul Gaston, *The New South Creed* (1970); Richard Gray, *Writing the South: The Idea of an American Region* (1986); J. Morgan Kousser, *The Shaping of Southern Politics: Suffrage Restriction and Establishment of the One Party South* (1974); J. Morgan Kousser and James McPherson, eds., *Region, Race, and Reconstruction* (1982); Lawrence Larsen, *The Rise of the Urban South* (1985); Raymond B. Nixon, *Henry W. Grady: Spokesman of the New South* (1969); David M. Potter, *The South and the Concurrent Majority* (1972); Charles R. Wilson, *Baptized in Blood: The Religion of the Lost Cause, 1865–1920* (1980); C. Vann Woodward, *The Origins of the New South* (1951); C. Vann Woodward, *Tom Watson: Agrarian Rebel* (1938).

The Southern Economy and Race

David Carlton, *Mill and Town in South Carolina, 1880–1920* (1982); Pete Daniels, *Breaking the Land: The Transformation of Cotton, Tobacco, and Rice Cultures Since 1880* (1985); Steven Hahn, *The Roots of Southern Populism: Yeoman Farmers and the Transformation of the Georgia Upcountry, 1850–1890* (1983); Louis T. Harlan, *Booker T. Washington* (1972), and *Booker T. Washington: The Wizard of Tuskegee* (1983); Robert Higgs, *Competition and Coercion: Blacks in the American Economy, 1865–1890* (1977); J. M. McPherson, *The Abolitionist Legacy: From Reconstruction to the NAACP* (1975); August Meier, *Negro Thought in America, 1880–1915: Racial Ideologies in the Age of Booker T. Washington* (1963); Howard Rabinowitz, *Race Relations in the Urban South, 1865–1890* (1978); Roger Ransom and Richard Sutch, *One Kind of Freedom: The Economic Consequences of Emancipation* (1977); Donald Spivey, *Schooling for the New Slavery: Black Industrial Education* (1978); J. F. Stover, *The Railroads of the South* (1955); Edward Wheeler, *Uplifting the Race: The Black Minister in the New South, 1865–1902* (1986); Joel Williamson, *The Crucible of Race: Black-White Relations in the American South Since Emancipation* (1984), and *After Slavery* (1965); C. Vann Woodward, *The Strange Career of Jim Crow* (3rd rev. ed., 1974); Gavin Wright, *Old South, New South* (1986).

Opening of the West

Walton Bean, *California* (1978); Ray A. Billington, *Westward Expansion* (1967); Thomas D. Clark, *Frontier America* (rev. ed., 1969); Robert Hine, *The American West* (2d, rev. ed., 1984); Paul Hutton, ed., *Soldiers West: Biographies from the Military Frontier* (1987); Howard Lamar, *The Reader's Encyclopedia of the American West* (1977), and *The Far Southwest, 1846–1912* (1966); Gerald McFarland, *A Scattered People: An American Family Moves West* (1985); Leo Marx, *The Machine in the Garden* (1964); Donald W. Meinig, *The Southwest: Three People in Geographical Change, 1600–1970* (1971); Frederick Merk, *History of the Westward Movement* (1978); Roderick Nash, *Wilderness and the American Mind* (3rd ed., 1982); Earl Pomery, *The Pacific Slope* (1968); Wallace Stegner, *Beyond the Hundredth Meridian: John Welsey Powell and the Second Opening of the West* (1954); Henry Nash Smith, *Virgin Land* (1950); Donald Worster, *Rivers of Empire: Water, Aridity and the Growth of the American West* (1985).

The Peoples of the West

Rudolfo Acuna, *Occupied America: A History of Chicanos* (1981); Ralph Andrist, *The Long Death: The Last Days of the Sioux Nation* (1964); Robert Athearn, *In Search of Canaan: Black Migration in Kansas, 1879–1880* (1978); Gunther Barth, *Bitter Strength: A History of the Chinese in the United States, 1850–1870* (1964); Gretchen Bataille and Charles Silet, *The Pretend Indians: Images of Native Americans in the Movies* (1980); Beverly Beeton, *Women Vote in the West: The Woman Suffrage Movement, 1869–1896* (1986); Thomas Berger, *Little Big Man* (1964); Robert Berkhofer, Jr., *The White Man's Indian* (1978); Dee Brown, *Bury My Heart at Wounded Knee: An Indian History of the American West* (1970); Dee Brown, *The Gentle Tamers: Women of the Old West* (1958); Edward Curtis, *The North American Indian* (1972); David Dary, *Cowboy Culture* (1981); Everett Dick, *Sod House Frontier* (1954); Carol Fairbanks, *Prairie Women: Images in American and Canadian Fiction* (1986); John Mack Faragher, *Women and Men on the Overland Trail* (1979); Christine Fisher, ed., *Let Them Speak for Themselves: Women in the American West, 1849–1900* (1977); Joe B. Frantz and Julian Choate, *The American Cowboy: The Myth and Reality* (1955); Julie Roy Jeffrey, *Frontier Women: The Trans-Mississippi West, 1840–1880* (1979); Alvin Josephy, *The Indian Heritage in America* (1969); William Katz, *The Black West* (1971); Polly W. Kaufman, *Women Teachers on the Frontier* (1984); William Leckie, *The Buffalo Soldiers: A Narrative History of the Negro Cavalry* (1967); Frederick Luebke, *Ethnicity on the Great Plains* (1980); Robert Mardock, *Reformers and the American Indian* (1971); M. S. Meier and Feliciano Rivera, *The Chicanos: A History of the Mexican Americans* (1972); Sandra Myres, *Western Women and the Frontier Experience, 1880–1915* (1982); James S. Olsen and Raymond Wilson, *Native Americans in the Twentieth Century* (1984); Nell Painter, *The Exodusters: Black Migration to Kansas after Reconstruction* (1976); Paul Prucha, *American Indian Policy in Crisis* (1976); Harriet and Fred Rochlin, *Pioneer Jews: A New Life in the Far West* (1984); Mari Sandoz, *Cheyenne Autumn* (1954); William Savage, *The Cowboy Hero: His Image in American History and Culture* (1979), and as ed., *Cowboy Life* (1975); Kent Steckmesser, *The Western Hero in History and Legend* (1965);

Elinor Pruitt Stewart, *Letters of a Woman Homesteader* (1913, 14); Joanna Stratton, *Pioneer Women: Voices of the Kansas Frontier* (1981); John Tebbel and Keith Jennison, *The American Indian Wars* (1960); Robert Utley, *High Noon in Lincoln: Violence on the Western Frontier* (1987); Robert Utley, *The Indian Frontier of the American West, 1846–1890* (1984), and *Frontier Regulars: The United States Army and the Indian, 1866–1891* (1974); Sylvia Van Kirk, *Many Tender Ties: Women in Fur Trade Society* (1983); Wilcomb Washburn, *The Indian in America* (1975).

The Western Economy
Lewis Atherton, *Cattle Kings* (1961); Gunther Barth, *Instant Cities* (1975); Edward Dale, *The Range Cattle Industry* (rev. ed., 1969); David Dary, *Entrepreneurs of the Old West* (1986); Robert Dykstra, *The Cattle Towns* (1968); Gilbert Fite, *The Farmer's Frontier* (1966); Paul Gates, *History of Public Land Development* (1968); William Greever, *The Bonanza West: The Story of the Western Mining Rushes* (1963); Gene M. Gressley, *Bankers and Cattlemen* (1966); Robert West Howard, *The Great Iron Trail: The Story of the First Transcontinental Railroad* (1963); Donald Jackson, *Gold Dust* (1980); Richard Lingenfelter, *The Hardrock Miners: A History of the Mining Labor Movement in the American West, 1863–1893* (1974); Rodman Paul, *Mining Frontiers of the Far West, 1848–1880* (1963); Mari Sandoz, *Old Jules* (1962); Mari Sandoz, *The Buffalo Hunters: The Story of the Hide Men* (1978); Fred A. Shannon, *The Farmer's Last Frontier, 1860–1897* (1945); J. M. Skaggs, *The Cattle Trailing Industry* (1973); George R. Taylor and Irene Neu, *The American Railroad Network, 1861–1890* (1956); Mark Twain, *Roughing It* (1872); James Ward, *Railroads and the Character of America, 1820–1887* (1986); Walter Prescott Webb, *The Great Plains* (1931); Mark Wyman, *Hard Rock Epic: Western Miners and the Industrial Revolution, 1860–1910* (1979).

CHAPTER 21

General Studies
James Bryce, *The American Commonwealth*, 2 vols. (1888); Sean Cashman, *America and the Gilded Age* (1984); John Dobson, *Politics in the Gilded Age* (1978); Harold Faulkner, *Politics, Reform, and Expansion, 1890–1900* (1959); Richard Hofstader, *The Age of Reform: From Bryan to FDR* (1955); Nancy Eleanor Flexner, *Century of Struggle: The Women's Rights Movement in the United States* (1959); Morton Keller, *Affairs of State: Public Life in Late 19th Century America* (1977); H. Wayne Morgan, *From Hayes to McKinley* (1969); H. Wayne Morgan, ed., *The Gilded Age* (1970); Stephen Skowronek, *Building a New American State: The Expansion of National Administrative Capacities* (1982).

Ideology and Politics
Kenneth Davison, *The Presidency of Rutherford B. Hayes* (1972); Margaret Forster, *Significant Sisters: The Grassroots of Active Feminism, 1839–1939* (1986); Lewis Gould, *The Presidency of William McKinley* (1981); David C. Hammack, *Power and Society: Greater New York at the Turn of the Century* (1982); S. P. Hirshson,

Farewell to the Bloody Shirt: Northern Republicans and the Southern Negro, 1877–1893 (1962); Richard Jensen, *The Winning of the Midwest: Social and Political Conflict, 1888–1896* (1971); David Jordan, *Roscoe Conkling of New York* (1971); Paul Kleppner, *The Cross of Culture: A Social Analysis of Midwestern Politics* (1970), and *The Third Electoral System, 1853–1892: Voters, Parties, and Political Cultures* (1979); Robert Marcus, *Grand Old Party: Political Structure in the Gilded Age* (1971); Robert McCloskey, *American Conservatism in the Age of Enterprise* (1951); Michael McGerr, *The Decline of Politics: The American North, 1865–1928* (1988); Allan Nevins, *Grover Cleveland: A Study in Courage* (New York, 1932); Arnold Paul, *Conservative Crisis and the Rule of Law: Attitudes of Bar and Bench, 1887–1895* (1969); Allan Peskin, *Garfield* (1978); Thomas Reeves, *Gentlemen Boss: The Life of Chester Alan Arthur* (1975); David Rothman, *Politics and Power: The United States Senate, 1869–1901* (1966); R. Hal Williams, *Years of Decision: American Politics in the 1890s* (1978).

Protest and Reform
Geoffrey Blodgett, *The Gentle Reformers* (1966); William Dick, *Labor and Socialism in America* (1972); John Diggins, *The American Left in the Twentieth Century* (1973); Ari Hoogenboom, *Outlawing the Spoils: A History of the Civil Service Movement, 1865–1883* (1961); John Laslett, *Labor and the Left* (1970); Charles Lofgren, *The Plessy Case: A Legal-Historical Interpretation* (1987); Walter Nugent, *Money and American Society* (1968); John Sproat, *The Best Men: Liberal Reformers in the Gilded Age* (1968); Irwin Unger, *The Greenback Era: A Social and Political History of American Finance, 1865–1879* (1964).

Populism
Peter Argersinger, *Populism and Politics: William Alfred Peffer and the People's Party* (1974); Lawrence Goodwyn, *Democratic Promise: The Populist Movement in America* (1976); Steven Hahn, *The Roots of Southern Populism: Yeoman Farmers and the Transformation of the Georgia Upcountry* (1983); Sheldon Hackney, *Populism to Progressivism in Alabama* (1969); John Hicks, *The Populist Revolt* (1931); Robert McMath, *Populist Vanguard* (1975); Bruce Palmer, *Man Over Money* (1980); Norman Pollack, *The Populist Response to Industrial America* (1962); Theodore Saloutos, *Farmer Movements in the South, 1865–1933* (1960); Barton Shaw, *The Wool-Hat Boys: Georgia's Populist Party* (1984); C. Vann Woodward, *Tom Watson, Agrarian Rebel* (1938), and *The Origins of the New South* (1972); Allan Weinstein, *Prelude to Populism: Origins of the Silver Issue* (1970).

The Depression of 1893 and the Election of 1896
Paolo Coletta, *William Jennings Bryan: Political Evangelist* (1964); Robert F. Durden, *The Climax of Populism: The Election of 1896* (1965); Ray Ginger, *Altgeld's America* (1958); Paul W. Glad, *McKinley, Bryan, and the People* (1964), and *The Trumpet Soundeth* (1960); Charles Hoffman, *The Depression of the Nineties: An Economic History* (1970); J. Rogers Hollingsworth, *The Whirligig of Politics: The Democracy of Cleveland and Bryan* (1963); Stanley Jones, *The Presidential Election of 1896* (1964); Louis Koenig, *Bryan* (1971); Samuel McSeveney, *The Politics of Depression* (1972).

CHAPTER 22

General

Richard Bannister, *Social Darwinism* (1979); Robert Beisner, *From the Old Diplomacy to the New, 1865–1900* (1975); Charles Campbell, *The Transformation of American Foreign Relations, 1865–1900* (1976), and *From Revolution to Rapprochement: The United States and Great Britain, 1783–1903* (1974); Richard Challener, *Admirals, Generals and American Foreign Policy, 1889–1914* (1973); John Dobson, *America's Ascent: The United States Becomes a Great Power, 1880–1914* (1978); John Lewis Gaddis, *Russia, the Soviet Union, and the United States* (1978); John A. S. Grenville and George Young, *Politics, Strategy, and American Diplomacy* (1967); Richard Hofstadter, *Social Darwinism in American Thought* (rev. ed., 1959); Ronald Jensen, *The Alaska Purchase and Russian-American Relations* (1970); David Pletcher, *The Awkward Years* (1962); Emily Rosenberg, *Spreading the American Dream* (1982); Tom Terrill, *The Tariff, Politics, and American Foreign Policy, 1874–1901* (1973); Mira Wilkins, *The Emergence of the Multinational Enterprise* (1970); William A. Williams, *The Tragedy of American Diplomacy* (rev. ed., 1962).

The Question of Imperialism

David Anderson, *Imperialism and Idealism: American Diplomats in China, 1861–1898* (1986); William Becker, *The Dynamics of Business-Government Relations* (1982); Robert L. Beisner, *Twelve Against Empire* (1968); Phillip Darby, *Three Faces of Imperialism: British and American Approaches to Asia and Africa, 1870–1970* (1987); Philip S. Foner, *The Spanish-Cuban-American War and the Birth of American Imperialism*, 2 vols., (1972); Frank Friedel, *The Splendid Little War* (1958); Willard Gatewood, Jr., *Black Americans and the White Man's Burden, 1898–1903* (1975); Kenneth Hagan, *American Gun-Boat Diplomacy, 1877–1889* (1973); David Healy, *U.S. Expansionism* (1970); Michael Hunt, *Ideology and U.S. Foreign Policy* (1987); Walter LaFeber, *The New Empire* (1963); Frederick Merk, *Manifest Destiny and Mission in American History* (1963); Wolfgang Mommsen and Jurgen Osterhammel, eds., *Imperialism and After* (1986); H. Wayne Morgan, *America's Road to Empire: The War With Spain and Overseas Expansion* (1965); Thomas J. Osborne, *Empire Can Wait: American Opposition to Hawaiian Annexation, 1893–1898* (1981); Ernest Paolino, *The Foundations of American Empire* (1973); Thomas Paterson, ed., *Imperialism and Anti-Imperialism* (1973); Bradford Perkins, *The Great Rapprochement* (1968); Julius Pratt, *The Expansionists of 1898* (1936); Tony Smith, *The Pattern of Imperialism: The United States, Great Britain and the Late Industrializing World Since 1815* (1982); Richard Turk, *The Ambiguous Relationship: Theodore Roosevelt and Alfred Thayer Mahan* (1987).

The United States and Asia

David Anderson, *Imperialism and Idealism: American Diplomacy in China, 1861–1898* (1985); Warren Cohen, *America's Response to China* (rev. ed., 1980); Michael Hunt, *The Making of a Special Relationship: The United States and China to 1914* (1983); Jane Hunter, *The Gospel of Gentility: American Women Missionaries in Turn-of-the-Century China* (1984); Akira Iriye, *Across the Pacific* (1967) and *Pacific Estrangement: Japanese and*

American Expansion, 1897–1911 (1972); Yur-Bok Lee and Wayne Patterson, eds., *One Hundred Years of Korean-American Relations, 1882–1982* (1986); Ernest May and John Fairbanks, eds., *America's China Trade in Historical Perspective* (1986); Glenn May, *Social Engineering in the Philippines* (1980); Thomas McCormick, *China Market: America's Quest for Informal Empire, 1893–1901* (1968); Charles Neu, *The Troubled Encounter* (1975); Peter Stanley, *A Nation in the Making: The Philippines and the United States* (1974); Randall Stross, *The Hard Earth: American Agriculturalists on Chinese Soil, 1898–1937* (1986); James Thomson, Peter Stanley, and John Perry, *Sentimental Imperialists: The American Experience in East Asia* (1981); Robert Welch, Jr., *Response to Imperialism: The United States and the Philippine-American War, 1899–1902* (1979); Marilyn B. Young, *Rhetoric of Empire: American China Policy, 1895–1901* (1968).

The United States and the Americas

Robert Brown, *Canada's National Policy, 1883–1900* (1964); Kenneth Bourne, *Britain and the Balance of Power in North America, 1815–1908* (1967); Walter LaFeber, *Inevitable Revolutions: The United States in Central America* (rev. ed., 1984); Lester Langley, *The Banana Wars* (1983), and *The United States and the Caribbean, 1900–1970* (1980); Louis Perez, Jr., *Cuba under the Platt Amendment, 1902–1934* (1986), and *Cuba Between Empires, 1878–1902* (1983); Dexter Perkins, *The Monroe Doctrine, 1867–1907* (1937); Ramon Ruiz, *Cuba* (1968); Karl Schmitt, *Mexico and the United States, 1821–1973* (1974); Josefina Vazquez and Lorenzo Meyer, *The United States and Mexico* (1985).

CHAPTER 23

General Studies

John Chambers II, *The Tyranny of Change: America in the Progressive Era, 1900–1917* (1980); Arthur Ekrich, *Progressivism in America* (1974); Lewis Gould, ed., *The Progressive Era* (1974); Richard Hofstader, *The Age of Reform: From Bryan to FDR* (1955); Gabriel Kolko, *The Triumph of Conservatism* (1963); Arthur Link and Richard L. McCormick, *Progressivism* (1983); William O'Neill, *The Progressive Years* (1975); James Weinstein, *The Corporate Ideal in the Liberal States, 1900–1918* (1969); Robert Wiebe, *Businessmen and Reform: A Study of the Progressive Movement* (1962).

The Progressive Impulse

Daniel Aaron, *Men of Good Hope: A Story of American Progressives* (1951); Richard Abrams, *The Burdens of Progress* (1978); Robert H. Bremner, *From the Depths: The Discovery of Poverty in the United States* (1956); David Chalmers, *The Social and Political Ideas of the Muckrakers* (1964); Clarke Chambers, *Paul U. Kellog and the Survey* (1971); Robert Crunden, *Ministers of Reform: The Progressives' Achievements in American Civilization, 1889–1920* (1982); Charles Forcey, *The Crossroads of Liberalism: Croly, Weyl, Lippmann and the Progressive Era, 1900–1925* (1961); William Hutchinson, *The Modernist Impulse in American Protestantism* (1976); Roy Lubove, *The Professional Altruist: The Emergence of Social Work as a Career, 1880–1930* (1965); D. W. Marcell, *Progress and Pragmatism: James,*

Dewey, Beard and the American Idea of Progress (1974); Daniel Nelson, *Frederick W. Taylor and the Rise of Scientific Management* (1980); David Noble, *The Progressive Mind, 1890–1917* (rev. ed., 1981); Morton White, *Social Thought in America: The Revolt Against Formalism*, (1949); Harold Wilson, *McClure's Magazine and the Muckrakers* (1970).

Social Reform and Minority Rights
Allen F. Davis, *American Heroine: The Life and Legend of Jane Addams* (1973), and *Spearheads of Reform: The Social Settlements and the Progressive Movement, 1890–1919* (1967); Louis Harlan, *Separate and Unequal: Public School Campaigns and Racism in the Southern Seaboard States, 1900–1915* (1968); Charles F. Kellogg, *NAACP: A History of the National Association for the Advancement of Colored People, 1909–1920* (1967); Roy Lubove, *The Progressives and the Slums: Tenement House Reform in New York City* (1962); James McPherson, *The Abolitionist Legacy: From Reconstruction to the NAACP* (1975); David Musto, *The American Disease: Origins of Narcotics Control* (1973); Elliot M. Rudwick, *W.E.B. DuBois* (1968); James Timberlake, *Prohibition and the Progressive Campaign* (1963).

Women
Paula Baker, *Gender and the Transformation of Politics: Public and Private Life in New York, 1870–1930* (1989); Nancy F. Cott, *The Grounding of Modern Feminism* (1987); Nancy Dye, *As Equals and Sisters: Feminism, the Labor Movement, and the Women's Trade Union League of New York* (1980); Linda Gordon, *Woman's Body, Woman's Right: A Social History of Birth Control* (1976); David Kennedy, *Birth Control in America: The Career of Margaret Sanger* (1970); Aileen Kraditor, *Ideas of the Woman Suffrage Movement* (1965); Ellen Lagemann, *A Generation of Women: Education in the Lives of Progressive Reformers* (1979); David Morgan, *Suffragists and Democrats: The Politics of Woman Suffrage in America* (1972); William O'Neil, *Divorce in the Progressive Era* (1967); Ruth Rosen, *The Lost Sisterhood: Prostitutes in America, 1900–1918* (1982); Rosalind Rosenberg, *Beyond Separate Spheres: Intellectual Roots of Modern Feminism* (1982).

Education, the New Professionalism, and Entertainment
Burton Bledstein, *The Culture of Professionalism* (1976); Lawrence Cremin, *The Transformation of the School: Progressivism in American Education* (1961); John DiMeglio, *Vaudeville U.S.A.* (1973); Lewis Erenberg, *Steppin' Out: New York Nightlife and the Transformation of American Culture, 1890–1930* (1981); James Farrell, *Inventing the American Way of Death, 1830–1920* (1980); Thomas Haskell, *The Emergence of Professional Social Science* (1977); Bruce Kuklick, *The Rise of American Philosophy* (1977); Martin Laforse and James Drake, *Popular Culture and American Life: Selected Topics in the Study of American Popular Culture* (1981); Robert Sklar, *Movie-Made America: A Social History of the American Movies* (1975); Paul Starr, *The Social Transformation of American Medicine* (1982); David Tyack and Elizabeth Hansot, *Managers of Virtue: Public School Leadership in America, 1820–1980* (1982); Lawrence Vesey, *The Emergence of the American University* (1970).

Local and State Reform
Richard Abrams, *Conservatism in a Progressive Era: Massachusetts Politics, 1900–1912* (1964); John Buenker, *Urban Liberalism and Progressive Reform* (1973); James Crooks, *Politics and Progress: The Rise of Urban Progressivism in Baltimore, 1895–1911* (1968); Dewey Grantham, *Southern Progressivism: The Reconciliation of Progress and Tradition* (1983); Melvin Holli, *Reform in Detroit: Hazen S. Pingree and Urban Politics* (1969); Jack Kirby, *Darkness at Dawning: Race and Reform in the Progressive South* (1972); Richard L. McCormick, *From Realignment to Reform: Political Change in New York State, 1893–1910* (1981); George Mowry, *The California Progressives* (1951); Bradley Rice, *Progressive Cities: The Commission Government Movement in America, 1901–1920* (1977); Jack Tager, *The Intellectual as Urban Reformer: Brand Whitlock and The Progressive Movement* (1968); David P. Thelen, *The New Citizenship: Origins of Progressivism in Wisconsin* (1972), and *Robert LaFollette and the Insurgent Spirit* (1976).

National Politics and Public Policy
Donald Anderson, *William Howard Taft* (1973), John Blum, *The Republican Roosevelt* (1954); John Blum, *Woodrow Wilson and the Politics of Morality* (1954); John Milton Cooper, Jr., *The Warrior and the Priest: Woodrow Wilson and Theodore Roosevelt* (1983); John Gable, *The Bull Moose Years* (1978); Alexander George and Juliette George, *Woodrow Wilson and Colonel House: A Personality Study* (1956); Lewis Gould, *Reform and Regulation: American Politics, 1900–1916* (1978); Samuel Hays, *Conservation and the Gospel of Efficiency: The Progressive Conservation Movement, 1890–1920* (1959); James Holt, *Congressional Insurgents and the Party System* (1969); Arthur Link, *Woodrow Wilson*, 5 vols. (1947–1965), and *Woodrow Wilson and the Progressive Era, 1910–1917* (1954); Albro Martin, *Enterprise Denied: Origins of the Decline of American Railroads, 1897–1917*, David McCullough, *Mornings on Horseback* (1981); Michael McGerr, *The Decline of Popular Politics: The American North, 1865–1928* (1986); Edmund Morris, *The Rise of Theodore Roosevelt* (1979); George Mowry, *The Era of Theodore Roosevelt* (1958); James Penick, *Progressive Politics and Conservation: The Ballinger-Pinchot Affair* (1968); Harold Pinkett, *Gifford Pinchot: Private and Public Forester* (1970); Edwin Weinstein, *Woodrow Wilson: A Medical and Psychological Biography* (1981); Craig West, *Banking Reform and the Federal Reserve, 1863–1923* (1977); Clifton Yearley, *The Money Machines* (1970).

CHAPTER 24

General
Paul Abrahams, *The Foreign Expansion of American Finance and Its Relationship to Foreign Economic Policies of the United States, 1907–1921* (1976); Robert Beisner, *From the Old Diplomacy to the New, 1865–1900* (1975); John Dobson, *America's Ascent: The United States Becomes a Great Power, 1880–1914* (1978); Morrell Heald and Lawrence Kaplan, *Culture and Diplomacy* (1977); Peter Karsten, *The Naval Aristocracy* (1972); Robert Osgood, *Ideals and Self-Interest in America's Foreign Relations* (1953); Emily Rosenberg, *Spreading the American Dream: American Economic and Cultural Expansion, 1890–1945* (1982); Robert

Schulzinger, *American Diplomacy in the Twentieth Century* (1984); Tom Terrill, *The Tariff, Politics, and American Foreign Policy, 1874–1901* (1973); Rubin Weston, *Racism and U.S. Imperialism, 1865–1946* (1971); Mira Wilkins, *The Emergence of the Multinational Enterprise* (1970).

Roosevelt, Taft, and Wilson
Howard K. Beale, *Theodore Roosevelt and the Rise of America to World Power* (1956); David Burton, *Theodore Roosevelt: Confident Imperialist* (1968); Robert W. Cherney, *A Righteous Cause: The Life of William Jennings Bryan* (1985); Richard H. Collin, *Theodore Roosevelt, Culture, Diplomacy, and Expansion* (1985); John Cooper, Jr., *Walter Hines Page* (1977); Lloyd Gardner, *Wilson and Revolutions, 1913–1921* (1976); *William Jennings Bryan: Missionary Isolationist* (1983); Arthur Link, *Wilson: The Diplomatist* (1957) and *Woodrow Wilson: Revolution, War, and Peace* (1979); Frederick Marks III, *Velvet on Iron: The Diplomacy of Theodore Roosevelt* (1979); Ralph E. Minger, *William Howard Taft and United States Foreign Policy* (1975).

Asia, the Pacific, and Latin America
Warren Cohen, *America's Response to China* (rev. ed., 1980); Akira Iriye, *Pacific Estrangement: Japanese and American Expansion, 1897–1911* (1972); Jerry Israel, *Progressivism and the Open Door* (1971); David Healy, *Gunboat Diplomacy in the Wilson Era: The U.S. Navy in Haiti, 1915–1916* (1976); Walter LaFeber, *The Panama Canal* (1978); Lester Langley, *Struggle for the American Mediterranean* and *The United States and the Caribbean, 1900–1970* (1980); Glenn May, *Social Engineering in the Philippines* (1980); Robert McClellan, *The Heathen Chinese: A Study of American Attitudes Toward China* (1971); David McCullough, *The Path Between the Seas: The Creation of the Panama Canal, 1870–1914* (1977); Dana Munro, *Intervention and Dollar Diplomacy in the Caribbean, 1900–1920* (1964); Charles Neu, *The Troubled Encounter* (1975); Robert Smith, *The United States and Revolutionary Nationalism in Mexico, 1916–1932* (1972); Peter Stanley, *A Nation in the Making: The Philippines and the United States, 1899–1921* (1974).

From Neutrality to War
Thomas Baily and Paul Ryan, *The Lusitania Disaster* (1975); John Coogan, *The End of Neutrality: The United States, Britain, and Maritime Rights, 1899–1915* (1981); John Cooper, *The Vanity of Power: American Isolationism and the First World War* (1969); Patrick Devlin, *Too Proud to Fight: Woodrow Wilson's Neutrality* (1974); Ross Gregory, *The Origins of American Intervention in the First World War* (1977); Burton Kaufman, *Efficiency and Expansion: Foreign Trade Organization in the Wilson Administration* (1974); Roland Marchand, *The American Peace Movement and Social Reform* (1973); Ernest May, *The World War and American Isolationism, 1914–1917* (1959); Jeffrey Safford, *Wilsonian Maritime Diplomacy* (1977).

The First World War Abroad
Arthur Barbeau and Henri Florette, *The Unknown Soldiers: Black American Troops in World War I* (1974); Edward Coffman, *The War to End All Wars: The American Military Experience in World War I* (1968); Paul

Fussell, *The Great War and Modern Memory* (1975); John Gifford, *The Citizen Soldiers* (1972); Otis Graham, *The Great Campaigns* (1971); Maurine Greenwald, *Women, War, and Work* (1980); N. Gordon Levin, Jr., *Woodrow Wilson and World Politics: America's Response to War and Revolution* (1968); Laurence Stallings, *The Doughboys: The Story of the AEF, 1917–1918* (1963); Frank Vandiver, *The Life and Times of John J. Pershing*, 2 vols. (1977).

The Homefront
Valerie Conner, *The National War Labor Board: Stability, Social Justice, and the Voluntary State in World War I* (1983); Robert Cuff, *The War Industries Board: Business Government-Relations During World War I* (1973); Carol Gruber, *Mars and Minerva: World War I and the Uses of Higher Learning in America* (1975); Ellis Hawley, *The Great War and the Search for Modern Order* (1979); Robert Haynes, *A Night of Violence: The Houston Riot of 1917* (1976); David Kennedy, *Over Here: The First World War and American Society* (1980); Seward Livermore, *Politics Is Adjourned: Woodrow Wilson and the War Congress, 1917–1918* (1966); Frederick Luebke, *Bonds of Loyalty: German Americans and World War I* (1974); Paul Murphy, *World War I and the Origins of Civil Liberties* (1979); Jordan Schwarz, *The Speculator: Bernard M. Baruch in Washington, 1917–1965* (1981); Barbara Steinson, *American Women's Activism in World War I* (1982); Stephen Vaughn, *Holding Fast the Inner Lines: Democracy, Nationalism, and the Committee on Public Information* (1979); James Weinstein, *The Decline of Socialism in America, 1912–1923* (1967).

Versailles
Thomas Bailey, *Woodrow Wilson and the Great Betrayal* (1945), and *Woodrow Wilson and the Lost Peace* (1944); Robert Ferrell, *Woodrow Wilson and World War I* (1985); Inga Floto, *Colonel House at Paris* (1980); John Gaddis, *Russia, the Soviet Union, and the United States* (1978); Lloyd Gardner, *Safe for Democracy: The Anglo-American Response to Revolution, 1913–1923* (1984); Arno Mayer, *Politics and Diplomacy of Peacemaking* (1965); Charles Mee, Jr., *The End of Order, Versailles, 1919* (1980); Ralph Stone, *The Irreconcilables: The Fight Against the League of Nations* (1970); Ralph Stone, *The Irreconcilables* (1970).

Aftermath
David Brody, *Labor in Crisis* (1965); Stanley Coben, *A. Mitchell Palmer* (1963); Stanley Cooperman, *World War I and the American Mind* (1970); Roberta Feuerlicht, *Justice Crucified* (1977); Robert Murray, *The Red Scare* (1955); Burl Noggle, *Into the Twenties* (1977); Stuart Rochester, *American Liberal Disillusionment in the Wake of World War I* (1977); Francis Russell, *A City in Terror* (1975); William Tuttle, Jr., *Race Riot: Chicago in the Red Summer of 1919* (1970); Stephen Ward, ed., *The War Generation: Veterans of the First World War* (1975).

CHAPTER 25

General Studies
Frederick Lewis Allen, *Only Yesterday: An Informal History of the 1920s* (1931); John Braeman et al., ed.,

Change and Continuity in Twentieth Century America: The 1920s (1968); John Hicks, *The Republican Ascendancy, 1921–1933* (1960); Isabel Leighton, ed., *The Aspirin Age* (1949); William Leuchtenburg, *The Perils of Prosperity, 1914–1932* (1958); Donald McCoy, *Coming of Age* (1973); Geoffrey Perrett, *America in the Twenties* (1982); Arthur Schlesinger, Jr., *The Crisis of the Old Order* (1957); David Shannon, *Between the Wars: America, 1919–1940* (1979).

Economics, Business, and Labor

Irving Bernstein, *The Lean Years: A History of the American Worker, 1920–1933* (1960); David Brody, *Steelworkers in America* (1960), and *Workers in Industrial America* (1980); Alfred Chandler, *Strategy and Structure: Chapters in the History of American Inustrial Enterprise* (1962); Ed Cray, *Chrome Colossus: General Motors and Its Times* (1980); Gilbert Fite, *George Peek and the Fight for Farm Parity* (1954); James Flink, *The Car Culture* (1975); Louis Galambos, *Competition and Cooperation* (1966); James Gilbert, *Designing the Industrial State* (1972); Allan Nevins and Frank Hill, *Ford*, 3 vols. (1954–1963); Jim Potter, *The American Economy Between the Wars* (1974); John Rae, *American Automobile* (1965), and *The Road and the Car in American Life* (1971); George Soule, *Prosperity Decade* (1947); Keith Sward, *The Legend of Henry Ford* (1948); Leslie Woodcock Tentler, *Wage Earning Women: Industrial Work and Family Life in the United States, 1900–1930* (1979); Bernard Weisberger, *The Dream Maker* (1979) [about Will Durant, President of General Motors]; Robert Zieger, *Republicans and Labor, 1919–1929* (1969).

Mass Society and Mass Culture

Erick Barnouw, *A Tower of Babel: A History of American Broadcasting in the United States to 1933* (1966); Daniel Boorstin, *The Americans: The Democratic Experience* (1973); Paul Carter, *Another Part of the Twenties* (1977); Robert Creamer, *Babe* (1974); Kenneth Davis, *The Hero: Charles A. Lindbergh* (1954); Stuart Ewing, *Captains of Consciousness* (1976); Robert Lynd and Helen Lynd, *Middletown: A Study in Modern Culture* (1929); Roland Marchand, *Advertising the American Dream: Making Way for Modernity, 1920–1940* (1985); Lary May, *Screening Out the Past* (1980); Leonard Mosley, *Lindbergh: A Biography* (1976); Otis Pease, *The Responsibilities of American Advertising* (1959); Daniel Pope, *The Making of Modern Advertising* (1983); Randy Roberts, *Jack Dempsey, The Manassa Mauler* (1979); Philip Rosen, *The Modern Stentors: Radio Broadcasting and the Federal Government, 1920–1933* (1980); Robert Sklar, *Movie-Made America: A Cultural History of American Movies* (1975).

High Culture

Carlos Baker, *Hemingway* (1956); Malcolm Cowley, *Exile's Return* (1934); Robert Crunden, *From Self to Society: Transition in Modern Thought, 1919–1941* (1972); Frederick Hoffman, *The Twenties* (1949); Arthur Mizner, *The Far Side of Paradise* (1951); Roderick Nash, *The Nervous Generation: American Thought, 1917–1930* (1969), Mark Shorer, *Sinclair Lewis* (1961); Marvin Singleton, *H.L. Mencken and the "American Mercury" Adventure* (1962); Edmund Wilson, *The Twenties* (1975).

Women, Youth, and Minorities

Lois Banner, *American Beauty* (1983); William Chafe, *The American Women: Her Changing Social, Economic, and Political Roles, 1920–1970* (1972); David Cronon, *Black Moses: The Story of Marcus Garvey* (1955); Paula Fass, *The Damned and Beautiful: American Youth in the 1920s* (1977); Linda Gordon, *Woman's Body, Woman's Right: A Social History of Birth Control in America* (1976); Nathan Huggins, *Harlem Renaissance* (1971); J. Stanley Lemons, *The Woman Citizen: Social Feminism in the 1920s* (1973); David Lewis, *When Harlem Was in Vogue* (1981); Glenna Matthews, *"Just a Housewife!" The Rise and Fall of Domesticity in America* (1987); Wilson Moses, *The Golden Age of Black Nationalism, 1850–1925* (1988); Arnold Rampersad, *The Life of Langston Hughes*, 2 vols. (1986–1988); Ricardo Romo, *East Los Angeles: History of a Barrio* (1983); Lois Scharf, *To Work and to Wed* (1980); Alan Spear, *Black Chicago* (1967); Joe Trotter, *Black Milwaukee: The Making of an Industrial Proletariat* (1985); Theodore Vincent, *Black Power and the Garvey Movement* (1971); Winifred Wandersee, *Women's Work and Family Values, 1920–1940* (1981).

Political Fundamentalism

David Burner, *The Politics of Provincialism* (1968); David Chalmers, *Hooded Americanism: The History of the Ku Klux Klan* (1965); Norman Clark, *Deliver Us from Evil* (1976); Robert Divine, *American Immigration Policy* (1957); Norman Furniss, *The Fundamentalist Controversy, 1918–1933* (1954); Ray Ginger, *Six Days or Forever? Tennessee v. John Scopes* (1958); Joseph Gusfeld, *Symbolic Crusade* (1963); John Higham, *Strangers in the Land: Patterns of American Nativism, 1860–1925* (1955); Kenneth Jackson, *The Ku Klux Klan in the City, 1915–1930* (1967); Don Kirschner, *City and Country: Rural Responses to Urbanization in the 1920s* (1970); George Marsden, *Fundamentalism and American Culture* (1980); Andrew Sinclair, *Prohibition: The Era of Excess* (1962); William Wilson, *Coming of Age: Urban America, 1915–1945* (1974).

Politics, Public Policy, and the Election of 1928

Kristi Andersen, *The Creation of a Democratic Majority* (1979); Paula Edler, *Governor Alfred E. Smith: The Politician as Reformer* (1983); James Giglio, *H. M. Daugherty and the Politics of Expediency* (1978); Oscar Handlin, *Al Smith and His America* (1958); Ellis Hawley, *Herbert Hoover as Secretary of Commerce: Studies in New Era Thought and Practice* (1974); Robert Himmelberg, *The Origins of the National Recovery Administration: Business, Government, and the Trade Association Issue, 1921–1933* (1976); J. Joseph Huthmacher, *Massachusetts People and Politics, 1919–1933* (1959); Alan Lichtman, *Prejudice and the Old Politics* (1979); Richard Lowitt, *George Norris*, 2 vols. (1971); Donald McCoy, *Calvin Coolidge* (1967); Robert Murray, *The Harding Era* (1969), and *The Politics of Normalcy* (1973); Burl Noggle, *Teapot Dome* (1962); Elisabeth Perry, *Belle Moskowitz: Feminine Politics and the Exercise of Power in the Age of Alfred E. Smith* (1987); George Tindall, *The Emergence of the New South* (1967); Eugene Trani and David Wilson, *The Presidency of Warren G. Harding* (1977).

CHAPTER 26

General Studies

Frederick Lewis Allen, *Since Yesterday* (1939); Lester Chandler, *America's Greatest Depression, 1929–1941* (1970); John Garraty, *The Great Depression: An Inquiry into the Causes, Course, and Consequences of the Worldwide Depression of the Nineteen Thirties as Seen by Contemporaries and in the Light of History* (1987); Charles Kindleberger, *The World in Depression* (1973); Robert McElvaine, *The Great Depression: America, 1929–1941* (1984); Broadus Mitchell, *Depression Decade* (1947); Arthur Schlesinger, Jr., *The Crisis of the Old Order* (1957).

The Great Crash and the Origins of the Great Depression

Milton Friedman and Ana Schwartz, *The Great Contraction* (1965); John Galbraith, *The Great Crash* (1988); Susan Kennedy, *The Banking Crisis of 1933* (1973); Robert Sobel, *The Great Bull Market: Wall Street in the 1920s* (1968); Peter Temin, *Did Monetary Forces Cause the Great Depression?* (1976); Gordon Thomas and Max Morgan-Witts, *The Day the Bubble Burst: The Social History of the Wall Street Crash of 1929* (1979).

Depression Life

Edward Anderson, *Hungry Men* (1935); Robert Angell, *The Family Encounters the Depression* (1936); Ann Banks, *First Person America* (1980); Caroline Bird, *The Invisible Scar* (1966); The Federal Writers' Project, *These Are Our Lives* (1939); John Garraty, *Unemployment in History: Economic Thought and Public Policy* (1978); Mirra Komarovsky, *The Unemployed Man and His Family* (1940); Robert Lynd and Helen Lynd, *Middletown in Transition* (1937); Robert McElvaine, ed., *Down & Out in the Great Depression* (1983); H. Wayne Morgan, *Drugs in America: A Social History, 1800–1980* (1981); David Musto, *The American Disease, Origins of Narcotics Control* (rev. ed., 1988); Lois Scharf, *To Work and to Wed: Female Employment, Feminism, and the Great Depression* (1980); Studs Terkel, *Hard Times: An Oral History of the Great Depression* (1970); Tom Terrill and Jerrold Hirsch, eds., *Such as Us: Southern Voices of the Thirties* (1978); Winifred Wandersee, *Women's Work and Family Values, 1920–1940* (1981); Susan Ware, *Holding Their Own: American Women in the 1930s* (1982); Jeane Westin, *Making Do: How Women Survived the '30s* (1976).

Ethnicity and Race

Rodolfo Acuna, *Occupied America* (rev. ed., 1981); Ralph Bunche, *The Political Status of the Negro in the Age of FDR* (1973); Dan Carter, *Scottsboro: A Tragedy of the American South* (1969); Sarah Deutsch, *No Separate Refuge: Culture, Class, and Gender on an Anglo-Hispanic Frontier in the American Southwest, 1880–1940* (1987); Abraham Hoffman, *Unwanted Mexican-Americans in the Great Depression* (1974); Richard Polenberg, *One Nation Divisible: Class, Race, and Ethnicity in the United States Since 1938* (1980); Bernard Sternsher, ed., *The Negro in Depression and War* (1969); Robert Weisbrot, *Father Divine and the Struggle for Racial Equality* (1983); Nancy Weiss, *The National Urban League* (1974); Raymond Wolters, *Negroes and the Great Depression* (1970).

Depression Culture

Daniel Aaron, *Writers on the Left* (1961); James Agee, *Let Us Now Praise Famous Men* (1941); Andrew Bergman, *We're in the Money: Depression America and Its Films* (1971); Eileen Eagan, *Class, Culture and the Classroom* (1981); Neal Gabler, *An Empire of Their Own: How the Jews Invented Hollywood* (1988); Richard Pells, *Radical Visions and American Dreams* (1973); John Steinbeck, *The Grapes of Wrath* (1939); William Stott, *Documentary Expressionism and Thirties America* (1973); Warren Susman, *Culture as History: The Transformation of American Society in the Twentieth Century* (1984); Twelve Southerners, *I'll Take My Stand: The South and the Agrarian Tradition* (1937).

Radicalism and Protest

Irving Bernstein, *The Lean Years: A History of the American Worker, 1920–1933* (1960); Roger Daniels, *The Bonus March* (1971); John Hevener, *Which Side You On? The Harlan County Coal Miners, 1931–1939* (1978); Harvey Klehr, *The Heyday of American Communism: The Depression Decade* (1983); Donald Lisio, *The President and Protest: Hoover, Conspiracy, and the Bonus Riot* (1974); Mark Naison, *Communists in Harlem During the Depression* (1983); Theodore Saloutos and John Hicks, *Twentieth Century Populism: Agrarian Protest in the Middle West, 1900–1939* (1951); John Shover, *Cornbelt Rebellion: The Farmers' Holiday Association* (1965).

The Hoover Years

David Burner, *Herbert Hoover: A Public Life* (1979); Martin Fausold, *The Presidency of Herbert C. Hoover* (1985); Martin Fausold and George Mazuzun, eds, *The Hoover Presidency* (1974); George Nash, *The Life of Herbert Hoover* (1983); James Olson, *Herbert Hoover and the Reconstruction Finance Corporation* (1977); Albert Romasco, *The Poverty of Abundance: Hoover, The Nation, the Depression* (1965); Elliot A. Rosen, *Hoover, Roosevelt, and the Brains Trust: From Depression to New Deal* (1977); Jordan Schwarz, *The Interregnum of Despair* (1970); Joan Hoff Wilson, *Herbert Hoover: Forgotten Progressive* (1975).

CHAPTER 27

General Studies

John Braeman et al., *The New Deal*, 2 vols. (1975); Paul Conkin, *The New Deal* (1967); Otis Graham, Jr., *Encore for Reform: The Old Progressives and the New Deal* (1967); Barry Karl, *The Uneasy State* (1983); William Leuchtenburg, *Franklin D. Roosevelt and the New Deal* (1963); Robert McElvaine, *The Great Depression: America, 1929–1941* (1984); Gerald Nash, *The Great Depression and World War II* (1979); Harvard Sitkoff, ed., *Fifty Years Later: The New Deal Evaluated* (1985).

Franklin and Eleanor

James Burns, *Roosevelt: The Lion and the Fox* (1956); Kenneth Davis, *FDR*, 2 vols. (1972–1986); Frank Freidel, *Franklin D. Roosevelt*, 4 vols. (1952–1973); Joseph Lash, *Eleanor and Franklin* (1971); Ted Morgan, *FDR: A Biography* (1985); Eleanor Roosevelt, *This Is My Story* (1937), and *This I Remember* (1949); Lois Scharf, *Eleanor Roosevelt: First Lady of American Liberalism* (1987); Arthur Schlesinger, Jr., *The Age of Roosevelt*, 3 vols. (1957–1960); Rexford Tugwell, *The Democratic Roosevelt: A Biography of Franklin D. Roosevelt* (1957); Geoffrey Ward, *Before the Trumpet: Young Franklin Roosevelt* (1985), and *A First Class Temperament: The Emergence of Franklin Roosevelt* (1989).

The New Dealers
Michael Beschloss, *Kennedy and Roosevelt: The Uneasy Alliance* (1980); John Blum, *From the Morgenthau Diaries*, 3 vols. (1959–1965); Harold Ickes, *The Secret Diaries of Harold L. Ickes*, 3 vols. (1953–1954); Peter Irons, *The New Deal Lawyers* (1982); Joseph Lash, *Dealers and Dreamers: A New Look at the New Deal* (1988); Katie Lochheim, ed., *The Making of the New Deal: The Insiders Speak* (1983); George Martin, *Madame Secretary: Frances Perkins* (1976); George McJimsey, *Harry Hopkins: Ally of the Poor and Defender of Democracy* (1987); Raymond Moley, *After Seven Years* (1939); Frances Perkins, *The Roosevelt I Knew* (1946); Samuel Rosenman, *Working for Roosevelt* (1952); Jordan Schwarz, *Liberal: Adolf A. Berle and the Vision of an American Era* (1987); Robert Sherwood, *Roosevelt and Hopkins: An Intimate History* (1948); Bernard Sternsher, *Rexford Tugwell and the New Deal* (1964); Susan Ware, *Partner and I: Molly Dewson, Feminism, and New Deal Politics* (1987).

Recovery and Reform
Bernard Belush, *The Failure of the NRA* (1975); Ellis Hawley, *The New Deal and the Problems of Monopoly* (1966); Barry Karl, *Executive Reorganization and Reform in the New Deal* (1963); Mark Leff, *The Limits of Symbolic Reform: The New Deal and Taxation, 1933–1939* (1984); Thomas McCraw, *TVA and the Public Power Fight* (1970); James Olson, *Saving Capitalism: The RFC and the New Deal, 1933–1940* (1988); Michael Parrish, *Securities Regulation and the New Deal* (1970); Richard Polenberg, *Reorganizing Roosevelt's Government* (1966); Albert Romasco, *The Politics of Recovery: Roosevelt's New Deal* (1983).

Agriculture
Sidney Baldwin, *Poverty and Politics: The Rise and Decline of the Farm Security Administration* (1967); David Conrad, *The Forgotten Farmers: The Story of Sharecroppers in the New Deal* (1965); Richard Kirkendall, *Social Scientists and Farm Politics in the Age of Roosevelt* (1966); Paul Mertz, *The New Deal and Southern Rural Poverty* (1978); W. D. Rowley, *M. L. Wilson and the Campaign for Domestic Allotment* (1970); Walter Stein, *California and the Dust Bowl Migration* (1973); Van Perkins, *Crisis in Agriculture* (1969); Donald Worster, *Dust Bowl: The Southern Plains in the 1930s* (1979).

Relief and the Rise of the Semi-Welfare State
Searle Charles, *Minister of Relief* (1963) [about Harry Hopkins]; Paul Conkin, *FDR and the Origins of the Welfare State* (1967) and *Tomorrow a New World* (1971); Phoebe Cutler, *The Public Landscape of the New Deal* (1986); Richard Lowitt and Maurine Beasley, eds., *One Third of a Nation: Lorena Hickok Reports on the Great Depression* (1981); Roy Lubove, *The Struggle for Social Security* (1968); Jerre Mangione, *The Dream and the Deal: The Federal Writers' Project, 1935–1943* (1972); Jane deHart Matthews, *The Federal Theater, 1935–1939* (1967); Richard McKinzie, *The New Deal for Artists* (1973); Francis O'Connor, ed., *Art for the Millions: Es-*

says from the 1930s by Artists and Administrators of the WPA Federal Art Project* (1973); Karen Becker Orhn, *Dorothea Lange and the Documentary Tradition* (1980); Marlene Park and Gerald Markowitz, *Democratic Vistas: Post Offices and Public Art in the New Deal* (1984); John Salmond, *The Civilian Conservation Corps* (1967); Bonnie Schwartz, *The Civil Works Administration, 1933–1934* (1984).

Dissent and Protest
Alan Brinkley, *Voices of Protest: Huey Long, Father Coughlin, and the Great Depression* (1982); Donald Grubbs, *Cry from Cotton: The Southern Tenant Farmers Union and the New Deal* (1971); Abraham Holzman, *The Townsend Movement* (1963); Glen Jeansonne, *Gerald L. K. Smith: Minister of Hate* (1988); R. Alan Lawson, *The Failure of Independent Liberalism, 1930–1941* (1971); Leo Ribuffo, *The Old Christian Right: The Protestant Far Right from the Great Depression to the Cold War* (1983); Charles Tull, *Father Coughlin and the New Deal* (1965); T. Harry Williams, *Huey Long* (1969); Frank Warren, *Liberals and Communism: The "Red Decade" Revisited* (1966), and *An Alternative Vision: The Socialist Party in the 1930s* (1976); George Wolfskill, *Revolt of the Conservatives: A History of the American Liberty League, 1934–1940* (1962).

Labor
Jerold Auerbach, *Labor and Liberty: The La Follette Committee and the New Deal* (1966); John Barnard, *Walter Reuther and the Rise of the Auto Workers* (1983); Irving Bernstein, *Turbulent Years: A History of the American Worker, 1933–1941* (1969); Melvyn Dubofsky and Warren Van Tine, *John L. Lewis: A Biography* (1977); Sidney Fine, *Sit-Down: The General Motors Strike of 1936 1937* (1969); Peter Friedlander, *The Emergence of a UAW Local* (1975); August Meier and Elliott Rudwick, *Black Detroit and the Rise of the UAW* (1979); David Milton, *The Politics of U.S. Labor: From the Great Depression to the New Deal* (1980); Ronald Schatz, *The Electrical Workers* (1983).

New Deal Politics
John Allswang, *The New Deal in American Politics* (1978); Frank Freidel, *FDR and the South* (1965); J. Joseph Huthmacher, *Senator Robert Wagner and the Rise of Urban Liberalism* (1968); James Patterson, *Congressional Conservatism and the New Deal* (1967), and *The New Deal and the States* (1969); William Leuchtenburg, "The Origins of Franklin D. Roosevelt's 'Court Packing' Plan," in Philip Kurland, ed., *The Supreme Court Review* (1966).

Minorities
Laurence Kelly, *The Assault on Assimilation: John Collier and the Origins of Indian Policy Reform, 1920–1954* (1983); John Kirby, *Black Americans in the Roosevelt Era: Liberalism and Race* (1980); Carey McWilliams, *North from Mexico* (1949); Donald Parman, *The New Deal and the Navajoes* (1976); Kenneth Philp, *John Collier's Crusade for Indian Reform, 1920–1934* (1977); Francis Prucha, *The Indians in American Society: From the Revolutionary War to the Present* (1985); Mark Reisler, *By the Sweat of Their Brow: Mexican Immigrant Labor in the United States, 1900–1940* (1976); Harvard Sitkoff, *A New Deal for Blacks* (1978); Raymond Walters,

Negroes and the Great Depression: The Problem of Economic Recovery (1970); Nancy Weiss, *Farewell to the Party of Lincoln: Black Politics in the Age of FDR* (1983); Robert Zangrando, *The NAACP Crusade Against Lynching* (1980).

CHAPTER 28

Diplomacy Before the War
Selig Adler, *The Uncertain Giant* (1965); Thomas Buckley, *The United States and the Washington Naval Conference, 1921–1922* (1970); Charles Chatfield, *For Peace and Justice: Pacifism in America, 1914–1941* (1971); Warren Cohen, *Empire Without Tears: American Foreign Relations, 1921–1933* (1988); Frank Costigliola, *Awkward Dominion: American Political, Economic, and Cultural Relations with Europe, 1919–1933* (1985); Charles DeBenedetti, *The Peace Reform Movement in American History* (1980), and *Origins of the Modern American Peace Movement, 1915–1929* (1978); Roger Dingman, *Power in the Pacific: The Origins of Naval Arms Limitation, 1914–1922* (1976); Robert Ferrell, *Peace in Their Time* (1952), and *American Diplomacy in the Great Depression* (1970); Peter Filene, *Americans and the Soviet Experiment, 1917–1933* (1967); John Lewis Gaddis, *Russia, the Soviet Union, and the United States* (1978); Akira Iriye, *After Imperialism: The Search for a New Order in the Far East, 1921–1931* (1965); Harold Josephson, *James T. Shotwell and the Rise of Internationalism in America* (1976); Melvyn Leffler, *The Elusive Quest* (1979); Elting E. Morison, *Turmoil and Tradition* (1964) [on Henry Stimson]; Arnold Offner, *The Origins of the Second World War* (1975); Stephen Rabe, *The Road to OPEC: U.S. Relations with Venezuela, 1919–1976* (1982); Raymond Sontag, *A Broken World, 1919–1939* (1971); Robert Schulzinger, *The Wise Men of Foreign Affairs: A History of the Council on Foreign Relations* (1984); Adam Ulam, *Expansion and Coexistence: Soviet Foreign Policy from 1917 to 1973* (rev. ed., 1974); Joan Hoff Wilson, *American Business and Foreign Policy, 1920–1933* (1968), and *Herbert Hoover* (1975).

The Roosevelt Era and the Coming of World War II
Dorothy Borg, *The United States and the Far Eastern Crisis of 1933–1938* (1964); James MacGregor Burns, *Roosevelt: The Lion and the Fox* (1956); Robert Dallek, *Franklin D. Roosevelt and American Foreign Policy, 1932–1945* (1979); Robert Divine, *The Reluctant Belligerent* (2d ed., 1979); Herbert Feis, *The Road to Pearl Harbor* (1950); John Findling, *Close Neighbors, Distant Friends: United States-Central American Relations* (1987); Lloyd Gardner, *Economic Aspects of New Deal Diplomacy* (1964); Irwin Gellman, *Good Neighbor Diplomacy* (1979); Betty Glad, *Key Pittman: The Tragedy of a Senate Insider* (1986); Patrick Headen, *Roosevelt Confronts Hitler: America's Entry into World War II* (1987); Warren Kimball, *The Most Unsordid Act: Lend Lease, 1939–1941* (1969); Walter LaFeber, *Inevitable Revolutions: The United States in Central America* (1983); Douglas Little, *Malevolent Neutrality: The United States, Great Britain, and the Origins of the Spanish Civil War* (1985); Lorenzo Meyer, *Mexico and the United States in the Oil Controversy, 1917–1942* (1977); Arthur Morse, *While Six Million Died* (1968); Gordon Prange, *At Dawn We Slept* (1981); David Reynolds, *The Creation of the Anglo-American Alliance,* *1937–1941* (1982); John Toland, *Infamy* (1982); Jonathan Utley, *Going to War with Japan, 1937–1941* (1985); Roberta Wohlstetter, *Pearl Harbor: Warning and Decision* (1962); Bryce Wood, *The Making of the Good Neighbor Policy* (1961); David Wyman, *The Abandonment of the Jews* (1984).

War and Strategy
John Dower, *War Without Mercy: Race and Power in the Pacific War* (1986); David Eisenhower, *Eisenhower at War, 1943–1945* (1986); B. H. Liddell Hart, *History of the Second World War* (1970); Max Hastings, *OVERLORD: D-Day and the Battle of Normandy* (1984); Akira Iriye, *Power and Culture: The Japanese-American War, 1941–1945* (1981); D. Clayton James, *The Years of MacArthur, 1941–1945* (1975) and (with Anne Sharp Wells), *A Time for Giants: Politics of the American High Command During World War II* (1987); Eric Larabee, *Commander in Chief: Franklin Delano Roosevelt, His Lieutenants, and Their War* (1987); William Manchester, *American Caesar* (1979); Samuel Eliot Morison, *The Two Ocean War* (1963); Bernard C. Nalty, *Strength for the Fight: A History of Black Americans in the Military* (1986); Forrest Pogue, *George C. Marshall*, 3 vols. (1963–1975); Ronald Schaffer, *Wings of Judgment: American Bombing in World War II* (1985); Michael Sherry, *The Rise of American Air Power* (1987); Bradley Smith, *The Shadow Warriors: O.S.S. and the Origins of the C.I.A.* (1983); Ronald Spector, *The Eagle Against the Sun: The American War With Japan* (1985); James Stokesbury, *A Short History of World War II* (1980).

War and Diplomacy
Henry Blumenthal, *Illusion and Reality in Franco-American Diplomacy, 1914–1945* (1982); Russell Buhite, *Decision at Yalta* (1986); James MacGregor Burns, *Roosevelt: The Soldier of Freedom* (1970); Winston Churchill, *The Second World War*, 6 vols. (1948–1953); Diane Shaver Clemens, *Yalta* (1970); Robert Divine, *Roosevelt and World War II* (1969); Herbert Feis, *Roosevelt, Churchill, Stalin: The War They Waged and the Peace They Sought* (1957); Fraser J. Harbutt, *The Iron Curtain: Churchill, America, and the Origins of the Cold War* (1986); George Herring, *Aid to Russia, 1941–1946* (1977); Warren Kimball, ed., *Churchill and Roosevelt: The Complete Correspondence, 1939–1945* (1984); Gabriel Kolko, *The Politics of War* (1968); William Roger Louis, *Imperialism at Bay: The United States and the Decolonization of the British Empire, 1941–1945* (1978); Mark H. Lytle, *The Origins of the Iranian-American Alliance, 1941–1953* (1987); William Hardy McNeill, *America, Britain, and Russia* (1953); David Painter, *Oil and the American Century: The Political Economy of U.S. Foreign Oil Policy, 1941–1954* (1986); Keith Sainsbury, *Roosevelt, Stalin, Churchill, and Chaing Kai Shek, 1943: The Moscow, Cairo, and Tehran Conferences* (1985); Martin Sherwin, *A World Destroyed: The Atomic Bomb and the Grand Alliance* (1975); Gaddis Smith, *American Diplomacy During the Second World War, 1941–1945* (2d ed., 1985); Michael B. Stoff, *Oil, War, and American Security: The Search for a National Policy on Foreign Oil, 1941–1947* (1980); Christopher Thorne, *Allies of a Kind: The United States, Great Britain, and the War Against Japan, 1941–1945* (1978); David Wyman, *The Abandonment of the Jews: America and the Holocaust, 1941–1945* (1984).

CHAPTER 29

Organizing for War

John M. Blum, "V" Was for Victory: Politics and American Culture During World War II (1976); David Brinkley, Washington Goes to War (1988); Bruce Catton, The War Lords of Washington (1948); George Flynn, The Mess in Washington: Manpower Mobilization in World War II (1979); Philip Funginiello, The Challenge to Urban Liberalism: Federal-City Relations During World War II (1978); Mark Harris et al., The Homefront (1984); Philip Knightly, The First Casualty (1975); Clayton Koppes and Gregory Black, Hollywood Goes to War (1987); Richard Lingeman, Don't You Know There's a War On? The American Home Front, 1941–1945 (1970); Gerald Nash, The American West Transformed: The Impact of the Second World War (1985); Geoffrey Perrett, Days of Sadness, Years of Triumph: The American People, 1939–1945 (1973); Richard Polenberg, War and Society: The United States, 1941–1945 (1972); Studs Terkel, "The Good War:" An Oral History of World War II (1984); Harold Vatter, The American Economy in World War II (1985); Allan Winkler, The Politics of Propaganda: The Office of War Information, 1942–1945 (1978).

Workers and Women at War

Karen T. Anderson, Wartime Women: Sex Roles, Family Relations, and the Status of American Women During World War II (1981); Matthew Baigall and Julia Williams, eds., Artists Against War and Fascism (1986); M. Joyce Baker, Images of Women on Film: The War Years, 1941–1945 (1981); James Foster, The Union Politic: The C.I.O. Political Action Committee (1975); Sherna Berger Gluck, Rosie the Riveter Revisited: Women, the War, and Social Change (1987); John Harris, The Right to Manage (1982); Susan Hartmann, The Home Front and Beyond: American Women in the 1940s (1982); Maurice Isserman, Which Side Were You On? The American Communist Party During the Second World War (1982); Paul Koistinen, The Hammer and the Sword: Labor, the Military, and Industrial Mobilization, 1920–1945 (1979); Nelson Lichtenstein, Labor's War at Home (1982); Ruth Milkman, Gender at Work: The Dynamics of Job Segregation by Sex During World War II (1987).

Minorities and the War

A. Russell Buchanan, Black-Americans in World War II (1977); Dominic Capeci, Jr., Race Relations in Wartime Detroit (1984), and The Harlem Race Riot of 1943 (1977); Richard Dalfiume, Desegregation of the U.S. Armed Forces (1969); Lee Finkel, Forum for Protest: The Black Press During World War II (1975); Mauricio Mazon, The Zoot Suit Riots (1984); Phillip McGuire, ed., Taps for a Jim Crow Army: Letters from Black Soldiers in World War II (1982); Patrick Washburn, A Question of Sedition: The Federal Government and the Investigation of the Black Press During World War II (1986); Neil Wynn, The Afro-American and the Second World War (1976).

Internees and Refugees

Robert Abzug, Inside the Vicious Heart: Americans and the Liberation of the Nazi Concentration Camps (1985); Richard Breitman and Alan Kraut, American Refugee Policy and European Jewry, 1933–1945 (1987); Commission on Wartime Relocation and Internment of Civilians, Personal Justice Denied (1982); P. Scott Corbett, Quiet Passages: The Exchange of Civilians Between the United States and Japan during World War II (1987); Roger Daniels, Concentration Camps U.S.A. (1971); Leonard Dinnerstein, America and the Survivors of the Holocaust (1982); Richard Drinnon, Keeper of Concentration Camps: Dillon S. Myer and American Racism (1987); Masayo Umezawa Duus, Unlikely Liberators: The Men of the 100th and 442nd (1987); Bill Hosokawa, Nisei (1969); Peter Irons, Justice at War: The Story of the Japanese American Internment Cases (1983); Deborah Lipstadt, Beyond Belief: The American Press and the Coming of the Holocaust, 1933–1945 (1986); Michi Weglyn, Years of Infamy: The Untold Story of America's Concentration Camps (1976); David Wyman, The Abandonment of the Jews (1984); Norman Zucker and Naomi Flink Zucker, The Guarded Gate: The Reality of American Refugee Policy (1987).

Atoms and the End of WW II

Gar Alperovitz, Atomic Diplomacy (rev. ed., 1985); Nuel Davis, Lawrence and Oppenheimer (1969); Robert Donovan, Conflict and Crisis (1977); Herbert Feis, Between War and Peace: The Potsdam Conference (1960); Herbert Feis, The Atomic Bomb and the End of World War II (2d ed., 1966); John L. Gaddis, The United States and the Origins of the Cold War (1971); John Gilkenson, Jr., Gathering Rare Ores: The Diplomacy of Uranium Acquisition, 1943–1954 (1987); John Hersey, Hiroshima (1946); Richard Hewlett and Oscar Anderson, The New World (1962); Dan Kurzman, Day of the Bomb: Countdown to Hiroshima (1986); Vojtech Mastny, Russia's Road to the Cold War (1979); Thomas Paterson, On Every Front: The Making of the Cold War (1979); Richard Rhodes, The Making of the Atomic Bomb (1986); Lisle Rose, After Yalta (1973); Martin Sherwin, A World Destroyed (1975).

CHAPTER 30

The Postwar Era

Erik Barnouw, Tube of Plenty: The Evolution of American Television (1975); Paul Boyer, By the Bomb's Early Light (1986); Serge Gilbaut, How New York Stole the Idea of Modern Art (1983); James Gilbert, Another Chance (1981); James Gilbert, A Cycle of Outrage (1986); Eric Goldman, The Crucial Decade and After (rev. ed., 1960); Alonzo Hamby, The Imperial Years (1976); Kenneth Jackson, Crabgrass Frontier: The Suburbanization of the United States (1985); Landon Jones, Great Expectations: America and the Babyboom Generation (1980); Richard Kluger, Simple Justice: The History of the Brown v. Board of Education and Black America's Struggle for Equality (1975); George Lipsitz, Class and Culture in Postwar America (1981); David Marc, Demographic Vistas (1984); James O'Connor, ed., American History/American Television (1983); William O'Neill, American High (1986); Richard Pells, The Liberal Mind in a Conservative Age (1985); Dana Polan, Power and Paranoia: History, Narrative, and the American Cinema, 1940–1950 (1986); Richard Polenberg, One Nation Divisible (1980); Leila Rupp and Verta Taylor, Survival in the Doldrums: The American Women's Rights Movement, 1945 to the 1960s (1987); Mark Silk, Spiritual Politics: Religion and America Since World War II (1988);

Jules Tygiel, *Baseball's Great Experiment: Jackie Robinson and His Legacy* (1983).

The Cold War in the West
Dean Acheson, *Present at the Creation* (1969); Stephen Ambrose, *The Rise to Globalism* (3rd ed., 1983); Robin Edmonds, *Setting the Mold: The United States and Great Britain, 1945–1950* (1986); Richard Wightman Fox, *Reinhold Niebuhr: A Biography* (1985); Lawrence Freedman, *The Evolution of Nuclear Strategy* (1983); Richard Freeland, *The Truman Doctrine and the Origins of McCarthyism* (1970); John L. Gaddis, *The United States and the Origins of the Cold War* (1972), *Strategies of Containment* (1982), and *The Long Peace: Inquiries into the History of the Cold War* (1987); Lloyd Gardner, *Architects of Illusion* (1970); David Green, *The Containment of Latin America* (1971); Gregg Herken, *The Winning Weapon* (1980); Michael Hogan, *The Marshall Plan: America, Britain, and the Reconstruction of Western Europe, 1947–1952* (1987); Fred Kaplan, *The Wizards of Armageddon* (1983); Laurence Kaplan, *The United States and NATO* (1984); George Kennan, *Memoirs*, 2 vols. (1967, 1972); Bruce Kuniholm, *The Origins of the Cold War in the Near East* (1980); Walter LaFeber, *America, Russia, and the Cold War* (5th ed., 1985); Mark H. Lytle, *The Origins of the Iranian-American Alliance, 1941–1953* (1987); Robert Messer, *The End of an Alliance* (1982); Aaron D. Miller, *Search for Security* (1980); James Miller, *The United States and Italy, 1940–1950* (1986); Thomas Paterson, *On Every Front* (1979); Robert Pollard, *Economic Security and the Origins of the Cold War* (1985); Ronald Pruessen, *John Foster Dulles* (1982); Cheryl Rubenberg, *Israel and the American National Interest* (1986); Gaddis Smith, *Dean Acheson* (1972); Hugh Thomas, *Armed Truce: The Beginnings of the Cold War, 1945–1946* (1987); Dan Tschirgi, *The Politics of Indecision* (1983); Adam Ulam, *The Rivals* (1971); Immanuel Wexler, *The Marshall Plan Revisited* (1983); Lawrence Wittner, *American Intervention in Greece, 1943–1949* (1982); Daniel Yergin, *Shattered Peace* (1977).

The Cold War in Asia
Robert Blum, *Drawing the Line: The Origin of the American Containment Policy in East Asia* (1982); Warren I. Cohen, *America's Response to China* (2d ed., 1980); Ronald Caridi, *The Korean War and American Politics* (1969); Bruce Cummings, *The Origins of the Korean War* (1980), and as ed., *Child of Conflict: The Korean-American Relationship, 1943–1953* (1983); William Head, *America's China Sojourn* (1983); Gary Hess, *The United States' Emergence as a Southeast Asian Power, 1940–1950* (1987); Akira Iriye, *The Cold War in Asia* (1974); Burton Kaufman, *The Korean War* (1986); Charles Neu, *The Troubled Encounter: The United States and Japan* (1975); Michael Schaller, *The United States and China in the Twentieth Century* (1979); Michael Schaller, *The American Occupation of Japan: The Coming of the Cold War to Asia* (1985); John W. Spanier, *The Truman-MacArthur Controversy and the Korean War* (1959); William Stueck, Jr., *The Road to Confrontation* (1981); Christopher Thorne, *Allies of a Kind* (1978); Nancy Tucker, *Patterns in the Dust: Chinese-American Relations and the Recognition Controversy, 1949–1950* (1983).

The Domestic Cold War
Michael Belknap, *Cold War Political Justice: The Smith Act, the Communist Party, and American Civil Liberties* (1977); David Caute, *The Great Fear* (1978); Larry Ceplair and Steven Englund, *The Inquisition in Hollywood* (1983); Robert Griffin, *The Politics of Fear* (1970); Stanley I. Kutler, *The American Inquisition: Justice and Injustice in the Cold War* (1982); Robert Lamphere and Tom Shachtman, *The FBI-KGB War* (1986); Victor Navasky, *Naming Names* (1980); William O'Neill, *A Better World: Stalinism and the American Intellectuals* (1983); Michael Oshinsky, *A Conspiracy So Immense: The World of Joe McCarthy* (1983); Ronald Radosh and Joyce Radosh, *The Rosenberg File* (1983); Thomas Reeves, *The Life and Times of Joe McCarthy* (1982); Paul Rogin, *The Intellectuals and McCarthy* (1969); Richard Rovere, *Senator Joe McCarthy* (1959); Nora Sayre, *Running Time: Films on the Cold War* (1982); Nancy Lynn Schwartz, *The Hollywood Writers' War* (1982); Ellen Shrecker, *No Ivory Tower: McCarthyism and the Universities* (1984); Peter Steinberg, *The Great "Red Menace:" United States Prosecution of American Communists, 1947–1952* (1984); Athan Theoharis, *Seeds of Repression: Harry S Truman and the Origins of McCarthyism* (1971); Allen Weinstein, *Perjury: The Hiss-Chambers Case* (1978); Robert Williams, *Klaus Fuchs: Atom Spy* (1987).

The Truman Administration
Jack Ballard, *The Shock of Peace: Military and Economic Demobilization after World War II* (1983); William Berman, *The Politics of Civil Rights in the Truman Administration* (1970); Barton Bernstein, ed., *Politics and Policies of the Truman Administration* (1970); Richard Dalfiume, *Desegregation of the U.S. Armed Forces* (1969); Robert Donovan, *Conflict and Crisis* (1977) and *Years of Tumult* (1982); Andrew Dunar, *The Truman Scandals and the Politics of Morality* (1984); Robert Ferrell, *Harry S Truman and the Modern American Presidency* (1983); Donald Fixico, *Termination and Relocation: Federal Indian Policy, 1945–1960* (1986); Alonzo Hamby, *Beyond the New Deal* (1973); Alton Lee, *Truman and Taft-Hartley* (1966); Maeva Marcus, *Truman and the Steel Seizure* (1977); Norman Markowitz, *The Rise and Fall of the People's Century: Henry A. Wallace and American Liberalism, 1941–1948* (1973); Allen Matusow, *Farm Politics and Policies in the Truman Years* (1967); Donald McCoy, *The Presidency of Harry S Truman* (1984); Donald McCoy and Richard Ruetten, *Quest and Response: Minority Rights and the Truman Administration* (1973); Merle Miller, *Plain Speaking* (1973); Richard Miller, *Truman: The Rise to Power* (1986); Allen Yarnell, *Democrats and Progressives: The 1948 Presidential Election as a Test of Postwar Liberalism* (1974).

CHAPTER 31

General
James Gilbert, *Another Chance* (1981); Eric Goldman, *The Critical Decade and After, 1945–1960* (1960); Godfrey Hodgson, *America in Our Time* (1976); Martin Jezer, *The Dark Ages: Life in the United States, 1945–1960* (1982); William Leuchtenberg, *A Troubled Feast* (1979); Peter Lewis, *The Fifties* (1977); Douglas Miller and Marion Nowak, *The Fifties: The Way We Really*

Were (1977); Ronald Oakley, *God's Country: America in the 1950s* (1986); William O'Neill, *American High* (1986).

American Life and Culture
Erik Barnouw, *Tube of Plenty* (1975); Daniel Bell, *The End of Ideology* (1960); Carl Belz, *The Story of Rock* (2d ed., 1972); Victoria Byerly, *Hard Times Cotton Mill Girls* (1986); Paul Carter, *Another Part of the Fifties* (1983); William Chafe, *The American Woman, 1920–1970* (1972); Bruce Cook, *The Beat Generation* (1970); Richard Davies, *The Age of Asphalt* (1975); Carl Degler, *At Odds* (1980); John D'Emillio and Estelle Freedman, *Intimate Matters: A History of Sexuality in America* (1988); James Flink, *The Car Culture in America* (1973); Betty Friedan, *The Feminine Mystique* (1963); John Kenneth Galbraith, *The Affluent Society* (1958); Herbert Gans, *The Levittowners* (1967); James Gilbert, *A Cycle of Outrage* (1986); Charlie Gillett, *The Sound of the City: The Rise of Rock and Roll* (1970); Will Herberg, *Protestant-Catholic-Jew* (1956); Thomas Hine, *Populux* (1986); Kenneth Jackson, *Crabgrass Frontier* (1985); David Marc, *Demographic Vistas* (1984); Mary McAuliffe, *Crisis on the Left* (1978); C. Wright Mills, *The Power Elite* (1956) and *White Collar* (1951); George Nash, *The Conservative Intellectual Movement in America* (1976); Richard Pells, *The Liberal Mind in a Conservative Age* (1985); David Potter, *People of Plenty* (1956); David Riesman, *The Lonely Crowd* (1950); Gaye Tuchman et al., eds., *Hearth and Home: Images of Women in the Mass Media* (1978); Ed Ward et al., *Rock of Ages: The Rolling Stone History of Rock and Roll* (1986); Carol Warren, *Madwives: Schizophrenic Women in the 1950s* (1987); William Whyte, *The Organization Man* (1956).

Foreign Policy in the Eisenhower Era
Stephen Ambrose, *Ike's Spies: Eisenhower and the Espionage Establishment* (1981); Richard Barnet, *Intervention and Revolution* (rev. ed., 1972); Blanche W. Cook, *The Declassified Eisenhower* (1981); Chester Cooper, *The Lion's Last Roar: Suez, 1956* (1978); Robert Divine, *Eisenhower and the Cold War* (1981), and *Blowin' in the Wind: The Nuclear Test Ban Debate, 1954–1960* (1978); Townsend Hoopes, *The Devil and John Foster Dulles* (1973); Richard Immerman, *The CIA in Guatemala* (1982); Madeline Kalb, *The Congo Cables: The Cold War in Africa from Eisenhower to Kennedy* (1982); Burton Kaufman, *Trade and Aid: Eisenhower's Economic Policy* (1982); Richard Melanson and David Mayers, eds., *Reevaluating Eisenhower: American Foreign Policy in the 1950s* (1987); Kermit Roosevelt, *Counter-Coup* (1979,80); Stephen Schlesinger and Steven Kinzer, *Bitter Fruit* (1981); Richard Welch, Jr., *Response to Revolution: The United States and the Cuban Revolution, 1954–1961* (1985); Mira Wilkins, *The Maturing of Multinational Enterprise* (1974).

Civil Rights
Numan Bartley, *The Rise of Massive Resistance: Race and Politics in the South during the 1950s* (1969); Jack Bloom, *Class, Race, and the Civil Rights Movement* (1987); James Duram, *Moderate Among Extremists: Dwight D. Eisenhower and the School Desegregation Crisis* (1981); David Garrow, *Bearing the Cross* (1986); Vincent Harding, *There is a River: The Black Struggle for Freedom in America* (1981); Elizabeth Huckaby, *The Crisis at Central High: Little Rock 1957–1958* (1980); Richard Kluger, *Simple Justice* (1975); Anthony Lewis et al., *Portrait of a Decade* (1964); August Meier and Elliott Rudwick, *Core: A Study in the Civil Rights Movement, 1942–1968* (1975); Stephen Oates, *Let the Trumpet Sound: The Life and Times of Martin Luther King, Jr.* (1982); Bernard Schwartz, *Inside the Warren Court* (1983); C. Vann Woodward, *The Strange Career of Jim Crow* (3rd ed., 1974); Juan Williams, *Eyes on the Prize: America's Civil Rights Years, 1954–1965* (1987).

Domestic Politics
Stephen Ambrose, *Eisenhower the President* (1984); Alexander Bickel, *Politics and the Warren Court* (1965); Piers Brendon, *Ike* (1986); Larry Burt, *Tribalism in Crisis: Federal Indian Policy, 1953–1961* (1982); Barbara Clowse, *Brainpower for the Cold War: The Sputnik Crisis and the National Defense Education Act of 1958* (1981); Donald Fixico, *Termination and Relocation: Federal Indian Policy, 1945–1960* (1986); Fred Greenstein, *The Hidden Hand Presidency: Eisenhower as Leader* (1982); Robert Heilbroner, *The Limits of American Capitalism* (1965); Joann Krieg, ed., *Dwight D. Eisenhower: Soldier, President, and Statesman* (1987); David W. Reinhard, *The Republican Right Since 1945* (1983); Elmo Richardson, *The Presidency of Dwight D. Eisenhower* (1979); Mark Rose, *Interstate: Express Highway Politics, 1941–1956* (1979); Michael Straight, *Trial by Television* (1954); Herbert Vatter, *The U.S. Economy in the 1950s* (1963); Gary Wills, *Nixon Agonistes* (1970).

CHAPTER 32

General
Todd Gitlin, *The Sixties* (1987); Richard Goodwin, *Remembering America: A Voice from the Sixties* (1988); Godfrey Hodgson, *America in Our Time* (1976); Landon Y. Jones, *Great Expectations: America and the Baby Boom Generation* (1981); Allen Matusow, *The Unraveling of America: A History of Liberalism in the 1960s* (1984); Lawrence Wright, *The New World: Growing Up in America, 1960–1984* (1988).

The Counterculture and New Left
Serge Denisoff, *Great Day Coming: Folk Music and the American Left* (1971); Morris Dickstein, *The Gates of Eden*; Joan Didion, *Slouching Towards Bethlehem* (1968), and *White Album* (1979); Todd Gitlin, *The Whole World Is Watching: The Mass Media in the Making and Unmaking of the New Left* (1981); Paul Goodman, *Growing Up Absurd* (1960); Maurice Isserman, *If I Had a Hammer . . . : The Death of the Old Left and the Birth of the New Left* (1987); Judy Kaplan and Linn Shapiro, *Red Diaper Babies: Children on the Left* (1985); Kenneth Kenniston, *The Uncommitted* (1965); Lawrence Lader, *Power on the Left* (1979); Martin Lee and Bruce Shlain, *Acid Dreams: The CIA, LSD, and the Sixties Rebellion* (1985); Dennis McNally, *Desolate Angel: Jack Kerouac, the Beat Generation, and America* (1979); William O'Neill, *Coming Apart* (1971); Theodore Roszak, *The Making of a Counter Culture* (1969); Stanley Rothman and S. Robert Lichter, *Roots of Rebellion* (1982); Kirkpatrick Sale, *SDS* (1973); Anthony Scaduto, *Bob Dylan* (1971); Philip Slater, *The Pursuit of Loneliness* (1970); Students for a Democratic Society, *The Port Huron Statement* (1962); Hunter Thompson, *Hell's Angels*

(1967) and *Fear and Loathing in Las Vegas* (1971); Ed Ward et al., *Rock of Ages: The Rolling Stone History of Rock and Roll* (1986); Tom Wolfe, *Electric Kool-Aid Acid Test* (1968).

Civil Rights and Black Power
Michael Belknap, *Federal Law and Southern Order: Racial Violence and Constitutional Conflict in the Post-Brown South* (1987); Derrick Bell, *And We Are Not Saved: The Elusive Quest for Racial Justice* (1987); Jack Bloom, *Class, Race, and the Civil Rights Movement* (1987); Taylor Branch, *Parting the Waters* (1988); Carl Brauer, *John F. Kennedy and the Second Reconstruction* (1980); Stokely Carmichael and Charles Hamilton, *Black Power* (1967); Clayborne Carson, *In Struggle: SNCC and the Black Awakening of the 1960s* (1981); William Chafe, *Civilities and Civil Rights* (1980) and *The Unfinished Journey* (1986); Joe Feagin and Harlan Hahn, *Ghetto Revolts* (1973); David Garrow, *Bearing the Cross* (1986) and *The FBI and Martin Luther King* (1981); Vincent Harding, *There is a River: The Black Struggle for Freedom in America* (1981); Otto Kerner et al., *The Report of the National Advisory Commission on Civil Disorders* (1968); Steven Lawson, *Black Ballots* (1976) and *In Pursuit of Power* (1985); Malcolm X (with Alex Haley), *The Autobiography of Malcolm X* (1966); August Meier and Elliott Rudwick, *Core: A Study in the Civil Rights Movement, 1942–1968* (1975); Stephen Oates, *Let the Trumpet Sound: The Life and Times of Martin Luther King, Jr.* (1982); Bernard Schwartz, *Inside the Warren Court* (1983); Harvard Sitkoff, *The Struggle for Black Equality, 1954–1980* (1981); Juan Williams, *Eyes on the Prize: America's Civil Rights Years, 1954–1965* (1987); Harris Wofford, *Of Kennedy and Kings* (1980); Eugene Wolfenstein, *The Victims of Democracy: Malcolm X and the Black Revolutionaries* (1981).

The Kennedys and Lyndon Johnson
Robert Caro, *The Years of Lyndon Johnson: The Path to Power* (1982); Paul Conkin, *Big Daddy from the Pedernales: Lyndon Baines Johnson* (1986); Ronnie Dugger, *The Politician* (1982); Jim Heath, *Decade of Disillusionment* (1975); Henry Hurt, *Reasonable Doubt: An Investigation into the Assassination John F. Kennedy* (1985); Lyndon Johnson, *Vantage Point* (1971); Doris Kearns, *Lyndon Johnson and the American Dream* (1976); Bruce Miroff, *Pragmatic Illusions* (1976); Herbert Parmet, *Jack* (1980), and *JFK—The Presidency of John F. Kennedy* (1983); Arthur Schlesinger, Jr., *The Thousand Days* (1965), and *Robert Kennedy and His Times* (1978); Earl Warren et al., *The Report of the Warren Commission* (1964); Theodore White, *The Making of the President, 1960* (1961).

Politics and Foreign Policy in the Kennedy-Johnson Era
Henry Aaron, *Politics and the Professors* (1978); Graham Allison, *Essence of Decision: Explaining the Cuban Missile Crisis* (1971); James Anderson and Jared Hazelton, *Managing Macroeconomic Policy: The Johnson Presidency* (1986); Desmond Ball, *Politics and Force Levels: The Strategic Missile Program of the Kennedy Administration* (1980); Warren Cohen, *Dean Rusk* (1980); Hugh Graham Davis, *Uncertain Trumpet* (1984); Greg Duncan, *Years of Poverty, Years of Plenty* (1984); Robert Haveman, ed., *A Decade of Federal Antipoverty Pro-*

grams (1977); Walter LaFeber, *America, Russia, and the Cold War, 1945–1984* (5th ed., 1985); Sar Levitan and Robert Taggart, *The Promise of Greatness* (1976); Richard Mahoney, *JFK: Ordeal in Africa* (1983); Walter McDougall, *...The Heavens and the Earth: A Political History of the Space Age* (1985); Charles Murray, *Losing Ground: American Social Policy, 1950–1980* (1984); Thomas Noer, *Cold War and Black Liberation: The United States and White Rule in Africa, 1948–1968* (1985); Francis Fox Piven and Richard Cloward, *Regulating the Poor* (1971); Emmette Redford and Richard McCulley, *White House Operations: The Johnson Presidency* (1986); Gerald Rice, *The Bold Experiment: JFK's Peace Corps* (1985); Glenn Seaborg, *Kennedy, Khrushchev, and the Test Ban* (1981); R. B. Smith, *An International History of the Vietnam War: The Kennedy Strategy* (1985); Tom Wicker, *JFK and LBJ* (1968); Bryce Wood, *The Dismantling of the Good Neighbor Policy* (1985); Peter Wyden, *The Bay of Pigs* (1979).

CHAPTER 33

The United States and the Vietnam War

Loren Baritz, *Backfire: A History of How American Culture Led Us into Vietnam and Made Us Fight the Way We Did* (1985); Larry Berman, *Planning a Tragedy* (1982); William Broyles, *Brothers in Arms: A Journey From War to Peace* (1986); Richard Dean Burns and Milton Leitenberg, eds., *The Wars in Vietnam, Cambodia, and Laos, 1945–1982* (1984); Larry Cable, *Conflict of Myths: The Development of American Counterinsurgency Doctrine and the Vietnam War* (1986); Francis Fitzgerald, *Fire in the Lake* (1972); Leslie Gelb and Richard Betts, *The Irony of Vietnam: The System Worked* (1979); Mike Gravel et al., *The Pentagon Papers*, (1975); David Halberstam, *The Best and the Brightest* (1972) and *The Making of a Quagmire* (rev. ed., 1987); George Herring, *America's Longest War* (2d ed., 1986); George Kahin, *Intervention: How America Became Involved in Vietnam* (1986); Stanley Karnow, *Vietnam* (1983); Gabriel Kolko, *Anatomy of a War* (1985); Andrew Krepinevich, Jr., *The Army and Vietnam* (1986); Guenter Lewy, *America in Vietnam* (1978); Kathryn Marshall, *In the Combat Zone: An Oral History of Women in the Vietnam War, 1966–1975* (1987); Tim Page, *Nam* (1983); Bruce Palmer, Jr., *The 25-Year War* (1984); Archimedes Patti, *Why Viet Nam?* (1983); Norman Podhoretz, *Why We Were in Vietnam* (1982); Al Santoli, *Everything We Had: An Oral History of the Vietnam War by Thirty Three American Soldiers Who Fought It* (1981); Neil Sheehan, *A Bright Shining Lie: John Paul Vann and America in Vietnam* (1988); Ronald Spector, *The United States Army in Vietnam* (1983); Shelby Stanton, *Rises and Fall of an American Army: U.S. Ground Forces, Vietnam, 1965–1973* (1985) and *Green Berets at War* (1985); Harry Summers, Jr., *On Strategy: A Critical Analysis of the Vietnam War* (1981); Wallace Terry, *Bloods: An Oral History of the Vietnam War by Black Veterans* (1984); William Turley, *The Second Indochina War: A Short Political and Military History* (1986).

Dissent Against the War

William Berman, *William Fulbright and the Vietnam War* (1988); Eugene Brown, *William Fulbright: Advise and Dissent* (1984); David Caute, *The Year of the Barri-*

cades, 1968 (1988); Gloria Emerson, *Winners and Losers* (1976); David Farber, *Chicago '68* (1988); Todd Gitlin, *The Sixties* (1987); Myra MacPherson, *Long Time Passing: Vietnam and the Haunted Generation* (1984); Norman Mailer, *Armies of the Night* (1968) and *Miami and the Siege of Chicago* (1969); James Miller, *Democracy Is in the Streets* (1987); Thomas Powers, *Vietnam: The War at Home* (1973); Herbert Schandler, *The Unmaking of a President: Lyndon Johnson and Vietnam* (1977); Melvin Small, *Johnson, Nixon, and the Doves* (1988); William Strauss, *Chance and Circumstance* (1978); Irwin Unger, *The Movement* (1974); Lawrence Wittner, *Rebels Against War: The American Peace Movement, 1933–1983* (1984); Nancy Zaroulis and Gerald Sullivan, *Who Spoke Up? American Protest Against the War in Vietnam* (1984).

The Nixon Presidency Before Watergate
Richard Barnet, *The Giants: Russia and America* (1977); Fawn Brodie, *Richard Nixon* (1981); John Erlichman, *Witness to Power* (1982); Raymond Garthoff, *Détente and Confrontation: American-Soviet Relations from Nixon to Reagan* (1985); Seymour Hersh, *The Price of Power: Kissinger in the Nixon White House* (1983); Henry Kissinger, *The White House Years* (1979) and *Years of Upheaval* (1982); Robert Litwack, *Détente and the Nixon Doctrine* (1984); Morris Morley, *The United States and Chile* (1975); Roger Morris, *Uncertain Greatness: Henry Kissinger and American Foreign Policy* (1977); Daniel Patrick Moynihan, *The Politics of a Guaranteed Income* (1973); Richard Nixon, *RN* (1978); Leon Panetta and Peter Gall, *Bring Us Together: The Nixon Team and the Civil Rights Retreat* (1971); William Safire, *Before the Fall* (1975); William Shawcross, *Sideshow: Nixon, Kissinger, and the Destruction of Cambodia* (1978); Robert Sutter, *The China Quandary* (1983); Theodore White, *The Making of the President, 1968* (1969); Gary Wills, *Nixon Agonistes* (1970).

Minorities: Background and Politics
Rodolfo Acuna, *Occupied America* (2d ed., 1981); Mario Barerra, *Race and Class in the Southwest* (1979); John Burma, ed., *Mexican-Americans in the United States* (1970); Albert Camarillo, *Hispanics in a Changing Society* (1979); Tony Castro, *Chicano Power* (1974); Vine Deloria, *Behind the Veil of Broken Treaties* (1974); Patrick Gallagher, *The Cuban Exile* (1980); Hazel W. Hertzberg, *The Search for an American Indian Identity: Modern Pan-Indian Movements* (1971); Peter Iverson, *The Navajo Nation* (1981); Virginia Sanchez Korrol, *From Colonia to Community* (1983); Darcy McNickle, *Native American Tribalism* (1973); Joan Moore and Harry Pachon, *Hispanics in the United States* (1985); Joan Moore et al., *Homeboys* (1978); Roger Nichols, *The American Indian: Past and Present* (3rd ed. 1986); James Olsen and Raymond Wilson, *Native Americans in the Twentieth Century* (1984); A. Petit, *Images of Mexican American in Fiction and Film* (1980); Thomas Sanders and Walter Peek, *Literature of the American Indian* (1976); Ronald Taylor, *Chavez and the Farm Workers* (1975); Dennis Tedlock and Barbara Tedlock, eds., *Teachings from the American Earth: Indian Religion and Philosophy* (1975); Arnulfo Trejo, ed., *The Chicanos: As We See Ourselves* (1979); Karl Wagenheim, *Puerto Rico: A Profile* (1975).

CHAPTER 34

American Society and the Economy in the 1970s
Richard Barnet, *The Lean Years* (1980); John Blair, *The Control of Oil* (1976); Barry Bluestone and Bennett Harrison, *The Deindustrialization of America* (1982); Peter Calleo, *The Imperious Economy* (1982); Peter Carroll, *It Seemed Like Nothing Happened: The Tragedy and Promise of America in the 1970s* (1982); Peter Clecak, *America's Quest for an Ideal Self* (1983); Barry Commoner, *The Politics of Energy* (1979); Jim Hougan, *Decadence: Radical Nostalgia, Narcissism, and Decline in the 1970s* (1975); Christopher Lasch, *The Culture of Narcissism* (1978); J. Anthony Lukas, *Common Ground: A Turbulent Decade in the Lives of Three American Families* (1986); Martin Melosi, *Coping with Abundance: Energy and Environment in Industrial America* (1985); John Schwarz, *America's Hidden Success* (rev. ed., 1988); Robert Sherrill, *The Oil Follies of 1970–1980* (1983); Lester Thurow, *The Zero-Sum Society* (1980).

Environmentalism
Rachel Carson, *Silent Spring* (1962); Barry Caspar and Paul Wellstone, *Powerline* (1981); Barry Commoner, *The Closing Circle* (1971); Albert Cowdry, *This Land, This South: An Environmental History* (1983); Thomas Dunlap, *DDT: Scientists, Citizens, and Public Policy* (1981); Edith Efron, *The Apocalyptics* (1984); Sam Hays, *Beauty, Health, and Permanence: Environmental Politics in the United States, 1955–1985* (1987); Ronald Inglehart, *The Silent Revolution* (1977); Ian McHarg, *Design with Nature* (1969); Daniel Martin, *Three Mile Island* (1980); Lester Milbrath, *Environmentalists: Vanguard for a New Society* (1984); Ralph Nader and John Abbotts, *The Menace of Atomic Energy* (1977); Roderick Nash, *Wilderness and the American Mind* (3rd ed., 1982); Marc Reisner, *Cadillac Desert: The American West and Its Disappearing Water* (1986); Robert Stobaugh and Daniel Yergin, eds., *Energy Future* (1979); James Trefethen, *An American Crusade for Wildlife* (1975); Thomas Whiteside, *The Pendulum and the Toxic Cloud* (1979); Donald Worster, *Rivers of Empire: Water Aridity, and the Growth of the American West* (1985).

Feminism, Sexual Politics, and the Family
Rae Andre, *Homemakers: The Forgotten Workers* (1981); Judith Barwick, *In Transition: How Feminism, Sexual Liberation, and the Search for Self-Fulfillment Have Altered America* (1979); Peter Berger and Bridgett Berger, *The War Over the Family: Capturing the Middle Ground* (1983); Mary Frances Berry, *Why ERA Failed: Politics, Women's Rights, and the Amending Process of the Constitution* (1986); Caroline Bird, *Born Female: The High Cost of Keeping Women Down* (1969); Susan Brownmiller, *Against Our Will: Men, Women, and Rape* (1975); William Chafe, *Women and Equality: Changing Patterns in American Culture* (1977); Robert Coles and Geoffrey Stokes, *Sex and the American Teenager* (1985); Angela Davis, *Women, Race, and Class* (1981); Barbara Deckard, *The Women's Movement* (1975); Carl Degler, *At Odds* (1980); John D'Emilio, *Sexual Politics, Sexual Communities: The Making of a Homosexual Minority in the United States, 1940–1970* (1983); John D'Emilio and Estelle Freedman, *Intimate Matters: A History of Sexuality in America* (1988); Andrea Dworkin, *Right-Wing*

Women (1983); Barbara Ehrenreich, *The Hearts of Men: American Dreams and the Flight From Commitment* (1983); Susan Estebrook, *If All We Did Was to Weep at Home: A History of White Working-Class Women in America* (1979); Sara Evans, *Personal Politics: The Roots of Women's Liberation in the Civil Rights Movement and the New Left* (1979); Lillian Faderman, *Surpassing the Love of Men* (1979); Shulamith Firestone, *The Dialectic of Sex: The Case for the Feminist Revolution* (1970); Jo Freeman, *The Politics of Women's Liberation* (1975); Victor Fuchs, *How We Live: An Economic Perspective on Americans from Birth to Death* (1983); Carol Gilligan, *In Another Voice: Psychological Theory and Women's Development* (1982); Germaine Greer, *The Female Eunuch* (1972); Alice Kessler Harris, *Out to Work* (1982); Judith Hole and Ellen Levine, *The Rebirth of Feminism* (1971); Louis Kapp Howe, *Pink Collar Workers: Inside the World of Women's Work* (1977); Gloria Hull et al., *But Some of Us Are Brave: Black Women Studies* (1982); Morton Hunt, *Sexual Behavior in the 1970s* (1974); Elizabeth Janeway, *Cross Sections from a Decade of Change* (1983); Jonathan Katz, ed., *Gay American History* (1976); Linda Kerber and Jane Matthews, eds., *America: Refocusing the Past* (1981); Christopher Lasch, *Haven in a Hostile World* (1979); Kate Millett, *Sexual Politics* (1970); Steven Mintz and Susan Kellogg, *Domestic Revolutions: A Social History of American Family Life* (1988); Robin Morgan, ed., *Sisterhood Is Powerful: An Anthology* (1970); Helen Rogan, *Mixed Company: Women in the Modern Army* (1981); La Frances Rodgers-Rose, ed., *The Black Woman* (1980); Sheila Rothman, *Woman's Proper Place* (1978); Nancy Seifer, *Nobody Speaks for Me: Self-Portraits of American Working-Class Women* (1976); Gloria Steinem, *Outrageous Acts and Everyday Rebellions* (1983); Nancy Wolloch, *Women and the American Experience* (1984).

Watergate
Richard Ben-Veniste and George Frampton, *Stonewall* (1978); John Dean, *Blind Ambition* (1976); J. Anthony Lukas, *Nightmare: The Underside of the Nixon Years* (rev. ed., 1988); Richard Nixon, *RN: The Memoirs of Richard Nixon* (1978); Arthur Schlesinger, Jr., *The Imperial Presidency* (1973); Jonathan Schell, *The Time of Illusion* (1975); John Sirica, *To Set the Record Straight* (1979); Theodore White, *Breach of Faith* (1975); Bob Woodward and Carl Bernstein, *All the President's Men* (1974), and *The Final Days* (1976).

Politics and Diplomacy in the Ford-Carter Years
Zbigniew Brzezinski, *Power and Principle* (1983); Jimmy Carter, *Keeping the Faith* (1982); Rosalynn Carter, *First Lady from Plains* (1984); Terry Deibel, *Presidents, Public Opinion, and Power: The Nixon, Carter, and Reagan Years* (1987); Gerald Ford, *A Time to Heal* (1979); Millicent Gates and Bruce Geelhoed, *The Dragon and the Snake: An American Account of the Turmoil in China, 1976–1977* (1986); Robert Hartman, *Palace Politics* (1980); Michael Hogan, *The Panama Canal in American Politics* (1986); Henry Jackson, *From the Congo to Soweto: U.S. Foreign Policy Toward Africa Since 1960* (1982); Hamilton Jordan, *Crisis* (1982); Walter LaFeber, *The Panama Canal* (rev. ed., 1989); Clark Mollenhoff, *The President Who Failed* (1980); Richard Pipes, *U.S.-Soviet Relations in the Era of Détente* (1981); William Quandt, *Camp David* (1986); Stephen Rabe, *The Road to OPEC: U.S. Relations with Venezuela, 1919–1976* (1982); R. K. Ramazani, *The U.S. and Iran* (1982); A. James Reichley, *Conservatives in an Age of Change: The Nixon and Ford Administrations* (1981); Kirkpatrick Sale, *Power Shift* (1975); Gary Sick, *All Fall Down* (1985); Gaddis Smith, *Morality, Reason, and Power* (1986); Robert Sutter, *The China Quandary* (1983); Strobe Talbot, *Endgame* (1979); Seth Tillman, *The U.S. in the Middle East* (1982); Cyrus Vance, *Hard Choices* (1983).

CHAPTER 35

Contemporary American Society
Robert Bellah et al., *Habits of the Heart: Individualism and Commitment in American Life* (1985); Thomas Edsall, *The New Politics of Inequality* (1984); Michael Goldfield, *The Decline of Organized Labor in the United States* (1987); Michael Harrington, *The New American Poverty* (1984); Jonathan Kwitny, *The Crimes of Patriots: A True Tale of Dope, Dirty Money, and the CIA* (1987); Frank Levy *Dollars and Dreams: The Changing American Income Distribution* (1987); Jane Mansbridge, *Why We Lost the ERA* (1986); David Marc, *Demographic Vistas: Television in American Culture* (1984); Robert McElvaine, *The End of the Conservative Era: Liberalism After Reagan* (1987); Michael Piore and Charles Sabal, *The Second Industrial Divide: Possibilities for Prosperity* (1987); Frances Fox Piven and Richard Cloward, *The New Class War* (1982); Robert Sklar, *Prime Time* (1980); Robert Spitzer, *The Right to Life Movement and Third Party Politics* (1987); Peter Steinfels, *The Neo-Conservatives* (1979); Studs Terkel, *The Great Divide* (1988); John Woodridge, *The Evangelicals* (1975).

The Reagan Presidency
Frank Ackerman, *Reaganomics* (1982); Stephen Cimbala, *The Reagan Defense Program* (1986); Joan Claybrook, *Retreat from Safety: Reagan's Attack on American Health* (1984); Robert Dallek, *Ronald Reagan: The Politics of Symbolism* (1984); Michael Deaver, *Behind the Scenes* (1987); Ronnie Duggar, *On Reagan* (1983); Rowland Evans and Robert Novak, *The Reagan Revolution* (1981); Jonathan Lash, *A Season of Spoils: The Story of the Reagan Administration's Attack on the Environment* (1984); Robert Lekachman, *Greed Is Not Enough* (1983); Jane Mayer and Doyle McManus, *Landslide: The Unmaking of the President, 1984–1988* (1988); Austin Ranney, ed., *The American Elections of 1984* (1985); Richard Reeves, *The Reagan Detour* (1985); Donald Regan, *For the Record* (1988); Larry Speakes, *Speaking Out* (1988); Paul Stares, *Space and National Security* (1987); David Stockman, *The Triumph of Politics: The Inside Story of the Reagan Revolution* (1986); Gary Wills, *Reagan's America* (1987).

Foreign Policy in the 1980s
Lawrence Barrett, *Gambling with History* (1984); Tom Barry et al., *The Other Side of Paradise: Foreign Control in the Caribbean* (1984); Karl Bermann, *Under the Big Stick* (1985); Raymond Bonner, *Weakness and Deceit: U.S. Policy and El Salvador* (1984); Tom Buckley, *Violent Neighbors* (1984); Bradford Burns, *At War with Nicaragua* (1987); Leslie Cockburn, *Out of Control* (1987); Christopher Coker, *The United States and South*

Africa, 1968–1985 (1986); Stephen Emerson, *Secret Warriors* (1988); Carl Feldbaum and Ronald Bee, *Looking the Tiger in the Eye: Confronting the Nuclear Threat* (1988); Roy Gutman, *Banana Diplomacy* (1988); Alexander Haig, Jr., *Caveat: Realism, Reagan, and Foreign Policy* (1984); Jerry Hough, *The Struggle for the Third World* (1986); Bruce Jentleson, *Pipeline Politics: The Complex Political Economy of East-West Trade* (1986); Walter LaFeber, *Inevitable Revolutions* (2d ed., 1984); David Martin and John Wolcott, *Best Laid Plans* (1988); Morris Morley, *The Imperial State and Revolution* (1987); Robert Pastor, *Condemned to Repetition: The United States and Nicaragua* (1987); Stephen Randall, *U.S. Foreign Oil Policy, 1919–1984* (1985); Jonathan Schell, *The Fate of the Earth* (1982); Lars Schoultz, *National Security and U.S. Policy Toward Latin America* (1987); Strobe Talbott, *Deadly Gambits: The Reagan Administration and the Stalemate in Nuclear Arms Control* (1984), and *The Russians and Reagan* (1984); Sanford Ungar, *Africa* (1985); Thomas Walker, ed., *Reagan Versus the Sandinistas* (1987); Bob Woodward, *Veil: The Secret Wars of the CIA* (1987).

Minority Relations and the New Immigration
Ken Auletta, *The Underclass* (1982); John Crewden, *The Tarnished Door: The New Immigrants and the Transformation of America* (1983); Roger Daniels et al., eds., *Japanese-Americans: From Relocation to Redress* (1986); Leonard Dinnerstein and David Reimers, *Ethnic Americans* (2d ed., 1982); Reynolds Farley and Walter Allen, *The Color Line and the Quality of Life in America* (1987); Douglas Glasgow, *The Black Underclass* (1980); Stanford Lyman, *Chinese Americans* (1974); Joan Moore and Harry Pachon, *Hispanics in the United States* (1985); Adolph Reed, *The Jesse Jackson Phenomenon: The Crisis of Purpose in Afro-American Politics* (1986); David Reimers, *Still the Golden Door: The Third World Comes to America* (1985); The Staff of the *Chicago Tribune, The American Millstone: An Examination of the Nation's Permanent Underclass* (1986); Shih-Shan Henry Tsai, *The Chinese Experience in America* (1986); William J. Wilson, *The Declining Significance of Race: Blacks and Changing American Institutions* (2d ed., 1980).

PHOTO CREDITS

CHAPTER 17

603 Winslow Homer, "A Visit from the Old Mistress," 1876. Oil on canvas, 18″ × 24⅛″. National Museum of American Art, Smithsonian Institution. Gift of William T. Evans; **607-L** Library of Congress; **607-R** U.S. Army Military History Institute, Carlisle Barracks, Penna.; **609** Library of Congress; **610** The Library Company of Philadelphia; **616** Library of Congress; **618** Library of Congress; **623** Courtesy of the New York Historical Society, New York City; **625** Richard Norris Brooke, "A Pastoral Visit, Virginia." In the collection of The Corcoran Gallery of Art, Museum Purchase, Gallery Fund; **629** The Valentine Museum of the Life and History of Richmond, Cook Collection; **631-L** Courtesy of the American Antiquarian Society; **631-R** Sophic Smith Collection, Smith College; **633** The Granger Collection; **636** Rutherford B. Hayes Presidential Center; **638** United States Senate, Committee on Rules and Administration; **639** Library of Congress, Division of Rare Books and Manuscripts; **642** The Bettmann Archive; **643** Courtesy of The British Library, London.

CHAPTER 18

647 The Granger Collection; **649** Library of Congress; **651** The Bettmann Archive; **652** The Margaret Woodbury Strong Museum, Rochester, N.Y.; **654** Culver Pictures; **657** Library of Congress; **666** Courtesy of Exxon; **669** Lee Boltin Picture Library; **674** Courtesy of the Metropolitan Life Insurance Company, N.Y.; **678** Collection of Lee Baxandall.

CHAPTER 19

683 Theodore Groll, German, 1857–1913: "Washington Street, Indianapolis at Dusk," 1892–95. Oil on canvas, 76″ × 98½″. Copyright 1989 Indianapolis Museum of Art. Gift of a Couple of Old Hoosiers; **684** Library of Congress; **685** "Cliff Dwellers," 1913. George Wesley Bellows, United States, 1882–1925. Oil on canvas, 39½″ × 41½″. Los Angeles County Museum of Art, Los Angeles County Funds; **692** National Archives. Photo courtesy Rudolph Vetter/Interpretive Photography; **694** Courtesy of the New York Public Library, Astor, Lenox, and Tilden Foundations; **698** Milwaukee Art Museum, Layton Art Collection; **700** *Good Housekeeping*, March 1, 1889; **702** The Margaret Woodbury Strong Museum, Rochester, N.Y.; **707** Staten Island Historical Society; **711** Museum of Art, Rhode Island School of Design, Joseph Metcalf and Walter H. Kimball Funds.

GENERATIONS OF THE REPUBLIC

714-L The Fine Arts Museum of San Francisco. Gift of Mr. and Mrs. John D. Rockefeller, 3rd; **714-C** Milwaukee County Historical Society; **714-R** Courtesy of the Museum of Modern Art, N.Y. Museum Purchase; **715-L** Library of Congress; **715-C** University of Oregon Library; **715-R** Library of Congress; **716-L** The Bettmann Archive; **716-C** Museum of the City of New York; **716-R** Minneapolis Institute of Arts; **717-L** Tuskegee University Archives, Chester Higgins Collection; **717-C** Ashfield Historical Society, Howes Brothers Photograph; **717-R** Ashfield Historical Society, Howes Brothers Photograph.

CHAPTER 20

719 Idaho State Historical Society; **721** Courtesy of the New York Public Library; **723** Robert P. Coggins Collection of Southern American Art; **727** Brown Brothers; **735** Library of Congress; **742** National Anthropological Archives, Smithsonian Institution; **746** Henry E. Huntington Library and Art Gallery; **748** Courtesy, Wichita Art Museum, the Roland P. Murdock Collection; **753** Nebraska State Historical Society, Solomon D. Butcher Collection; **754** Greeley Municipal Museum.

CHAPTER 21

759 Courtesy of the New York Historical Society, New York City; **760** Culver Pictures; **761** Library of Congress; **763** Chicago Historical Society; **765** Bancroft Library; **769** Library of Congress; **770** California State Library; **775** The Kansas State Historical Society, Topeka, Kans. **779** Courtesy, Dover Publications, N.Y.; **782** Museum of American Political Life, University of Hartford, Conn.; **783** Library of Congress; **787** Library of Congress.

CHAPTER 22

791 Tsuneo Tambu Collection, Yokohama, Japan. Photo courtesy Laurie Platt Winfrey, Inc.; **792** "Bugler." *Colliers*, September 10, 1898, p. 13. Courtesy of the New York Public Library; **797** Fred Pansing, "Naval Parade," August 20, 1898. Oil on canvas. Courtesy of the Museum of the City of New York; **803** Library of Congress (both); **806** Hawaii State Archives; **813** Library of Congress; **816** Library of Congress (both); **819** New York Public Library, Lewis Hine Collection.

CHAPTER 23

823 Library of Congress (detail); **824** Brown Brothers; **825** "The Four Suffragettes." *Colliers*, 1912. Courtesy of the New York Public Library; **829** Culver Pictures; **833** San Diego Historical Society, Ticor Collection; **837** The Henry E. Huntington Library, San Marino, Calif.; **840** Drawing by Charles Dana Gibson. Dover Publications; **844-L** Brown Brothers; **844-R** Library of Congress; **845** Library of Congress; **850** Culver Pictures; **856** Edmund Charles Tarbell, 1862–1938. "Thomas Woodrow Wilson," 1921. Oil on canvas, 46″ × 36 1/4″. NPC.65.42. National Portrait Gallery, Smithsonian Institution. Transfer from the NMAA; gift of the City of New York through the National Art Committee.

CHAPTER 24

861 George Luks. "Armistice Night." 1918. Oil on canvas, 37″ × 68 3/4″. Collection of Whitney Museum of American Art. Anonymous gift. 54.58; **864** Theodore Roosevelt Collection, Harvard College Library;

871 Brown Brothers; 876 Trustees of the Imperial War Museum, London (both); 881 National Archives; 883 U.S. Military Academy, West Point Museum Collection; 885 National Archives, U.S. War Department; 891 WPA mural by Earl Lonsbury. "Battle Engagement," WPA Photo Collection. Archive of American Art, Smithsonian Institution; 892 Trustees of the Imperial War Museum, London; 896 Brown Brothers; 898 Collection of Albert Craig; 899 Bildarchiv Preussischer Kulturbesitz.

CHAPTER 25

903 Western Illinois University Art Gallery/Museum; 904 The Bettmann Archive; 908 From the Collections of Henry Ford Museum & Greenfield Village; 911 Gerrit Beneker, American, 1882–1934. "Portrait of Homer White." Collection of the Canton Art Institute, Canton, O.; 913 *American Quarterly*, Vol. 10, 1958, p. 419; 914 Library of Congress; 916 The Bettmann Archive; 919 Lief Neandross, "The Roxy Theater." Watercolor. Courtesy of the Rambusch Co., N.Y.; 922 The Bettmann Archive; 927 Paul Cadmus, "To the Lynching!" 1935. Pencil and watercolor on paper, 20 1/2″ × 15 3/4″. Collection of Whitney Museum of American Art. Purchase 36.32; 931 UPI/Bettmann Newsphotos.

GENERATIONS OF THE REPUBLIC 5

936-L Idaho State Historical Society, Photo #60-139.13; 936-C Library of Congress, Arnold Genthe Collection; 936-R Ashfield Historical Society Museum, Howes Brothers Photograph; 937-L Alice Lloyd College Photo Archives, Astor Dobson Collection; 937-C Richard Samuel Roberts Collection; 937-R Culver Pictures; 938-L Laura Gilpin, "Farnsworth-Hazelhurst Wedding," 1926, 79.130/97. Courtesy Amon Carter Museum, Ft. Worth, Tex. Copyright 1981; 938-C Library of Congress; 938-R Library of Congress; 939-L Library of Congress; 939-C Library of Congress; 939-R Wayne Miller/ Magnum.

CHAPTER 26

941 Library of Congress (both); 946 *Vanity Fair*, October 1933. Courtesy of the New York Public Library; 950 Brown Brothers; 953 Library of Congress; 957 UPI/ Bettmann Newsphotos; 958 Photofest; 960 Library of Congress; 961 Library of Congress; 962 Library of Congress; 966 United States Air Force.

CHAPTER 27

975 Franklin D. Roosevelt Library; 976-T Franklin D. Roosevelt Library; 976-B Elizabeth Olds, "Miner Joe," 1937. National Museum of American Art, Smithsonian Institution; 978 UPI/Bettmann Newsphotos; 982 Library of Congress; 986 UPI/Bettmann Newsphotos; 987 Peter Hopkins, "Riot at Union Square, March 6, 1930," 1947. Courtesy of the Museum of the City of New York; 993 The Bettmann Archive; 1001 Tom Lea, "Back Home: Pleasant Hill, Mo., 1865." National Archives; 1003 Library of Congress.

CHAPTER 28

1009 National Archives; 1010-T AP/Wide World; 1010-B United States Marine Corps Historical Center; 1015 UPI/Bettmann Newsphotos; 1021 UPI/Bettmann Newsphotos; 1029 United States Marine Corps, Defense Department; 1031 AP/Wide World; 1032 Jacob Law-

rence, "War Series: Shipping Out," 1947. Egg tempera on composition board, 20″ × 16″. Collection of Whitney Museum of American Art. Gift of Mr. And Mrs. Roy R. Neuberger. 51.7; 1037 United States Coast Guard; 1039 B. Anthony Stewart, 1951. National Geographic Society.

CHAPTER 29

1047 Franklin D. Roosevelt Library; 1051 William Strout, LIFE MAGAZINE, copyright TIME Inc.; 1055 Courtesy Du Pont, Inc.; 1056 Library of Congress; 1058 Library of Congress; 1061 Library of Congress; 1065 UPI/Bettmann Newsphotos; 1069 UPI/Bettmann Newsphotos; 1072 National Archives, United States Army Signal Corps; 1076 Brian Brake/Photo Researchers; 1078 *Colliers*, May 3, 1947. Courtesy Library of Congress; 1079 Andy Hernandez/Picture Group.

CHAPTER 30

1083 J.R. Eyerman, LIFE MAGAZINE, copyright TIME Inc.; 1088 United States Navy, Courtesy Harry S Truman Library; 1089 Copyright 1946, TIME Inc. Reprinted by permission; 1090 AP/Wide World; 1099 Museum of Modern Art, Film Stills Archive, N.Y.; 1105 The Bettmann Archive; 1116 AP/Wide World.

CHAPTER 31

1119 Copyright 1959 by Norman Rockwell. Reproduced by permission of the Norman Rockwell Estate. Photo courtesy of Mike Cluff; 1121 Courtesy Cadillac Motor Cars (both); 1123 Elliott Erwitt/Magnum; 1127 Russell R. Klein House. Kentfield, Calif. From *Architectural Record*, Vol. 121, No. 6, May 1957; 1132 Eve Arnold/ Magnum; 1139 United Press Associations; 1141 AP/ Wide World; 1146 Burt Glinn/Magnum; 1149 The Bettmann Archive.

CHAPTER 32

1153 Fred Ward/Black Star; 1154 Drawing by Ruby. *Children in Crisis: A Study of Courage and Fear* by Robert Coles. © 1964–67 by Robert Coles. By permission of Little, Brown and Company; 1158 The Bettmann Archive; 1164 AP/Wide World; 1169 Charles Moore/ Black Star; 1171 UPI/Bettmann Newsphotos; 1172 UPI/ Bettmann Newsphotos; 1173 Michael Alexander/Black Star; 1174 From Richard Harwood and Haynes Johnson, *Lyndon*, 1973. Washington Post Books, Praeger Publishers. Reprinted with permission; 1180 Friedel/Black Star; 1184 UPI/Bettmann Newsphotos.

GENERATIONS OF THE REPUBLIC

1188-L Courtesy of James West Davidson; 1188-C Spencer Museum of Art, University of Kansas, Gift of Marion Palfi (1917–1978); 1188-R David S. Strickler/Picture Cube; 1189-L Courtesy of Christine Leigh Heyrman; 1189-C Courtesy of Michael B. Stoff; 1189-R Courtesy of William E. Gienapp; 1190-L Bruce Davidson/Magnum; 1190-C Courtesy of Mark H. Lytle; 1190-R Leonard Freed/Magnum; 1191-L Burk Uzzle/Picture Group; 1191-C Burt Glinn/Magnum; 1191-R Arthur Glauberman/Photo Researchers.

CHAPTER 33

1193 Tim Page; 1194 John Folio/Valley News Dispatch; 1197-T Co Rentmeester/TIME-LIFE Pictures; 1197-C James Pickerell/Black Star; 1197-B Tim Page; 1198-L

Index

Page numbers in *italic* refer to illustrations, tables, and charts. Page numbers followed by "*n.*" (e.g., 1160*n.*) refer to footnotes. Book titles and Supreme Court cases are listed, respectively, under "Books" and "Supreme Court, U.S."

ABOUT THE AUTHORS

JAMES WEST DAVIDSON received his Ph.D. from Yale University. A historian who has pursued a full-time writing career, he is the author of numerous books, among them *After the Fact: The Art of Historical Detection* (with Mark H. Lytle), *The Logic of Millennial Thought: Eighteenth-Century New England*, and *Great Heart: The History of a Labrador Adventure* (with John Rugge).

WILLIAM E. GIENAPP has a Ph.D. from the University of California, Berkeley. He is Professor of History at the University of Wyoming, where he was the 1988–1989 Seibold Professor. In 1988 he was given the Avery O. Craven Award for his work, *The Origins of the Republican Party, 1852–1856*. Currently he is at work on *Abraham Lincoln and Civil War America*.

CHRISTINE LEIGH HEYRMAN is Associate Professor of History at Brandeis University. She received a Ph.D. in American Studies from Yale University and is the author of *Commerce and Culture: The Maritime Communities of Colonial Massachusetts, 1690–1750*. Her professional activities include serving on the Editorial Board of the *Journal of American History* and as Council Secretary for the Institute of Early American History and Culture.

MARK II. LYTLE, who was awarded a Ph.D. from Yale University, is Professor of History and Environmental Studies and Chair of the American Studies Program at Bard College. He is also Director of the Master of Arts in Teaching Program at Bard. His publications include *The Origins of the Iranian–American Alliance, 1941–1953* and *After the Fact: The Art of Historical Detection* (with James West Davidson). In 1989 he received the Horace Kidger Award of the New England History Teachers Association. He is now at work on *The Uncivil War: America in the Vietnam Era*.

MICHAEL B. STOFF is Associate Professor of History at the University of Texas at Austin, where he directs the honors program in history. The recipient of a Ph.D. from Yale University, he wrote *Oil, War, and American Security: The Search for a National Policy on Foreign Oil, 1941–1947* and the forthcoming *Manhattan Project: A Documentary Introduction to the Development and Use of the Atomic Bomb*.